**To be renewed or returned on or before the date marked below:**

| | |
|---|---|
| -5 OCT 1995 | 17 DEC 2008 |
| 31 Oct 1995 | 12 MAY 2010 |
| 23 FEB 1998 | 04 JUL 2013 |
| 27 OCT 1998 | 5/7/17 |
| 24 Nov 1998 | |
| 25 OCT 1999 | |
| 29 DEC 1999 | |
| -5 DEC 2003 | |
| 2 Jan 04 R | |

**PLEASE ENTER ON LOAN SLIP:**

AUTHOR: DEVALENTINE

TITLE: FOOT AND ANKLE DISORDERS IN CHILDREN

# Foot and Ankle Disorders in Children

# Foot and Ankle Disorders in Children

Edited by

## Steven J. DeValentine, D.P.M.

Past Clinical Assistant Professor
Department of Surgery
California College of Podiatric Medicine
San Francisco, California

Chief
Department of Podiatric Surgery
Kaiser Permanente Medical Center
South Sacramento, California

Churchill Livingstone
New York, Edinburgh, London, Melbourne, Tokyo

**Library of Congress Cataloging-in-Publication Data**

Foot and ankle disorders in children / edited by Steven J.
  DeValentine
        p.  cm.
    Includes bibliographical references and index.
    ISBN 0-443-08698-2
    1. Foot—Abnormalities.  2. Ankle—Abnormalities.  3. Pediatric
orthopedics.  I. DeValentine, Steven J.
    [DNLM: 1. Ankle—abnormalities. 2. Foot Deformities—in infancy &
childhood.  3. Foot Deformities—therapy.  WE 883 F687]
RD781.F573  1992
618.92'097585—dc20
DNLM/DLC
for Library of Congress                                    91-34009
                                                              CIP

**© Churchill Livingstone Inc. 1992**

Distributed in the United Kingdom by Churchill Livingstone, Robert Stevenson
House, 1–3 Baxter's Place, Leith Walk, Edinburgh EH1 3AF, and by associated com-
panies, branches, and representatives throughout the world.

Accurate indications, adverse reactions, and dosage schedules for drugs are provided
in this book, but it is possible that they may change. The reader is urged to review
the package information data of the manufacturers of the medications mentioned.

The Publishers have made every effort to trace the copyright holders for borrowed
material. If they have inadvertently overlooked any, they will be pleased to make the
necessary arrangements at the first opportunity.

Acquisitions Editor: *Leslie Burgess*
Production Designer: *Jill Little*
Production Supervisor: *Jeanine Furino*

Printed in the United States of America

First published in 1992     7 6 5 4 3 2 1

*To my family,*
*whose patience, understanding,*
*and constant encouragement*
*have made this work possible.*

*To my wife, Sandra,*
*and my children,*
*David, Jonathan, and Ashley.*

*And to my parents,*
*Joseph J. DeValentine and Pauline A. DeValentine.*

# Contributors

**Alan S. Banks, D.P.M.**
Faculty, The Podiatric Institute; Director, Podiatric Medical Education and Residency Training, Northlake Regional Medical Center, Tucker, Georgia

**Timothy J. Blakeslee, D.P.M.**
Podiatrist, Department of Podiatric Surgery, Kaiser Permanente Medical Center, South Sacramento, California

**Louis J. Caputo, D.P.M.**
Chief, Podiatric Medicine Department, El Camino Hospital, Mountain View, California; Staff Podiatrist, Sunnyvale Medical Clinic, Sunnyvale, California

**Gershon Chaimsky, M.D.**
Senior Orthopaedic Surgeon, Department of Orthopaedic Surgery, Hadassah University Hospital, Jerusalem, Israel

**Paul D. Dayton, D.P.M.**
Podiatrist, Department of Podiatric Surgery, Kaiser Permanente Medical Center, San Jose, California

**Steven J. DeValentine, D.P.M.**
Past Clinical Assistant Professor, Department of Surgery, California College of Podiatric Medicine, San Francisco, California; Chief, Department of Podiatric Surgery, Kaiser Permanente Medical Center, South Sacramento, California

**Michael S. Downey, D.P.M.**
Associate Professor and Chairman, Department of Surgery, Pennsylvania College of Podiatric Medicine; Faculty, Podiatry Institute, Philadelphia, Pennsylvania

**James P. Fagan, D.P.M.**
Program Director, Podiatric Surgical Residency Program, Kaiser Hospital; Chief, Department of Podiatric Surgery, Kaiser Permanente Medical Center, Oakland, California

**Flair D. Goldman, D.P.M.**
Clinical Associate Professor, Department of Anatomy, California College of Podiatric Medicine, San Francisco, California; Chief, Department of Podiatric Surgery, Kaiser Permanente Medical Center, Santa Clara, California

## Donald R. Green, D.P.M.
Clinical Instructor, Department of Orthopedics, University of California, San Diego, School of Medicine, La Jolla, California; Faculty, The Podiatry Institute, Tucker, Georgia; Former Chairman and Professor, Department of Surgery, Pennsylvania College of Podiatric Medicine, Philadelphia, Pennsylvania

## Cheryl Hanson, D.P.M., Ph.D.
Staff Physician, Department of Podiatric Surgery, Kaiser Permanente Medical Center, Sacramento, California

## Geoffrey S. Heard, D.P.M.
Joseph Oloff Surgical Fellow; Clinical Assistant Professor, Department of Surgery, California College of Podiatric Medicine, San Francisco, California

## Stephen L. Kaufman, M.D.
Associate Clinical Professor, Department of Pediatrics, University of California Medical Center, San Francisco, California

## Kevin A. Kirby, D.P.M.
Assistant Professor of Biomechanics, California College of Podiatric Medicine, San Francisco, California; Podiatric Biomechanics Consultant, Kaiser Permanente Medical Center; Private Practice, Pacific Health Center, Sacramento, California

## Thomas K. Koch, M.D.
Associate Professor of Clinical Neurology and Pediatrics, Department of Neurology and Pediatrics, Division of Child Neurology, University of California, San Francisco, School of Medicine, San Francisco, California

## Patrick A. Landers, D.P.M.
Private Practice, Cuyahoga Falls, Ohio

## Karen G. Lo, D.P.M.
Chief Podiatric Surgical Resident, Cleveland Foot Clinic and Affiliated Hospitals, Cleveland, Ohio

## Lauri McDaniel, D.P.M.
Associate Professor, Department of Podiatric Medicine, California College of Podiatric Medicine, San Francisco, California; Podiatrist, Department of Podiatric Surgery, Kaiser Permanente Medical Center, Hayward, California

## Sheila G. Moore, M.D.
Assistant Professor, Department of Radiology, Stanford University School of Medicine, Palo Alto, California

## Joan Oloff, D.P.M.
Private Practice, Los Gatos, California

## Lawrence M. Oloff, D.P.M.

Dean for Academic Affairs, Associate Professor, Department of Surgery, Co-Director, Special Problems Clinic, California College of Podiatric Medicine, San Francisco, California; Assistant Clinical Professor, Department of Dermatology, Stanford University School of Medicine, Palo Alto, California

## Shlomo Porat, M.D., M.Ch.Orth.

Senior Lecturer, Department of Orthopaedic Surgery, Hebrew University Medical School; Chief, Pediatric Orthopaedic Surgery Service, Hadassah University Hospital, Jerusalem, Israel

## Laurence Rubin, D.P.M.

Private Practice, Richmond, Virginia

## John M. Schuberth, D.P.M.

Attending Staff, Department of Orthopedic/Podiatric Surgery, Kaiser Permanente Medical Center; Clinical Associate Professor, Department of Surgery, California College of Podiatric Medicine, San Francisco, California

## Barry L. Scurran, D.P.M.

Chief, Department of Podiatric Surgery, and Chief, Medical Staff Education, Kaiser Permanente Medical Center, Hayward, California; Clinical Associate Professor, Department of Surgery, California College of Podiatric Medicine, San Francisco, California; Clinical Instructor, Stanford University School of Medicine, Palo Alto, California

## James L. Shively, M.D.

Department of Orthopaedic Surgery, Kaiser Hospital, Oakland, California

## Jeffrey E. Shook, D.P.M.

Podiatric Surgical Resident, New Jersey University of Medicine and Dentistry, East Newark, New Jersey

## Stephen H. Silvani, D.P.M.

Clinical Assistant Professor, Department of Podiatric Surgery, California College of Podiatric Medicine, San Francisco, California; Chief, Department of Podiatric Surgery, Kaiser Permanente Medical Center, Walnut Creek, California

## Thomas F. Smith, D.P.M.

Board of Trustees, The Podiatry Institute, Tucker, Georgia; Acting Chief of Podiatry, Veterans Administration Medical Center, Augusta, Georgia

## Clint M. Thorton, D.P.M.

Joseph Oloff Surgical Fellow; Assistant Professor, Department of Surgery, California College of Podiatric Medicine, San Francisco, California

## Ronald L. Valmassy, D.P.M.

Professor and Former Chairman, Department of Podiatric Biomechanics, California College of Podiatric Medicine, San Francisco, California

## Anvar M. Velji, M.D.

Associate Clinical Professor, Department of Medicine, University of California, Davis, School of Medicine, Davis, California; Chief, Division of Infectious Diseases, Kaiser Permanente Medical Center, South Sacramento, California

## Calvin Wheeler, M.D.

Clinical Instructor, Department of Pediatrics, University of California, San Francisco, School of Medicine, San Francisco, California; Subchief, Pediatric Neurology, Department of Neurology, Kaiser Permanente Medical Center, Hayward, California

## Kent K. Wu, M.D.

Senior Surgeon, Bone Joint Center, Henry Ford Hospital, Detroit, Michigan

## Gerard V. Yu, D.P.M.

Associate Professor and Former Chairman, Department of Surgery, Ohio College of Podiatric Medicine/Cleveland Foot Clinic and Affiliated Hospitals; Chief, Division of Podiatry, Department of Surgery, Meridia Huron Hospital, East Cleveland, Ohio

# Preface

*Foot and Ankle Disorders in Children* has been written as a resource text for the practicing podiatric surgeon. Those foot and ankle surgeons with a particular interest in children's extremity disorders will find within the pages of the book detailed technical information about the management of a variety of pediatric foot and ankle problems from the simple and commonplace to the exotic and rare.

The book is divded into six major sections: Principles; Congenital Deformities; Developmental Disorders; The Foot and Ankle in Neuromuscular Disease; Trauma in Children; and Metabolic Bone Disorders and Tumerous Conditions. Section I provides an overview of functional anatomy and physiology, physical and neurologic examination, and diagnostic imaging in children. The focus of this section is the differences between the pediatric and the adult examination. Section II provides an extensive overview of the most common congenital foot, ankle, and lower extremity problems that are seen from infancy to skeletal maturity. Section III discusses the nonsurgical and surgical management of many of the most common types of pediatric "walk-in"-type problems, including torsional problems, pes valgus, hallux valgus, digital deformities, and other miscellaneous conditions. Section IV discusses conservative and surgical management of neuromuscular disorders; Section V provides, detailed, up-to-date information on the management of all types of foot and ankle injuries. Finally, the section on Metabolic Bone Disorders and Tumerous Conditions provides an overview of management of these types of metabolic problems with emphasis on the differences between children and adults. An extensive reference list categorized by subject is provided at the end of each chapter, should the reader desire a more in-depth discussion of any subject; additional suggested readings are also often provided.

All children are special. They deserve our best and most conscientious effort. It is my sincere hope that this book will contribute to the podiatrist's ability to enhance the quality of life of children with foot and ankle disorders.

*Steven J. DeValentine, D.P.M.*

# Acknowledgments

My sincere thanks to all the contributing authors who helped to bring this work to fruition so that all clinicians who treat foot and ankle disorders in children will benefit from their combined knowledge, experience, and dedication to teaching.

A special acknowledgment goes to Celeste Wardin, who provided most of the original illustrations for this text. Her work is a valuable addition to the book.

A special thank you to Cathy Landrum, who has provided her talented assistance in the development of this and other related projects.

# Contents

# VI. METABOLIC BONE DISORDERS AND TUMEROUS CONDITIONS

# 1

# Functional Developmental Anatomy and Physiology of the Lower Extremity

CHERYL HANSON

The child's musculoskeletal system differs appreciably from that of the adult in terms of its anatomic, physiologic, and biomechanical characteristics. As a result, pediatric musculoskeletal injury patterns, as well as the child's healing response to injury and elective operative intervention, may also vary significantly from what would be expected in the adult. Appropriate surgical and nonsurgical management of pediatric lower extremity disorders must be based upon a thorough knowledge of these differences. This chapter will attempt to provide the reader with a brief overview of the basic anatomic, physiologic, and biomechanical characteristics of the pediatric lower extremity musculoskeletal system, with emphasis on those areas that differ most significantly from the corresponding areas in the skeletally mature patient. The reader is referred to any of the more detailed anatomic texts for a thorough review of the embryology and gross anatomy of the lower extremity.

## LOWER EXTREMITY DEVELOPMENT

### Embryology

The embryonic period consists of the first seven postovulatory weeks.[1] The lower limb buds, which form slightly later than the upper limb buds, appear somewhere between the third and fifth embryonic weeks.[2-8] The lower limb buds begin lateral to the fifth lumbar and first sacral myotomes.[6] The arrangements of spinal nerves to the lower extremities is segmental and is established in response to the development of myotomes.[9] The lumbosacral plexus bifurcates to form a ventral division destined to supply flexor musculature, and a dorsal division to innervate the extensor muscles.[6]

Initially, the prospective plantar surface of the lower limb starts out directed cephalad. This later rotates; by the sixth embryonic week approximately 90 percent of the anticipated inward rotation has taken place and the plantar surfaces of the feet as well as the posterior leg surfaces face toward the midsagittal plane of the body.[7] Congenital deformities of the foot occur prior to the seventh embryonic week, when the structural and skeletal components are determined.[10]

The fetal period begins with the eighth embryonic week. At this time the foot is in 90 degrees of equinus and adducted. The foot becomes supinated and is externally rotated relative to the leg. Then, early in the fourth month, the foot pronates into a position of midsupination. Although pronatory changes will continue through the fetal period, some degree of supination may persist after birth.[7]

The central portion of the limb bud is composed of primitive undifferentiated mesenchymal cells, which are able to differentiate into muscle, hyaline cartilage, and the cartilaginous precursor of bone. As this cartilaginous precursor of a tubular bone increases in size, the central portion is invaded by a blood vessel, which brings higher oxygen concentration to the cells. This vessel becomes the nutrient artery for the bone and will initiate the process of ossification.

Ossification of the foot begins early in the fetal period. The foot, or tarsus, first appears as a mesenchymal condensation at 5 to 6 weeks. Within a few days chondrification begins centrally. The individual bones of the foot chondrify in a definite sequence: the second to fourth metatarsals first, followed by the cuboid and fifth metatarsal. The navicular bone is the last tarsal bone to chondrify. In the digits chondrification proceeds in a proximal to distal direction. Ligaments and tendons also differentiate in a proximal to distal direction.[7]

Although ossification of the foot does not occur during the embryonic period proper, the synovial joints begin to develop as "interzones" between the various elements.[1] From the sixth week of embryonic life, active intrauterine movement of the limbs is essential to the normal embryonic development of synovial joints.[5]

## Ossification

As the cartilage model of a long bone is invaded by blood vessels, osteogenesis occurs. The transformation from cartilaginous precursor to ossified unit occurs via two discrete processes, intramembranous and endochondral ossification. These two basic types of bone formation refer only to the primary pattern of development of each individual structural unit. Subsequent growth of any particular bone may involve discrete, juxtaposed, or interspersed areas of both basic patterns within the same bone.[8] The central portion of the long bone is the first region to exhibit endochondral ossification. A bony collar develops around the midshaft of the cartilage model accompanied by vascular invasion and resultant formation of the so-called primary ossification center. At a later time, frequently postnatally, there is further vascular invasion of the chondroepiphysis and formation of secondary ossification centers at the ends of the bone. This type of bone formation is referred to as *endochondral* ossification. As bone replaces the initial cartilage model, surface periosteum forms, adding width to the enlarging bone. Future latitudinal growth of the diaphysis and metaphysis involves periosteal apposition and endosteal absorption, maintaining a relatively constant cortical thickness.

Growth cartilage cells are nourished by diffusion of nutrients through the matrix. Nutrients, derived from the joint fluid as a result of pressure diffusion accomplished by the movement of opposing joint surfaces, will penetrate the epiphysis to a limited extent. Deeper layers of the epiphysis are supplied from the bony centrum itself. At the longitudinal growth plate, blood vessels that enter the epiphysis penetrate the bony end plate and terminate as capillaries in the underlying growth cartilage matrix.[10]

Initially the ossification process extends at relatively equal rates toward each end of the bone. Only postnatally is there a significant difference in the rates of growth of each epiphysis and physis. As the primary ossification center approaches each cartilaginous end, selected areas of the cartilage increasingly resemble the physis. This process usually occurs by the end of the third or beginning of the fourth gestational month. As the individual bone elongates and widens in the metaphyses by the normal process of endochondral ossification, extensive remodeling occurs through the endochondral process of cell division and osseous replacement at the physis. The initially formed membranous bone is remodeled to create the lamellar bone characteristic of mature cortical bone.[11]

It is the persistence of the cartilaginous layer known as the *growth plate* or *physis* that enables both latitudinal and longitudinal growth of bone to occur. Latitudinal growth occurs by cell division and intercellular matrix expansion within the physis (interstitial growth) and by cellular addition peripherally at the zone of Ranvier (appositional growth). Once the ossification center has expanded to the epiphyseal margin, relatively minor damage to the periphery of the physis may lead to formation of an osseous bridge, severely limiting growth potential both latitudinally and longitudinally.[11] If no damage occurs to the physis during development, this layer eventually disappears and growth ceases. At that time epiphyseal and metaphyseal vascular channels grow across the physeal plate, establishing a bony fusion of the primary and secondary ossification centers.[12]

*Physiologic epiphysiodesis* is this normal replacement of the physis. Initially small osseous bridges form between the epiphyseal ossification center and the metaphysis. The process is complete when the cartilaginous physis has been totally replaced by osseous tissue. Epiphysiodesis occurs earlier in girls than in boys. We now know that each physis has its own pattern of closure and that this contributes to specific patterns of injury during fractures. As a general rule, epiphysiodesis begins centrally and proceeds centrifugally. However, the distal tibial physis closes in the middle and medial regions first and laterally later. Vascular invasion of the tarsus, heralding the approach of ossification, first begins in the talus.[1]

Ossification in the foot begins in the tips of the distal phalanges and then advances proximally. Soon after, periosteal bone collars are formed, first around the metatarsal shafts and later around the proximal and middle phalanges. The primary centers of ossification of the second and third metatarsals appear in the ninth week of fetal life, whereas those of the fourth and fifth metatar-

sals do not appear until the tenth week. Physes are initially present at both ends of the metatarsals and phalanges, but the secondary center develops at only one end. The other physis will degenerate. The active secondary centers of ossification of the lesser four metatarsals develop distally. The epiphyses of the lesser four metatarsals fuse with the diaphyses between the ages of 16 and 18 years. The fifth metatarsal develops an additional secondary center of ossification at the proximal, lateral portion of the base, where the peroneus brevis muscle inserts. This process may become increasingly evident between 9 and 14 years of age and is often mis-

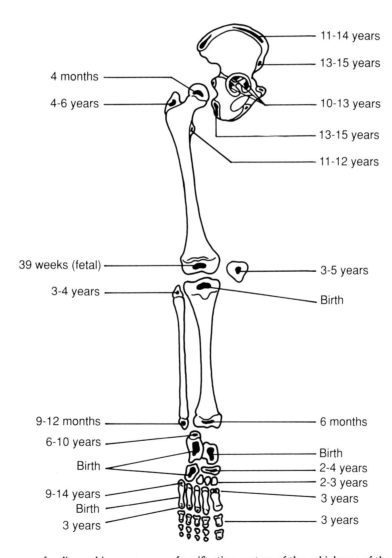

**Fig. 1-1.** Average age of radiographic appearance of ossification centers of the ephiphyses of the lower extremity.

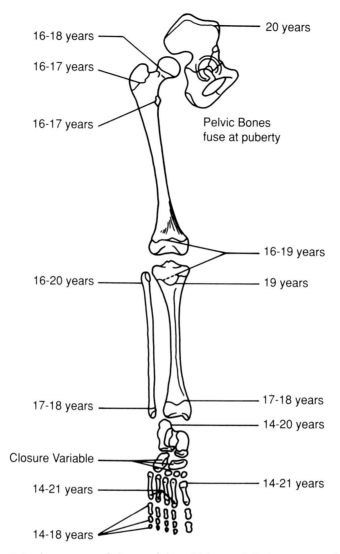

**Fig. 1-2.** Average age of closure of the ephiphyses of the lower extremity.

taken for an avulsion fracture. (It traverses the tubercle in a direction almost parallel to the long axis of the shaft and does not extend proximally into the metatarsocuboid joint or medially into the joint between the fourth and fifth metatarsals; this orientation usually distinguishes it from the transverse or oblique orientation of fifth metatarsal base fractures.)

Avulsion of the base of the fifth metatarsal is relatively common in children, although it can also be confused with the os vesalianum, a normal sesamoid.[4] The primary ossification center of the first metatarsal is visible during

the twelfth week of fetal life. Its secondary center of ossification, located proximally, appears between 3 and 4 years of age and fuses with the diaphysis between 16 and 18 years of age. A pseudoepiphysis occasionally may be formed at the distal end of the first metatarsal.[13] Ossification of the medial and lateral sesamoids of the first metatarsophalangeal joint usually takes place between 12 and 14 years of age.

Ossification of the small bones of the foot begins with a central primary ossification center and proceeds outward from the center in a circumferential manner using

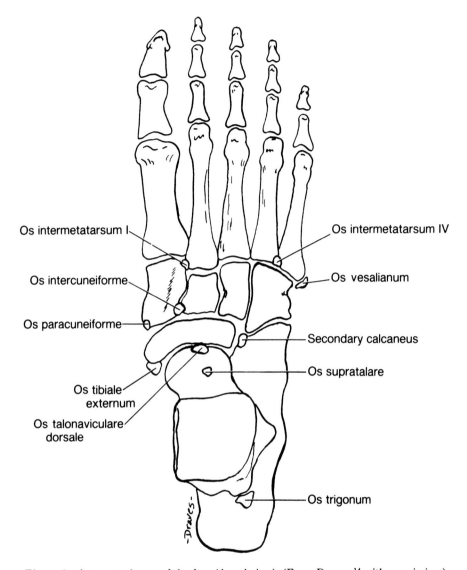

**Fig. 1-3.** Accessory bones of the foot (dorsal view). (From Draves,[14] with permission.)

the pre-existing cartilage template. At birth, ossification centers of the calcaneus, talus, and cuboid are usually present, in addition to those of the phalanges and metatarsals. Secondary ossification centers will appear pre- or post-natally depending on the bone and individual variability. Figure 1-1 shows the average age of appearance of centers of ossification of the epiphyses in the lower limb, and Figure 1-2 shows the average age of closure of these same epiphyses.

The calcaneus is the first tarsal bone to begin ossification. Its primary ossification center appears between the fifth and sixth fetal months.[1,4] A secondary center of ossification, the apophysis will begin to ossify at 4 to 6 years of age in girls and at 5 to 9 years of age in boys. It will fuse to the body of the calcaneus at about 16 years in the female and at about 20 years in the male. Ossification of this secondary center may be irregular and should not be mistaken for a fracture. The cortical shell of the calcaneus will continue to remodel during growth in response to dynamic weight-bearing stresses. In the young child the cortex is cartilaginous and imparts additional protective resilience to the bone, making calcaneal fractures relatively uncommon. The largely cartilaginous nature of the child's calcaneus, combined with the increased elasticity of the child's bone, probably dissipates the applied forces throughout the foot and leg without concentrating it on the calcaneus.[4]

The talus is the second tarsal bone to ossify, usually at about the eighth fetal month. It may, however, ossify postnatally.[4] A secondary ossification center may also form at the posterior aspect of the talus and become radiographically visible between the ages 8 and 12. Talar fractures are relatively rare in children because a greater proportion of the immature talus is composed of cartilage, which is very elastic, and pediatric spongiosa bone is capable of absorbing much greater force than adult spongiosa bone.[3] The child has a more flexible blood supply to the talus, which is provided by branches from the anterior tibial, perforating peroneal, and posterior tibial arteries. Therefore, avascular necrosis is rarely a complication of talar fractures in children. The lower incidence of avascular necrosis is probably due to the talus being composed primarily of cartilage with a relatively small proportion of ossified bone.[3] Since the sinus tarsi is the entry point for much of the blood supply to the talus and calcaneus, minimal dissection should be performed in this region during surgical procedures.

Midfoot ossification begins with ossification of the cuboid bone at or near birth. The average age for ossification of the lateral cuneiform bone is 4 to 20 months; the medial cuneiform ossifies at about 2 years and the intermediate cuneiform at about 3 years. The navicular is the last tarsal bone to appear and ossifies between the second and the fifth year. A secondary ossification center may also form at the navicular tuberosity and become radiographically visible between 8 and 12 years of age.

Accessory ossicles and sesamoid bones may cause confusion in the differential diagnosis of chip fractures, especially in the midfoot region. Knowledge of their normal location facilitates this differentiation. In addition, radiographs should be evaluated for smooth cortical borders versus irregular fractured edges. The os tibiale externum (accessory tarsal navicular or prehallux), which is a secondary ossification center for the navicular and may persist as a separate accessory bone, is present in about 10 percent of the population.[13] The os trigonum extends from the posterior aspect of the talus adjacent to the groove for the flexor hallucis longus tendon. (Figures 1-3 to 1-5 illustrate the most common accessory and sesamoid bones of the foot as described by Draves.[14])

The primary ossification center of the tibia appears at the ninth week of fetal life. Toward the eighth or ninth fetal month, the proximal epiphysis of the tibia begins to ossify. The proximal tibial tubercle begins to ossify between 7 and 11 years. The distal tibial epiphysis appears between the sixth and tenth months of postnatal life, and the distal tibial ossification center appears between the second and third year of life.[15] The medial malleolus begins to ossify at 7 years in girls and at 8 years in boys. By 14 to 15 years the entire distal epiphysis, including the malleolus, is ossified, and between 16 and 18 years it unites with the metaphysis. The medial malleolus occasionally develops a separate secondary center of ossification, which can mimic a fracture. Epiphysiodesis of the distal tibial physis initially involves the medial portion. The distal tibial growth plate closes from medial to lateral over a 1½ year period between 13 and 18 years of age.[16,17]

In the fibula the primary ossification center appears in the tenth week of fetal life. The distal epiphysis appears between the eleventh and eighteenth postnatal months, and the upper epiphysis begins to ossify between 2 and 5 years. The distal fibula develops an ossification center during the second and third years.[15,16] Both fibular epiphyses will fuse with the diaphysis between 18 and 22 years of age.

## Growth

The skeletal system does not develop at a constant rate from fetus to adult. There is a relative acceleration during early childhood, followed by another acceleration during the adolescent growth spurt.

Growth of the foot, in particular, starts during the embryonic period. According to Gould et al.[18] who monitored foot growth in children under 5 years of age via measurement of changes in shoe size, "under 15 months of age, growth necessitated ½ size footwear change in less than 2 months; from 15 months to 2 years of age, ½ size increase occurred every 2 to 3 months; from 2 to 3 years of age, ½ size change every 3 to 4 months; and from 3 to 5 years of age, ½ size change every 4 months." This reflects a sharply decreasing rate of foot growth from infancy through 5 years of age. Then, from 5 to 12 years of age in girls and from 5 to 14 years of age in boys, the average increase in the length of the foot is 0.9 cm per year. This rate of growth decreases markedly after 12 years of age in girls and after 14 years of age in boys,

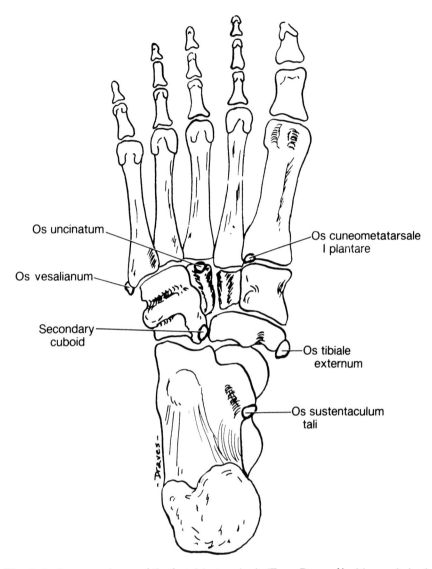

**Fig. 1-4.** Accessory bones of the foot (plantar view). (From Draves,[14] with permission.)

until the foot attains its mature length at the average age of 14 years in girls and 16 years in boys.[1,19] The tibia attains its mature length at age 15 in girls and 17 in boys.[20]

Figure 1-6 shows the relative growth contributions of the various physes of the lower extremity. Proximal epiphyses usually account for a greater percentage of extremity growth than distal epiphyses. This assumes clinical importance when trying to predict potential limb length discrepancies following physeal injuries.

Physeal injuries of the foot are far less likely to cause significant length disturbance or functional impairment than growth plate injuries of the leg, owing in part to the foot's relatively slow growth after age 5. Also, completion of foot growth occurs earlier than completion of leg growth. The foot has achieved almost 50 percent of its mature length by age 1 year in girls and 1½ years in boys, as compared with 50 percent of the mature length at 3 years for the femur and tibia. The average foot has achieved 96 percent of its total length in girls and 88

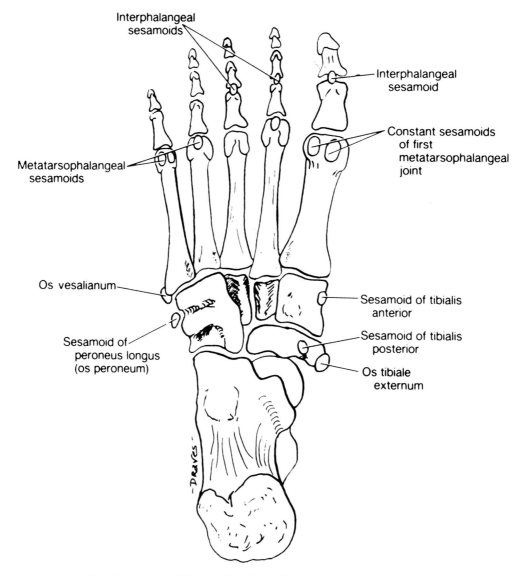

**Fig. 1-5.** Sesamoid bones of the foot. (From Draves,[14] with permission.)

percent of its total length in boys by 12 years.[3] Thus factors that might disturb growth and ultimate length of the foot or of an individual bone in the foot would be proportionately less important in the older child than for similar growth mechanism injuries to the femur or tibia.[13] Since the foot matures earlier than the tibia, factors that inhibit growth in the leg of a child (e.g., vascular conditions, muscle weakness) would ultimately affect the length of the foot proportionately less than the length of the tibia.

Bone growth is influenced by both systemic and local factors (see Table 1-1). Systemic factors influencing growth include genetics, nutrition, hormones, and infection.[3,15] Muscle forces likewise play an important role in modulating growth. Cartilage growth is stimulated by hormones such as thyroxin, growth hormone, sulfatin factor, and testosterone.[8,21] Testosterone initially stimulates the physis to undergo rapid cell division and widening during the growth spurt (anabolic effect) but eventually manifests a slowdown of growth and consolidation

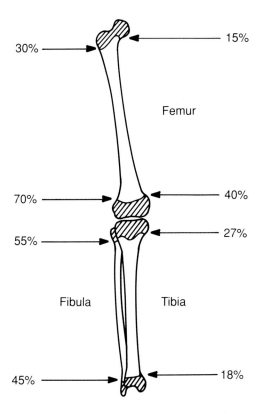

30% — 15%

Femur

70% — 40%

55% — 27%

Fibula   Tibia

45% — 18%

**Fig. 1-6.** Growth contributions of the physes of the lower extremity. The percentage of growth contribution to the individual bone is represented by the left column of numbers. The percentage of growth contribution to the entire lower extremity is represented by the right column.

**Table 1-1. Factors Affecting Epiphyseal Growth**

| Factor | Effect on Growth |
|--------|------------------|
| Systemic: | |
| Genetic | ↑ ↓ |
| Nutrition | ↑ ↓ |
| Growth hormone (GH) | ↑ GH → gigantism |
| | ↓ GH → dwarfism |
| Thyroid hormone (TH) | ↑ TH → ↑ rapidity |
| | ↓ TH → cretinism |
| Androgens | ↑ Growth → eventual closure |
| Estrogens | ↑ Growth → early closure |
| Local | |
| Compression | Slight ↑ → ↑ growth |
| | Large ↑ → ↓ growth |
| Nearby fracture | ↑ growth |
| Infection | ↓ |
| Injury | ↓ |
| Interference with circulation | ↓ |

(From DeValentine,[3] with permission.)

of the cartilage (androgenic effect).[11] Estrogen appears to have a greater effect on stimulating growth of already differentiated osseous tissue and may actually slow cartilage growth, either primarily or secondarily, by affecting the subchondral plates on either side of the physis.[8,11] While estrogen stimulates an increase in growth rate of girls during adolescence, it also results in early physeal closure, causing girls to be shorter than boys at maturity.[3] Maximal length of the long bones in girls is attained at earlier skeletal and chronological ages than it is in boys. Within about 2 years after the onset of puberty and the elaboration of estrogen, female growth ceases.[15] Estrogen given supplementally will also stimulate an initial growth spurt, but early closure quickly follows, causing a reduction in total longitudinal growth. Testosterone has a similar initial effect on growth, but it simultaneously increases the production of bone and will eventually close

the male physeal plate.[15] During the first year of life, fractures are relatively rare in children. The development of multiple, severe fractures during that time may be the first indication of metabolic disorders or skeletal dysplasia.

Intrinsic factors such as disruption of the mechanical constraints of the periosteal sleeve or increased vascularity, both of which accompany metaphyseal and diaphyseal fractures, may play an influential role in longitudinal bone growth.[11] Fractures of the metaphysis or diaphysis of long bones, without epiphyseal involvement, may result in temporary stimulation of longitudinal growth, due at least in part to the hyperemia associated with fracture healing. Chronic inflammation producing hyperemia has a similar effect, whereas atrophy, disuse (as with immobilization), and malnutrition may be associated with decreased growth rates.[10] Local factors that can decrease the rate of growth include partial growth arrest secondary to injury, vascular insult, or osteomyelitis.[15] Infection or trauma that alters the blood supply or damages the growth plate can influence final bone growth. Burns that extend down to the zone of Ranvier and the peripheral growth plate can cause growth impairment and subsequent angular deformity if not complete disruption.[21] Irradiation has also been shown to impair physeal growth, the changes being proportional to the quantity of radiation delivered and inversely proportional to age at the time of treatment.[22]

Local factors can also influence differential growth within a single epiphysis. For example, small increases in compression will stimulate physeal growth, while large increases in compression can retard physeal growth.[15] Previous research has demonstrated that cyclic weight-bearing in an eccentric pattern can stimulate growth on the compression side of the physis.[23] Within a physiologic range, increasing tension or compression accelerates growth; however, beyond the physiologic limits of either, growth may be significantly decreased or even stopped. These principles are referred to as the *Heuter-Volkmann law* of cartilage growth.[11] Clinically, these forces can be appreciated in the spontaneous correction of angular deformities such as genu valgum or genu varum. The normal fluctuations in rate of physeal growth, as influenced by the compression forces of genu varum or genu valgum positions, are illustrated in Figure 1-7. Pauwels[23] demonstrated that the growth plate responds eccentrically to changes in pressure and will, through selective growth in different regions, attempt to reorient itself perpendicular to the major joint reaction forces across the physis.

Since similar physiologic processes are involved in bone growth and bone healing, it is not surprising to find the same extrinsic and intrinsic factors to be influential. Factors promoting bone healing include growth hormone, various thyroid hormones, calcitonin, insulin, vitamins A and B in physiologic doses, anabolic steroids, chondroitin sulfate, hyaluronidase, certain types of electrical current, low-dosage hyperbaric oxygenation, and exercise.[25-29] Factors that appear to retard bone healing are corticosteroids, diabetes, endocrinopathies, high doses of certain vitamins (e.g., A and D), anemia, unusual chemicals, denervation, irradiation, high-dosage hyperbaric oxygenation, some antibiotics, and anticoagulants.[24,25-29] The degree of trauma, as well as the degree of immobilization, influences the rate of healing following a fracture.

## ANATOMY AND PHYSIOLOGY OF GROWING BONE

The *diaphysis* constitutes the major portion of the cortical osseous structure of a long bone. It develops primarily through periosteal and intramembranous osseous tissue apposition on the original endochondral model, as well as endosteal remodeling and bone formation.[8] At birth, the diaphysis consists primarily of laminar (fetal, woven) bone lacking in haversian systems.[11] The *metaphyses*, located at each end of the diaphysis, are characterized by decreased cortical thickness and increased amounts of trabecular bone, comprising both primary and secondary spongiosa.[8,11] The metaphyseal cortex is also more porous. Periosteum is more firmly attached to the metaphyses than it is to the diaphysis. The *epiphyses*

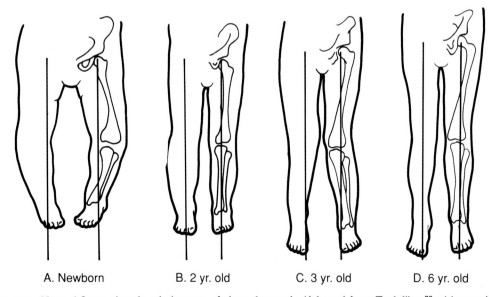

A. Newborn          B. 2 yr. old          C. 3 yr. old          D. 6 yr. old

**Fig. 1-7.** Normal fluctuations in relative rate of physeal growth. (Adapted from Tachdjian,[39] with permission.)

are completely cartilaginous at birth, except for that of the distal femur. During development this cartilage model is gradually replaced by bone, leaving only articular cartilage at skeletal maturity.

## The Physis

The *growth plate* or *physis* is the site of both longitudinal and latitudinal expansion of the bone. Anatomically, the growth plate (Fig. 1-8) can be divided into several zones or layers of cells, embedded in a matrix of ground substance composed of collagen fibers in chondroitin sulfate. Beginning at the epiphyseal end of the physis, there is a subchondral plate of bone through which blood vessels pass to supply blood to the growth plate layers. Germinal cells of the articular cartilage are nourished by diffusion from synovial fluid rather than receiving a direct blood supply. Although the layers or zones of the physis have been variously named,[3,5,10] the essential description of these layers remains the same.

The layer of chondrocyte cells nearest the epiphysis is embedded in abundant matrix. Within this zone of growth[10] (or proliferative zone or resting/germinal cell layer[3]), cells of the germinal layer multiply and grow, and hyaline intercellular matrix is produced. The next layer of cells is composed of cells undergoing rapid mitosis and is referred to as the *zone of proliferation*.[3] The resting and dividing cells are intimately associated with blood

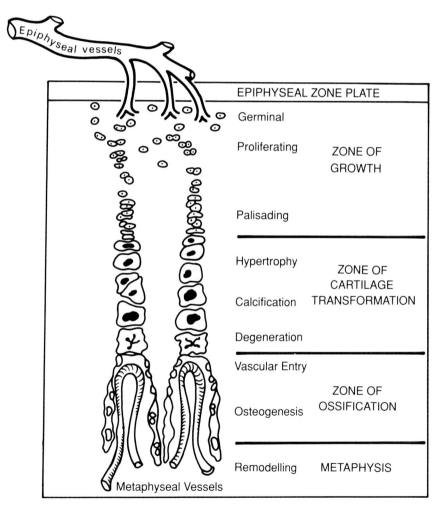

**Fig. 1-8.** Model of the growth plate and zones of growth.

vessels of the epiphysis. The third layer of cells is composed of chondrocytes undergoing hypertrophy to as much as five times their normal size and is appropriately referred to as the *zone of hypertrophy*.[3] This enlargement is accompanied by a reduction of matrix between the lacunae. In the fourth layer, the *zone of ossification,* hypertrophic cells begin to disintegrate in conjunction with the calcification of the surrounding cartilage matrix. The disintegration of the hypertrophic cells results in invasion of the metaphyseal blood vessels and increased local oxygen tension, thereby promoting ossification of the matrix ground substance. The invading metaphyseal vessels deposit osteoid on the calcified cartilage columns. Injuries involving the zone of ossification have a relatively minor impact on growth.

The region between the zone of hypertrophying cells and the zone of ossifying cells appears to be the structurally weakest part of the physis because of the reduced concentration of cementing ground substance and is therefore the most likely to be involved in physeal fractures. Although classical physeal disruption takes place in this plane, Bright et al.[30] have shown experimentally that physeal fractures may take a circuitous route through other layers of the physis as often as 50 percent of the time. Provided the layers of proliferating and hypertrophying cells remain attached to the epiphysis with its epiphyseal blood supply undisturbed, there is unlikely to be any growth disturbance.[3] However, the possibility of growth disturbance should be considered with any physeal injury.

The strength of the epiphyseal plate stems externally from reinforcement by the periosteum and internally from the mamillary processes (undulations in the growth plate). The periosteum in children is both thicker and stronger than in adults. The growth plate structure makes it most resistant to traction and least resistant to torsion. The undulations in the growth plate help to resist shear stresses.

Compression (or pressure) epiphyses, located primarily at the ends of long bones, are associated with longitudinal growth of bone, while traction epiphyses are more involved with the eventual shape of bone.[15] Traction epiphyses are nonarticular. The calcaneal apophysis and tibial tuberosity are prime examples of traction epiphyses.

Injuries to the physis are frequently referred to as epiphyseal injuries; however, as pointed out by Banks,[3] this is a misnomer because it is not epiphyseal damage, but rather physeal damage, that may cause growth arrest.

## Bone

The external surface of the *periosteum* provides the attachment of most muscle fibers along the metaphysis and diaphysis. This structure allows coordinated growth of bone and muscle units.[11] Sharpey's fibers, collagen connections between tendon or ligament and cortical bone, develop with progressive skeletal maturation. According to Ogden, "these differing and developing interrelationships between soft tissue and chondro-osseous components are major factors in the tendency toward soft tissue/bone interface avulsion in the adult and intra-osseous failure in a child."[8]

Developing bone initially has fewer lamellar components and a relatively greater porosity than mature bone. The porous nature of a child's bone allows failure not only in tension but also in compression, resulting in the characteristic complete or incomplete fractures that occur.[10] Bone tissue with an irregular, relatively unorganized pattern of collagen orientation and lacunar distribution has been termed *woven bone* (fibrous, nonlamellar).[11] It is generally found in areas of endochondral ossification and at sites of tendinous or ligamentous attachments and is eventually replaced by mature lamellar bone. It is also characteristic of the initial bone formation within fracture callus. *Trabecular bone* consists of a three-dimensional lattice of woven osseous plates and columns and may be found throughout the developing skeleton.[11] It is progressively oriented, organized, and transformed to mature lamellar bone to provide maximal strength with use of minimal osseous material. *Laminar bone* is the characteristic layered bone of the initial diaphyseal and metaphyseal cortices.[11] *Lamellar bone* is mature, more biologically responsive bone, characterized by collagen fibrils running in different directions in each of the multiple lamellae.[11] The strongest bone is circumferential lamellar bone, followed in descending order of strength by primary laminar, secondary haversian, and woven bone.[8]

Bone generally remodels in response to the normal physiologic stresses of body weight, muscle activity, joint motion, and intrinsic controls such as the periosteum.[11] Physiologic remodeling depends upon endochondral and periosteal (appositional) bone formation and integrated resorption. It is generally accepted that the straightening of the deformity caused by a malunited fracture is due mainly to variable apposition and resorption at the fracture site (Wolff's law).[11] Wolff's law suggests that bone is deposited in areas subjected to stress and is resorbed in areas of minimal stress. Bone remodeling occurs because of simultaneous osteoblastic deposition of bone on one surface and osteoclastic resorption on the opposite surface.

During the growing years, bone deposition exceeds bone resorption. The remodeling capacity of a deformity caused by a fracture or epiphyseal injury is a function of three factors: (1) age of the child; (2) distance of the fracture from the bone end; and (3) amount of angulation.[11,32] Each of these factors must be considered in determining the acceptability of fracture position pre- or postreduction. Minimal angular deformities (15 degrees or less) may resolve spontaneously if at least 1 to 2 years of growth remain.[3] Rotational deformities *cannot* be expected to remodel. In general, some remodeling will usually occur in children with 2 or more years of growth ahead, with fractures nearer the growth plate (ends of the bone), and in children with deformities in the plane of movement of the joint.[11,32,33] Remodeling will not help: (1) displaced intra-articular fractures; (2) fractures in the middle of a bone shaft that are significantly shortened, angulated, or rotated; (3) displaced fractures with the axis of displacement perpendicular to the plane of movement; or (4) displaced fractures crossing the growth plate at right angles.[33]

## Vascular Supply

Developing bone is known to be extremely vascular. The periosteum contains numerous small vessels that play a role in osteogenesis. The endosteal surfaces of both the metaphysis and the diaphysis receive blood via the nutrient artery, and the epiphysis receives blood from vessels penetrating through the cartilage. Epiphyseal and metaphyseal blood supplies are considered to be functionally and anatomically separate (see Fig. 1-9).

The physis receives its blood supply from three different sources: epiphyseal vessels, metaphyseal vessels, and perichondral vessels. Each of these systems is essentially end-arterial. This pattern changes with bony maturation. As the secondary center of ossification enlarges to form a subchondral plate, small vessels from the

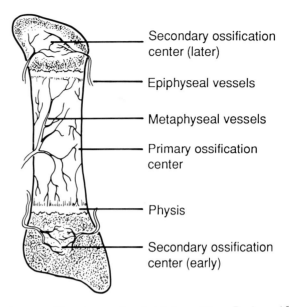

Secondary ossification center (later)

Epiphyseal vessels

Metaphyseal vessels

Primary ossification center

Physis

Secondary ossification center (early)

**Fig. 1-9.** Vasculature of pediatric bone (From Rockwood,[38] with permission.)

epiphyseal circulation penetrate the plate to supply the germinal layer of the physis. These vessels retain an end-arterial pattern. The net effect of this type of circulatory pattern is that anything that compromises even a part of the epiphyseal circulation, temporarily or permanently, can affect physeal zones of growth that are associated with those vessels. Since all epiphyses in the foot and ankle are extra-articular, the epiphyseal blood supply to the physis is rarely disrupted with physeal injuries. Meanwhile, the perichondral vascular network provides peripheral circulation to the epiphysis, physis, and metaphysis. The most important branches supply the zone of Ranvier. Disruption of these vessels can interfere with appositional growth at the periphery of the physis. On a longer-term basis, this may result in eccentric growth and premature, localized epiphysiodesis. It is important to avoid stripping the perichondrium and periosteum near the physis during surgery in order to protect the blood supply and lessen the chances of growth arrest. The nutrient artery supplies the metaphyseal side of the growth plate. Interruption of the metaphyseal circulation has no significant effect on chondrogenesis.

When the germinal layer ceases its division and growth, the physeal plate narrows, and the invading metaphyseal vessels eventually penetrate the plate and establish vascular channels across the physis. Ossification and complete bony union between the primary and secondary ossification centers eventually result.[15]

## Cartilage, Ligaments, and Soft Tissue

Since chondrocytes require very little oxygen for their metabolism but are dependent on the diffusion of nutrients from the synovial fluid, the two most important factors in the optimal nutrition of articular cartilage are a healthy synovial membrane to produce the synovial fluid and adequate "circulation" of this fluid through the matrix to reach the chondrocytes. Nutrition of the cartilage is enhanced by joint motion. Immobilization of a joint, especially if prolonged, leads to stasis of synovial fluid and to disuse atrophy of the cartilage.[5] Synovial fluid has the dual function of nourishing the articular cartilage and lubricating the joint surfaces.

It has been theorized that hyaline articular cartilage arises by differentiation from the same cartilaginous precursor cells that form the physis and the epiphysis. Once formed, however, hyaline cartilage will not undergo ossification.[3] As pointed out by Bennett et al., "unlike bone, the differentiated hyaline cartilage comprising the joint surfaces, and probably, the relatively undifferentiated hyaline cartilage of the epiphyses, appear to have a limited ability to repair or regenerate."[34] If nearly anatomic reduction is achieved following intra-articular fractures, the thin scar of fibrocartilage that forms is believed to have little significance for normal joint function. However, if there is a significant gap following reduction, the fibrocartilage may not be able to withstand normal wear and tear and may contribute to early degenerative changes.

The cartilaginous epiphyseal plate is weaker than bone and ligamentous structures and therefore more likely than the ligaments to fail during the years of skeletal development.[16] Ligament injuries and joint dislocation become more common with the attainment of skeletal maturity. The growth plate, however, has a higher elastic modulus than the fibrous periosteum. Because only shearing and avulsion forces can separate the epiphysis, fractures through bone are more common in childhood than epiphyseal separations.[10]

*Tendon* or *ligament* injuries are rare prior to complete skeletal maturation. Since tendons derive their major blood supply from the mesotenon, disruption of this blood supply may cause the tendon to degenerate. The ligaments and joint capsule usually attach directly and densely into the epiphyseal perichondrium and zone of Ranvier. Although ligaments exhibit greater laxity in children than in adults, the capsule and ligaments are relatively more resistant to stress than the adjacent bone and cartilage.[32] The laxity of developing ligaments allows a greater degree of distortion without failure of ligaments in children; however, this laxity decreases with age, and the ligament becomes increasingly susceptible to rupture. Ogden has indicated that "the basis of both tendinous and ligamentous healing is sufficient anatomical reapproximation to allow bridging with collagen and fibroblastic tissue, and the subsequent reorientation of the collagen to re-establish the tensile strength."[11] If a tendon is injured, the damaged tendon ends, as compared with osseous fracture surfaces, do not contribute significantly to the initial healing process.[35] Instead there is fibroblastic infiltration from the surrounding soft tissues. The reparative capacity of the child's tendon is much greater than that of the adult's.[15]

## BIOMECHANICAL PROPERTIES OF GROWING BONE

Mature (adult) bone is physiologically and mechanically in a relatively static state compared with immature (pediatric) bone.[3] Modes of failure within bone will vary with the degree of chondro-osseous maturation. Under normal conditions there are four basic types of stress in developing bones: tension (elongation), compression, shear, and torsion. Physiologic stress, in the form of compression and tension, appears necessary for the continued orderly development of growth plates. Within a physiologic range increases in either compression or tension will accelerate growth, but beyond physiologic limits growth may be either impaired or stopped entirely. When stress forces are increased beyond physiologic limits, the deformation that results is a function of both the magnitude of force exerted and the rate of loading.

Trauma to longitudinal growth plates may be caused by any combination of these forces. Tension and compression stresses are applied in a longitudinal direction; shear stresses are applied at oblique angles; and rotational force produces torsional stresses. The plate is least resistant to torsion and most resistant to traction.[10] Research suggests that the epiphysis can probably be displaced as much as 0.5 mm before any gross separation begins.[8] Bright et al.[30] noted that shear cracks in the growth plate are seen when the load applied to the plate is 50 percent of that necessary to separate the plate.

The periosteum, which is attached directly in the zone of Ranvier at both ends of the developing long bone, is only loosely attached to the diaphysis and metaphysis. This periosteal sleeve functions as an intrinsic tensile restraint. The increased density of the periosteum around the physeal periphery provides increased resistance to shear and tensile failure at the physis. Additionally, the physeal periosteum blends into the epiphyseal perichondrium and joint capsule, which further enhances the strength of the growth plate.

As noted by DeValentine, "extrinsic factors such as magnitude, direction, and rate of application of force are important in determining the location and way in which bone or physis will fail."[3] Intrinsic characteristics of developing bone and cartilage, such as energy-absorbing capacity, elasticity, fatigue strength, and density, can also influence the response of these tissues to potentially injurious forces. Each of these characteristics goes through changes during skeletal maturation. Bright and Elmore[36] showed that the viscoelasticity of physeal cartilage is dependent on rate of loading. The greater elasticity ascribed to immature bone is probably a function of its lower density (greater porosity). Children's bone can thus tolerate a greater degree of deformation than mature bone. Compact adult bone fails in tension only, whereas the more porous nature of a child's bone allows failure in compression as well.[37] The increasing size of the secondary center of ossification affects the energy-absorbing capacity of the physis and contributes to the greater incidence of physeal injuries in older children. Increasing diaphyseal and metaphyseal cortical width and the development of primary and secondary osteons affect the modulus of elasticity and relative density and thereby cause different fracture patterns.[8] For example, greenstick fractures may be seen in immature bone rather than the complete fractures seen in mature bone.

The strength of the physis is a function of cytoarchitectural type, cellular arrangement, and intercellular cartilaginous matrix. In the first two physeal zones abundant cartilage matrix intrinsically strengthens the physis. The third zone, consisting of hypertrophic chondrocytes and decreased quantities of matrix, has been shown experimentally to be the weakest portion of the epiphyseal plate. This weakness occurs with respect to shearing, bending, and tension but not compression stresses. The fourth zone is reinforced by calcification but is still weaker than the first and second zones.[11] The ability of the physis to resist separation and shear stress is increased by the mountainous convolutions and small interdigitating mamillary processes that increase its surface area. Despite the biomechanical data that have been accumulated and clinical studies that have indicated the physis to be the weakest link in the immature skeletal unit, only about 15 to 20 percent of all fractures in children actually occur through the growth plate.[15]

The region of trabecular formation in the metaphysis also contributes to physeal strength. However, the thin, fenestrated metaphyseal cortex makes this portion of the bone susceptible to injuries, such as compression or torus fractures, which are not usually seen in adults. Since the epiphysis is primarily cartilaginous, it functions as a limited shock absorber. Therefore, fracture-producing forces are transmitted more directly into the metaphysis, resulting in torus fractures. It appears that enlargement of the epiphyseal ossification center reduces the resiliency and shock-absorbing capability of the epiphysis, resulting in more direct transmission of deforming forces into the growth plate.[21] Since the growth plate is a potentially weaker region, it may be sheared through the third and fourth cellular zones. The metaphysis of immature long bones is composed of a loosely woven spongiosa bone that has greater porosity, vascularity, and elasticity than mature bone. This spongiosa bone also acts as a shock absorber. The junction of the metaphyseal and diaphyseal bone is relatively resistant to fracture as compared with adjacent regions of bone because the cortex becomes thicker and osteonal remodeling takes place here.

Throughout most of childhood, the periosteum is thicker, more osteogenic, and more resistant to disruption than similar tissue in adults.[32] The periosteum is more easily separated from bone in children, so it often remains partially intact following a fracture and may lessen the degree of displacment. In addition to greater thickness and strength, the periosteum in children also produces callus more quickly and in greater amount than in adults.

In summary, the developing skeleton is undergoing active, often rapid, growth and remodeling. Therefore pediatric fractures heal rapidly, nonunion is rare, overgrowth may occur, and some angular deformities may spontaneously correct.[32] From a biomechanical perspective there are numerous differences between the immature and the mature skeleton. Major changes undergone by developing bone are increases in the density of the cortex and changes in the proportions of trabecular (endosteal) and cortical bone in the diaphysis, metaphysis, and epiphysis. Porosity is greater in immature bone and may play a role in stopping fracture propagation. Comminuted fractures are uncommon in children. In children cortical bone has a greater capacity for plastic deformation prior to failure and will often buckle rather than break. This is a compression type of bone failure.[32] Plastic deformation is essentially an irreversible deformation. Clinically, this suggests that bone can sustain permanent damage even though no gross fracture or decrease in load-carrying capacity is noted.[8]

# REFERENCES

1. Tachdjian MO: Introduction. p. 1. In The Child's Foot. WB Saunders, Philadelphia, 1985
2. Salter RS: Specific fractures and joint injuries in children. p. 427. In Textbook of Disorders and Injuries of the Musculoskeletal System. 2nd Ed. Williams & Wilkins, Baltimore, 1983
3. DeValentine SJ: Foot and ankle fractures in children. p. 473. In Scurran BL (ed): Foot and Ankle Trauma. Churchill Livingstone, New York, 1989
4. Gross RH: Fractures and Dislocations of the Foot. p. 1043. In Rockwood CA Jr, Wilkins KE, King RE (eds): Fractures in Children. Vol 3. JB Lippincott, Philadelphia, 1984
5. Salter RS: Normal structure and function of musculoskeletal tissues. p. 5. In Textbook of Disorders and Injuries of the Musculoskeletal System, 2nd Ed. Williams & Wilkins, Baltimore, 1983
6. Sarrafian SK: Anatomy of the foot and ankle. JB Lippincott, Philadelphia, 1983
7. McCarthy DJ: Anatomy. p. 3. In McGlamry ED (ed): Fundamentals of Foot Surgery. Williams & Wilkins, Baltimore, 1987
8. Ogden JA: Anatomy and physiology of skeletal development. p. 16. In Skeletal injury in the Child. Lee & Febiger, Philadelphia, 1982
9. Arey LB: Developmental Anatomy. 7th Ed. WB Saunders, Philadelphia, 1974
10. Siffert RS, Feldman DJ: Trauma to the child's foot and ankle, including growth plate and epiphyseal injuries. p.
11. Ogden JA: The uniqueness of growing bones. p. 1. In Rockwood CA Jr, Wilkins KE, King RE (eds): Fractures in Children. Vol. 3. JB Lippincott, Philadlphia, 1984
12. Brighton C: Structure and function of the growth plate. Clin Orthop 136:22, 1978
13. Ogden JA: Foot. p. 621. In Skeletal Injury in the Child. Lea & Febiger, Philadelphia, 1982
14. Draves DJ: Anatomy of the Lower Extremity. Williams & Wilkins, Baltimore, 1986
15. Bright RW: Physeal injuries. p. 87. In Rockwood CA Jr, Wilkins KE, King RE (eds): Fractures in Children. Vol. 3. JB Lippincott, Philadelphia, 1984
16. Ogden JA: Tibia and Fibula. p. 555. In Skeletal Injury in the Child. Lea & Febiger, Philadelphia, 1982
17. Kleiger B, Barton J: Epiphyseal ankle fractures. Bull Hosp Jt Dis Orthop Inst 25:240, 1964
18. Gould N, Moreland M, Trevino S et al: Foot growth in children age one to five years. Foot Ankle: 10:211, 1990
19. Blais MM, Green WT, Anderson M: Lengths of the growing foot. J Bone Joint Surg [Am] 38A:998, 1956
20. Anderson, M, Green WT: Lengths of the femur and tibia: norms derived from orthoroentgenograms of children from 5 years of age until epiphyseal closure. Am J Dis Child 75:279, 1968
21. Rose S, Bradley TR, Nelson JF: Factors influencing the growth of epiphyseal cartilage. Aust J Exp Biol Med Sci 44:57, 1966
22. Ogden JA: Injury to the growth mechanisms, p. 59. In Skeletal Injury in the Child. Lea & Febiger, Philadelphia, 1982
23. Ryoppy, S, Karahaju EO: Alteration of epiphyseal growth by an experimentally produced angular deformity. Acta Orthop Scandi 45:290, 1974
24. Pauwels E: Über die mechanische Bedeutung der groberen Kortikalisstruktur beim normal und patlogisch verbogenen Rohrenknochen. Anat Nachr 1:53, 1950
25. Burger M, Sherman BS, Sobel AE: Observations on the influence of chondroitin sulfate on the rate of bone repair. J Bone Joint Surg [Br] 44:675, 1962
26. Herbsman H et al: The influence of systemic factors on fracture healing. J Trauma 6:75, 1966
27. Herold HZ, Tadmor A: Chondroitin sulfate in treatment of experimental bone defects. Isr J Med Sci 5:425, 1969
28. Herold HZ, Mobel TA, Tadmor A: Cartilage extract in treatment of fractures in rabbits. Acta Orthop Scand 40:317, 1969
29. Lack CH: Proteolytic activity and connective tissue. Br Med Bull 20:217, 1964
30. Bright RW, Burstein AH, Elmore SM: Epiphyseal-plate

cartilage. A biomechanical and histological analysis of failure modes. J Bone Joint Surg [Am] 56:688, 1974

31. Banks AS: Epiphyseal Injuries. p. 964. In McGlamry ED (ed): Comprehensive Textbook of Foot Surgery. Vol 2. Williams & Wilkins, Baltimore, 1987

32. Ogden JA: General Principles. p. 3. In Skeletal Injury in the Child. Lea & Febiger, Philadelphia, 1982

33. Rang M: Fracture care is a game of chess. p. 26. In Children's Fractures. JB Lippincott, Philadelphia, 1983

34. Bennett GA, Baur W, Maddock SJ: A study of the repair of articular cartilage. Am J Pathol 8:499, 1932

35. Clark CR, Ogden JA: Prenatal and postnatal development of the human knee joint meniscus. Trans Orthop Res Soc 6:225, 1981

36. Bright RW, Elmore SM: Physical properties of epiphyseal plate cartilage. Surg Forum 19:463, 1968

37. Rang M: Children are not just small adults. p. 1. In Children's Fractures. JB Lippincott, Philadelphia, 1983

38. Rockwood C: Fractures in Children. p. 91 JB Lippincott, Philadelphia; 1984

39. Tachdjian, MO: Pediatric Orthopedics. WB Saunders, Philadelphia, 1972

## SUGGESTED READINGS

Aitken AP: Fractures of the epiphysis. Clin Orthop 41:19, 1965

Carothers CO, Crenshaw AH: Clinical significance of a classification of epiphyseal injuries at the ankle. Am J Surg 89:879, 1955

Dale GC, Harris WR: Prognosis in epiphysis separation. An experimental study. J Bone Joint Surg [Br] 40:116, 1958

Dias LS, Tachdjian MJ: Physeal injuries of the ankle in children. Clin Orthop 136:230, 1978

Foucher M: De la divulsion des epiphyses. Cong Med France, Paris, 1:63, 1863

Lauge-Hansen N: Fractures of the ankle: 2 Combined experimental surgical and experimental roentgenologic investigations. Arch Surg 60:957, 1950

Ogden JA: Injury to the growth mechanisms of the immature skeleton. Skeletal Radiol 6:237, 1981

Ogden JA: Biology of chondro-osseous repair. p. 111. In Skeletal Injury in the Child. Lea & Febiger, Philadelphia, 1982

Ogden JA: Radiologic aspects. p. 41. In Skeletal Injury in the Child. Lea & Febiger, Philadelphia, 1982

Poland J: Traumatic Separation of the Epiphyses. Smith, Elder & Co., London, 1898

Rang M: Ankle. p. 308. In Children's Fractures. JB Lippincott, Philadelphia, 1983

Rang M: Foot. p. 323. In Children's Fractures. JB Lippincott, Philadelphia, 1983

Rang M: Fractures with vascular damage. p. 37. In Children's Fractures. JB Lippincott, Philadelphia, 1983

Rang M: Fractures in special circumstances. p. 51. In Children's Fractures. JB Lippincott, Philadelphia, 1983

Rang M: Soft-tissue injuries. p. 70. In Children's Fractures. JB Lippincott, Philadelphia, 1983

Rang M: Injuries of the epiphysis, the growth plate, and the perichondral ring. p. 10. In Children's Fractures. JB Lippincott, Philadelphia, 1983

Salter RS: Reactions of musculoskeletal tissues to disorders and injuries. p. 25. In Textbook of Disorders and Injuries of the Musculoskeletal System. 2nd Ed. Williams & Wilkins, Baltimore, 1983

Salter RS: Common normal variations. p. 101. In Textbook of Disorders and Injuries of the Musculoskeletal System. 2nd Ed. Williams & Wilkins, Baltimore, 1983

Salter RS: Congenital abnormalities. p. 113. In Textbook of Disorders and Injuries of the Musculoskeletal System. 2nd Ed. Williams & Wilkins, Baltimore, 1983

Salter RS: Disorders of epiphyses and epiphyseal growth. p. 285. In Textbook of Disorders and Injuries of the Musculoskeletal System. 2nd Ed. Williams & Wilkins, Baltimore, 1983

Salter RS: The general principles and specific methods of musculoskeletal treatment. p. 75. In Textbook of Disorders and Injuries of the Musculoskeletal System. 2nd Ed. Williams & Wilkins, Baltimore, 1983

Salter RB, Harris MD: Injuries involving the epiphyseal plate. J Bone Joint Surg 45:587, 1963

Weber BC: Treatment of Fractures in Children and Adolescents. Springer-Verlag, New York, 1980

# 2

# General Examination of the Infant and Child

*STEPHEN L. KAUFMAN*

A basic knowledge of pediatrics is essential for the clinician who treats lower extremity musculoskeletal disorders in children. Podiatric consultation may be requested for congenital anomalies such as polydactyly, syndactyly, metatarsus adductus, or clubfoot in the nursery, or for toeing-in, bowed legs, knock knee, etc. in the older child. Knowledge of normal development is necessary to reassure parents that time will resolve the apparent problem or to explain the reasons for intervention. Many abnormalities seen in adults originate in childhood. Only with a thorough knowledge of pediatrics can the evolution of the problem be understood and many of the difficulties be prevented through education and early treatment.

Podiatric care of children will include surgery. Perioperative care, including reducing a child's anxiety, use of appropriate anesthetic agents, and the postoperative management of pain, infection, and fluid therapy is imperative to minimize pediatric operative morbidity.

Podiatrists may be the first health care professionals to see a child who has been physically abused. Good interview technique is essential and dependent upon knowledge of a child's comprehension at various ages. The ability to distinguish patterns of abuse from normal bruising and bruising secondary to blood dyscrasias may be life-saving.

## GROWTH AND DEVELOPMENT

A child is not a miniature adult but an evolving organism whose nutritional requirements, laboratory values, drug dosages, and disease entities vary by size and age. An awareness of the dynamics of normal growth and development is essential for an accurate evaluation of a child. Growth refers to aspects of maturation that can be measured, while development describes changes in function.

## Growth

An average newborn is 20 inches long; body length increases to 30 inches at age 1 and 34 inches at age 2. (Length is measured horizontally, height vertically. There is a small but measurable difference between these modalities.) An average child grows 3 inches per year from age 2 to 6 and 2 inches per year from 7 to puberty. Prior to puberty there is less than a 2-inch differential between the median heights of boys and girls. In girls, the adolescent growth spurt is concomitant with the onset of puberty and subsides after menarche. Final height is about 2 inches more than height at menarche. In boys, growth acceleration begins approximately 2 years after the onset of puberty and continues until age 18 (Figs. 2-1 and 2-2).

Body proportions are age-related and are measured as the ratio of the upper segment (crown to symphysis pubis) to the lower segment (symphysis pubis to floor). In the newborn the ratio is about $1.7:1$, by 10 years it is $1:1$, and during adolescence it is $0.95:1$.

Also, the normal newborn has more variability in weight than in height. Average birth weight is 7½ pounds (range 5½ to 10), doubling by 5 months, tripling at 1 year, and quadrupling by 2 years. Thereafter until the onset of puberty, normal weight gain is 4 to 5 pounds yearly. Rapid weight gain accompanies the adolescent growth spurt.

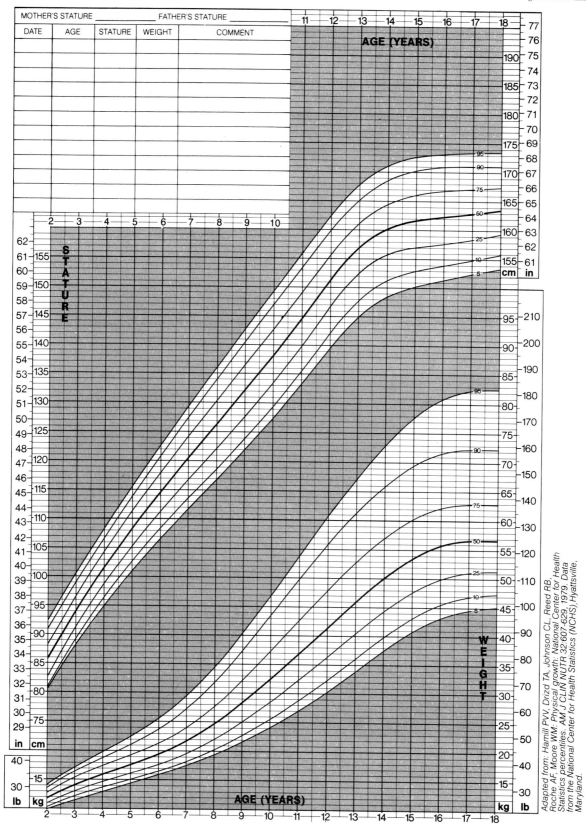

NAME _____ RECORD # _____

**Fig. 2-1.** Physical growth percentiles for girls 2 to 18 years.

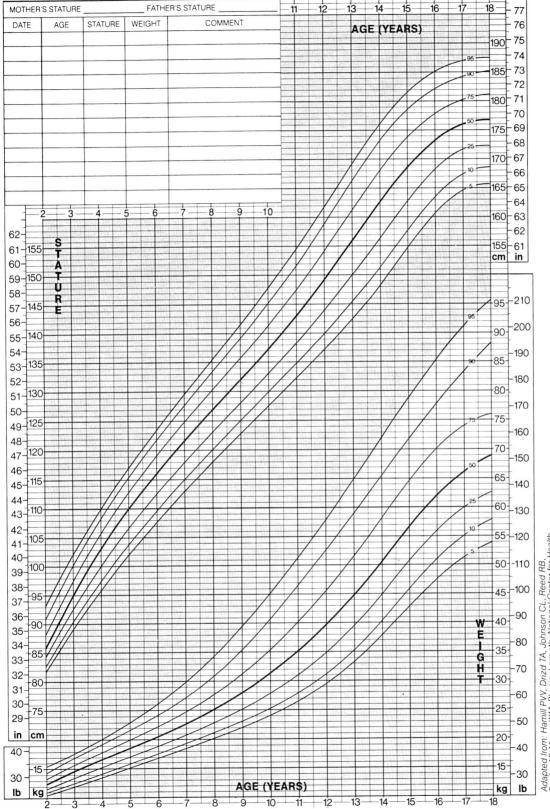

MOTHER'S STATURE _____ FATHER'S STATURE _____

| DATE | AGE | STATURE | WEIGHT | COMMENT |
|------|-----|---------|--------|---------|
|      |     |         |        |         |
|      |     |         |        |         |
|      |     |         |        |         |
|      |     |         |        |         |
|      |     |         |        |         |
|      |     |         |        |         |
|      |     |         |        |         |

AGE (YEARS)

STATURE

WEIGHT

AGE (YEARS)

Adapted from: Hamill PVV, Drizd TA, Johnson CL, Reed RB, Roche AF, Moore WM. Physical growth: National Center for Health Statistics percentiles. AM J CLIN NUTR 32:607-629, 1979. Data from the National Center for Health Statistics (NCHS), Hyattsville, Maryland.

© 1982 Ross Laboratories

**Fig. 2-2.** Physical growth percentiles for boys 2 to 18 years.

Table 2-1. **Chronology of Human Dentition**

### Primary or Deciduous Teeth

| | Calcification | | Eruption | | Shedding | |
|---|---|---|---|---|---|---|
| | Begins at | Complete at | Maxillary | Mandibular | Maxillary | Mandibular |
| Central incisors | 5th Fetal month | 18–24 Months | 6–8 Months | 5–7 Months | 7–8 Years | 6–7 Years |
| Lateral incisors | 5th Fetal month | 18–24 Months | 8–11 Months | 7–10 Months | 8–9 Years | 7–8 Years |
| Cuspids (canines) | 6th Fetal month | 30–36 Months | 16–20 Months | 16–20 Months | 11–12 Years | 9–11 Years |
| First molars | 5th Fetal month | 24–30 Months | 10–16 Months | 10–16 Months | 10–11 Years | 10–12 Years |
| Second molars | 6th Fetal month | 36 Months | 20–30 Months | 20–30 Months | 10–12 Years | 11–13 Years |

### Secondary or Permanent Teeth

| | Calcification | | Eruption | |
|---|---|---|---|---|
| | Begins at | Complete at | Maxillary | Mandibular |
| Central incisors | 3–4 Months | 9–10 Years | 7–8 Years | 6–7 Years |
| Lateral incisors | Maxillary, 10–12 months | 10–11 Years | 8–9 Years | 7–8 Years |
| | Mandibular, 3–4 months | | | |
| Cuspids (canines) | 4–5 Months | 12–15 Years | 11–12 Years | 9–11 Years |
| First premolars | 18–21 Months | 12–13 Years | 10–11 Years | 10–12 Years |
| Second premolars | 24–30 Months | 12–14 Years | 10–12 Years | 11–13 Years |
| First molars | Birth | 9–10 Years | 6–7 Years | 6–7 Years |
| Second molars | 30–36 Months | 14–16 Years | 12–13 Years | 12–13 Years |
| Third Molars | Maxillary, 7–9 years | 18–25 Years | 17–22 Years | 17–22 Years |
| | Mandibular, 8–10 years | | | |

Adapted from chart prepared by P.K. Losch, who carried out radiographic assays of the jaws of 1,000 children in metropolitan Boston in 1942 at the Harvard School of Dental Medicine and provided the data for this chart. (From Vaugn VC III, McKay RJ: Nelson Textbook of Pediatrics. 10th Ed. WB Saunders, Phildelphia; 1975, with permission.)

The head circumference of a newborn is 13 to 14 inches, increasing to 18 inches at 1 year and 19 inches by 2 years. The posterior fontanelle closes between 2 and 4 months, the anterior fontanelle by 14 months. Failure of the head to grow is caused either by early fusion of the sutures and premature closure of the fontanelles or by inadequate brain development. After 2 years, changes in head size are less important except in specific disease states.

Teething is highly irregular with respect to both age and order of eruption. In general, the first tooth appears at 6 months, and the other teeth erupt according to the following rule: the number of teeth equals age in months minus 6. There are 20 teeth in the primary dentition, and they typically appear in the following order: two lower central incisors, four upper incisors, two lower lateral incisors, four first molars, four canines, and last, four second molars. The loss of the primary dentition begins between 6 and 7 years, and the permanent teeth erupt in similar fashion (Table 2-1).

## Development

*Development* refers to change in function and in children is complex, multifaceted, and strongly influenced by innate and environmental factors. The fetus responds to environmental forces in utero. Alcohol, nicotine, other drugs, both legal and illegal, maternal illness, fever, radiation, placental inadequacy, immunologic problems, trauma, uterine space abnormalities, and perhaps maternal anxiety all may have negative effects on the fetus. Recent studies suggest the maternal voice and music heard repetitively in utero increase the infant's attention to these sounds after birth.

A child's development can be subdivided into sensory, fine and gross motor coordination, language, and social aspects. One useful method of quantitation is the Denver Development Screening Test (Fig. 2-3). This test has its greatest value in charting a child's rate of progress and should not be used as an intelligence test.

The term *intelligence* is misleading; its frequent use

**Fig. 2-3.** Denver Developmental Screening Test. (From Frankenburg WK, Dodds JB: J Pediatr 71:181, 1967, with permission.)

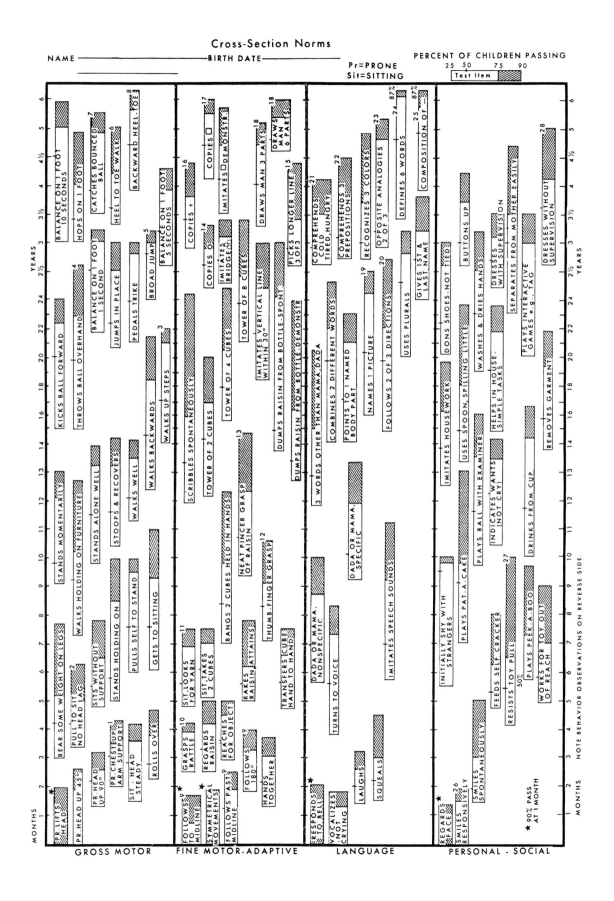

Cross-Section Norms

NAME ———————— BIRTH DATE ————————

Pr=PRONE
Sit=SITTING

PERCENT OF CHILDREN PASSING

25 50 75 90

Test Item

GROSS MOTOR

FINE MOTOR-ADAPTIVE

LANGUAGE

PERSONAL-SOCIAL

as a synonym for abstract ability creates inappropriate expectations for the child. More accurately, a child may be considered to have a group of intelligences, including abstract, memory, motor, verbal, social, and musical. By this approach a profile of a child's capacities is developed and ideally lends itself to the structuring of an educational milieu tailored to the individual's strengths and weaknesses. Developmental assessment requires a thorough knowledge of normality and variability. A normal child is often precocious in one area and delayed in another. Prediction of future development in early childhood, except in extreme situations or in the presence of known disease entities, is very inaccurate.

Evaluation of the sensorium in small children is important but difficult to accomplish. Although children are capable of responding to auditory stimuli before birth, severe hearing loss is frequently not diagnosed until 2 to 3 years of age and moderate loss until 3 to 4 years. Parents often misinterpret a child's hearing ability because of response to nonverbal stimuli such as body language and vibration. Hearing loss must be considered in any child with speech delay. Other causes of retarded speech include developmental delay, palatal abnormalities, relatively nonverbal households, and a bilingual environment.

Infants have vision at birth, including rudiments of tracking. Nystagmus, strabismus, cataracts, glaucoma, ptosis, and retinal abnormalities can interfere with visual perception. Prompt diagnosis is important if vision and depth perception are to be preserved. Olfactory sense is present at birth, and within the first week of life infants can distinguish their mother's breast pad from that of another lactating woman. The newborn also has the capacity to feel and to respond to tactile stimulation, including temperature changes and pain. Although an infant is unable to communicate verbally, there is no reason to ignore pain management during and after traumatic procedures.

Rapid acquisition of speech is a startlingly swift phenomenon. An infant attends to the human voice and coos in response by 8 weeks, laughs out loud by 16 weeks, and forms polysyllabic sounds by 28 weeks. Words (i.e., sounds symbolic of an object) develop at about 9 months, and the average 1-year-old speaks three words. Language development proceeds rapidly, with 10 words by 18 months and hundreds of words and rudimentary three-word sentences by 2 years. After age 2 attention is directed not only to speech acquisition but also to enunciation and problems such as stuttering and stammering.

Social development occurs according to an innate timetable modified by environmental influences. A social smile is present by 6 weeks and responsive laughter by 4 months. Fear of strangers and clinging to parents is apparent at 7 to 9 months. Temper tantrums are common in the second year of life. Parents and teachers are important role models for the child in establishing sexual identification and self-esteem. Sexual identification is normally established by 2 years. Children are capable of cooperating in toilet training around age 2. Parallel play occurs at age 3 and cooperative play at age 4. School readiness is variable and dependent not only on the ability to learn to read and write but on physical size, fine motor skills, social skills, linguistic ability, and self-esteem. Toward the end of childhood there is a strong tendency to form unisexual groups whose mutual support helps the child deal with early pubertal changes and social expectations.

Adolescence is a transition between childhood and maturity. Despite variability of onset and rapid physical changes, the sequence of events is remarkably constant. A generally accepted method of classifying physical changes of puberty has been depicted and described by Tanner (Figs. 2-4 and 2-5, Appendixes 2-1 and 2-2).

In boys the onset of pubertal changes begins about age 12 with testicular enlargement and thinning of the scrotum, followed 6 months later by the appearance of pubic hair. Phallic enlargement begins 12 to 18 months after testicular enlargement. A growth spurt occurs 2 to 2½ years after the onset of sexual changes and averages about 11 inches. The entire sequence is completed within 4½ years. Development of facial and axillary hair is erratic and dependent on hereditary factors. Transient gynecomastia is frequently seen in boys early in puberty.

In girls the onset of puberty is heralded by the appearance of breast buds between ages 10 and 11. It is common for breasts to develop neither simultaneously nor symmetrically. The development of pubic hair is similar to that in boys except that in 16 percent of girls pubic hair precedes the onset of breast budding. In contradistinction to its timing in boys, the growth spurt is concomitant with the beginning of puberty. Menarche occurs 2 to 2½ years after the appearance of breasts. The average girl grows 1 to 4 inches postmenarche, and the majority of this growth is completed in 2 years. Dur-

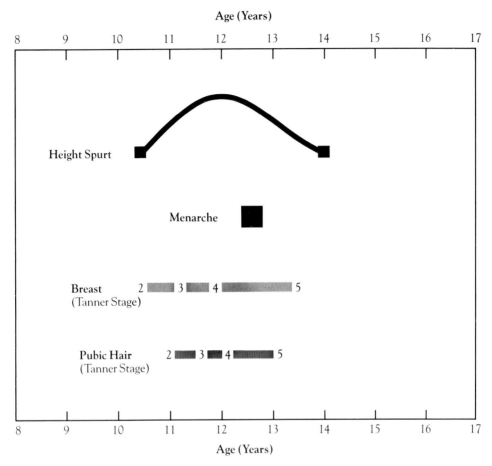

**Fig. 2-4.** Sequence of pubertal events, average American girl. (From Johnson TR, Moore WM, Jeffries JE: Children Are Different: Developmental Physiology. 2nd Ed. Ross Laboratories, Columbus, OH, 1978, with permission.)

ing the first year menses are usually anovulatory and irregular.

## NUTRITION

Dietary allowances as recommended by the Food and Nutrition Board of the National Academy of Sciences and the National Research Council are listed in Table 2-2. In most instances breast milk is the best source of nutrition for infants, providing sufficient calories and water for the first 6 months of life. Although breast milk is low in iron, there are substances in the milk that markedly enhance iron absorption as compared with artificial formulas.

Breast-fed infants should need no supplements; however, dark-skinned infants with limited exposure to sunlight, need a vitamin D supplement. Breast milk is high in cholesterol, which is important for normal development of the central nervous system. Other advantages of breast milk include reduction in infant allergies and partial protection from viral and bacterial infection. The value of breast milk is influenced by maternal diet and drug use. Formula feeding is an acceptable substitute for breast feeding in areas where good sanitation exists. Inability to thrive on cow's milk formulas may be due to allergy or to lactose intolerance. In those infants, a soy or protein hydrolysate formula can be used, and lactose can be replaced with another carbohydrate.

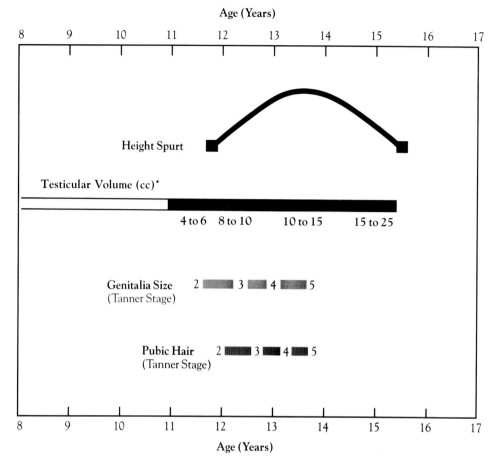

**Fig. 2-5.** Sequence of pubertal events, average American boy. (From Johnson TR, Moore WM, Jeffries JE: Children Are Different: Developmental Physiology. 2nd Ed. Ross Laboratories, Columbus, OH 1978, with permission.)

The daily fluid consumption of a healthy infant is 10 to 15 percent of body weight. Intake requirement varies with exercise, weight, external and body temperature, respiratory rate, and urine specific gravity.

Caloric requirements are 100 to 200 kcal/kg/day for the first year and decrease by about 10 kcal/kg/day for each succeeding 3-year period, with the exception of the accelerated growth period in adolescence. Physical activity uses 15 to 25 kcal/kg/day with peaks of 50 to 80 kcal/kg/day with maximal exertion. Normally less than 10 percent of food energy is lost in stool.

Protein requirements are between 2 and 3.5 g/kg/day in infancy and gradually decrease throughout childhood. Proteins are broken down to amino acids prior to absorption from the gastrointestinal tract. There are 24 amino acids in food, of which 9 are essential in infant nutrition: threonine, valine, leucine, isoleucine, lysine, tryptophan, phenylalanine, methionine, and histidine. The absence of any of these places the child in a negative nitrogen balance.

Carbohydrates are the major source of energy for the child. The infant has a poor capacity for storage and is therefore more vulnerable to hypoglycemia. After infancy a healthy diet includes 55 percent carbohydrates, 30 percent fat, and 15 percent protein. Preferably the majority of carbohydrates should be complex rather than simple sugars. Although lactose intolerance is very common, especially in black and Asiatic adults, it is infrequent in childhood.

Fats are essential to the health of a growing child, and

## Table 2-2. Dietary Allowances[a]

| Individual | Age (yr) | Weight (kg) | Weight (lb) | Height (cm) | Height (in) | Protein (g) | Vitamin A (µg RE)[b] | Vitamin D (µg)[c] | Vitamin E (mg α-TE)[d] | Vitamin C (mg) | Thiamin (mg) | Riboflavin (mg) | Niacin (mg NE)[e] | Vitamin B6 (mg) | Folacin (µg)[f] | Vitamin B12 (µg) | Calcium (mg) | Phosphorus (mg) | Magnesium (mg) | Iron (mg) | Zinc (mg) | Iodine (µg) |
|---|---|---|---|---|---|---|---|---|---|---|---|---|---|---|---|---|---|---|---|---|---|---|
| Infants | 0.0–0.5 | 6 | 13 | 60 | 24 | kg × 2.2 | 420 | 10 | 3 | 35 | 0.3 | 0.4 | 6 | 0.3 | 30 | 0.5[g] | 360 | 240 | 50 | 10 | 3 | 40 |
|  | 0.5–1.0 | 9 | 20 | 71 | 28 | kg × 2.0 | 400 | 10 | 4 | 35 | 0.5 | 0.6 | 8 | 0.6 | 45 | 1.5 | 540 | 360 | 70 | 15 | 5 | 50 |
| Children | 1–3 | 13 | 29 | 90 | 35 | 23 | 400 | 10 | 5 | 45 | 0.7 | 0.8 | 9 | 0.9 | 100 | 2.0 | 800 | 800 | 150 | 15 | 10 | 70 |
|  | 4–6 | 20 | 44 | 112 | 44 | 30 | 500 | 10 | 6 | 45 | 0.9 | 1.0 | 11 | 1.3 | 200 | 2.5 | 800 | 800 | 200 | 10 | 10 | 90 |
|  | 7–10 | 28 | 62 | 132 | 52 | 34 | 700 | 10 | 7 | 45 | 1.2 | 1.4 | 16 | 1.6 | 300 | 3.0 | 800 | 800 | 250 | 10 | 10 | 120 |
| Males | 11–14 | 45 | 99 | 157 | 62 | 45 | 1,000 | 10 | 8 | 50 | 1.4 | 1.6 | 18 | 1.8 | 400 | 3.0 | 1,200 | 1,200 | 350 | 18 | 15 | 150 |
|  | 15–18 | 66 | 145 | 176 | 69 | 56 | 1,000 | 10 | 10 | 60 | 1.4 | 1.7 | 18 | 2.0 | 400 | 3.0 | 1,200 | 1,200 | 400 | 18 | 15 | 150 |
|  | 19–22 | 70 | 154 | 177 | 70 | 56 | 1,000 | 7.5 | 10 | 60 | 1.5 | 1.7 | 19 | 2.2 | 400 | 3.0 | 800 | 800 | 350 | 10 | 15 | 150 |
|  | 23–50 | 70 | 154 | 178 | 70 | 56 | 1,000 | 5 | 10 | 60 | 1.4 | 1.6 | 18 | 2.2 | 400 | 3.0 | 800 | 800 | 350 | 10 | 15 | 150 |
|  | 51+ | 70 | 154 | 178 | 70 | 56 | 1,000 | 5 | 10 | 60 | 1.2 | 1.4 | 16 | 2.2 | 400 | 3.0 | 800 | 800 | 350 | 10 | 15 | 150 |
| Females | 11–14 | 46 | 101 | 157 | 62 | 46 | 800 | 10 | 8 | 50 | 1.1 | 1.3 | 15 | 1.8 | 400 | 3.0 | 1,200 | 1,200 | 300 | 18 | 15 | 150 |
|  | 15–18 | 55 | 120 | 163 | 64 | 46 | 800 | 10 | 8 | 60 | 1.1 | 1.3 | 14 | 2.0 | 400 | 3.0 | 1,200 | 1,200 | 300 | 18 | 15 | 150 |
|  | 19–22 | 55 | 120 | 163 | 64 | 44 | 800 | 7.5 | 8 | 60 | 1.1 | 1.3 | 14 | 2.0 | 400 | 3.0 | 800 | 800 | 300 | 18 | 15 | 150 |
|  | 23–50 | 55 | 120 | 163 | 64 | 44 | 800 | 5 | 8 | 60 | 1.0 | 1.2 | 13 | 2.0 | 400 | 3.0 | 800 | 800 | 300 | 18 | 15 | 150 |
|  | 51+ | 55 | 120 | 163 | 64 | 44 | 800 | 5 | 8 | 60 | 1.0 | 1.2 | 13 | 2.0 | 400 | 3.0 | 800 | 800 | 300 | 10 | 15 | 150 |
| Pregnant |  |  |  |  |  | +30 | +200 | +5 | +2 | +20 | +0.4 | +0.3 | +2 | +0.6 | +400 | +1.0 | +400 | +400 | +150 | [h] | +5 | +25 |
| Lactating |  |  |  |  |  | +20 | +400 | +5 | +3 | +40 | +0.5 | +0.5 | +5 | +0.5 | +100 | +1.0 | +400 | +400 | +150 | [h] | +10 | +50 |

[a] The allowances are intended to provide for individual variations among most normal persons in the United States under usual environmental stresses. Diets should be based on a variety of common foods to provide other nutrients for which human requirements have been less well defined.

[b] Retinol equivalents. 1 retinal equivalent = 1 µg retinol or 6 µg β-carotene.

[c] As cholecalciferol. 10 µg cholecalciferol = 400 IU of vitamin D.

[d] α-tocopherol equivalents. 1 mg d-α tocopherol = 1 α-TE.

[e] 1 NE (niacin equivalent) is equal to 1 mg of niacin or 60 mg of dietary tryptophan.

[f] The folacin allowances refer to dietary sources as determined by Lactobacillus casei assay after treatment with enzymes (conjugases) to make polyglutamyl forms of the vitamin available to the test organism.

[g] The recommended dietary allowance for vitamin B12 in infants is based on average concentration of the vitamin in human milk. The allowances after weaning are based on energy intake (as recommended by the American Academy of Pediatrics) and consideration of other factors, such as intestinal absorption.

[h] The increased requirement during pregnancy cannot be met by the iron content of habitual diets in the United States nor by the existing iron stores of many women; therefore, the use of 30 to 60 mg of supplemental iron is recommended. Iron needs during lactation are not substantially different from those of nonpregnant women, but continued supplementation of the mother for 2 to 3 months after parturition is advisable to replenish stores depleted by pregnancy.

(From Forbes, 1985, as adapted from Committee on Dietary Allowances and Food and Nutrition Board: Recommended Dietary Allowances. 9th Ed. National Academy of Sciences, Washington, 1980, with permission.)

cholesterol is necessary for normal development of the nervous system. After infancy a large proportion of the fats should be polyunsaturated. While diet is important, most children with marked hypercholesterolemia have a genetic basis for their disease.

Adequate amounts of vitamins and minerals are necessary for normal growth and development. It is rare in the United States for a healthy child on a typical diet to suffer from a deficiency or an excess. Thus despite a multimillion dollar vitamin industry, a normal child does not require supplementation. Fluoride is an exception in areas where the water supply is not fluoridated or in families that drink only bottled water. The addition of fluoride to water reduces dental cavities by between 35 and 50 percent, but excess fluoride causes mottling of the teeth.

# HISTORY

Obtaining a complete history is the most important element in the diagnosis of disease in children. A thorough knowledge of normal variation is essential because the presentation of many diseases is dependent upon race, gender, and age. Diseases are dynamic processes, and the evolution of symptoms is more important than their static description. Because young children are developmentally inarticulate and adolescents voluntarily inarticulate, a history is often obtained from a parent, which entails the danger of distortion or misrepresentation of the patient's problem. With adolescents the history of the present illness as obtained separately from patient and parent often reveals discrepancies that are useful in diagnosis.

A complete history can be obtained by subdividing it into the following categories: (1) informant; (2) chief complaint; (3) present illness; (4) past history; (5) family history; (6) social history.

## Informant

The informant may be the child, parent, other adult, school authority, or a doctor's note. A comment on the reliability of the informant is pertinent.

## Chief Complaint

The chief complaint should be a direct quote from the informant. Logical assumptions or paraphrasing by the interviewer leads to distortion. If feasible, the child

should be asked directly why he or she was brought to the clinician.

## Present Illness

The history of the present illness includes the genesis of the problem and its evolution through time. In some cases a portion of the family history or social history may need to be included. The child's health prior to the onset of the problem should be recorded and the initial symptoms dated and timed. This is followed by the progression of the disease and the sequence and timing of new symptoms. Factors that alleviate or aggravate the symptoms should be included, as well as what medications have been taken and to what effect. Informants should be allowed to express their opinions as to the etiology of their problems. The astute clinician asks questions that reveal significant details not considered relevant by informants. Pertinent negative information is an important aspect of the present illness.

## Past History

The past history is a complete medical picture of the child exclusive of the present illness. Sometimes information uncovered in the past history will later be found relevant to the present illness. The past history originates with the pregnancy and includes maternal parity, presence of sexually transmitted disease, and risk factors for hepatitis B and the acquired immunodeficiency syndrome (AIDS).

Abnormalities in the intrauterine environment may be significant in understanding pathology that may not become apparent for months or years. Drugs ingested during the pregnancy — legal or illegal, prescription or over-the-counter, including nicotine and alcohol — should be noted. Maternal illnesses, especially fevers, preeclampsia, surgery, trauma, autoimmune disorders, blood incompatibilities, uterine spacial abnormalities, and poly- or oligohydramnios should be listed; the infant's presentation (e.g., breech or vertex), maternal anesthesia or analgesia during labor, and type of delivery should be described; and the Apgar score (Table 2-3) at 1 and 5 minutes of age should be recorded.

## Nutrition

Children who are small for gestational age, dysmature, or hypoglycemic in the neonatal period may have had intrauterine nutritional deficiency. A nutritional history includes whether the child was breast- or bottle-fed, type

Table 2-3. **Apgar Score of Newborn Infant**

| | Sign | Score | | |
|---|---|---|---|---|
| | | 0 | 1 | 2 |
| **A** | Appearance (color) | Blue; pale | Body pink; extremities blue | Completely pink |
| **P** | Pulse (heart rate) | Absent | Below 100 | Over 100 |
| **G** | Grimace (reflex irritability in response to stimulation of sole of foot) | No response | Grimace | Cry |
| **A** | Activity (muscle tone) | Limp | Some flexion of extremities | Active motion |
| **R** | Respiration (respiratory effort) | Absent | Slow; irregular | Good strong cry |

of formula, age of weaning, dates of solid food introduction, appetite, current diet, and vitamin supplementation. Known or suspected food allergies and intolerances should be listed.

## Development

Development information pertinent to the history has been covered in the section on growth and development.

## Immunizations

The completeness of immunizations not only is important for disease prevention but also serves as a clue to the degree of parental concern. Any abnormal reactions to vaccines should be recorded, including skin tests for tuberculosis and, in the case of foreign-born children, whether and when they received bacille Calmette-Guérin (BCG) vaccine.

## Previous Illnesses

Enumerate all previous illnesses, including contagious diseases, by age, severity, complications, and sequelae. List previous hospitalizations, surgical procedures, fractures, and accidents by date and diagnosis.

## Allergies

An accurate allergic history is difficult to obtain. Many symptoms such as rash, diarrhea, recurrent pneumonia, sinusitis, bronchitis, and headache may have an allergic etiology unrecognized by the informant. Alternatively, symptoms ascribed to allergy may have a different cause.

## Personality

Children can only be understood in the context of their school and family. Inquire about relationships with parents and siblings and the quality of interrelationship with peers. Record traits such as thumb-sucking, enuresis, encopresis, tics, tantrums, withdrawal, and aggressivity.

In the older child review drug use, including cigarettes and alcohol, and sexual activity.

## Review of Systems

Much of this material has been recorded in previous sections and need not be repeated. This section serves as a recapitulation and by approaching the material in a different way enhances the completeness and accuracy of the history.

*Neuromuscular:* Head trauma; concussion; loss of consciousness; seizures; headache; ataxia; postural deformities; hyperactivity; attention span; school performance; deterioration of intellectual, memory, or motor skills; muscle tone and strength

*Head:* Size and shape

*Eyes:* Position, size, visual acuity, strabismus, infection

*Nose:* Shape, discharge, sneezing, stuffiness, epistaxis

*Ears:* Shape, position, hearing, infection, discharge

*Mouth and throat:* Number and condition of teeth, gum problems, throat infections, quality of speech, mouth breathing, snoring, shape of palate and uvula, fetis oris

*Respiratory:* Chronic or recurrent cough, croup, bronchitis, pneumonia, wheezing, chest pain, exposure to tuberculosis, previous chest radiograph

*Cardiovascular:* Hypertension, murmurs, exercise tolerance, cyanosis, dyspnea, syncope

*Gastrointestinal:* Appetite and digestion, diarrhea, constipation, type and color of stool, abdominal pain, jaundice, encopresis

*Urinary:* Infections, frequency, urgency, dysuria, enuresis, polydipsia, polyuria, hematuria, character of stream

*Genital:* Structural abnormalities, rashes, discharges, sexually transmitted disease, contraception, trauma, menarche, dysmenorrhea, description of menses

*Skin and appendages:* Rashes, birthmarks, scars, injuries, condition of nails, color, and texture of hair

*Endocrine:* Abnormalities of linear growth, obesity, failure to thrive, diabetes, eating disorders, goiter, thyroid disease, hirsutism, sexual development

*Hematologic:* Anemias, including iron deficiency, sickle cell, and thalassemia; bruising; hemorrhage

*Extremities:* Structural abnormalities, including polydactyly or syndactyly, joint function, pain, clumsiness, limp

### Family History

The child is the genetic product of the parents. Growth, development, congenital anomalies, and inherited diseases can only be understood by obtaining a thorough family history. Record parental ages, occupations, heights, weights, sexual development, and significant illnesses. Include the obstetric and psychological history of the parents. Detail age, sex, growth, development, and illnesses of siblings. Add relevant information about maternal and paternal grandparents and relatives with potentially inheritable conditions. Review the family history for tuberculosis, diabetes, convulsive disorders, cancer, hypertension, strokes, heart disease, liver or kidney disorders, allergy, infertility, mental retardation, and emotional instability. Permit the informant the opportunity to add additional information about the family that may be significant.

### Social History

Both nature and nurture are inextricably intertwined in shaping the child. Parents and siblings are usually the most important role models for the developing ego. Thus, composition of the family, ages, education, and socioeconomic level are essential components for understanding the child. Marital status and degree of dysharmony within the household may reveal potential for physical or emotional abuse, sexual molestation, or neglect. Inquire about expectations of the parents with regard to behavior, school performance, and future of the child. Record parental behavior as evidenced during the interview and attitudes concerning smoking, drinking, drugs, and discipline.

## PHYSICAL EXAMINATION

The physical examination of the child is a screening procedure, with emphasis on those areas of likely pathology suggested by the history. Modern medicine has made a host of valuable laboratory and imaging techniques available to the clinician. These tests are never a substitute for a careful physical examination. Careful record keeping is essential because that which is not written is assumed not to have been done. Blood pressure, fundoscopic, rectal, and vaginal examinations are performed selectively with consideration of the age of the patient and the nature of the problem.

The physical examination begins with observation of the child during the interview. Alertness, relationship with parents, hyperactivity, speech, gait, tics, skin color, and signs of distress can be noted prior to the formal examination. Children's fearfulness can be modified by approaching them slowly, being flexible as to whether they lie or sit on the examining table or remain on a parent's lap, talking to them in a gentle manner, and engaging them in a brief nonthreatening game (e.g., blowing out the otoscope light). Most errors are due to that which is not seen rather than to that which is misinterpreted. The child should be undressed completely, although this can be done in stages, and older children should be permitted the modesty of a gown. Adolescents should be asked whether they wish a parent or friend in the room or prefer privacy.

## Routine Measurements

Vital signs need to be obtained. Record oral or rectal temperatures on all sick children. Axillary temperatures are unreliable. Measure the pulse when the child is relaxed. Evaluate rate, regularity, and quality, and record the location where the pulse was obtained. Note the rate, regularity, and depth of respirations and the presence of stridor or wheezing. Obtain an accurate blood pressure by using a cuff that measures two-thirds to three-quarters of the upper arm. Record the pressure yearly on all children over 4 years. Hypertension cannot be diagnosed by a single measurement.

Height and weight without clothes should be recorded for all children and the values plotted on a standard growth graph. Head circumference is measured regularly until age 2 and if relevant to the presenting problem. General appearance includes race, nutritional status, size for age, sensorium, overt evidence of illness, alertness, facial expression, nature of cry or speech, and cooperativeness.

## Head and Neck

Inspect the head for size, shape, bossing, and hair distribution. Palpate the fontanelles and sutures in the sitting position. Note the presence of craniotabes, and auscultate for bruits. Observe the face for symmetry, proportions, weakness, depth of nasolabial folds, distance between nose and mouth, hypertelorism, and low-set ears, and percuss for sinus tenderness.

Examine the eyes for shape, (microphthalmus, Mongolian slant, epicanthal folds) exophthalmos, enophthalmos, ptosis, discharge, lacrimation, and strabismus. Evaluate pupillary size and shape, presence of anisocoria or coloboma, and reaction to light and accommodation. Look for scleral jaundice and corneal opacities. After age 4 routinely evaluate visual fields, visual acuity, and fundi.

Inspection of the ears begins with the position and size of the pinnae. For examination of the tympanic membrane with an otoscope, the auricle should be pulled backward and downward in the young child and backward and upward in the older child. Any discharge in the ear canal and mobility, color, landmarks, and perforations of the tympanic membrane should be noted. Gross hearing should be checked frequently and detailed audiometric testing done after age 4.

Observe the shape of the nose, the patency of nares, and the presence of discharge or epistaxis, and visualize mucous membranes and turbinates. Allergic children often have a horizontal crease across the ridge of the nose.

Observe the lips for thinness, shape, fissures, clefts, color, and sores, and note the presence of fetis oris. Describe the shape of palate and uvula. Note size and color of tongue, length and position of frenulum, color, hypertrophy, bleeding or ulcers of gums, and condition of buccal mucosa. Evaluate teeth for number, primary or secondary dentition, arrangement, and caries. Examine tonsils for size, inflammation, exudation, and crypts, and note the color of the tonsillar pillars. Examine the pharynx for hypertrophic lymphoid tissue, evidence of postnasal drip, and size of the epiglottis. Evaluate the voice for hoarseness, grunting, stridor, nature of cry, and quality of speech.

Observe the neck for position, flexibility, swellings, and webbing. Palpate for adenopathy, cysts, position of trachea, and size, nodularity, and consistency of thyroid.

## Thorax and Abdomen

The thorax should be examined for sternal shape, size and position of nipples, breasts, clavicles, and scapulae. Note contour of chest, rate and regularity of respirations, and the presence of retractions, pulsations, tachypnea, or dyspnea.

The lungs should be percussed for dullness and auscultated for adequacy of air exchange, ronchi, rales, and wheezes. Describe the nature of cough if present.

Inspect the heart for location and intensity of the apical beat, precordial bulge, and pulsations; palpate for thrills and vessel pulsations; percuss heart borders; and auscultate for rhythm, rate, character, and quality of heart sounds. Murmurs should be described as systolic or diastolic and by their intensity, pitch, duration, and transmission.

Observe the contour of the abdomen and the presence of distension, venous engorgement, visible peristalsis, musculature, scars, hernias, and abnormalities of the umbilicus. Percuss for a fluid wave, shifting dullness, and organ size. Palpate the liver and spleen for size and the abdominal wall for tenderness, rigidity, or rebound. Compare femoral and radial pulses simultaneously.

## Genitalia and Rectum

In the male genitalia note whether the penis is circumcised and if not, the retractability of the foreskin. Also note the size and position of the meatal opening, size, and the shape and consistency of the testes and scrotum. Distinguish between an undescended testicle and a retractile one.

Inspect the female genitalia for labial abnormalities, hymeneal aperture, vaginal opening, and clitoral size and shape. Note any discharge or evidence of sexual abuse. Use Tanner staging (Table 5-8) to describe pubic hair, breast development, and genital maturity.

Observe the rectum for fissures, hemorrhoids, or prolapse. Palpate only for specific indications. Note sphincter tone, masses, tenderness, and presence of stool in ampulla. Examine stool on gloved finger.

## Skin, Lymph Nodes, and Back

The skin is the largest organ. Most diseases of the skin can be diagnosed by inspection, and many systemic diseases have identifiable skin manifestations. Examine the skin for color, turgor, edema, birth marks, bleeding, bruises, striae, and rashes.

Lymph nodes should be evaluated for location, size, sensitivity, mobility, consistency, fluctuation, and whether they are discrete or matted. When palpating lymph nodes, pay particular attention to suboccipital, preauricular, anterior and posterior cervical, submaxillary, sublingual, axillary, supraclavicular, epitrochlear, and inguinal areas.

The spine and back should be observed for posture,

scoliosis, kyphosis, mobility, and pilonidal cyst or dimple. Palpate for tenderness over the spine and at the cardio-vascular angle.

## Extremities and Hips

The extremities should be inspected for deformity, asymmetry, stance, gait, temperature, muscle mass, tone, and edema. Joints are evaluated for swelling, redness, pain, limitation of motion, and nodules. Note abnormalities of hands and feet such as polydactyly, clubbing, simian lines, clinodactyly, syndactyly, nail deformities, splinter hemorrhages, tibial torsion, pronation of feet, metatarsus adductus, and flatfoot. Shoe wear is a useful indication of a child's gait and balance. The normal foot of the infant appears abnormal if judged by adult standards. It is fatter and wider, with an indistinct longitudinal arch and no transverse arch.

Congenital hip dysplasia is a common anomaly, which must be diagnosed early if a successful outcome is to be anticipated. The incidence varies with sex, race, maternal hormones, and inheritance and is commonly associated with oligohydramnios, breech delivery, torticollis, metatarsus adductus, and calcaneal valgus (Table 2-4).

The Ortelani test is a click palpated and sometimes heard when the hip of a newborn is reduced by placing it in an abducted, flexed position, while the Barlow test is a provocative test, which actively dislocates an unstable hip. The Ortelani is positive in all newborns with dysplastic hips but in only 15 percent of children with this condition beyond the age of 6 months. Limited abduction of the hip is minimal at birth but is present in 86 percent of such infants by 6 months. Apparent inequality in leg length or skin folds is often a useful clue to the diagnosis. Clinical signs of hip dysplasia between 2 months and 2 years include limited abduction, shortening of the thigh, Galleazzi's sign, Trendelenburg's sign, asymmetric skin folds, and a waddling gait. When hip dysplasia is suspected either by physical examination or because of an associated anomaly, the best confirmatory test is ultrasound. A stable hip at birth may dislocate later, especially in children with abnormal muscle tone. Failure to diagnose and treat hip dysplasias early results in serious hip problems in adulthood in 60 percent of cases.

Table 2-4. **Incidence of Breech Delivery**

| | |
|---|---|
| All breech deliveries | 7% |
| Metatarsus adductus | 2% |
| Torticollis | 20% |

Pigeon toe, or toeing-in, may be caused by femoral or tibial torsion or metatarsus adductus. The former conditions generally correct spontaneously whereas the latter requires treatment. If the metatarsus adductus is flexible, correction can be achieved by passive stretching or shoes with straight lasts. If a fixed deformity is present, serial casting is necessary.

## Neuromuscular System

The neuromuscular examination of the child is dependent on age and cooperation. Cerebral function is evaluated by level of consciousness; behavior; memory; orientation; auditory, visual, and verbal comprehension; and performance of skilled motor acts. Testing of cerebellar function consists of looking for ataxia, incoordination, spontaneous or intention tremor, nystagmus, slurred speech, or abnormal posture. The motor component includes muscle size, tone, consistency, strength, myotonic contractions, fasciculations, tremors, resistance to passive movement, and involuntary movement. Deep reflexes include those of the biceps, triceps, radial, knee, and ankle muscles and are measured on a scale from absent to sustained clonus. Superficial reflexes include those of the cremasteric, abdominal, plantar, and gluteal muscles. Abnormal reflexes such as Hoffmann's, Babinski, Kernig, and Brudzinski's should be sought.

## Special Considerations in the Newborn

Examination of the newborn differs in several ways from that of the older child. The physician should approach the child only after becoming acquainted with the maternal history and details of the pregnancy and delivery. Emphasis should be placed on a search for congenital anomalies, delivery trauma, and congenitally acquired infections.

Evaluate the infant's height and weight in relation to gestational age. In small infants determine whether the child is premature or small for gestational age, using parameters such as reflexes, height/weight ratio, breast hypertrophy, foot creases, and ear cartilage. Note the Apgar score at 1 and 5 minutes after birth.

Newborn skin is often ruddy and mottled, with lanugo hair over the shoulders and back. Vernix caseosa, milia, capillary hemangiomata, mongolian spots, and scattered petechiae are frequently seen. The shape of the head may be distorted by overlapping sutures, caput succedaceum, or cephalohematomas. The head should be palpated for fusion of sutures and the presence of anterior and posterior fontanelles and the eyes examined for a red reflex bilaterally. The clavicle is the most commonly fractured bone, and such fractures can usually be diagnosed by palpation. Any abnormality of the lower extremities should alert the examiner to the possibility of hip dysplasia. However, many apparent abnormalities in the lower extremities are only transient results of intrauterine positioning. Fixed positional abnormalities are never normal. The nails of a newborn are rudimentary. The presence of syndactyly, polydactyly, or clinodactyly may be clues to serious underlying defects. If an infant is seen soon after birth, the number of vessels in the umbilical cord should be noted. Genital abnormalities, defects in three or more organ systems, or specific abnormalities known to be associated with a chromosomal disorder require a prompt karyotype determination.

# PERIOPERATIVE CARE

## Preparation for Surgery

Hospitalization is a traumatic experience for children. In children over age 3, anxiety can be reduced by a clear, concise explanation of the purpose of surgery, probable sequence of events, likelihood of pain or discomfort related to tests or procedures, and nature of anesthesia. Children are comforted by bringing objects from home that are invested with positive emotion, such as a favorite blanket or stuffed animal. A good hospital needs empathetic personnel familiar with children and facilities for parents to remain with their child overnight. Parents are encouraged to maintain an attitude of confidence and cheerfulness. The anesthetist should visit the child and parents prior to surgery and the child should be given preanesthetic medications that will permit transportation to the operating suite in a light sleep.

A thorough history should be obtained, but certain aspects deserve special attention. Recent exposure to infectious disease, especially chickenpox, may result in contamination of an operating room or an entire ward. A past history of wheezing or recurrent laryngotracheobronchitis may influence the approach to airway management or drug use. Bleeding tendency, response to previous surgeries, and anesthetic agents, exercise tolerance, drug reactions, and abnormal weight loss are also important. Medications such as cortisone, antiepileptics,

and sedatives may alter response to anesthesia. The time of the last meal should be noted because of the danger of aspiration during anesthetic induction. A family history of bleeding disorder, hemoglobinopathy, or abnormal reaction to muscle relaxants is important.

A thorough physical examination should be made, with special emphasis on the presence of infectious disease, vital signs (including height and weight), cardiovascular system, and loose teeth. Small, narrow nares filled with secretions, tonsillar or adenoidal hypertrophy, or protruding maxilla may predispose the child to upper airway obstruction after sedation or induction. A normal child needs a minimal amount of laboratory studies prior to surgery. Generally a complete blood count and a urinalysis will suffice. Syphilis screening and chest radiography are not needed routinely. If indicated by history, bleeding time, blood urea nitrogen, creatinine, electrolytes, $Pa_{O_2}$, $Pa_{CO_2}$, and blood pH may be helpful.

Scheduled surgery should be postponed if the child presents with significant anemia (e.g., hemoglobin less than 9 g/dl or hematocrit less than 27 percent. A current respiratory infection or recent exposure to infectious disease is also a reason to postpone elective surgery.

Infants may have regular formula or breast milk up to 4 hours prior to surgery unless there is a problem with gastrointestinal motility. Older children should have no milk or solids for 12 hours, although sweetened fruit juice may be given 4 to 8 hours prior to surgery.

Even when immediate surgery is necessary, a brief delay is essential, to stabilize the child. In hypotonic or isotonic dehydration, correction with intravenous fluids should be carried out by using Ringer's lactate or normal saline at the rate of 10 to 20 ml/kg/h for the first 1 to 2 hours and after the child has voided twice, adding potassium, 20 mEq/L, and switching to half-normal saline. Hypertonic dehydration is less common, and the deficit must be replaced more slowly if seizures are to be avoided. If the child is hypotensive or shocky, 3 to 5 percent of body weight should be added as plasma or albumin. If shock persists, whole blood may be required. These guidelines need to be revised hourly depending on the status of the individual child.

High fever causes children to respond poorly to general anesthesia. Rectal acetaminophen and surface cooling with a water blanket are effective means of lowering body temperature. Surgery may commence when rectal temperature is below 39°C, and cooling should cease at 38°C.

Prophylactic antibiotics are used when there is a sig-

Table 2-5. **Antibiotic Prophylaxis**

| Drug | Dosage | Timing |
|------|--------|--------|
| Ampicillin | 50 mg/kg, IM or IV | ½ hour pre- and 8 hours postsurgery |
| Gentamicin | 1.5–2 mg/kg, IM or IV | ½ hour pre- and 8 hours postsurgery |
| Vancomycin | 20 mg/kg IV | ½ hour pre- and 8 hours postsurgery |
| Penicillin V | 1 g PO | 1 hour presurgery |
| | 0.5 g PO | 6 hours postsurgery |
| Penicillin, aqueous | 50,000 U/kg IV or IM | 30–60 minutes presurgery |
| | 25,000 U/kg IV or IM | 6 hours postsurgery |

nificant risk of postoperative infection or the result of infection could be catastrophic or as dictated by the underlying condition of the child, the nature of the surgery, and the type of wound. In clean wounds, antibiotics are used only if the child is immunosuppressed, a prosthetic device is to be installed, or infection is present at a site distant from the wound; in neonates only when a major body cavity is entered and in open heart surgery. Contaminated, dirty, or infected wounds such as those associated with an open fracture should receive prophylaxis. General prophylaxis for contaminated wounds consists of ampicillin plus gentamicin. Vancomycin can be substituted for gentamicin. In children with pre-existing heart disease the drug of choice is penicillin (Table 2-5).

Children usually require preanesthetic drugs. Both the drug and the dosage varies with age (Table 2-6). Intraoperatively, fluid and electrolyte balance must be maintained and fluid losses replaced. Maintenance for most children is calculated to be 1,500 ml/m². If blood loss is greater than 15 percent (newborns have 90 ml/kg, older children 75 ml/kg), transfusion is indicated. Transfused blood should be less than 4 days old because older blood tends to be hyperkalemic, acidotic, and depleted of clotting factors. Children and especially infants are subject to

hypothermia and need to have their temperature monitored during surgery.

## Postoperative Care

Following surgery small children should be placed on a warmed bed on their side or abdomen. Children, especially under age 6, who have been intubated may develop subglottic edema. Treatment consists of intravenous fluids, humidified oxygen, and bronchodilator aerosols. Adequacy of pulmonary air exchange can be measured by $Pa_{O_2}$ and $Pa_{CO_2}$ determinations. Infants and nonverbal children can experience pain, which is accompanied by physiologic and behavioral changes. Cardiopulmonary signs include decreased $P_{O_2}$, and increased heart rate, blood pressure, intracranial pressure, and pulmonary vascular resistance. Catecholamine release increases, leading to elevated free fatty acids, hyperglycemia, and metabolic acidosis. Behavioral changes include increased motor activity, crying, and grimacing. Treatment may involve use of local anesthetic agents, acetaminophen, codeine, morphine, or fentanyl. Nonsteroidal anti-flammatory drugs are contraindicated because of their effect on bilirubin metabolism and platelet activity. Sedatives have no analgesic effect and may mask airway obstruction or potentiate respiratory insufficiency.

Table 2-6. **Preanesthetic Drugs**

| Age | Drug | Dosage |
|-----|------|--------|
| 0–6 months | Atropine | 0.02 mg/kg |
| 6–12 months | Atropine + | |
| | Pentobarbital | 3–4 mg/kg; maximum dose 120 mg |
| 12+ months | Scopolamine + | 0.02 mg/kg |
| | Pentobarbital + | |
| | Morphine or | 0.05–0.1 mg/kg; maximum dose 10 mg |
| | Meperidine | 1–2 mg/kg; maximum dose 100 mg |

## SUGGESTED READINGS

Apgar V et al: Evaluation of the newborn infant—second report. JAMA 168:1985, 1958

Behrman RE, Vaughan VC (eds): Nelson Textbook of Pediatrics. 11th Ed. WB Saunders, Philadelphia, 1987

Coleman M (ed): Neonatal Neurology. University Park Press, Baltimore, MD, 1981

Coleman SS: Congenital Dysplasia and Dislocation of the Hip. CV Mosby, St. Louis, 1978

Copeland KC: Variations in Normal Sexual Development. Pediatr Rev 8(2):Aug. 1986

Copeland KC, Brockman RR, Rauh JL (eds): Assessment of Pubertal Development. Ross Laboratories, Columbus, 1986

Davis JA, Dobbing J: Paediatrics. 2nd Ed. University Park Press, Baltimore, 1981

Ferguson AB Jr (ed): Orthopedic Surgery in Infancy and Childhood. 5th Ed. Williams & Wilkins, Baltimore, 1981

Forbes GB (ed): Pediatric Nutrition Handbook. 2nd Ed. American Academy of Pediatrics, Elk Grove Village, IL, 1985

Gordin P: MDs urged to address infant pain more aggressively. Pediatric News 24(2):5, 1990

Johnson TR, Moore WM, Jeffries JE: Children are Different: Developmental Physiology. Ross Laboratories, Colombus, 1978

Iattanzi WE: Simplifying the Approach to Fluid Therapy. Contemp Pediatr 6:72, Feb. 1989

Modern Nutrition in Health and Disease. 7th Ed. Lea & Febiger, Philadelphia, 1988

Peter G: Report of the Committee on Infectious Diseases. 21st Ed. American Academy of Pediatrics, Elk Grove Village, IL, 1988

Rudolph AM (ed): Textbook of Pediatrics. 18th Ed. Appleton & Lange, East Norwalk, CT, 1987

Shwartz MW et al: Principles and Practice of Clinical Pediatrics. Year Book Medical Publishers, Chicago, 1987

Silver HK, Kempe HC, Bruyn HB, Fulginitti VA: Handbook of Pediatrics. 15th Ed. Lange Medical Publications, Los Altos, CA, 1980

Tanner JM: Growth at Adolescence. 2nd Ed. Blackwell Scientific Publications, Oxford, 1962

Tanner JM: Growth and endocrinology of the adolescent. In Gardner II (ed): Endocrine and Genetic Diseases of Childhood and Adolescents. 2nd Ed. WB Saunders, Philadelphia, 1975

# Appendix 2-1. Typical Progression of Female Pubertal Development.

## Pubertal development in size of female breasts.

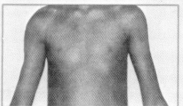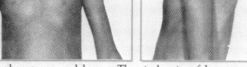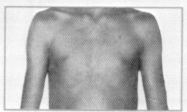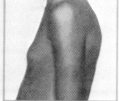

**Stage 1.** The breasts are preadolescent. There is elevation of the papilla only.

**Stage 2.** Breast bud stage. A small mound is formed by the elevation of the breast and papilla. The areolar diameter enlarges.

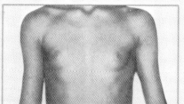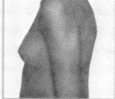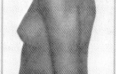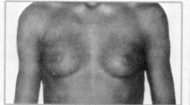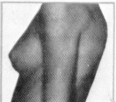

**Stage 3.** There is further enlargement of breasts and areola with no separation of their contours.

**Stage 4.** There is a projection of the areola and papilla to form a secondary mound above the level of the breast.

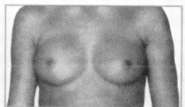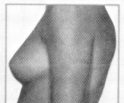

**Stage 5.** The breasts resemble those of a mature female as the areola has recessed to the general contour of the breast.

## Pubertal development of female pubic hair.
### Stage 1. There is no pubic hair.

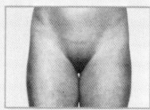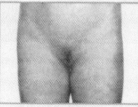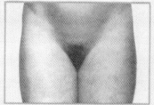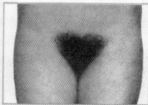

**Stage 2.** There is sparse growth of long, slightly pigmented, downy hair, straight or only slightly curled, primarily along the labia.

**Stage 3.** The hair is considerably darker, coarser, and more curled. The hair spreads sparsely over the junction of the pubes.

**Stage 4.** The hair, now adult in type, covers a smaller area than in the adult and does not extend onto the thighs.

**Stage 5.** The hair is adult in quantity and type, with extension onto the thighs.

(From Johnson TR, Moore WM, Jeffries JE: Children Are Different: Physiology. 2nd Ed. Ross Laboratories, Columbus, OH, 1978, with permission.)

# Appendix 2-2. Typical Progression of Male Pubertal Development

## Pubertal development in size of male genitalia.

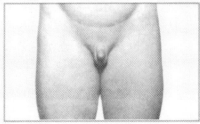 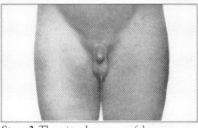 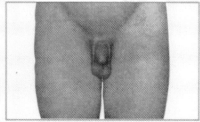

**Stage 1.** The penis, testes, and scrotum are of childhood size.

**Stage 2.** There is enlargement of the scrotum and testes, but the penis usually does not enlarge. The scrotal skin reddens.

**Stage 3.** There is further growth of the testes and scotum and enlargement of the penis, mainly in length.

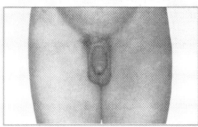 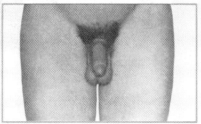

**Stage 4.** There is still further growth of the testes and scrotum and increased size of the penis, especially in breadth.

**Stage 5.** The genitalia are adult in size and shape.

## Pubertal development of male pubic hair.

**Stage 1.** There is no pubic hair.

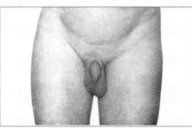 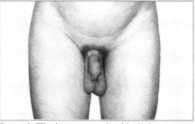

**Stage 2.** There is sparse growth of long, slightly pigmented, downy hair, straight or only slightly curled, primarily at the base of the penis.

**Stage 3.** The hair is considerably darker, coarser, and more curled. The hair spreads sparsely over the junction of the pubes.

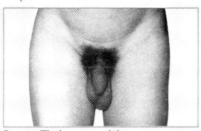 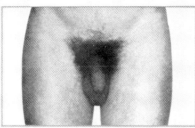

**Stage 4.** The hair, now adult in type, covers a smaller area than in the adult and does not extend onto the thighs.

**Stage 5.** The hair is adult in quantity and type, with extension onto the thighs.

(From Johnson TR, Moore WM, Jeffries JE: Children Are Different: Physiology. 2nd Ed. Ross Laboratories, Columbus, OH 1978, with permission.)

# 3

# Neurologic Examination of the Infant and Child

*CALVIN WHEELER*

The neurologic examination should be problem-oriented, and each examination should be designed by the historical facts. The neurologic history provides an organized and systematic record of data, from which a differential diagnosis is established. Consideration must be given to the possible site of disordered function and the nature of the lesion. Establishing the correct diagnosis leads to the ideal management of the musculoskeletal problem in the infant or child.

## THE NEUROLOGIC HISTORY

The neurologic history is of utmost importance in arriving at the correct diagnosis and must begin with the chief complaint or central problem. With the newborn infant and young child, the history must be obtained from the parent, other adults who reside in the home, or other observers. Some 3- to 4-year-olds may provide accurate answers to simple questions. Preschool and school-age children are often able to provide important observations concerning their problem. Once the examiner has an understanding of the chief complaint, subsequent history and conversation should be directed toward streamlining diagnostic possibilities. The physician must determine whether the potential pathologic process involves a focal lesion or a more generalized or diffuse disease process and must determine the tempo of the symptoms and whether or not it represents a progressive disease (Table 3-1). Following establishment of the chief complaint, a more detailed history, including present illness, past history, family history, and social history should be recorded. Pregnancy, gestational, parturitional, and perinatal details may be important. Maternal diseases and medications administered during pregnancy should also be recorded.

During the history gathering session the initial stages of the examination begin through observation of the infant or child sitting either on a parent's lap or in a chair beside the parent. Many postural abnormalities and deformations begin in utero. Biomechanical forces are important in the morphogenesis of muscles, ligaments, cartilage, and bone. It has also been observed that constraining and restraining forces on the fetal body for a sufficient time do produce modifications of the body habitus. The forces of uterine compression, intrauterine compression, and extrauterine compression are most significant during the latter part of the second and the third trimester. While diseases of the central and peripheral nervous systems and congenital muscle diseases may cause generalized hypotonia, the deformations occur because of fetal susceptibility to extrinsic deforming forces. An infant may present with a pattern of deformation that may include metatarsus adductus, dislocatable hips, tibia bowing, hyperflexed hips, hyperextended knees (genu recurvatum), or multiple foot deformities. Foot deformities are extremely common and may include calcaneal valgus, metatarsus adductus, various forms of equinovarus, and overlapping toes.

In *calcaneal valgus* the foot is maintained in a dorsiflexed and everted position and is usually flexible. The bones of the calcaneal valgus foot appear in near normal alignment. The term *metatarsus adductus* describes an adducted and usually supinated forefoot, with the heel

39

Table 3-1. **Classification of Neurologic Disorders by History**

Acute neurologic disorders
  Intoxications
  Animal and insect bites
  Head trauma
  Cerebrovascular disease
  Acquired metabolic encephalopathies
  Infections
  Postinfectious neurologic syndromes
  Acute increased intracranial pressure
  First episode of a recurrent neurologic disorder
  Hysteria
Episodic or relapsing neurologic disorders
  Seizures
  Migraine and other causes of headache
  Breath-holding spells
  Syncope
  Vertigo
  Substance abuse
  Inborn errors of metabolism
  Behavioral disorders
  Sleep disorders
Static nonprogressive neurologic disease
  Mental retardation
  Cerebral palsy
  Learning disabilities
  Behavior disorders
Progressive neurologic disease
  Inborn errors of metabolism
  Degenerative diseases
  Neurocutaneous syndromes
  Chronic infections
  Intracranial masses
  Chronic intoxication
  Neuromuscular diseases
  Psychiatric disorders

(From Evans OB: Manual of Child Neurology. Churchill Livingstone, New York, 1987, with permission.)

and ankle in normal position. This deformity may be mild and flexible or more rigid and less responsive to treatment. The equinovarus or clubfoot anomaly includes adduction and supination of the forefoot, heel varus, and equinus. Again, the deformity may be flexible with respect to the normal position or more rigid requiring more vigorous treatment. Overlapping toes generally involve a soft tissue element; however, if osseous elements are involved, corrective surgery may be necessary.

## Infant Development

Diseases affecting many different systems may have neurologic manifestations, or underlying neurologic disease may be exacerbated by many acute illnesses. It is important to have a full knowledge and understanding of normal development, neuroanatomy, neurophysiology,

and variations from normal development in order to correctly interpret the clinical findings in an infant or child (Fig. 3-1). The premature infant, so often hypotonic normally as compared with the full-term infant, may not have a fully and symmetrically developed Moro or startle reflex, which in the waking state is normally present from birth until the age of 3 months. An asymmetry in the reflex at any time is abnormal in the full-term infant and suggests a hemiparesis, brachial plexus injury, or spinal cord defect. The Moro (startle) reflex is elicited by either extending the infant's head or allowing the head to fall back 30 to 40 degrees into the examiner's hand. The first phase of the response is sudden extension and abduction of both arms with extension of the legs, followed by a slower adduction of the arms, often associated with tremor. Spontaneous leg posture should be observed; prolonged frog leg positioning suggests hypotonia. The lower extremities, elbows, and knees of these infants are abducted proximally.

The tonic neck response is elicited when the head is turned to either side with the infant supine and a resultant extension of the arm and leg is seen on the side to which the head is turned while the other arm and leg are generally flexed. An asymmetric tonic neck response is normally present at 2 to 6 months. An obligatory asymmetric tonic neck response is abnormal in this age range. Excessive opisthotonic posturing occurring spontaneously or responsively may be an early sign of cerebral palsy. Symmetric kicking of legs until age 4 months is normal, while continued symmetric kicking after this age suggests spastic diplegia.

By 2 months of age infants predominantly keep the hands fisted although intermittent spontaneous opening is observed. When prone, they often lift the head for several seconds. By 3 months hand fisting is decreased and the head is often lifted above the body plane while maintaining the truncal position on horizontal suspension. By 4 months infants can hold the head steady when supported in a sitting position, can reach for and grasp objects, and usually are able to bring them to the mouth. By 5 to 6 months infants are able to lift the head when supine, roll from prone to supine, and lift the head and chest from the prone position. No head lag is exhibited on pull to sit, and sitting is accomplished with support. By 7 to 8 months they should be able to sit in a tripod position without support, stand briefly, and reach out for objects and people. Infants should begin pulling themselves to sit and should sit well without support as well as stand and hold on by 9 to 10 months. By 11 to 12 months infants

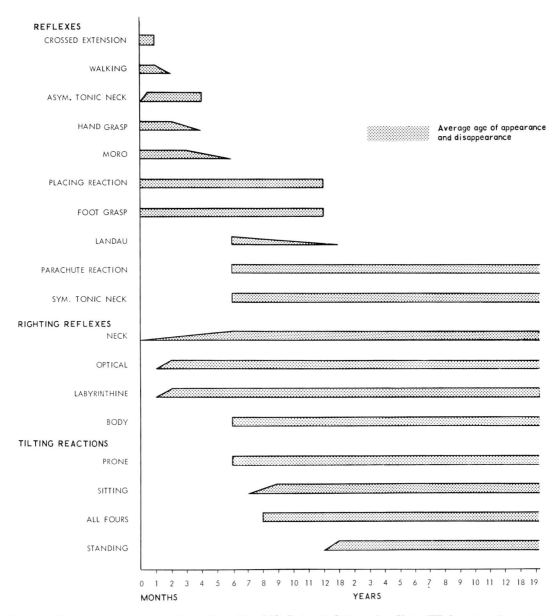

**Fig. 3-1.** Reflex maturation chart. (From Tachdjian, MO: Pediatric Orthopedics. Vol 1. WB Saunders, Philadelphia, 1972, with permission.)

should walk with assistance, creep well, and be involved in some complex task such as dressing assistance. Somewhat unstable but independent ambulation is seen at 13 to 15 months, and fine motor movement with scribbling should also be observed. By 18 months the milestone of climbing stairs with assistance, climbing onto chairs, and throwing a ball should be reached, and by 24 months, infants are generally able to run, walk up and down stairs alone, placing two feet on each step and balance well enough to kick a ball.

## THE NEUROLOGIC EXAMINATION

The neurologic examination begins with a general medical examination (Table 3-2). The skin is evaluated for neurocutaneous lesions and other stigmata that may be suggestive of underlying neural or musculoskeletal defects (Table 3-3). Abnormal facial features should also be noted.

When evaluating the head, eyes, ears, nose, and throat, the examiner measures the fronto-occipital circumference in addition to evaluating symmetry and looking for defects in the skull. The eyes, ears, and nose are evaluated for dysmorphic features, including those of symmetry and development. The mouth is evaluated for incomplete development and early signs of muscle disease. Neck development, posture, and spine alignment are evaluated. The presence of midline clefts, dimples,

Table 3-2. **Medical History for Neurologic Diseases**

Chief complaint

Present history
    Symptoms
    Onset
    Duration
    Progression
    Recurrence

Past history
    Perinatal history
        Pregnancy: duration, exposures, complications
        Labor: duration, monitoring, complications
        Delivery: presentation, Apgar scores, complications
        Neonatal course: hospital stay, complications
    Past medical illnesses
        Accidents and injuries
        Hospitalizations
        Acute infectious disorders and exposures
    Review of systems
    Immunizations
    Allergies
    Medications and dosages
    Environmental

Family history
    Neurologic and developmental disorders
    Other medical diseases and general health
    Causes of death
    Pedigree

Development

School performance
    Grades
    Academic and psychological testing
    Conduct

(From Evans OB: Manual of Child Neurology. Churchill Livingstone, New York, 1987, with permission.)

Table 3-3. **Neurologic Disorders with Cutaneous Abnormalities**

| Disorder | Abnormality |
|---|---|
| Neurofibromatosis | Café au lait patches<br>Axillary freckling<br>Subcutaneous nodules (neurofibromata) |
| Tuberous sclerosis | Amelanotic nevi<br>Subungual phakomas<br>Shagreen patch<br>Adenoma sebaceum |
| Sturge-Weber syndrome | Port wine angioma of the face |
| Incontinentia pigmenti | Early: macules, bullae<br>Late: brown, irregular macules<br>Resolution |
| Klippel-Trenaunay syndrome | Angiomas and limb hypertrophy |
| Linear sebaceous nevus | Midline nevus of face and scalp with yellow nodules |
| Sjögren-Larssen syndrome | Icthyosis |
| Fabry's disease | Periumbilical and groin angiokeratomas |
| Dermatomyositis | Maculopapular rash on extensor surfaces, heliotrope around eyes, "butterfly" rash on face |
| Ataxia telangiectasia | Conjunctival telangiectasia |
| Spina bifida | Midline hair patch, lipoma, dimple, or skin mark on back |
| Phenylketonuria | Eczema |
| Hartnup disease | Photosensitivity, pellagra rash |
| Biotinidase deficiency | Rash |
| Trichorrhexis nodosa (hair) | Arginosuccinicaciduria<br>Menkes syndrome |

(From Evans OB: Manual of Child Neurology. Churchill Livingstone, New York, 1987, with permission.)

sinus tracts, or abnormal hair growth may suggest underlying spinal deformities, which at times may be palpable. The extremities are observed for symmetry, posture, and movement pattern. Much information can be gained by watching the patient walk in a normal pattern as well as on the heels, on the toes, and in a tandem fashion. More subtle abnormalities may be seen by having the patient turn rapidly in walking, do a deep knee bend, and stand with feet together.

## Examination of the Infant

The examination of the full-term infant is best performed in two stages. The initial stage is performed with the infant recumbent and preferably awake, alert, and in an unobtrusive and comfortable environment. The pupils and palpebral fissures are evaluated for symmetry, as are the extraocular muscles producing movement of the eyes in all fields. Facial expression, eye closure, and response to auditory stimuli are then assessed. Normal newborn posture includes increased flexor tone, with arms and legs flexed and hands intermittently fisted in a symmetric manner. When the infant is prone, the flexed limb posture is generally maintained. Crawling movements and mild degrees of head turning may be observed.

The second phase of the examination is an interactive phase with active examination. Muscle tone can now be assessed through passive range of motion of the limbs at each joint, which also allows the physician to estimate muscle strength. During active handling, the presence or absence of clonus, as well as the deep tendon reflexes, can also be evaluated. Patella reflexes are more easily elicited followed by Achilles tendon and upper extremity reflexes. These may be more difficult to elicit in a newborn but should soon thereafter be reproducibly obtained. The degree of head control or presence of head lag is evaluated, as well as truncal control during ventral suspension. The plantar response in the newborn is often flexor and symmetric but may be extensor, and if symmetric, it may be a normal variant. Ankle clonus may be present in the newborn, with up to 12 beats obtained. Clonus tends to be more prominent in excited states, although sustained ankle clonus has pathologic significance and suggests critical spinal dysfunction. The cranial nerves may be further evaluated by the doll's eye maneuver to assess visual tracking and movement. Crying allows the examiner to evaluate the tone, volume, and pitch as well as tongue bulk, palatal anatomy, and facial symmetry. Infants with intact auditory function will often blink two to three times following loud noise stimuli.

## Examination of the Child

The approach to the neurologic examination of the child older than 2 years also varies with the age of the patient; however, the approach to the examination closely follows that used in younger children. Observation, confrontation, and game playing remain key tools in eliciting normal motor behavior as well as assessing abnormal function in this age group. In children beyond 4 years of age the neurologic examination assumes a more characteristic and formal pattern similar to that of the stereo-typed examination used in adolescent and adult patients. It remains most important to stay relaxed and to utilize behaviors and environments comfortable to the patient in order to obtain the best neurologic evaluation. While nervous system function is similar in infants and young children, the morphologic and physiologic immaturity in the younger age group produces variations in the normal response. It is therefore most important to be familiar with the variation in clinical expression as well as the time window of expression.

### Cranial Nerve Evaluation

Although the cranial nerve examination is carried out in an orderly fashion, it is often helpful to vary the examination according to the cooperation level of the child (Table 3-4). The function of cranial nerve I, the Olfactory nerve, is rarely involved in diseases of children but is easily tested by using simple and pleasant odors. The function of cranial nerve II, the optic nerve, is of great importance in a neurologic evaluation. Visual acuity and visual fields are often reliable in the school age child; however, gross behavioral responses are often utilized in the preschool child. In severely visually compromised infants and young children, greater accuracy is obtained by using the electrophysiologic examination or visual evoked responses. When evaluating cranial nerves III, IV, and VI, extraocular muscles are assessed through observation of visual tracking; lid elevation and pupillary reaction are

Table 3-4. **Cranial Nerve Examination**

| Cranial Nerve | Examination |
|---|---|
| I, Olfactory | Smell |
| II, Optic | Visual acuity and fields, pupillary light reflex |
| III, Oculomotor | Ocular motility (up, medially, down, and in), pupillary light reflex |
| IV, Trochlear | Ocular motility (down and out) |
| V, Trigeminal | Facial sensation, corneal reflex, mastication |
| VI, Abducens | Ocular motility (lateral) |
| VII, Facial | Facial expression |
| VIII, Vestibulocochlear | Hearing, balance |
| IX, Glossopharyngeal | Gag reflex, swallowing, phonation |
| X, Vagus | Palatal motility, phonation |
| XI, Accessory | Head turning, shoulder shrug |
| XII, Hypoglossal | Tongue protrusion |

(From Evans OB: Manual of Child Neurology. Churchill Livingstone, New York, 1987, with permission.)

also recorded. Cranial nerve V is evaluated by observing or obtaining a history of adequate chewing and intact facial sensation. An intact cranial nerve VII produces symmetric facial expression and appropriate taste. Cranial nerve VIII, the acoustic nerve, has an auditory and vestibular division. The child should be observed for appropriate understanding and response to auditory stimuli. An intact vestibular system contributes to balance and stability during rapid posture changes and rotation. Cranial nerves IX and X, the glossopharyngeal and vagus nerves, innervate the palate, pharynx, and larynx and contribute to a proper swallow, voice, and cry and a positive gag reflex. Cranial nerve XI, the spinal accessory nerve, is responsible for innervating the muscles required for head movements seen when the patient is in the upright as well as the prone position. Cranial nerve XII, the hypoglossal nerve, is responsible for tongue movement. The symmetry of the tongue is also evaluated for evidence of atrophy, fibrillation, and deviation from midline. Myotonia of the tongue can be detected by percussion.

## Motor Function

The extent to which the motor system is examined is largely directed by the clinical history. Muscle bulk is easily evaluated by observation. The presence of atrophy and fasciculations should also be noted. The muscles of the upper and lower extremities should be palpated for consistency and for evidence of muscle tenderness, nerve tenderness, nerve hypertrophy and myotonia. Muscle tone is assessed by the resistance of muscles to passive movement when the limb is relaxed and not under voluntary control. During examination of muscle tone, the degree of tension present on passive muscle stretching should be noted, as well as extensibility of the hand and range of motion of the joints. Muscle strength is resistance of muscles to active movement. In infants and small children the movement pattern is observed for asymmetry or unusual postures. The motor develop-

Table 3-5. **Muscle Strength Grades**

| |
|---|
| 0 = No muscle contraction |
| 1 = Trace muscle contraction |
| 2 = Active movement at joint, not against gravity |
| 3 = Active movement at joint against gravity |
| 4 = Active movement against resistance |
| 5 = Normal or full strength |

mental reflexes are also noted. In many children maximal strength cannot be assessed, and the examiner must rely on the execution of functional movements. A commonly used muscle strength grading system is outlined in Table 3-5. An attempt should be made to correlate patterns of muscle weakness to associated spinal innervation patterns (Table 3-6).

Muscle strength in the extremities is assessed by evaluating proximal and distal groups of muscles as well as individual muscles against resistance. Neck flexor and extensor strength is also tested against resistance. Weakness of proximal muscles is often associated with anterior horn cell disease, primary muscle disease, and some systemic diseases (Table 3-7). Neck flexor and extensor strength may also be affected by these disease processes. Neck flexor weakness is often recorded early in the course of inflammatory muscle disease and is delayed in muscular dystrophies. Distal weakness is characteristic of peripheral nerve disease, although myotonic dystrophy, distal myopathy, and monomelic myopathy may also be associated with distal weakness.

A proper interpretation of muscle weakness requires the examiner to ask: Is the process focal or diffuse? Are there associated changes in muscle tone? Are adventitious movements present? What is the degree of activity of the deep tendon reflexes? Are pathologic reflexes, including abnormal plantar responses, present? Other associated neurologic deficits or abnormalities are also important, such as the presence of dysmetria, body or head titubation, and ocular signs. A decrease in muscle tone is seen in anterior horn cell disease, peripheral nerve disease, myopathies, and cerebellar disease. Increased tone is noted in critical spinal dysfunction and in basal ganglia rigidity.

Deep tendon reflexes (muscle stretch reflexes) are generally easily obtained when the child is relaxed and cooperative. The biceps, triceps, brachioradialis, patellar, and Achilles tendon reflexes are commonly examined. The interpretation of deep tendon reflexes is important. Response may be described as normal, hyperactive, hypoactive, clonic, or absent and may be symmetric or asymmetric. A common grading system used to record deep tendon reflex response is provided in Table 3-8. The reflex elicited depends on striking the proper tendon and the force and velocity of the hammer. Each tendon reflex represents a spinal segmental level (Table 3-9). Hyperreflexia or clonic reflexes are seen in

Table 3-6. **Lower Extremity Muscle Innervation**

| Nerve | Anatomic Part | Muscle | Spinal Segment |
|---|---|---|---|
| Superior gluteal | Buttock | Gluteus medius | L4–S1 |
| | | Gluteus minimus | L4–S1 |
| | | Tensor fasciae latae | L4–S |
| Inferior gluteal | Buttock | Gluteus maximus | L4–S2 |
| Femoral | Thigh | Iliopsoas | L1–L3 |
| | | Sartorius | L2–L3 |
| | | Quadriceps femoris | L2–L4 |
| Obturator | Thigh | Pectineus | L2–L3 |
| | | Adductor Longus | L2–L3 |
| | | Gracilis | L2–L4 |
| | | Adductor brevis | L2–L4 |
| | | Obturator externus | L3–L4 |
| | | Adductor magnus | L3–L4 |
| Sciatic, tibial division | Thigh | Semitendinosus | L4–L5 |
| | | Biceps (long head) | S1–S2 |
| | | Semimembranosus | L4–S1 |
| | Popliteal space (tibial nerve) | Gastrocnemius | L5–S2 |
| | | Plantaris | L4–S1 |
| | | Popliteus | L4–S1 |
| | | Soleus | L5–S2 |
| | Leg | Tibialis posterior | L5–S1 |
| | | Flexor digitorum longus | L4–S1 |
| | | Flexor hallucis longus | L4–S1 |
| | Foot | Abductor hallucis | S1–S2 |
| | | Abductor digiti minimi | S1–S2 |
| | | Interossei dorsales | S1–S2 |
| Sciatic, peroneal division | Thigh | Biceps (short head) | L4–S1 |
| | Leg (deep peroneal nerve) | Tibialis anterior | L4–L5 |
| | | Extensor hallucis longus | L4–S1 |
| | | Extensor digitorum longus | L4–S1 |
| | | Peroneus tertius | |
| | Foot | Extensor digitorum brevis | L4–S1 |
| | Leg (superficial peroneus nerve) | Peroneus longus | L5–S1 |
| | | Peroneus brevis | L5–S1 |

(From Evans OB: Manual of Child Neurology. Churchill Livingstone, New York, 1987, with permission.)

critical spinal dysfunction. Hyporeflexia is commonly seen in myopathies and peripheral neuropathies. In myopathic diseases, reflexes may be normal early and absent later. In the peripheral neuropathies, reflexes may be depressed or absent depending on the severity of the process, the distal reflexes commonly being more severely affected. In anterior horn cell disease, the patellar reflexes are generally absent early on, while the remaining reflexes are normal. Cerebellar disease generally produces decreased muscle tone and may increase or decrease deep tendon reflexes depending on whether critical spinal dysfunction is associated.

It is felt that the response to plantar stimulation (cutaneous nociceptive stimulation of the lateral sole) has limited clinical usefulness as a screening reflex for neurologic disease in newborns. The plantar response, however, in all children with normal central nervous system function should be plantar-flexor in direction.

Table 3-7. **Patterns of Muscle Weakness and Neurologic Localization**

| Pattern | Neurologic Localization |
|---|---|
| Proximal, symmetric | Myopathies, spinal muscular atrophies |
| Distal, symmetric | Polyneuropathy |
| Unilateral (hemiparesis) | Contralateral cerebral cortex, internal capsule, brain stem, ipsilateral spinal cord |
| Unilateral bulbar, contralateral extremities | Brain stem |
| Paraparesis | Myelopathy, bilateral cortical or internal capsule |
| Monoparesis | Plexus, nerve root, peripheral nerve |

(From Evans OB: Manual of Child Neurology. Churchill Livingstone, New York, 1987, with permission.)

The method of stimulation is important as a sharp object might produce mostly a withdrawal response while too light a touch will produce no response. A key or similar object generally produces an appropriate stimulus and should be moved along the lateral aspect of the plantar aspect of the foot, beginning at the heel and moving up to the ball of the foot but staying lateral to the great toe. When a clear response is not observed, it is more helpful to record exactly the observed movements. In the normal response the first movement of the great toe is in the plantar-flexor direction. The classic Babinski reflex exhibits extension of the great toe with extension and fanning of the other toes. A positive Babinski reflex is also recorded when the first movement of the great toe is extensor and is followed by flexor movement, while the remaining toes show either no movement or flexion. A mute plantar response suggests severe sensory loss or paralysis of the foot. A withdrawal response may be seen in metabolic neuropathies or if an excessively sharp object is used. If the response to plantar stimulation is asymmetric (i.e., mute on one side and flexor on the

Table 3-8. **Grading of Reflexes**

| Grade | Reflex |
|---|---|
| 0 | Absent |
| 1 | Trace |
| 2 | Normal |
| 3 | Brisk |
| 4 | Clonus |

Table 3-9. **Innervation of Deep Tendon Reflexes**

| Tendon | Peripheral Nerve | Spinal Segment |
|---|---|---|
| Achilles | Sural | S1–S2 |
| Patellar | Femoral | L3–L4 |
| Biceps | Musculocutaneous | C5–C6 |
| Brachioradialis | Radial | C5–C6 |
| Triceps | Axillary | C6–C8 |

(From Evans OB: Manual of Child Neurology. Churchill Livingstone, New York, 1987, with permission.)

opposite side) other signs of neurologic disease should be looked for.

## Involuntary Movements

During the observation and interaction phase of the examination, adventitious or involuntary movements are analyzed (Table 3-10). Tremors are rhythmic alternating movements of small muscles or muscle groups and often involve the face and hands. Some occur when the involved muscles are quiet, while others occur during activity. Underlying systemic diseases must be considered, as well as cerebellar disease, trauma, and medications (e.g., valproic acid, lithium, caffeine, phenytoin, and the xanthenes). Dystonia is a fast and slow twisting movement of the trunk, head, and extremities, with very slow relaxation intervals. Most often these conditions are inherited, but they can follow traumatic and inflammatory diseases, mass lesions, and perinatal brain injury.

Athetosis is distinuished from dystonia by the smooth flow of posture from one position to another without sustained posturing of the limb. Athetoid movements tend to be accentuated during purposeful activity. Athe-

Table 3-10. **Involuntary Movements of Muscles**

| | |
|---|---|
| Fasciculations | Random contractions of groups of muscle fibers |
| Myokymia | Rhythmic, undulating contractions of groups of muscle fibers |
| Myoclonus | Random, single, shock-like contractions of muscles |
| Chorea | Random brief, repetitive contractions of muscles |
| Athetosis | Contractions of muscles that cause writhing movements |
| Tremor | Rhythmic contractions of muscles |
| Dystonia | Continuous contraction of opposing groups of muscles |
| Partial seizures | Coarse, semirhythmic contractions of groups of muscles |
| Tics | Stereotyped repetitive movements |

(From Evans OB: Manual of Child Neurology. Churchill Livingstone, New York, 1987, with permission.)

tosis involves a peculiar, writhing, irregular movement, with increased tone in the distal extremities. Lesions are commonly found in the basal ganglia and frequently follow birth injury. Chorea consists of rapid, involuntary, nonrhythmic, generalized jerks of various parts of the body. Movements occasionally "dance" from one joint to another and may involve facial grimacing and flexion-extension movements of the extremities. Myoclonus is an involuntary, repetitive, instantaneous, irregular contracture of a single muscle or group of muscles, which may also occur symmetrically, synchronically, or asymmetrically. Myoclonus is frequently associated with diffuse involvement of the brain, although on occasion it has been reported with localized lesions involving cerebellar outflow. Tics are rapid, involuntary, irregular, rotational movements that often resemble purposeful activity. They most often occur in muscles supplied by the motor cranial nerves (e.g., those of the shoulder, neck, and face). The movements are exacerbated by emotional stress and excitement. All these movement disorders disappear during sleep.

## Gait Evaluation

Evaluation of cerebellar function is an integral part of the examination of station and gait. When an older child is observed walking, one should watch for asymmetry of arm swing as well as for abnormal arm and hand posturing and instability of truncal muscles. During turning the examiner observes for extra steps. The child with proximal and calf muscle weakness would have difficulty rising completely on the tips of the toes and one with foot drop is unable to walk on the heels. Difficulty with tandem gait is seen with midline cerebellar lesions. Maintaining balance while doing deep knee bends also requires intact cerebellar function. The child with proximal muscle weakness has difficulty rising from a squatting position (Gowers sign). Walking on the lateral aspects of the feet often brings out hemiparetic posturing of an arm, suggesting subtle or remote upper motor neuron damage. A positive Romberg sign (swaying of the body with eyes closed, feet together, arms outstretched, palms facing ceiling, and fingers spread apart) is consistent with posterior column disease or a peripheral neuropathy. During this testing for Romberg sign a subtle hemiparesis may produce mild pronation of the affected arm, while a more involved hemiparesis will produce pronation followed by downward drift of the arm and at times by lateral movement of the arm. Cerebellar function may also be evaluated by repetitive finger tapping, foot tapping, finger to nose, and heel to shin movements and alternating pronation and supination of the hands and forearms. The cerebellar function is necessary for rhythm of movement and smooth execution of motor movement. Tremors associated with cerebellar disease are primarily present on intention or action.

Average gross motor milestones in older children would predict the ability to walk on tiptoes by 30 months, to balance on one foot and jump off the ground using both feet by 36 months, and to hop on one foot and throw a ball overhand by 48 months. Children may normally have an equinus gait or walk on their tiptoes for their first two walking years (generally from 1 to 3 years of age). The tiptoe gait may persist in a "habitual toe walker," or it may be associated with mild cerebral palsy. Some children also demonstrate congenital tight heel cords with restriction in dorsiflexion but normal stretch reflexes in the absence of other neurologic abnormalities. Cavus or high-arched feet may occur secondary to intrauterine position or they may be familial. The gradual development of a cavus foot in an older child suggests underlying degenerative disease such as Friedreich's ataxia, Charcot-Marie-Tooth disease, or developmental spinal abnormalities (Table 3-11). Flexible flatfoot becomes obvious when the developmental level of standing is reached and is a frequent occurrence. Patients with this condition often have an associated ligamentous laxity. Tight heel cords may also produce a secondary flatfoot. In infants the calcaneal valgus foot must be differentiated from the convex pes valgus deformity.

Many abnormalities of gait may be produced. Any lesion that disrupts the corticospinal innervation to limbs on one side of the body produces a spastic hemiplegic gait. Frequent observations include decreased arm swing and circumduction of the leg on the affected side and often a flexed posture of the arm with stress gait testing. A spastic paraplegic gait results from bilateral corticospinal tract involvement. Spasticity is seen in both lower extremities and often causes crossing of the legs, especially during attempts at weight-bearing. A cerebellar gait may arise from interruption of any of the many input systems to either midline cerebellar structures or cerebellar hemispheres. These patients often have an unsteady gait, they have difficulty with turns, and may veer in either direction. A waddling gait is seen in muscle disease and is suggestive of proximal weakness, espe-

**Table 3-11. Abnormalities of the Back and Extremities in Neurologic Disease**

| Examination | Sign | Neurologic Disease |
|---|---|---|
| Back | Scoliosis | Friedreich's ataxia |
| | | Neuromuscular diseases (many) |
| | | Spinal cord tumors |
| | | Neurofibromatosis |
| | | Syringomyelia |
| | | Congenital spinal anomalies |
| | Kyphosis | Mucupolysaccharidoses |
| | Mass | Spinal dysraphia with lipoma, myelocele, meningomyelocele |
| Extremities | Pes cavus | Friedreich's ataxia |
| | | Charcot-Marie-Tooth disease |
| | | Other neuropathies |
| | Joint contractures | Muscular dystrophies |
| | | Congenital myopathies |
| | | Arthrogryposis multiplex congenita |
| | | Dermatomyositis |
| | Joint laxity | Ehlers-Danlos syndrome |
| | Limb asymmetry | Hemiatrophy (parietal lobe injury) |
| | | Leg length (tethered cord, Klippel-Trenaunay syndrome) |
| | | Beckwith-Wiedemann syndrome |

(From Evans OB: Manual of Child Neurology. Churchill Livingstone, New York, 1987, with permission.)

cially of the gluteal muscle groups, which produces a side-to-side motion at the hips.

A steppage gait generally results from a peripheral neuropathy involving one or both legs, resulting in weakness of the distal muscles. Injury to or involvement of the peroneal nerve is a common finding associated with a peripheral neuropathy that makes walking difficult. The involved foot is usually lifted high above the ground to affect the swing-through phase of gait. An extrapyramidal gait often presents with a bradykinetic, festinating quality and with postures and movement suggestive of a Parkinson's syndrome. Limping is never normal. It may occur secondary to muscloskeletal pain or result from asymmetric muscle performance of the lower extremities. Limping may result from imbalances in pelvic and truncal musculature as well as from problems related to the knee, foot, and ankle. The knee normally flexes by about 70 degrees during the swing phase. Circumduction of the leg is necessary to clear the foot if knee flexion is restricted. Pelvic elevation is also necessary during this maneuver. An equinus contracture of the ankle will force the knee to hyperextend during the stance phase. A greater degree of knee flexion is required during the swing phase to clear the toes when the patient has foot drop or restricted ankle dorsiflexion.

Approximately 10 degrees of ankle dorsiflexion and 20 degrees of ankle plantar flexion are necessary for a normal gait. When plantar flexion is restricted, push-off is also restricted, and the forefoot and heel leave the floor simultaneously. Lack of foot dorsiflexion leaves the foot hanging during swing phase and requires a higher knee lift to follow through. Leg length measurements are important where indicated.

## NEURODIAGNOSTIC STUDIES

Following the history and complete neurologic examination, neurodiagnostic studies may be helpful. Indications for lumbar puncture seem to have decreased as newer evaluation techniques have become available. Lumbar puncture, however, remains invaluable to rule out infection and occult hemorrhage. Myelography also has been less often used with the advent of computed tomographic (CT) scanning and magnetic resonance imaging (MRI). The latter technique provides excellent visualization of the anatomy of the brain, spinal cord, and bone and produces no artifacts. Cerebral angiography (arteriography) is still the definitive procedure where suspicion remains of an occult blood vessel abnormality and often is used to assess the vascularity of a tumor or other mass lesion.

Skull, spinal, joint, and long bone radiographs continue to have limited usefulness. Digital vascular (subtraction) imaging may be used for the visualization of large vessels in their extracranial course. Electroencephalography (EEG) records the spontaneous electrical activity of the brain. It is used in assessing clinical seizures as well as for monitoring patients with severe state changes and possible cerebral inactivity.

Electromyography (EEG) records the electrical activity of muscle fibers through a needle electrode inserted into the muscle belly. Activity is noted during insertion of the needle as well as during the resting state. Abnormal spontaneous electrical activity may be recorded in the form of fasciculations, fibrillations, or positive sharp waves. Fasciculations are most often seen in chronic anterior horn cell disorders (e.g., amyotrophic lateral sclerosis). Fibrillations and positive sharp waves are detected 3 to 6 weeks following motor nerve injury. Re-innervation of denervated muscle fibers produces polyphasic motor units during volitional contraction. By localizing denervation changes among different muscles, the site of the lesion may be accurately localized. EMG studies may also serve a prognostic role following nerve injury.

Nerve conduction studies involve stimulating a motor or sensory nerve at different anatomic points and calculating the velocity of conduction of the propagated impulse. The fastest conducting fibers, the large myelinated nerve fibers, are recorded. Demyelination leads to a decrease in conduction velocity. This technique may detect entrapment neuropathies, differentiate demyelinating from axonal peripheral neuropathies, and assist in injury localization. However, small fiber neuropathies and predominantly axonal neuropathies may go undetected in a nerve conduction study.

Evoked potentials are recordings of the electrical activity in the central nervous system produced by stimulation of peripheral sensory receptors. Auditory stimuli, visual stimuli, and somatosensory evoked potentials may be obtained.

Muscle and nerve biopsy specimens are fragile and must be handled properly to obtain accurate and complete results. When performing these tests, one should have available histochemical, electron microscopic, biochemical, and enzymatic analyses and tissue culture where indicated. Special urine and blood tests are often invaluable in assessing metabolic, toxic, genetic, and degenerative disorders.

## SUMMARY

The neurologic examination of the infant and child is variable and dependent upon a thorough history and observations. The more complex and invasive tests should be reserved for the problem child. The more advanced tests are used to document or confirm clinical suspicions or findings and often as a baseline for long-term management.

# 4

# Diagnostic Imaging of the Pediatric Patient*

JOAN OLOFF
SHEILA G. MOORE

The world of diagnostic imaging is among the most rapidly evolving areas of medicine. These new techniques may play a role in the evaluation of the pediatric as well as the adult patient population. The plain film evaluation remains, however, the most common radiographic technique that is utilized in evaluation of the pediatric foot.

When evaluating pediatric radiographs, the clinician must have a thorough understanding of normal anatomy as well as of developmental patterns for that particular age. This chapter will review those normal developmental patterns and will also provide a review of different examples of pathology in the pediatric foot. With an increasing number of techniques available, the clinician may be confused as to the proper diagnostic workup for a particular pathology. This chapter will attempt to clarify the most appropriate use of these techniques.

## RADIOGRAPHIC ANATOMY
### Normal Ossification

Cartilaginous models of the tarsus form between the seventh and ninth weeks of gestation at which time ossification of the metatarsals and phalanges takes place. Ossification of the tarsal bones takes place later, at about 24 to 28 weeks of gestation. The only tarsal bones that are consistently ossified at birth are the talus and the calcaneus; however, they are incompletely ossified, and a

large portion of these bones remains cartilaginous. This is why large areas remain indiscernible on the radiograph of the pediatric foot. The reader is referred to Chapters 1 and 20 for a more extensive discussion of developmental skeletal anatomy.

As in the adult foot, a systematic approach to reading radiographs should be taken. Coleman[1] has suggested an easy, systematic approach to pediatric radiographs based on the following three important general observations of the ossification centers:

1. Presence and orderly appearance of ossification centers
2. Shape and size of visible ossification centers
3. Relationships of centers to each other

With respect to the first observation, any significant delay or alteration in the normal order of appearance of these ossification centers may be a sign of pathology (Fig. 4-1). The shape and size of the visible ossification centers should be evaluated next. Flattening and irregularity of multiple ossification centers may be indicative of a congenital dysplasia, such as epiphyseal dysplasia multiplex (Fig. 4-2). The relationships of ossification centers to each other are important because an alteration in the appearance of a single ossification center would suggest a local process. (Figs. 4-3 to 4-6).

There are several excellent accounts of the normal skeletal development of the foot (Table 4-1). The shafts of the metatarsals are ossified at birth, while their epiphyses are not. The epiphysis of the first metatarsal is proximal, and all the others are distal. The epiphysis may

---

* Pages 51–66 are adapted from Oloff,[18] with permission.

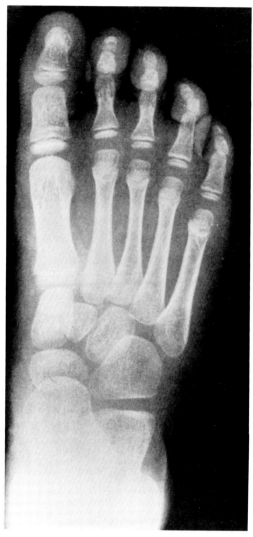

**Fig. 4-1.** Normal ossification centers. Note the presence and orderly appearance of both primary and secondary centers of ossification.

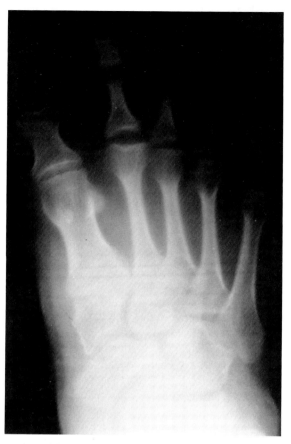

**Fig. 4-2.** Epiphyseal dysplasia multiplex. Flattening and irregularity of multiple ossification centers are indicative of a congenital dysplasia.

present at around 3 years of age and close at the age of about 15 to 20. This is true of the phalanges as well. The calcaneal apophysis is present at the age of about 8 to 10 years of age and fuses at the age of 16 to 20.

## Accessory Bones of the Foot

Accessory bones may be quite common in the foot. Chapter 17 provides an extensive discussion of accessory and sesamoid bones of the foot. It is essential that the clinician be familiar with the various accessory ossification centers in order to avoid misdiagnosing them as avulsion fractures. Accessory bones typically have a smooth, regular border, whereas fractures have an irregular outline. Accessory bones may develop a clinical significance of their own. Tachdjian has pointed out the clinical significance of two of the most common accessory bones of the foot, the os tibiale externum and the os trigonum.[2] The os tibiale externum, or accessory navicular, is described as being present in about 10 percent of children, eventually fusing to the main body of the navicular in 8 percent of adults. The typical location of this bone is proximal and plantar to the medial aspect of the navicular (Fig. 4-7). Kidner in 1929 was the first to recognize the relationship between this accessory bone and flatfoot deformities.[3] The pathologic attachment of

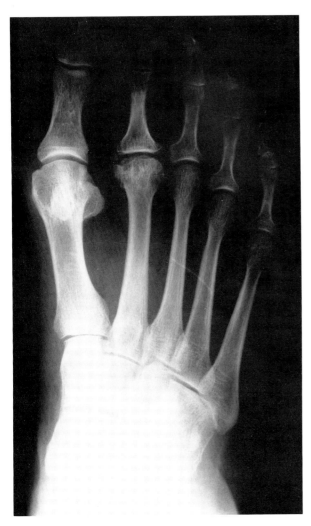

**Fig. 4-3.** Freiberg's infraction. An alteration in the appearance of a single ossification center is indicative of a local process. (Adapted from Oloff,[18] with permission.)

Table 4-1. **Normal Dates of Ossification**

| Location | Year Present | Year Fuses |
|---|---|---|
| Calcaneus | Birth | |
|     Apophysis | 8–10 years | 16–20 years |
| Talus | Birth | |
| Cuboid | Birth–6 months | |
| First cuneiform | 1½–2 years | |
| Second cuneiform | 2–2½ years | |
| Third cuneiform | 3–6 months | |
| Navicular | 3–4 years | |
| Metatarsals | Birth | |
|     Epiphysis | 1–3 years | 12–16 years |
|     Fifth metatarsal base Epiphysis | 9–13 years | 15 years |
| Phalanges | Birth | |
|     Epiphysis | 1–3 years | 12–15 years |

(From Oloff,[18] with permission.)

to remember that the normal epiphysis runs parallel to the long axis of the fifth metatarsal and the os vesalianum will therefore be oriented in a similar direction. Fractures in this area typically run more or less perpendicular to the long axis of the metatarsal.

Other accessory bones that may be seen include the os peroneum or peroneum sesamoid, which is located lateral and proximal to the cuboid. The os talonaviculare is located dorsally, overlying the talonavicular joint. Interphalangeal sesamoids are located plantarly and can be the source of a painful tyloma of the hallux. Care should be taken not to mistake accessory bones distal to the medial or lateral malleolus (the os subtibiale and the os subfibulare, respectively) for avulsion fractures.

It should be noted that plain film evaluation of sesamoid bones is usually sufficient in the pediatric patient population. In the older child or the adult patient if one is suspicious of degenerative changes between the sesamoid and the parent bone a computed tomography (CT) scan may provide useful information.

## RADIOGRAPHIC TECHNIQUES IN THE PEDIATRIC FOOT

In the infant modifications of standard radiographic techniques are necessary, since it is obviously not possible to perform the traditional weight-bearing examination in the prewalker. Radiographs should be taken in a simu-

the posterior tibial tendon to the os tibiale externum may cause the tendon to lose its mechanical leverage. The second accessory bone to which Tachdjian ascribes clinical significance is the os trigonum. This bone, located at the posterolateral aspect of the talus, is best visualized on the lateral radiograph of the foot.

The os vesalianum pedis is a third accessory bone commonly seen in the foot and is located at the lateral aspect of the base of the fifth metatarsal. This bone is easily confused with an avulsion fracture. It is important

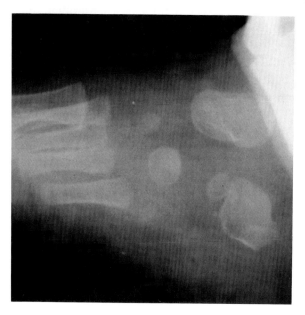
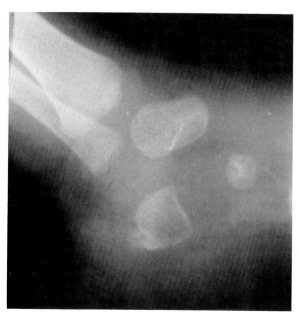

**Fig. 4-4.** Extra secondary areas of ossification, as in this calcaneus, may be seen as a normal variant. (Figure on right from Oloff,[18] with permission.)

lated weight-bearing position with a parent holding the child upright. Both feet may be radiographed simultaneously. It is not necessary to obtain oblique views unless trauma is suspected. In the older child, radiographs should be taken in the traditional weight-bearing angle, and base of gait positions. Once again, trauma should be evaluated by semi-weight-bearing or non-weight-bearing examinations. It is often useful to obtain radiographs bilaterally when evaluating suspected physeal injuries.

The relationships of osseous structures to one another are, in fact, a crucial part of interpreting pedal radiographs. Experience in evaluating the normal foot is a mandatory prerequisite for identifying pathology in the pediatric foot.[4] The following section will discuss radiographic evaluation of different types of pathology in children. Specific techniques that may be useful in evaluating these pathologies will be presented.[5]

# RADIOGRAPHIC EVALUATION OF METATARSUS ADDUCTUS

Metatarsus adductus is primarily a transverse plane pathologic condition and therefore is best evaluated on the dorsoplantar view. Certain angular relationships provide useful information for evaluating this deformity. The *metatarsus adductus angle,* formed by the intersection of the long axis of the second metatarsal with the perpendicular bisector of the lesser tarsus, defines the relationship of the metatarsals to the tarsus. Its normal value may range from 0 to 20 degrees.[2] In newborns angles as high as 35 degrees have been reported as being normal.[2] By the age of 1 year, however, these values could be reduced. This angle does not significantly change with pronation or supination. The *forefoot adductus angle,* formed by the intersection of the long axis of the second metatarsal with the long axis of the rearfoot, defines the relationship of the forefoot to the rearfoot. Since it includes the midtarsus, this angle will change greatly with pronation and supination. Its normal value ranges from 0 to 16 degrees. In the presence of a great deal of forefoot adduction, the metatarsus adductus deformity will be exaggerated.[6,7]

## Infant

Whether or not to obtain radiographs of the young pediatric patient with metatarsus adductus is a controversial point.[5] There are those who feel that treatment can be

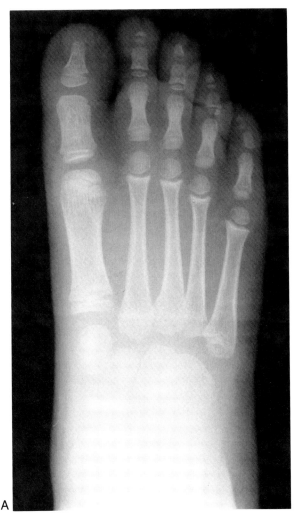

A

**Fig. 4-5. (A)** Kohler's disease. Flattening, irregularity, fragmentation, and sclerosis may all be radiographic signs of osteochondritis of the tarsal navicular. *(Figure continues.)*

rendered without the aid of radiographic examination. This is especially true in light of the fact that metatarsus adductus is a fairly simple clinical diagnosis. Nevertheless, we believe that there is a place for radiographic examination of these patients' feet for two main reasons: first, radiographs provide a useful baseline by which treatment can be judged, and second, radiographs help to monitor overcorrection of the midtarsal joint. This is seen as a rapid increase in cuboid abduction on the dorsoplantar view. Evidence of this should alert the clini-

cian that breakdown of the midtarsal joint is occurring and that treatment should be altered (Fig. 4-8).

## Older Child

In addition to the primary metatarsus adductus deformity, the older child may demonstrate evidence of compensation for this deformity. Since the primary deformity is located in the transverse plane, compensation occurs mainly in the transverse plane as well. They are both visualized best in the dorsoplantar view (Fig. 4-9). Compensation may occur at the subtalar joint and will be seen as an increase in the talocalcaneal angle (Kite's angle). Compensation may also occur at the midtarsal joint, as evidenced by a greater than 11-degree abduction of the cuboid upon the calcaneus.[8] The appearance of the compensated metatarsus adductus foot is commonly described as a *Z* or *serpentine* foot. It is interesting to note that there is very little compensation in the sagittal plane, and the lateral radiograph therefore does not usually demonstrate the severity of deformity in these children.

## RADIOGRAPHIC EVALUATION OF PES VALGUS DEFORMITIES
### Flexible Pes Valgus

Again, it is important to remember that radiographs for evaluation of the pediatric pes valgus foot should be obtained in the angle and base of gait to allow for ascertaining biomechanical information. Understanding of the normal biomechanical values is fundamental in the evaluation of this pathology.

**Dorsoplantar Radiographs**

The angle formed by the intersection of the longitudinal axis of the talus and the longitudinal axis of the calcaneus is called the talocalcaneal angle or Kite's angle. In infants and toddlers, the normal range for this angle is 30 to 50 degrees; this reduces to 15 to 30 degrees in children older than 5 years of age and remains the same for adults. Kite's angle will increase in pes valgus deformity because of medial talar deviation. In the flexible pes valgus foot, the longitudinal axis of the talus lies medial to the first metatarsal. Normally, it should pass through the first metatarsal. This medial deviation of the talus causes a

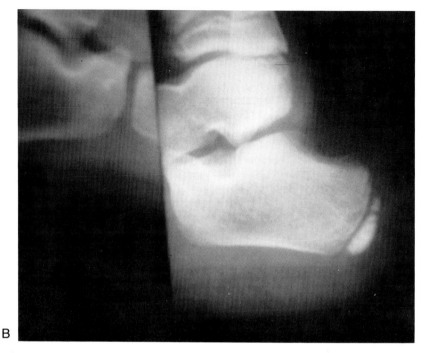

B

**Fig. 4-5** *(Continued).* **(B)** Sever's disease. It should be noted that irregularity, fragmentation, and sclerosis of the calcaneal apophysis may all be seen as normal variants. Sever's disease is not a radiographic diagnosis.

decrease in the articulation between the talar head and the navicular. Normally, approximately 70 to 75 percent of the talar head articulates with the navicular, but in the flexible pes valgus foot, this proportion usually decreases to less than 50 percent.

Another aspect of midtarsal joint pronation that can be seen on the dorsoplantar view is cuboid abduction. In the normal foot the lateral aspect of the calcaneus and the cuboid should fall on the same line, but in the flexible pes valgus foot there is typically a greater than 11-degree abduction of the cuboid on the calcaneus[9] (Fig. 4-10). This finding is more commonly seen in those flexible pes valgus feet that demonstrate transverse plane pathology. An example would be the previously discussed compensated metatarsus adductus deformity.

### Lateral Radiographs

The lateral view will be most impressive in those flexible pes valgus deformities that demonstrate pathology primarily in the sagittal plane (Fig. 4-11A). In children older than 5 years of age, the midtalar line should pass through the first metatarsal. In infants and very young children, the talar position deviates vertically, and the midtalar line falls plantar to the first metatarsal. The cyma line is the S-shaped curve that is formed by outlining the midtarsal joints (Fig. 4-11). In the flexible pes valgus foot there is typically an anterior break in this line, which is due to the anterior migration of the talus in these children. Further evidence of medial column pathology may be evidenced by a fault. This may be seen as sagging, which may occur between the talus and the navicular, the navicular and the medial cuneiform, or the medial cuneiform and the first metatarsal. Finally, the calcaneal inclination angle is usually decreased in these patients below the normal values of 15 to 25 degrees.

For evaluation of equinus in the pediatric pes valgus patient, a stress lateral radiograph should be considered (Fig. 4-11B). In the older child this is obtained by having the child flex the knee while placing full weight on the involved foot. It is important to make sure that the heel remains on the ground. In the infant a simulated stress

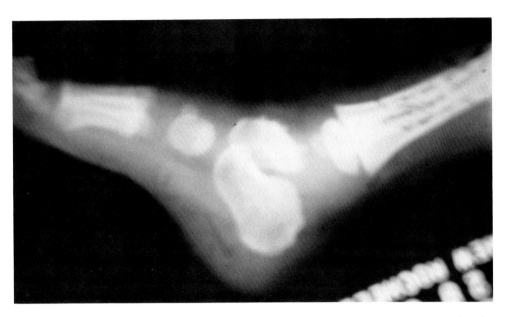

**Fig. 4-6.** Avascular necrosis of the talus in a young child. If any doubt exists, magnetic resonance imaging would provide the most sensitive examination for this pathology.

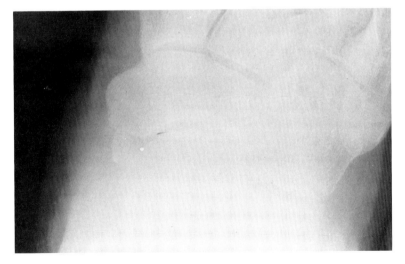

**Fig. 4-7.** Os tibiale externum. This accessory bone is present in about 10 percent of children, eventually fusing to the navicular in 8 percent of adults.

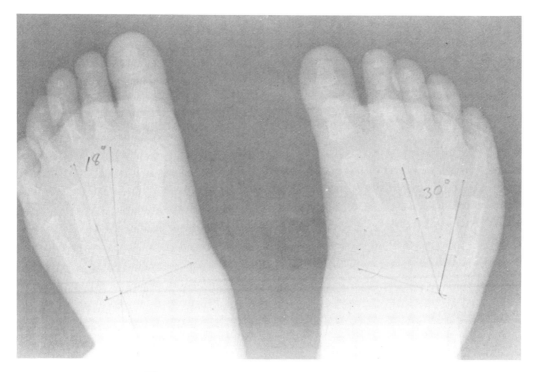

**Fig. 4-8.** Metatarsus adductus in the young child.

lateral view may be obtained by the examiner placing a board underneath the foot and applying a dorsiflexory stress on the foot through this board. If a soft tissue equinus is present, the examination may demonstrate an increase in midtarsal joint breakdown. Sagittal plane compensation may also occur elsewhere in the medial column. If equinus is secondary to an osseous block, the examiner will notice impingement of the dorsal head of the talus upon the anterior lip of the tibia. In the case of a long-standing osseous block, osteophytes on the dorsal head of the talus are usually present on the standard lateral radiograph. This is usually not seen prior to adolescence.

## Rigid Pes Valgus

### Tarsal Coalition

Radiographic evaluation of tarsal coalition is not usually a concern in the young child as these patients usually do not become symptomatic until adolescence. Tachdjian[2] has shown us that tarsal coalition is not acquired in adolescence; rather, coalitions remain cartilaginous prior to that stage of development.

The calcaneonavicular coalition is fairly common and rarely poses a diagnostic problem. The standard medial oblique radiograph of the foot usually demonstrates this coalition quite clearly (Fig. 4-12). In those cases in which there is a very close approximation between the calcaneus and the navicular, the possibility of a synchondrosis (cartilaginous coalition) or a syndesmosis (fibrous coalition) remains.

The talocalcaneal (subtalar) coalition is a second type of coalition that is commonly seen. The poor visualization of this joint on standard radiographs is the reason that this type of coalition may pose a greater diagnostic challenge. Coalition may occur at any of the three subtalar joint facets — namely the anterior, middle, and posterior facets — but the middle facet coalition is by far the most commonly seen. The lateral radiograph provides the first indication of a subtalar joint coalition. This view demonstrates secondary findings of coalition, which include: (1)

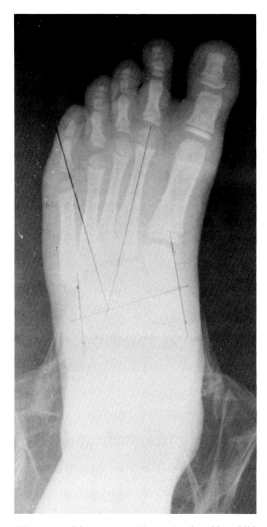

**Fig. 4-9.**  Metatarsus adductus in the older child.

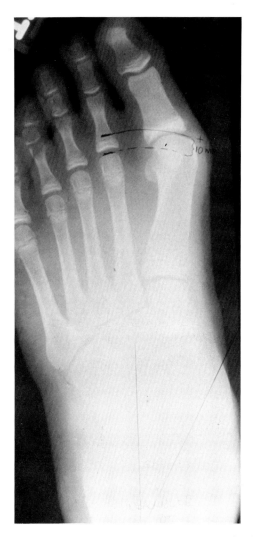

**Fig. 4-10.**  Flexible pes valgus. This dorsoplantar view illustrates the medial deviation of the talus. Midtarsal joint pronation is illustrated by the cuboid abduction.

talar beaking, usually on the talar side of the talonavicular joint; (2) blunting of the lateral process of the talus; and (3) loss of definition of the sinus tarsi region or posterior facet (Fig. 4-13). These secondary signs are usually not present until adolescence. Once they are demonstrated, the next step is to obtain Harris-Beath[10] views (Fig. 4-14, 4-15). These radiographs are taken with the patient standing on the film with knees flexed and with the x-ray tube placed behind the patient. Three radiographs are taken at 35, 45, and 55 degrees. This technique is used in an attempt to match the declination of the middle and posterior facets, which averages 45

degrees. In their original work Harris & Beath[10] recommended measuring declination of the middle facet first. This is not usually necessary. In the normal examination both the middle and posterior facets are present and parallel to each other; either complete obliteration or extensive angulation may be suggestive of a coalition. Confusion may occur because a long-standing flexible flatfoot deformity may also produce a severe angulation deformity of the middle facet.

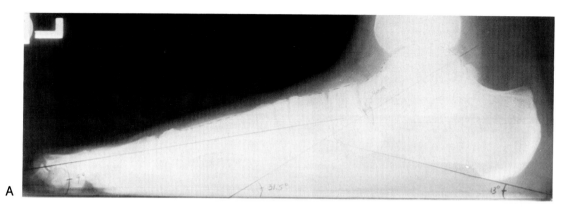

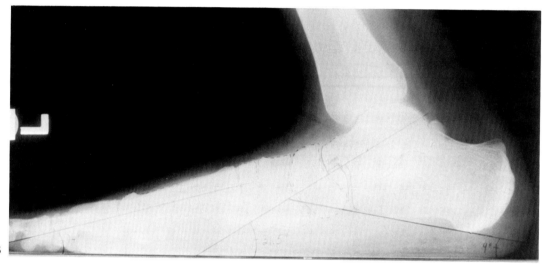

**Fig. 4-11.** Flexible pes valgus. **(A)** Lateral. The midtalar line falls plantar to the first metatarsal. The cyma line is broken 4 mm anteriorly. **(B)** Stress lateral. The stress lateral view evaluates the equinus deformity. Note the further decrease in the calcaneal inclination angle and the further break in the cyma line to 7 mm.

In those cases in which the diagnosis is questionable or surgical intervention is contemplated, further studies may be indicated. The gold standard for evaluation of subtalar coalition is CT (Fig. 4-16). It is best to image these feet in the coronal plane at 2 mm intervals. Images that are obtained at wider intervals may miss a subtle coalition. Sagittal re-formations may provide useful additional information for surgical planning. In our experience three-dimensional imaging has not provided sufficient additional information to justify its higher cost and loss of spatial resolution.

## Congenital Convex Pes Valgus

The fundamental pathology in the convex pes valgus deformity is the dislocation of the talonavicular joint,[2] specifically, a dorsal dislocation of the navicular upon the head of the talus. Plain films are extremely useful in the evaluation of this deformity.

The lateral radiograph of the foot best demonstrates the vertical talus deformity (Fig. 4-17); it is useful in differentiating the true dorsal dislocation of the navicular seen in vertical talus deformity from the flexible flatfoot

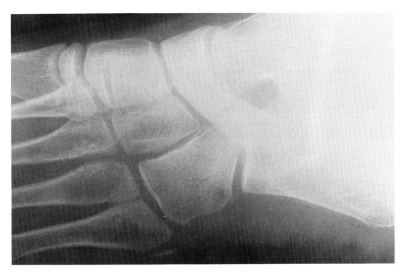

**Fig. 4-12.** The calcaneonavicular bar is readily diagnosed by the standard oblique projection of the foot.

deformity, in which more of an oblique talus is visualized. A second important finding on the lateral radiograph is a negative inclination of the calcaneus, which is due to the severe equinus deformity seen in these children. Additional plain film techniques may be necessary in infants or young children. As previously noted, the navicular is not normally ossified until around 3 or 4 years of age, and therefore it is difficult to differentiate the true vertical from the oblique talus in infants and very young children. As an aid to this diagnosis, the lateral radiograph may be taken in stressed plantar flexion (Fig. 4-18), with the examiner first stabilizing and then passively plantar-flexing the forefoot upon the rearfoot. In the flexible flatfoot deformity there will be a reduction of the talar declina-

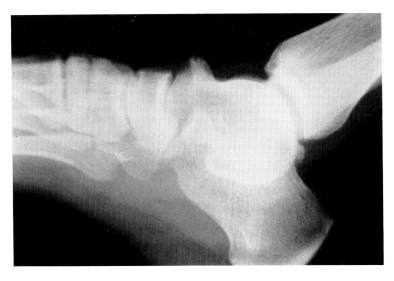

**Fig. 4-13.** Secondary changes of coalition that may be demonstrated on the lateral view include talar beaking, blunting of the lateral process of the talus, and loss of definition of the sinus tarsi.

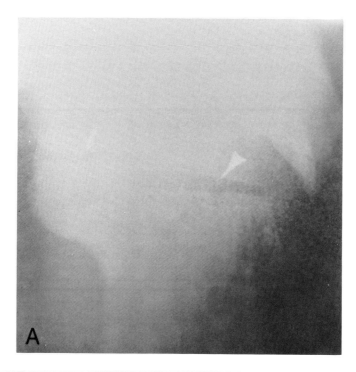

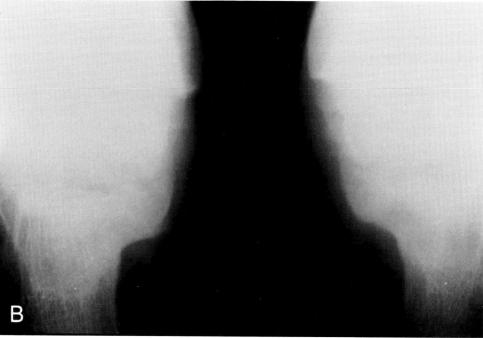

**Fig. 4-14.** Harris-Beath views. **(A)** This radiograph illustrates the normal presence and paralellism of the middle and posterior facets. **(B)** Note the angulation of the middle facets. This finding is not diagnostic of a coalition, as the longstanding flexible pes valgus may also show this adaptation.

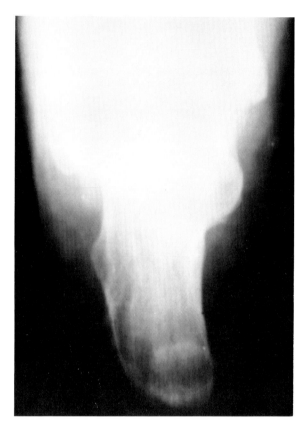

Fig. 4-15. Complete obliteration of the middle facet on this Harris-Beath view is diagnostic for a coalition.

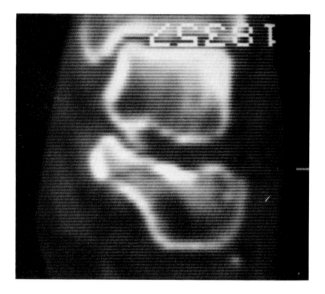

Fig. 4-16. CT scanning remains the most useful modality in the evaluation of tarsal coalitions. This reconstructed coronal view illustrates a subtle middle facet coalition.

tion; in fact, the midtalar line should fall within the upper one-third of the cuboid. In the convex pes valgus foot the talar position will become more vertical because of the rigid talonavicular dislocation. One should remember that this is a rigid deformity. This technique is crucial in infants, in whom clinical determination of flexibility is not reliable for differentiation of these complex pathologies.[7]

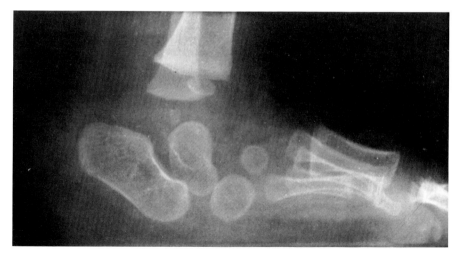

Fig. 4-17. Vertical talus. The lateral view best illustrates the vertical orientation of the talus. The negative calcaneal inclination should also be visualized.

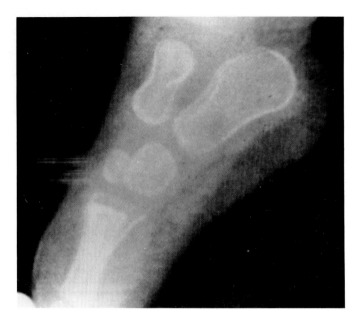

**Fig. 4-18.** Stress plantar flexion radiograph of a young child with flexible pes valgus. The talocalcaneal angle normalizes and the long axis of the talus falls into parallel alignment with the first metatarsal. In convex pes valgus the talus becomes more vertical with stress plantar flexion because of talonavicular dislocation.

Magnetic resonance imaging (MRI) provides an additional modality that may be used in the evaluation of congenital convex pes valgus. The unossified infant navicular, and therefore talonavicular, dislocation of convex pes valgus can be visualized on MRI. MRI should be reserved for children under age 4 with suspected convex pes valgus in whom plain and stress radiographs prove inconclusive.

## RADIOGRAPHIC EVALUATION OF CAVUS FEET

Plain film evaluation is sufficient in the evaluation of most cavus foot deformities. The lateral radiograph provides the greatest amount of information in these cases. The majority of the deformity lies in the sagittal plane, but it should be noted that frontal or transverse plane deformities may be a component of the overall deformity, in which case the dorsoplantar view may be more remarkable. The lateral view enables the clinician to delineate the level at which the deformity occurs. When the deformity occurs primarily in the hindfoot, the most prominent finding is the increase in the calcaneal inclination angle, which may approach 30 degrees or greater. The talocalcaneal angle is decreased[11] and the sinus tarsi becomes more prominent in these children. The talar declination angle also decreases so that the longitudinal axis of the talus falls dorsal to the first metatarsal bone. When the deformity occurs primarily in the forefoot, two primary types of pathology may be noted. In the anterior local type of cavus foot there is an increase in the declination of the first metatarsal, while the remaining metatarsal bones may appear normal. In the anterior global type of cavus foot all the metatarsals demonstrate an increased declination.

### Dorsoplantar Radiographs

As mentioned, the dorsoplantar view is more remarkable when there is evidence of a varus component to the deformity. One may notice an adduction of the forefoot and of the metatarsals (described in greater detail in the metatarsus adductus section of this chapter). The talocalcaneal, or Kite's angle decreases on this view. Digital deformities, such as claw toe, may be noticed in older children.

## Calcaneal Axial Radiographs

If a structural varus deformity of the calcaneus is suspected, a calcaneal axial radiograph may prove useful, especially in those cases in which a calcaneal osteotomy is contemplated. It is best to obtain this view with the patient in a weight-bearing position.

## Ankle Mortise Radiographs

Tachdjian points out the importance of excluding an ankle varus deformity in these patients.[2] An ankle mortise view should be obtained when there is a discrepancy between the clinical and radiographic findings. Again, this is most important when surgical intervention is contemplated.

## RADIOGRAPHIC EVALUATION OF TALIPES EQUINOVARUS DEFORMITY

The incidence of talipes equinovarus (clubfoot) deformity was found by Wynne-Davies to be 1.00 to 1.24 per 1,000 white births.[12] The incidence in first-degree relatives was noted to be 20 to 30 times as great. The pathologic anatomy involves a medial deviation of the navicular, cuboid, and calcaneus on the talus. The talus is three-quarters of its normal size. The majority of the talar deformity lies within the distal neck and head, and the angle between the head and neck and the body of the talus is decreased to 115 to 135 degrees (normal values are 150 to 160 degrees). The clinical findings of rearfoot varus, equinus, and forefoot adduction should be demonstrated radiographically. At a minimum, the required radiographs include a dorsoplantar view, a lateral view of the foot and ankle, and a stress lateral dorsiflexion view. The last view is necessary to evaluate the equinus deformity more accurately.

## Plain Film Radiographs

### Dorsoplantar View

The most significant finding on the dorsoplantar view is the superimposition of the talus and the calcaneus (Fig. 4-19), which results in a decrease in the talocalcaneal (Kite's) angle. The normal value for this angle is age-dependent: it is between 30 and 50 degrees, in infants,

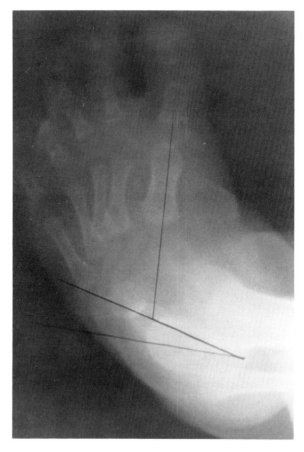

**Fig. 4-19.** Clubfoot (dorsoplantar view). The superimposition of the talus and the calcaneus is the most significant finding. The long axis of the talus lies lateral to the first metatarsal.

decreasing to 20 to 35 degrees in children older than 5 years. Values less than 20 degrees are consistent with hindfoot varus. In addition to the decrease in Kite's angle, the long axis of the talus will lie lateral to the first metatarsal. The medial displacement of the navicular will not be visible prior to its ossification, which may be further retarded in the clubfoot deformity. The adduction and varus of the forefoot are illustrated by the superimposition of the metatarsal bases.

### Lateral View

On the lateral view the talus and the calcaneus appear parallel, with no overlap of the anterior ends.[12] The normal superimposition of the metatarsals is absent owing to the forefoot inversion, and the first metatarsal appears most superior, also as a result of the forefoot deformity. The fibula is noted to be more posterior than normal, which is due to the external rotation required to stabilize the convex lateral border of the foot.

### Stress Lateral View

A lateral radiograph taken in stress dorsiflexion is essential to the thorough evaluation of the clubfoot deformity. In the infant this view is obtained by the examiner placing a dorsiflexion stress on the foot through a board placed beneath it. The examiner should be protected with lead gloves and an apron. In the older child this examination can be made with the patient in a weight-bearing position. In uncorrected clubfoot the calcaneus is locked in varus beneath the talus and the navicular is bound medially by soft tissue contractures. Therefore, on this view there is persistent equinus, which prevents the calcaneus from dorsiflexion.[12] Thus, the three signs of persistent clubfoot deformity on lateral radiographs are (1) no dorsiflexion of the calcaneus; (2) parallelism of the talus and calcaneus; and (3) no overlap of the anterior ends of the calcaneus and talus.

## Magnetic Resonance Imaging

The use of MRI in the evaluation of clubfoot deformity remains controversial. It is currently being used by some surgeons as an additional technique in the evaluation of this complex deformity. MRI provides a means to evaluate the aberrant tendonous and neurovascular anatomy in these cases. In addition, the medial displacement of the navicular may not be fully appreciated on conventional radiographs, as it may not yet be ossified. MRI provides a means of evaluating those structures not seen on the radiographs. In addition, MRI becomes particularly useful in evaluating those abnormalities of the spine that may be seen in conjunction with the clubfoot deformity.

## Corrected Clubfoot

Post-treatment radiographs are essential in the evaluation of the corrected clubfoot, unlike metatarsus adductus. Radiographic evidence of correction of all three components of the deformity should be demonstrated; the stress lateral view is particularly useful. These children often present with a persistent equinus deformity. In older children and adults one may notice a flattening of the dome of the talus following clubfoot correction. This

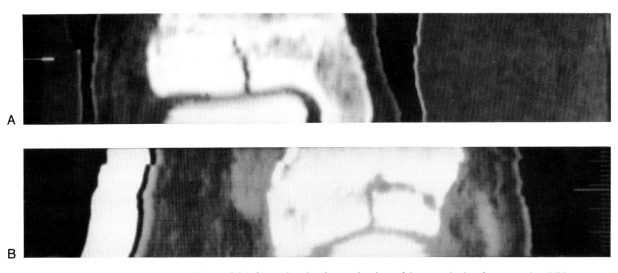

**Fig. 4-20.** CT scans may provide useful information in the evaluation of intra-articular fractures in children. **(A)** Coronal view illustrates the fracture line extending into the ankle joint. **(B)** Sagittal reconstruction illustrates the fracture line extending through the physis.

is a true flattening, which should be distinguished from the apparent flattening that can be seen when the leg is externally rotated. One consequence of treatment may be overcorrection, which can be so severe as to cause a rocker bottom foot. These children may demonstrate evidence of a dorsal subluxation or actual dislocation of the navicular upon the talus.

## RADIOGRAPHIC EVALUATION OF TRAUMA

The uniqueness of the growing skeleton should be appreciated by any clinician involved in the evaluation or treatment of fractures in children. Ogden[13] has identified basic patterns of children's fractures, which include longitudinal, transverse, oblique, spiral, impacted, comminuted, bowing, greenstick, torus, pathologic, and stress types. The younger the child at the time of injury, the greater the potential for growth disturbances later on. When appropriate, careful attention to anatomic reduction should be carried out. Fortunately, foot fractures in

early childhood are rare owing to the flexibility of the foot.

When assessing fractures in children, one must have a thorough understanding of the secondary ossification centers, (Chs. 1, 20). Comparison views of the uninvolved extremity may be useful in the evaluation of physeal trauma. When evaluating pediatric trauma, a minimum of two views at 90 degrees to each other should be obtained, and additional views such as obliques or axials may be obtained when necessary.

Occasionally additional modalities such as CT or MRI may be useful. CT remains the most useful technique when evaluating cortical bone and may provide useful information when evaluating displaced, comminuted fractures involving the physis. This is particularly true when evaluating complex fractures of the ankle joint in children (Fig. 4-20). MRI may have a role in the evaluation of subtle, marrow-replacing processes in children, which may include osteochondral dome fractures and avascular necrosis following skeletal trauma. Prior to obtaining either of these additional tests, the clinician should be certain of what information is needed and

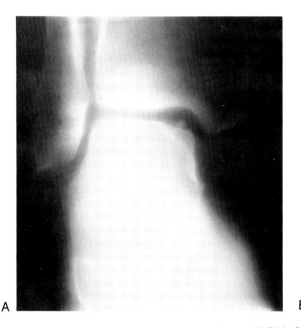
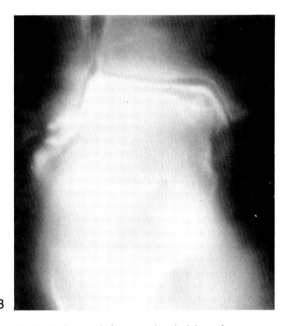

A

B

**Fig. 4-21.** Transchondral dome fracture of talus. **(A)** Plain film of ankle is diagnostic for transchondral dome fracture in this case. **(B)** Arthrography was advocated in the past to evaluate the integrity of the articular cartilage. This technique has largely been replaced by MRI.

which modality will be most likely to provide that information. Bone scanning has little use in the evaluation of skeletal trauma in children but may be useful when one is faced with questionable radiographs. Canale and Kelly[14] utilize serial bone scanning to determine when weight-bearing can be allowed following avascular necrosis of the talus.

Some have advocated use of MRI as a follow-up examination in all physeal injuries.[15] A fibrous bar may be a precursor of angular deformity.

## Transchondral Dome Fractures of the Talus (Osteochondritis Dissecans)

The etiology of osteochondral dome fractures of the talus is primarily traumatic. Symptomatology may vary from localized pain to a diffuse aching pain. This condition is characterized by articular cartilage injury, a subchondral fracture, and an attached subchondral bone fragment, which may become partially or completely separated from the underlying bone.

Plain films should be taken as an initial diagnostic screening procedure in these patients (Fig. 4-21). Necessary views include the anteroposterior, lateral, and mortise views of the ankle. Additional mortise views with the ankle in the plantar-flexed, neutral, and dorsiflexed positions may provide better visualization of these lesions.

Skeletal scintigraphy is also of limited value in the evaluation of osteochondral dome fractures, serving mainly as a screen in those cases in which either the presence or the location of pathology is in question.

CT scanning has remained the "gold standard" for evaluation of osteochondral dome fractures for several

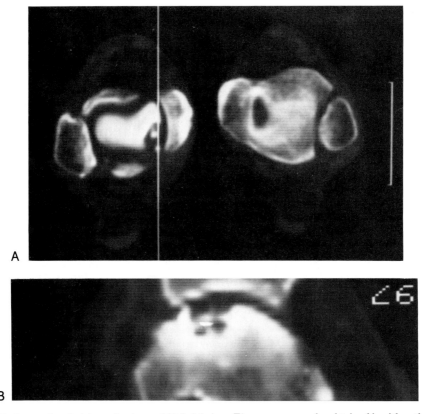

**Fig. 4-22.** CT of transchondral dome fractures. **(A)** Axial view: These scans may be obtained in either the axial or the coronal plane. This view illustrates a large posteromedial lesion. **(B)** Sagittal re-formations provide additional information, which may aid in guiding the surgical approach to these lesions. The articular cartilage may not be illustrated by this technique, however.

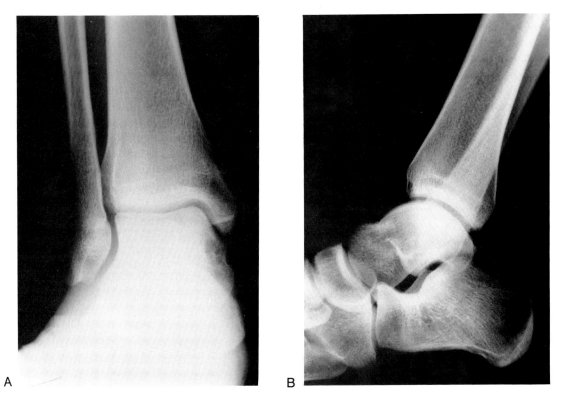

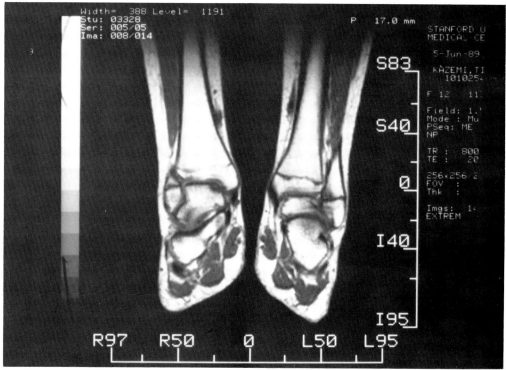

**Fig. 4-23.** Osteochondral dome fracture. **(A)** Plain film (ankle mortise) is suggestive of a radiolucency in the medial talar dome. **(B)** Lateral view is noncontributory in the evaluation of this lesion. **(C)** MRI is diagnostic for a transchondral dome fracture in the medial talar dome.

years (Fig. 4-22). Images are obtained in either the axial or coronal planes and are usually reformatted in the sagittal plane (Fig. 4-22B), which enables one to reconstruct a three-dimensional picture in order to determine the exact location and extent of the lesion. Image slices should be obtained within 2-mm sections to improve visualization of the lesion as well as improve the spatial resolution of the reformatted images. Studies have shown that CT stages these lesions more accurately than plain film examination.[16]

The use of MRI in evaluation of osteochondral dome fractures is increasing (Figs. 4-23 and 4-24). MRI is performed in both coronal and sagittal planes; since it is possible to obtain direct sagittal plane images, computer reformatting is not necessary. These images will allow for accurate assessment of the articular cartilage as well as the subchondral surface of bone. Partial volume artifacts are minimized by comparing the two imaging planes. Advantages of MRI over CT include ability to more accurately evaluate the articular cartilage and its potential usefulness in separating stable from loose lesions. Limitations of MRI include its lack of sensitivity in identifying loose bodies within the ankle joint.

## RADIOGRAPHIC EVALUATION OF TUMOR AND TUMOR-LIKE LESIONS

Standard radiography is the initial modality used in the evaluation of tumor and tumor-like lesions of the foot. Even in those cases in which the primary pathology appears to involve soft tissue, there may be secondary osseous changes that will aid in narrowing the differential diagnosis. The plain film evaluation should be performed in a non-weight-bearing position so as not to artificially alter the location or appearance of the lesion. Any further imaging modalities should be used prior to performing a biopsy, as a biopsy site may cause a false positive finding on a bone scan and MRI may overestimate the lesion size postbiopsy because hemorrhage and edema may be indistinguishable from tumor.

### Bone Tumors

#### Unicameral (Simple) Bone Cysts

Unicameral bone cyst is a common pediatric bone lesion, possibly resulting from disturbance of growth at the epiphyseal plate. There is a predilection for the metaphyseal region of bone. Simple bone cysts, 80 percent of which occur between the ages of 3 and 14 years and which occur in a 3:1 male/female ratio, are pathologically not neoplasms but cystic bony defects with thin fibrous tissue linings.

Radiographically, cysts are medullary, centrally located, and often confined to the metaphysis and immediately juxtaposed to the epiphyseal line. Rare extension to the epiphysis can be seen. A thin linear band of sclerotic bone will usually demarcate the cyst from normal surrounding medullary bone. During the latent stage the cyst can appear middiaphyseal in location and more oval in shape. Spontaneous fracture through a cyst may be accompanied by periosteal reaction, callous formation, and cortical thickening.

Plain film evaluation of unicameral bone cysts is usually sufficient. CT scanning may be useful in those cases in which a pathologic fracture may be suspected, but is not confirmed by standard radiographic techniques, particularly calcaneal lesions. The MRI appearance of simple bone cysts will reflect the stage and contents of the cyst. Regions are sharply demarcated by signal intensity from normal marrow. Simple bone cysts will be indicated by intermediate to low fluid signal intensity on $T_1$-weighted images and homogeneous bright signal intensity on $T_2$-weighted images (Fig. 4-25). There is, however, probably little role for MRI in the evaluation of simple bone cysts.

#### Aneurysmal Bone Cysts

Aneurysmal bone cyst is a non-neoplastic solitary lesion of bone. It is most frequently seen in adolescence, 75 percent of cases occurring before the age of 20. The patient usually presents with a nondescript pain, swelling, and limitation of motion. Aneurysmal bone cyst results from a sudden hemodynamic disturbance, such as a sudden vascular occlusion of the venous drainage of that segment of bone, or from the development of an arteriovenous shunt.

Radiographically an aneurysmal bone cyst can have four stages of development. The initial, or lytic phase, is seen as a well circumscribed ovoid area of rarefaction, which can be central, eccentric, or parosteal. The active growth phase is characterized by rapid destruction of bone and a subparosteal "blow-out" pattern. The mature stage, or stage of stabilization, is manifested by formation of a distinct peripheral bony shell, producing a char-

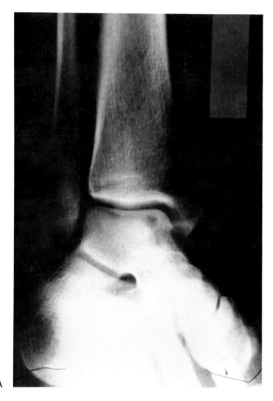

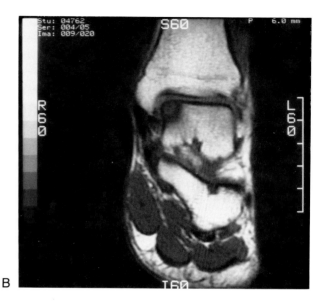

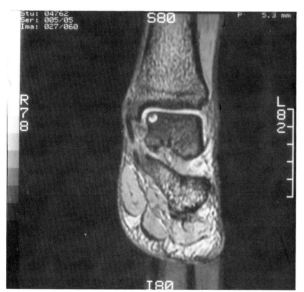

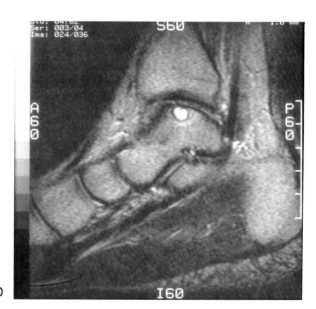

**Fig. 4-24.** Post-traumatic cyst. **(A)** Plain film is suggestive of a radiolucency in the medial talar dome. **(B)** $T_1$-weighted MRI is suggestive of a possible osteochondral dome fracture in the medial talar dome. **(C)** The $T_2$-weighted image demonstrates a high signal intensity, which suggests a fluid-filled cyst within the subcortical region of the talus. **(D)** The sagittal image confirms that the overlying cortex of this cyst remains intact. These post-traumatic cysts may actually represent precursors of frank osteochondral dome fractures. MRI provides an exquisitely sensitive means by which to evaluate the persistently painful post-traumatic ankle.

acteristic radiographic "soap bubble" appearance. During the healing phase, progressive calcification and ossification of the cyst and its eventual transformation to a dense bony mass with an irregular structure are seen.

MRI demonstrates a characteristic finding of a single or multiple fluid levels. This is thought to represent layered uncoagulated blood. The cysts are usually well demarcated from the surrounding, high-signal-intensity fatty marrow. When the diagnosis is uncertain after both a radiographic and an MR examination, a CT scan can be useful in identifying the thin cortical shell of the aneurysmal bone cyst as well as the fluid-fluid levels. The sensitivity and specificity of MRI versus CT in identifying these fluid-fluid levels have not been prospectively studied.

## Enchondroma

Enchondromas are slow-growing, usually asymptomic benign tumors composed of mature hyaline cartilage, which are centrally located within the medullary cavity of bone. They develop in the metaphysis, but can extend into the adjacent epiphysis and/or diaphysis. Solitary be-

nign enchondromas are common in children and may be seen in small bones such as the metatarsals and phalanges of the foot. Solitary lesions are the most common, but multiple unilateral enchondromas are seen in *Ollier's disease*. The condition of multiple enchondromas accompanied by multiple hemangiomas is referred to as *Maffucci syndrome*. Radiographically, enchondromas are round or oval radiolucent lesions with a sharp outline. Characteristic cartilaginous calcifications are seen. Plain film evaluation is usually sufficient in these patients.

## Fibroxanthoma (Nonossifying Fibroma)

Fibroxanthoma, nonossifying fibroma, and fibrous cortical defect are terms used to describe histologically similar lesions that occur in the metaphyseal region of bone[14] and are commonly encountered in the pediatric skeleton. Smaller lesions are usually less than 2 cm in diameter and are eccentrically located within the metaphysis. Radiographically, they are seen as a subtle loss of metaphyseal cortex. The margin is poorly defined in the early phases but is well defined with a thin rim of reactive bone in

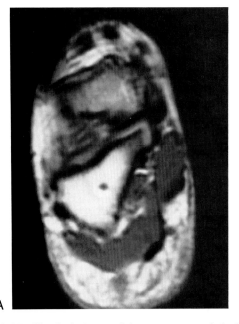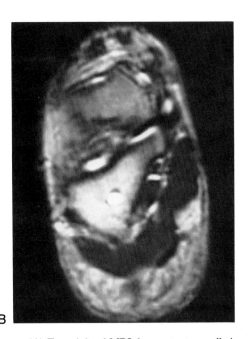

A          B

**Fig. 4-25.** Simple (unicameral) bone cyst; no pathologic fracture. **(A)** $T_1$-weighted MRI demonstrates well circumscribed lesion within the calcaneus. **(B)** $T_2$-weighted image demonstrates an increase in signal intensity suggestive of a fluid-filled cyst.

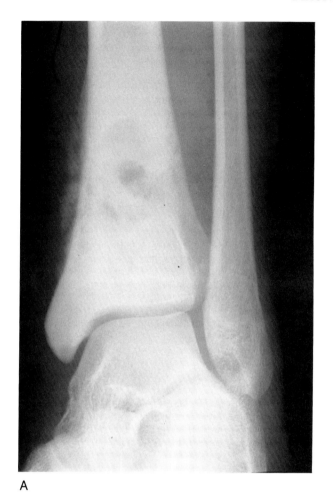

A

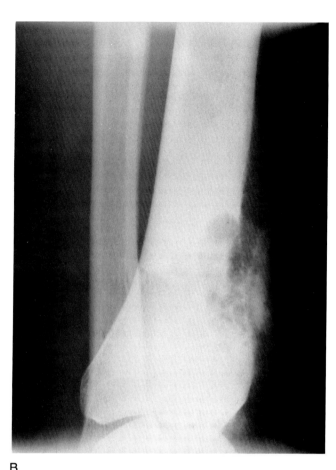

B

**Fig. 4-26.** Osteosarcoma of distal tibia. This lesion appears well circumscribed superiorly but poorly circumscribed inferiorly. The cortical break and extensive periosteal reaction are suggestive of a highly aggressive process.

older, regressing lesions. Spontaneous regression eventually occurs.

The larger, medullary fibroxanthoma (nonossifying fibroma) is a well defined osteolytic lesion involving the cortex and medullary cavity of the metaphysis and adjacent diaphysis of the long bone. Radiographically these lesions are metaphyseal and eccentrically located and may involve the entire diameter of the long bone. The inner boundary is usually well demarcated by a scalloped sclerotic border, and the cortex can be either thin or thickened and sclerotic. Pathologic fractures are uncommon but may occur.[17] Further diagnostic imaging is not usually indicated in these lesions.

### Osteoid Osteoma

The osteoid osteoma is a benign osteoblastic tumor, affecting mainly children and young adults; 76 percent of patients are between 5 and 25 years of age. The classic clinical presentation is that of a child who suffers nocturnal bone pain that is relieved by aspirin. Radiographically, an osteoid osteoma is an oval or round radiolucent lesion surrounded by a wide zone of sclerotic bone. The dense central osteoid nidus is eccentric and does not invade the soft tissues. In the long bones a nidus can be seen as a small lucency. Whether the nidus is lucent or dense may depend upon the age of the lesion, since increased density is more commonly found late in the disease. The lesion can be associated with intense cortical thickening, which varies with the child's age and the location of the lesion. When the plain film examination is nondiagnostic, CT or MRI may better delineate the osteoid nidus.

### Malignant Bone Tumors

Malignant bone tumors are relatively uncommon in the foot and ankle area in both adults and children. Radiographic signs of intramedullary bone destruction and tumor bone formation, cortical perforation, periosteal new bone formation, and extraosseous tumor extension are signs frequently associated with malignant bone tumors. The availability of newer, more sophisticated diagnostic imaging studies aids significantly in the evaluation of suspected lesions (Figs. 4-26 to 4-28). Biopsy is always necessary when a malignant lesion is suspected. Specific bone tumors are discussed in greater detail in Chapter 25.

## Soft Tissue Lesions

Plain film examination should always be the initial evaluation in all soft tissue lesions. Secondary invasion to the bony architecture may provide useful diagnostic information. MRI clearly is the modality of choice in evaluation of these lesions; once again, MRI should be performed prior to biopsy.

### Lipomas

Radiographically a lipoma appears as a clearly defined radiolucent soft tissue mass. There may or may not be calcification within the mass. On MRI lipomas are seen as well defined, circumscribed lesions. The signal intensity of the lesion mimics that of subcutaneous fat. There is typically a lack of surrounding soft tissue edema.

### Arteriovenous Malformation

An arteriovenous malformation is defined as a congenital lesion of dysplastic vascular origin, characterized by large feeding arteries causing decreased vascular resist-

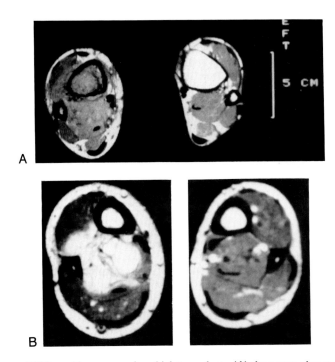

**Fig. 4-27.** Ewing's tumor. MRI provides a means by which to evaluate **(A)** the aggressive marrow-replacing properties, as well as **(B)** the aggressive soft tissue component of this tumor.

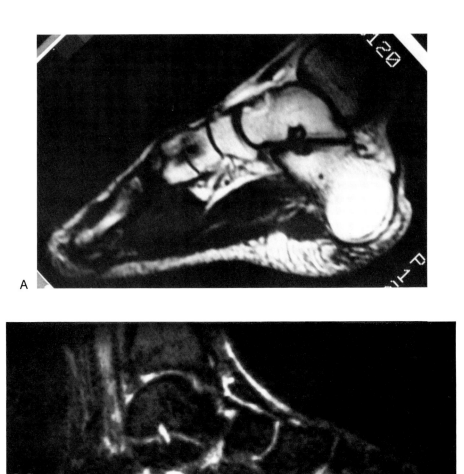

**Fig. 4-28.** Aggressive fibromatosis. (**A**) The $T_1$-weighted image illustrates abnormal mass plantar to the metatarsal bases. (**B**) A special fat suppression sequence (STIR) is helpful in highlighting this abnormality.

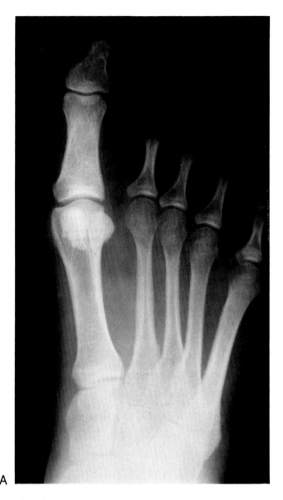

A

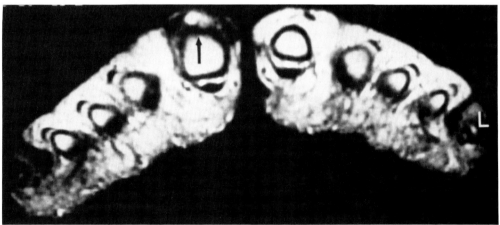

B

**Fig. 4-29.** Arteriovenous malformation in the foot. **(A)** Plain films illustrate the enlargement of the right hallux, which has occurred as a result of recurrent arteriovenous malformations since the age of 4 in this 21-year-old. **(B)** MRI is useful in localizing the AVM dorsal to the proximal phalanx, as well as in defining the normal marrow content of this abnormally enlarged bone. *(Figure continues.)*

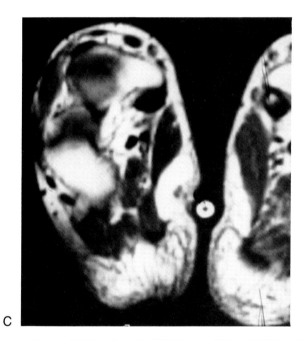
C

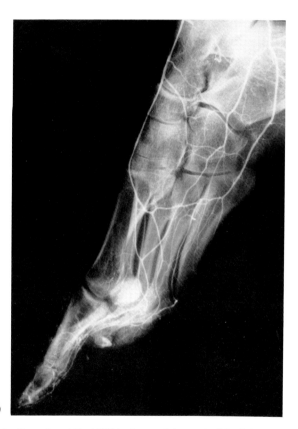
D

**Fig. 4-29** *(Continued).* **(C)** The sensitivity of MRI enabled detection of a subtle AVM in the medial aspect of the left heel, which had been initially missed with angiography (clinical suspicion prompted the further study). **(D)** Angiography remains necessary in these lesions, as embolization should be carried out prior to surgical resection.

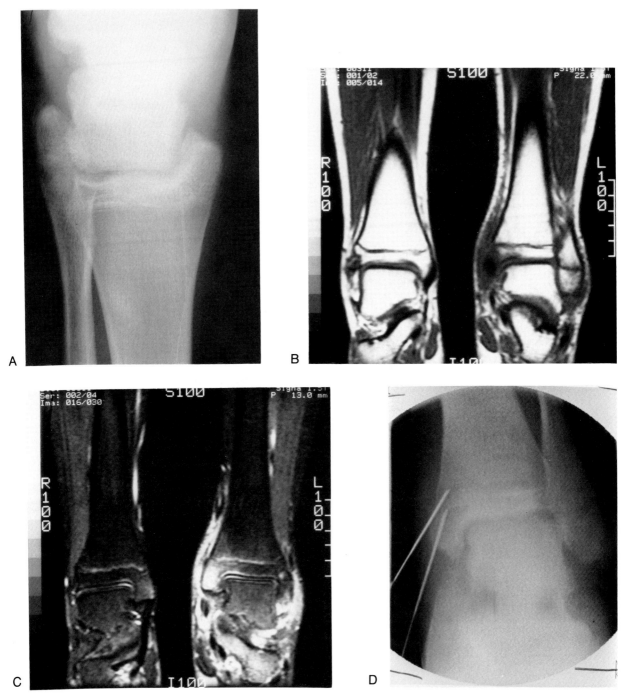

**Fig. 4-30.** Osteomyelitis. **(A)** Plain films demonstrate a very indistinct lucency in the distal metaphysis of the tibia. **(B)** A decrease in signal intensity at the level of the medial malleolus is detected on the $T_1$-weighted image. **(C)** An increase in signal intensity at the same location is detected on the $T_2$-weighted image. This combination of findings on MRI is highly suggestive of osteomyelitis. **(D)** Percutaneous needle biopsy confirmed the presence of osteomyelitis in the medial malleolus, as suggested by the MRI findings.

ance. It frequently presents as a complex network of arteriovenous communications, often referred to as a nidus. This nidus usually consists of multiple enlarged feeding arteries and draining veins. Arteriovenous malformations are almost always congenital, caused by a localized deficiency of capillary development. The lesion may present as a painful mass, which may or may not lead to a variety of conditions, including ulceration, hemorrhage, and infection.

Diagnostic angiography is useful in evaluation of these lesions. Conventional cut-film angiography provides superior spatial resolution which allows easier and more accurate measurement of the lesions. MRI may provide useful information in evaluation of arteriovenous malformations. One of us (J.O.) found MRI useful in detecting a lesion that was initially undetected by diagnostic angiography (Fig. 4-29).

## OSTEOMYELITIS

Hematogenous spread of infection is the most common cause of osteomyelitis in children; spread of infection by a puncture wound is also common. Significant bony destruction often does not appear on the radiograph until late in the second week of the disease. Radiographs can then be used to determine the location and extent of bone involvement and involucrum and sequestrum formation. Additional studies should be ordered when the clinician is suspicious of osteomyelitis.

Skeletal scintigraphy (gallium 67 citrate or indium 111 white blood cells and three-phase technetium 99m MDP scintigraphy) have been the most commonly used techniques for the detection of osteomyelitis. Scintigraphy is most useful for skeletal screening when the location of infection is unknown or when multiple sites of infection may be present. Comparison of MRI and scintigraphy shows that MRI is as accurate as radionuclide studies in the detection of osteomyelitis and is significantly more sensitive than the radionuclide techniques in detection of soft tissue infection. MRI may become increasingly preferred over scintigraphy in the evaluation of osteomyelitis since scintigraphy does not accurately define the full extent of infection, and separation of soft tissue and bone infection can be difficult.

MRI changes may be seen as early as a few hours after the seeding of an infection.[14] Marrow edema is seen as decreased signal intensity on $T_1$-weighted images, with signal intensity increases over time on $T_2$-weighted images. Special fat saturation and short TI inversion recovery (STIR) sequences will also demonstrate increased signal intensity (Fig. 4-30).

## REFERENCES

1. Coleman SS: Complex Foot Deformities in Children. Lea & Febiger, Philadelphia, 1983
2. Tachdjian MO: The Child's Foot. WB Saunders, Philadelphia, 1985
3. Tachdjian MO: Pediatric Orthopedics. WB Saunders, Philadelphia, 1972
4. Conway JJ, Cowell HR: Tarsal coalition, clinical significance in roentgenographic demonstration. Radiology 92:799, 1969
5. Simms G: Analytical radiography of clubfoot. J Bone Joint Surg [Br] 59:485, 1977
6. Lufted LB, Keats TE: Atlas of Roentgenographic Measurements. 3rd Ed. Year Book Medical Publishers, Chicago, 1972.
7. Osmond-Clark H: Congenital vertical talus. J Bone Joint Surg [Br] 38:33, 1936
8. Oloff-Solomon J: Radiographic evaluation in the pediatric patient. Clin Podiatr Med Surg 4:1, 1987
9. Jacobs A, Oloff LM, Visser H: Calcaneal osteotomy in the management of flexible and nonflexible flatfoot deformity: a preliminary report. J Foot Surg 20:2, 1981
10. Harris RI, Beath T: Etiology of peroneal spastic flatfoot. J Bone Joint Surg [Br] 30:624, 1948
11. Gamble FO, Yale I: Clinical Foot Roentgenology. RE Krieger, Huntington, NY, 1975
12. Turco VJ: Club Foot. Churchill Livingstone, New York, 1981
13. Ogden JA: The uniqueness of growing bones. In Rockwood CA Jr, Wilkins KE, King RE (eds): Fractures in Children. JB Lippincott, Philadelphia, 1984
14. Moore SG: Pediatric musculoskeletal imaging. In Start DD, Bradley WG (eds): Magnetic Resonance Imaging. CV Mosby, St. Louis, 1991
15. Jaramillo D, Hoffer FAC, Shapiro F et al: MR imaging of fractures of the growth plate. AJR 155:1261, 1990
16. Solomon MA, Gilula LA, Oloff LM: CT Scanning of the foot and ankle. 2. Clinical applications in review of the literature. AJR 146:1204, 1986
17. Beltran J, Simon DC, Levy M et al: Aneurysmal bone cysts: MR imaging at 1.5T. Radiology 158:689, 1986
18. Oloff J: Radiology of the foot in pediatrics. In Weissman SD (ed): Radiology of the Foot. Williams & Wilkins, Baltimore, 1989

## SUGGESTED READINGS

Ayeyre-Brook A: Congenital vertical talus. J Bone Joint Surg [Br] 49:618, 1967

Beltran J, McGhee RB, Shaffer PB et al: Experimental infections of the musculoskeletal system: evaluation with MR imaging and Tc-99m MDP and Ga-67 scintigraphy. Radiology 167:167, 1988

Beltran J, Noto AM, McGhee RB et al: Infections of the musculoskeletal system: high-field-strength MR imaging. Radiology 164:449, 1987

DeSmet AA, Fischer DR, Burnstein MI et al: Value of MR imaging in staging osteochondral lesions of the talus (osteochondritis dissecans): results in 14 patients. AJR 154:555, 1990

Feld R, Burk DL, McCue P et al: MRI of aggressive fibromatosis: frequent appearance of high signal intensity on $T_2$-weighted images. Magn Reson Imaging 8:583, 1990

Glass RBJ, Poznanski AK, Fisher MR et al: MR imaging of osteoid osteoma. J Comput Assist Tomogr 10:1065, 1986

Hoerr NL (ed): Radiographic Atlas of Skeletal Development of the Foot and Ankle. Charles C Thomas, Springfield, IL, 1962

Jaramillo D, Shapiro F, Hoffer FA et al: Posttraumatic growth-plate abnormalities: MR imaging of bony-bridge formation in rabbits. Radiology 175:767, 1990

Mason MD, Zlatkin MB, Esterhai JL et al: Chronic complicated osteomyelitis of the lower extremity: evaluation with MR imaging. Radiology 173:355, 1989

Mesgarzadeh M, Sapega AA, Bonakdarpour A et al: Osteochondritis dissecans: analysis of mechanical stability with radiography, scintigraphy and MR imaging. Radiology 165:775, 1987

Moore SG: MR precisely evaluates bone tumors: a practical approach to magnetic resonance evaluation of pediatric musculoskeletal tumors. Diagn Imaging 10:282, 1988

Moore SG, Berger P, Stanley P et al: Infectious, traumatic, mechanical, collagen and miscellaneous disorders of the musculoskeletal system. p. 913. In Cohen MD, Edwards MK (eds): Magnetic Resonance Imaging of Children. BC Decker, Philadelphia, 1990

Moore SG, Dawson KL: Tumors of the musculoskeletal system. p. 825. In Cohen MD, Edwards MK (eds): Magnetic Resonance Imaging of Children. BC Decker, Philadelphia, 1990

Nelson DW, DiPaola J, Colville M et al: Osteochondritis dissecans of the talus and knee: prospective comparison of MR and arthroscopic classifications. J Comput Assist Tomogr 14:804, 1990

Oloff J: Radiology of the foot in pediatrics. In Weissman SD (ed): Radiology of the Foot. Williams & Wilkins, Baltimore, 1989

Ozonoff MB: Pediatric Orthopedic Radiology. WB Saunders, Philadelphia, 197

Parker BR, Moore SG, Bleck EE: MR imaging of talipes.

Quinn SF, Murray W, Clark RA et al: MR imaging of chronic osteomyelitis. J Comput Assist Tomogr 12:113, 1988

Solomon MA, Gilula LA, Oloff LM: CT scanning of the foot and ankle. 1. Normal anatomy. AJR 146:92, 1986

Wells D & Oloff J: Radiographic Evaluation of osteochondral dome fractures. J Foot Surg 26 (3) May-June 1987

# 5

# Genetic Considerations in the Evaluation of Congenital Lower Extremity Disorders

*STEVEN J. DeVALENTINE*

Congenital conditions are, by definition, present at birth. Lower extremity deformities may be isolated or may be part of a more extensive syndrome. A thorough prenatal, postnatal, and family history should always be obtained, in an attempt to elucidate any genetic or environmental etiologic factors. The temptation to bypass a thorough history and complete physical examination of the infant or child in order to explore the more technical aspects of the extremity deformity should be avoided. Specific treatment of any given deformity may vary considerably depending upon long-term prognosis of the condition.

Many congenital foot and ankle anomalies are caused by genetic factors[1] (Table 5-1). A genetic condition can be defined as one that has the potential of being passed on to succeeding generations (inheritance). A basic knowledge of genetic principles of inheritance aids the clinician in establishing a more accurate diagnosis and in family counseling. One should be aware that just as congenital conditions may be genetic (polydactyly, syndactyly, cleft foot) or environmental (constriction bands), genetic conditions need not be present at birth (Charcot-Marie-Toothe disease, limb-girdle muscular dystrophy). Genetic conditions can be divided into three categories: (1)

disorders that exhibit mendelian patterns of inheritance; (2) chromosomal abnormalities; and (3) multifactorial conditions.[2]

Within the nucleus of all cells is found a dark-staining, amorphous, irregular material referred to as *chromatin*. At the time of cell division it separates and condenses into a finite number of chromosomes, which are constant in number and individually recognizable by shape for each species. Watson and Crick determined that each chromosome is composed of long strands of deoxyribonucleic acid (DNA) twisted into a double helical structure[3] (Fig. 5-1). The "crosspieces" of the double helix are composed of varying combinations of four nucleotide bases (cystosine, guanine, adenine, and thymine), which are paired. An almost infinite variation in the order of the nucleotide base pairs is possible. Small segments of nucleotide base pairs, which we label *genes,* are responsible for giving "orders" that regulate specific cell functions. Genes are not individually identifiable by laboratory techniques; however, each chromosome pair can be identified through cytogenetic laboratory analysis (Fig. 5-2). Each human cell has 46 individual chromosomes, 44 of which form 22 pairs, each pair being composed of

Table 5-1. **Major Genetic Disorders with Common Orthopedic Manifestations**

| Disease | Inheritance | Notes |
| --- | --- | --- |
| Achondroplasia | Dominant | Short-limbed dwarfism, with short proximal segment of limbs. Bulging frontal region of skull, flattened bridge of nose, small foramen magnum. Sometimes internal hydrocephalus. |
| Acrocephalosyndactyly (Apert syndrome) | Dominant | Deformity of skull with syndactyly of fingers and toes. |
| Acrocephalosyndactyly with polydactyly | Dominant | As above with polydactyly and progressive synostosis in the feet, hands, carpus, tarsus, cervical vertebrae, and skull. |
| Alkaptonuria | Autosomal recessive | Urine turns dark on standing and alkalinization, pigmentation of cartilage, disc calcification, and premature arthritis. |
| Brachydactyly | Dominant | Various types with shortening of one or more phalanges. |
| Calcaneonavicular fusion | Dominant, some cases only | — |
| Diaphysial aclasias (multiple exostoses) | Dominant | Exostoses typically at the growing ends of long bones, also in the hand. Occasional malignant change particularly in central tumors. |
| Diastrophic dwarfism | Autosomal recessive | Calcification of pinnae, scoliosis, foot and hand deformities, some cases cleft palate. |
| Dupuytren's contracture | Dominant | Typically in the hand. May affect plantar fascia. Also associated with knuckle pads. Onset usually in middle age. Association with epilepsy. |
| Ectrodactyly | Dominant | "Lobster claw" deformity of hand. |
| Ehlers-Danlos syndrome | Dominant | Marked joint laxity, lax skin, bruise easily, poor scar tissue. |
| Ellis-van Creveld syndrome (chondroectodermal dysplasia) | Autosomal recessive | Dwarfism, polydactyly, congenital heart defect, normal intelligence. |
| Engelmann's disease | Dominant sometimes | Gross thickening of the cortex of long bones. |
| Fanconi's anemia | Autosomal recessive | All marrow elements affected; pigmentation in the skin; heart and kidney malformations; radial club hand and thumb deformities. |
| Fanconi's syndrome (see Rickets) | — | — |
| Flexion contracture of fingers | Dominant sometimes | Usually affecting the little finger. |
| Gout | Dominant | — |
| Hemophilia (classical) | X-linked recessive | Recurrent hemarthroses lead to joint destruction in young adults. |
| Heart/hand syndrome (Tabatzik syndrome) | Dominant | Cardiac arrhythmia and malformation of upper extremities, particularly "stub thumb." |
| Homocystinuria | Autosomal recessive | Simulates Marfan syndrome but more commonly associated with mental retardation and epilepsy, which appear late in childhood; absence of joint laxity. |
| Hydrocephalus (due to congenital stenosis of aqueduct of Sylvius) | X-linked recessive (some cases) | Occurs alone without spina bifida or meningocele. Males only. |
| Joint laxity, familial | Dominant, some cases only | — |
| Madelung's deformity | Dominant | Also occurs in Turner syndrome. |
| Marfan syndrome | Dominant | Ectopia lentis, aortic aneurysm, excessive length of extremities (particularly distally), joint laxity, sometimes finger contractures. |
| Metaphysial dysostosis | Dominant, also recessive sometimes | Irregularity of the metaphysial ends of long bones. |
| Mucopolysaccharoidoses | | |
| Hurler syndrome (gargoylism) | Autosomal recessive | Progressive mental retardation, dwarfism, hepatosplenomegaly, and clouding of cornea. Chondroitin sulfate B and heparitin sulfate in the urine. |
| Hunter syndrome | X-linked recessive | As above but without corneal clouding and a slower course. Chondroitin sulfate B and heparitin sulfate in the urine. |

*Continued*

Table 5-1. *(continued)*

| Disease | Inheritance | Notes |
|---|---|---|
| Sanfilippo syndrome | Autosomal recessive | Severe mental defect, few skeletal changes. Heparitin sulfate only in the urine. |
| Morquio syndrome | Autosomal recessive | Dwarfism, not usually mental retardation, flattening of vertebral bodies, deformed femoral heads, keratosulfate in the urine. |
| Scheie syndrome | Autosomal recessive | Stiff joints, clouding of cornea, no mental retardation, chondroitin sulfate B in the urine. |
| Maroteaux-Lamy syndrome | Autosomal recessive | Osseous and corneal changes without mental retardation, chondroitin sulfate B in the urine. |
| Multiple epiphysial dysplasia | Dominant | Maldevelopment of many epiphyses leading to premature osteoarthritis. |
| Muscular dystrophy | | |
|    Duchenne's | X-linked recessive | Onset in early childhood. Formerly called pseudohypertrophic type. Males only. |
|    Resembling Duchenne's | Autosomal recessive | Both sexes affected. |
|    Limb-girdle | Autosomal recessive | Onset in adult life. |
|    Facioscapulohumeral | Dominant | Adult onset, slow course. |
| Myositis ossificans progressiva (fibrodysplasia ossificans progressiva) | Dominant | Progressive extraskeletal ossification, usually starting in head, neck, and trunk, with short great toes and thumbs. |
| Nail-patella syndrome | Dominant | Dysplasia of nails, absent or small patellae, which lead to recurrent dislocations, iliac horns, sometimes dislocation of head of radius. Linked to ABO blood groups. |
| Neurofibromatosis (von Recklinghausen's disease) | Dominant | Café-au-lait spots, multiple neurofibromata, scoliosis, pseudarthrosis of the tibia, fibrous replacement of other bones sometimes. |
| Osteogenesis imperfecta (fragilitas ossium) | Dominant | Fragile bones, blue sclerotics, otosclerosis developing in the second or third decade, joint laxity in 45 percent of cases. |
| Osteopetrosis | Dominant and recessive types | Increased density and fragility of bones with encroachment on marrow cavities leading to severe anemia. |
| Osteopoikilosis | Dominant | "Spotted bones" near the ends. Of no clinical significance. |
| Polydactyly, postaxial | Dominant | Frequent in blacks. |
| Polydactyly, preaxial | No clear genetic basis | — |
| Pseudohypoparathyroidism (Albright's hereditary osteodystrophy) | Dominant, perhaps X-linked dominant | Symptoms of hypoparathyroidism without response to parathormone. Short usually third and fourth metacarpal and metatarsal bones, epilepsy, mental retardation. |
| Pycnodysostosis | Autosomal recessive | Bone sclerosis with fragility, wide cranial fontanelles, micrognathism, hypoplasia of clavicles, and osteolysis of terminal phalanges. |
| Radioulnar synostosis | Dominant sometimes | Also occurs in Klinefelter syndrome. |
| "Rickets" | | |
|    Hypophosphatasia | Autosomal recessive | Absent alkaline phosphatase. |
|    Organic aciduria | X-linked recessive | Amino-aciduria, alkaline urine, proteinuria, renal tubular acidosis. |
|    Renal tubular acidosis | Dominant | Inability to acidify urine. |
|    Hypophosphatemia (vitamin-D-resistant) | X-linked dominant | Disordered renal phosphate transport with decreased intestinal calcium ion absorption. |
|    Fanconi syndrome | Autosomal recessive | Glucosuria, aminoaciduria, and hyperphosphaturia. |
| Sickle cell anemia | Autosomal recessive | One of the hemoglobinopathies with generalized osteoporosis, aseptic necrosis and multiple infarcts. |
| Spondyloepiphysial dysplasia | Dominant and X-linked | Delayed dwarfism; head and face not involved. |
| Symphalangism | Dominant | Fusion of distal or proximal interphalangeal joints. |
| Syndactyly | Dominant | Probably several different genes. |
| Thalassemia | Autosomal recessive | Osteoporosis, thickened trabeculae. |

(Modified from James,[1] with permission.)

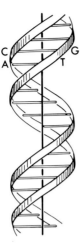

**Fig. 5-1.** A schematic representation of the double helix of DNA. The two ribbons represent the phosphate-sugar chains, and the horizontal bars represent the bonding between nucleotide base pairs. Small segments of base pairs, which we label genes, are responsible for giving the "orders" that regulate specific cell function. (From White et al.,[5] with permission.)

identical-appearing chromosomes. These chromosome pairs are referred to as *autosomes* and are numbered 1 to 22. The remaining pair constitutes the sex chromosomes. In the female the two chromosomes of this pair are identical-appearing and are labeled XX; in the male the two are very different in appearance and are labeled XY. The Y chromosome is much smaller than the X chromosome and has a very limited amount of genetic material. The egg and sperm form through cell division, with only one chromosome of each of the 23 chromosome pairs (23 of the 46 individual chromosomes) being transmitted to egg or sperm. The zygote is formed by union of the sperm and egg, which again creates 23 pairs of chromosomes (46 individual chromosomes). Each of the 23 pairs now contains one chromosome contributed by the father and one by the mother. If the zygote's sex chromosome pair is XX, the embryo will be female, and if it is XY, the embryo will be male.

Conditions that exhibit mendelian patterns of inheritance are characterized by an abnormality of only a single gene and cannot be identified by cytogenetic techniques. Patterns of transmission (inheritance) are dominant or recessive and can be autosomal or sex-linked. If a condition is expressed when only one of the two chromosomes in any pair has an abnormal gene, that condition is said to be *dominant*. If both chromosomes of any pair must have the same abnormal gene for the condition to be

expressed, it is called *recessive*. When the abnormal gene is located on the X chromosome, the condition is described as *X-linked* or *sex-linked*.

## MENDELIAN INHERITANCE PATTERNS

### Autosomal Dominant Inheritance

Autosomal dominant conditions tend to occur in each succeeding generation. When one parent has an abnormal gene on any autosomal chromosome, the condition will be expressed in the parent, and there is a 1 in 2 chance of each child being affected. Children who do not display the condition are genetically normal and therefore cannot pass it on. Autosomal dominant conditions affect both sexes equally and include polydactyly, syndactyly, brachydactyly, acrocephalosyndactyly, calcaneonavicular and talocalcaneal coalition, cleft foot, Marfan syndrome, osteogenesis imperfecta, multiple epiphyseal dysplasia, nail-patella syndrome, and von Recklinghausen's disease.

### Autosomal Recessive Inheritance

A child who expresses an autosomal recessive condition must have received one autosomal chromosome from each parent with the same abnormal gene. Each parent must therefore be affected or a carrier. In many instances both parents are clinically normal but are carriers; in this situation 1 in 4 children will express the condition, 2 in 4 will carry the trait (clinically normal), and 1 in 4 will be genetically and clinically normal. Autosomal recessive conditions affect both sexes equally and usually skip one or more generations. Conditions affecting the foot that are due to autosomal recessive inheritance patterns are much fewer in number than conditions due to autosomal dominant inheritance. They include diastrophic dwarfism (clubfoot), Carpenter syndrome (polysyndactyly), Smith Lemli-Opitz syndrome (syndactyly of the second and third toes), congenital insensitivity to pain (Charcot ankle), limb-girdle muscular dystrophy, sickle cell anemia, and thalassemia.[1,4]

### X-Linked Dominant Inheritance

X-linked (sex-linked) conditions are caused by one or more abnormal genes on an X chromosome(s). X-linked dominant conditions are expressed if the X chromosome

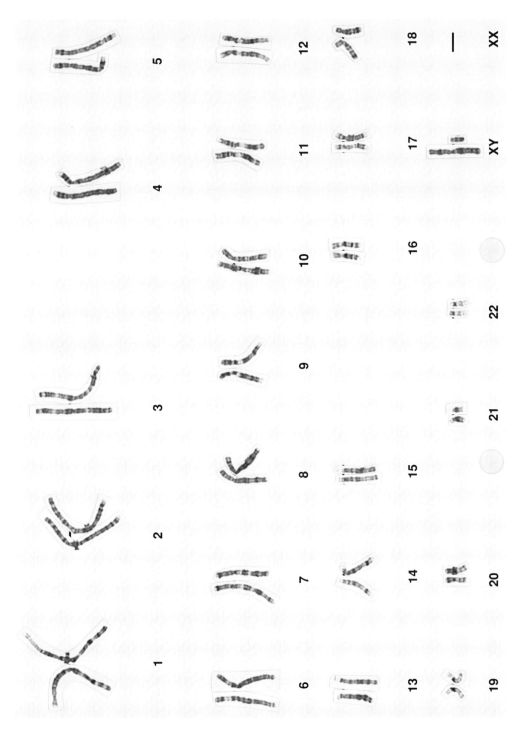

**Fig. 5-2.** A cytogenetic laboratory photograph of a 46XY karyotype of a normal male child. Each chromosome pair can be identified, matched, and compared for gross characteristics.

of a male child is affected or if either X chromosome of a female child is affected. Because the condition is dominant, one parent must exhibit the anomaly and the condition is passed from one generation to the next without skipping generations. Either sex may be affected, but X-linked dominant conditions differ from autosomal dominant conditions in that the affected male/female ratio is not equal. An affected mother has a 1 in 2 chance of having an affected son or daughter, whereas an affected father cannot pass the affected X chromosome to a son but will pass the abnormal X chromosome to all his daughters, who will each express the trait. Dominant X-linked conditions include vitamin D-resistant rickets and pseudohypoparathyroidism (brachymetatarsia).

## X-Linked Recessive Inheritance

In the X-linked recessive inheritance pattern the abnormal gene is also located on the X chromosome. Although the trait is recessive, the male child will exhibit it if he receives a single affected X chromosome from the mother. This will occur even if the father is clinically and genetically normal. In order for a female child to exhibit an X-linked recessive trait, the father must clinically exhibit the condition and the mother must at least carry the affected gene. A normal father and a carrier mother (both of whom are clinically normal) will have a 1 in 2 chance of having an affected son or a carrier daughter. An affected father and a normal mother cannot pass the condition to a son, but all daughters will be carriers. Consequently, X-linked recessive conditions tend to occur with a much higher frequency in males who receive the abnormal gene from a carrier mother. Duchenne's muscular dystrophy and classical hemophilia are examples.

## CHROMOSOMAL ABNORMALITIES

Chromosomal abnormalities occur primarily from failure of two paired chromosomes to separate during gamete formation (nondisjunction) or from fusion of a part of or all of one chromosome to another (translocation). The incidence of nondisjunction increases with increased maternal age (Down syndrome). The chromosomal morphology of the parents of such children is normal, and although the likelihood of their having more children

with chromosomal abnormalities may be higher than normal, this is not due to a gene defect. Translocation of a portion of one chromosome to another may be inherited, and thus a parent with this karyotype may have a 1 in 2 chance of each child being affected.

When a chromosome pair fails to separate during meiosis, one gamete receives 24 chromosomes [(46/2+1] and the other gamete receives 22 [(46/2)−1]. When these gametes (egg or sperm) join with other normal gametes during fertilization, one of the ensuing zygotes will have 47 chromosomes (3 of one type, or *trisomy*) and the other will have 45 chromosomes (1 of one type, or *monosomy*). Monosomic zygotes rarely survive. The trisomy syndromes of various chromosome pairs are identifiable via cytogenetic analysis and are usually associated with mental retardation and multiple congenital anomalies, including various foot and lower extremity anomalies. Convex pes valgus may be associated with trisomy 13 or trisomy 18.[3] Down syndrome (trisomy 21) children have a characteristic facial appearance, are mentally retarded, and often have flexible flatfoot.

As previously mentioned, the chromatin of active cells appears as an amorphous, dark-staining material under light microscopy. Chromosomes, however, form into readily identifiable pairs in dividing cells. The cytogeneticist is able to stimulate meiosis in certain cell types (lymphocytes, fetal cells that are shed into amniotic fluid) in a matter of days by growing them in tissue culture. These cells are then stained. The chromosomes can be examined under light microscopy and then photographed, enlarged, cut out, and mounted to create an individual record (Fig. 5-2). Children with multiple congenital anomalies should be evaluated by a pediatric geneticist and should have cytogenetic chromosome analysis.

## MULTIFACTORIAL CONDITIONS

The term *multifactorial inheritance* is used to describe conditions that do not exhibit strict mendelian patterns of transmission but do show definite familial tendencies. These anomalies are probably the result of nucleotide pattern abnormalities at multiple gene loci that work in combination to produce a clinical condition. The clinical expression of the condition is thought to exhibit a threshold phenomenon. If the number of gene abnormalities exceeds a certain level, the condition is exhibited. If the genetic threshold is not exceeded, the individual is clinically normal but is capable of genetically transmitting the condition to future generations. Environmental factors may also be important and may result in clinical expression of a condition at a lower genetic threshold than would be expected given a different environmental exposure. Clubfoot and congenital dislocated hip exhibit classical examples of multifactorial inheritance patterns. It is also likely that many clinical conditions such as clubfoot and pes planus may have diverse etiologies, which represent the spectrum from purely environmental to exclusively inherited, with a combination of factors in between.

## REFERENCES

1. James JIP: The orthopedic surgeon and research. J Bone Joint Surg [Br] 52B:14, 1970
2. Cowell HR: The genetics of foot disorders. Orthop Rev 2(8):55, 1978
3. Valentine GH: The chromosome disorders. JB Lippincott, Philadelphia, 1975
4. Wein BK, Cowell HR: Genetic considerations of foot anomalies in office practice. Foot Ankle 2(4):185, 1982
5. White A, Handler P, Smith EL: Principles of Biochemistry. 5th Ed. McGraw-Hill, New York, 1973, p 194

# 6

# Congenital Talipes Equinovarus

*STEVEN J. DeVALENTINE*
*TIMOTHY J. BLAKESLEE*

*Clubfoot* is a descriptive term generally applied to the clinical condition characterized by forefoot adduction and varus and equinus deformity of the hind foot (or entire forefoot and hind foot) (Fig. 6-1). The terms *clubfoot* and *talipes equinovarus* are used synonymously. The term *talipes* is derived from the Latin words *talus* (ankle) and *pes* (foot) and is often used in conjunction with descriptive terms that identify the direction that the malpositioned foot has assumed (e.g., talipes equinovalgus, talipes calcaneovalgus, talipes calcaneovarus). The word *equinus* describes the plantar-flexed or toe-pointed position characteristic of the equine hoof, and *varus* describes the inverted foot position.

The clubfoot condition has remained an enigma to surgeons for centuries. Testimony to the confusion that clubfoot evokes can readily be seen in the volumes of literature that have been and continue to be produced on this subject and the many striking disagreements contained within that literature. Some of this confusion, especially in the earlier literature, can undoubtedly be attributed to the fact that *clubfoot deformity* is a descriptive term that lumps together a group of morphologically similar but etiologically (and sometimes pathologically) different disorders. More recent authors have tried to clearly separate cases of congenital clubfoot in children into two groups, those that are secondary to another primary disease process (e.g., neurogenic disease or arthrogryposis) and those that are idiopathic. Most authors have assumed for study purposes that those children classified as having idiopathic clubfoot are a homogeneous group and therefore will respond to similar treatment in a like manner. The flaw in this assumption is twofold. First, the best evidence indicates that even so-called idiopathic clubfoot is probably produced by heterogeneous etiologic factors and thus may represent pathologically discordant conditions that will not respond equally to similar treatments. Second, in our experience some infants who are initially classified as having idiopathic clubfoot seem to have very subtle neurologic abnormalities which only become noticeable with later development and often are so subtle that a specific diagnosis is never made.

Also, traditionally there has been no lack of disagreement over the pathologic anatomy of clubfoot deformity. The medial and plantar angulation of the clubfoot talus and medial-plantar subluxation of the navicular about the talar head have long been well recognized and agreed upon. Earlier literature described an external torsional deformity of the tibia and fibula. More recently, use of sophisticated diagnostic techniques, such as magnetic resonance imaging (MRI) or three-dimensional computed tomography (CT) has suggested that although the head and neck of the talus are deviated in a plantar and medial direction, the talar body and trochlear talar surface may be slightly rotated externally within the ankle mortise as compared with the normal foot. An internal rotation of the entire foot on the talus around a longitudinal axis through the subtalar joint has also been documented by Bosch[1] and McKay[2] and confirmed by Simons and Sarrafian.[3] Good evidence also exists that the magnitude and the specific combination of pathologic deformities may vary significantly from one individual to the next.

It is important for the reader of clubfoot literature to keep in mind the variable and complex nature of this condition and the historical evolution of our knowledge concerning talipes equinovarus deformity. As E.H. Bradford stated in 1889[13]:

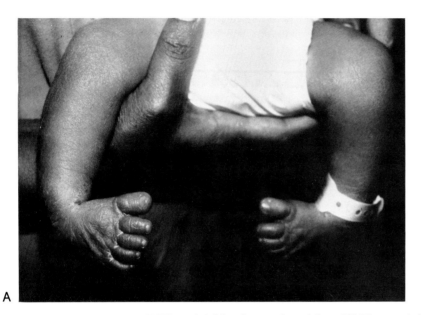
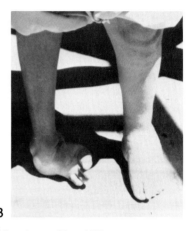

A  B

**Fig. 6-1.** **(A)** Bilateral clubfoot in a newborn infant. **(B)** Untreated clubfoot in an older child.

the literature on the treatment of clubfeet is, as a general rule, that of unvarying success. It is often as brilliant as an advertising sheet and yet in practice, there is no lack of half-cured or relapsed cases, sufficient evidence that methods of cure are not universally understood.

That statement could just as easily have been made by a contemporary surgeon. This chapter will be devoted to the diagnosis and treatment of congenital idiopathic clubfoot deformity, since this type probably includes the largest single group of reasonably similar clubfoot deformities. The surgical management of paralytic talipes equinovarus will be discussed in Chapter 19.

## HISTORY

Knowledge of the history of clubfoot is extensive, paralleling knowledge of the history of medicine. We know that clubfoot was recognized by most ancient civilizations. Ancient wall etchings in the tombs of Egyptian Pharaoh's depict individuals with clubfoot, and the mummy of the pharaoh Siptah ((Nineteenth Dynasty, circa 1210 B.C.) was found to have clubfoot deformity[4] (Fig. 6-2). Ancient Indian literature (Ajur-Veda, circa 1000 B.C.) contains the first known written description of clubfoot, recommending massage of the deformity, and

Hephaestus, the blacksmith of Olympus in Greek mythology, was represented in drawings as having bilateral clubfoot.[5] The ancient Aztecs also recognized clubfoot and treated it with splints made from cactus leaves. The pathologic anatomy of the clubfoot talus has been identified in a fifteenth century American Indian skeleton by Mann and Owsley.[6]

Hippocrates (about 300–400 B.C.), who is generally considered to be the father of Western medicine, also did not ignore clubfoot and other congenital orthopedic conditions in his writings. He recognized the difference between congenital and acquired clubfoot and proposed the first known etiologic theory, namely, that the deformity was caused by mechanical pressure in utero. He also recommended early treatment during infancy, with repeated manipulation and rigid bandaging, which is still consistent with modern principles of clubfoot therapy.[7]

The Dark Ages (about the sixth through the tenth centuries A.D.) and Middle Ages (eleventh through fifteenth centuries A.D.) added little to medical knowledge and nothing to the understanding or treatment of clubfooted children. In most societies clubfoot and other congenital deformities were considered marks of "divine discipline" or of the devil, and individuals with these conditions were ridiculed and made outcasts. With the Renaissance (fifteenth and sixteenth centuries) came a renewed interest in science and medicine and a greater

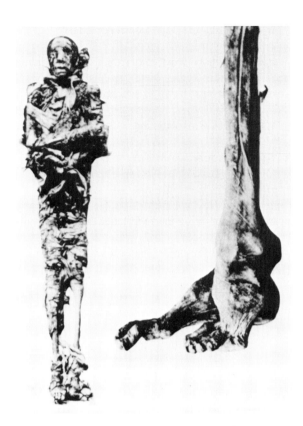

Fig. 6-2. Clubfoot deformity in the mummy of the Egyptian pharaoh Siptah (nineteenth dynasty, circa 1210 B.C.) (From the Egyption Museum, Cairo, Egypt, with permission.)

public acceptance of and some public aid for crippled children. Lorenz in 1782 first reported subcutaneous Achilles tenotomy in Frankfurt, and Guerin in 1838 reported using plaster of Paris bandaging in the treatment of clubfoot.[6] Antonio Scarpa in Italy in 1803 was the first to propose that osseous changes in clubfoot were secondary to soft tissue contracture.[8] Scarpa's work again encouraged the use of soft tissue release surgery. In Germany in 1831 Louis Stromeyer rediscovered the benefits of subcutaneous Achilles tenotomy in resistant cases and popularized this procedure among middle European physicians.[9] W. J. Little was probably Stromeyer's most noted patient. Little developed an equinovarus foot deformity subsequent to a childhood febrile illness and studied medicine in London with the specific purpose of discovering a treatment for his deformity. Stromeyer performed a successful Achilles tenotomy on Little and taught him the technique, which Little im-

ported to England, where he found considerable opposition since treatment of clubfoot was at the time considered outside the legitimate practice of surgery and was left to barber-surgeons. Little published his *Treatise on the Nature of Clubfoot and Analogous Distortions* in 1839 and became a pioneer in the field of orthopedic surgery.[5,10]

Although Hippocrates as early as 300 to 400 B.C. had recommended early treatment (manipulation and splinting) of clubfoot immediately after birth, this practice did not become commonplace until the late 1800s. Prior to that time treatment was routinely delayed until childhood or walking. During the late 1800s treatment of clubfoot became considerably more aggressive and even radical. This trend was promoted by the development of aseptic surgical technique by Lister in 1867, of the extremity tourniquet by Esmarch in 1873 and Cushing in 1904, and of radiography by Roentgen, as well as by the increasingly widespread use of general anesthesia. Many surgeons during the late nineteenth and early twentieth centuries used excochleation or rather indiscriminate resection of large bone wedges. Hugh Thomas (known for the Thomas splint, and Thomas wrench) and others recommended forcible manipulation. Many aggressive procedures of these types produced unfavorable results or high infection rates and led to the repopularization of nonoperative treatment by Hiram Kite.[11] Kite perfected the technique of gentle manipulation and stretching of the soft tissues in infants, followed by plaster of Paris casting, which is still used today.[12-14] He recognized that the ligaments and tendons of infants and children were often capable of withstanding greater tension than bone. Kite also recognized the importance of talocalcaneal position, and the angle between the talus and calcaneus as measured on radiographs is still referred to as *Kite's angle*. He was a strong proponent of nonoperative care and reported a very high (88 percent) success rate, which other clinicians have not been able to duplicate. This leads one to believe that either his talents were truly superior or his criteria for an acceptable result were less than that of other later observers.

From the middle of the twentieth century to the present there has again been an increasing trend toward early and more comprehensive surgical treatment which has been fostered by better understanding of the pathologic anatomy of clubfoot and by more sophisticated surgical and anesthetic techniques. Although various types of soft tissue release other than Achilles tenotomy had been recommended by early authors, including Phelps

(1890),[15] Codvilla (1906),[16] Brockman (1930),[17] Bost (1960),[18] Attenborough (1972),[19] and Goldner (1969),[20] a comprehensive approach to soft tissue release did not become popular until 1971 when Turco recommended his one-stage posteromedial soft tissue release.[21] Prior to that time most infants treated for clubfoot in the United States underwent a staged, piecemeal type of approach to clubfoot surgery, resulting in many cases in incomplete reduction of the deformity and high recurrence rates. A typical sequence in the treatment of a child with clubfoot prior to the popularization of Turco's one-stage release would be as follows: manipulation and casting without adequate reduction until several months of age; a second stage of isolated posterior release and incomplete reduction, followed by gradual recurrence of varus and equinus; and a third stage of medial release at 1 or 2 years of age, culminating in a stiff or partially corrected foot that might progress to fusion during adolescence. More recently McKay[2,22-24] and Simons[25,26] have recognized the subtalar and midtarsal rotational component of the deformity and have expanded Turco's concept to include circumferential release about the subtalar joint.

## INCIDENCE

Clubfoot is probably the most common pathologic congenital foot deformity. Most studies have reported the overall incidence at between 1 and 2 per 1,000 live births. However, a 1977 U.S. Public Health Service survey reported an incidence of 2.29 cases per 1,000 live births, which would make clubfoot one of the most common congenital anomalies found in the study.[27] The incidence of clubfoot has also been reported to vary considerably among different ethnic populations. Elegant studies of the Hawaiian population by Stewart[28] and Chung[29] showed the lowest incidence of congenital clubfoot in Asians (about 0.57 per 1,000 among the Chinese, Japanese, Indonesian, and Filipino populations) and the highest incidence in people of Polynesian descent (6.81 per 1000).[23] The incidence in the white population in Chung's study was 1.12 per 1,000, which closely matches that found in the British study by Wynne-Davies (1 per 1,000).[30] Clubfoot has also been reported to be more common among people of Middle Eastern, South African black (3.5 per 1000), and Mexican descent than in people of Anglo-Saxon descent.[31]

Most investigators have also reported a 2:1 to 2.5:1 male to female predominance.[29,30,32-35] In most studies 50 percent or more of patients exhibit bilateral involvement, and some studies have demonstrated a slightly greater predilection for right side involvement in unilateral cases.[29,32,35] Others have shown equal distribution of right and left side involvement.

## CLASSIFICATION

If one reviews the volumes of published literature regarding clubfoot, it is apparent that considerable controversy and differences of opinion persist. Owing to the varying degrees of morphologic severity and the complicated pathologic and etiologic factors, attempts at clubfoot classification have become complex. We have adapted an etiology-based classification system (Table 6-1) originally proposed by Hersh.[36]

## ETIOLOGY

The true cause of idiopathic clubfoot is unknown, although many theories have been proposed. When carefully examined, however, the evidence supporting each theory falls short on some vital point. The incidence of idiopathic clubfoot points to the existence of genetic factors, but the lack of a clear model of inheritance indicates that other factors are also involved. Three general hypotheses have been proposed based on (1) extrinsic factors affecting the embryo; (2) intrinsic and anatomic factors, and (3) heredity and environmental factors.

### Extrinsic Factors Affecting The Embryo

In the nineteenth century it was assumed that a strong emotional reaction in the mother during the early stages of pregnancy could disrupt the mother-embryo balance and produce an idiopathic clubfoot due to a central nervous system malfunction.[41,42] Fetal malposition and increased mechanical or hydrostatic intrauterine pressure have also been suggested[43-47] and rejected[48-50] as causes of idiopathic clubfoot. Common peroneal nerve paralysis induced by increased intrauterine pressure has also been suspected to be capable of causing this deformity.[51] The simultaneous occurrence of amniotic stric-

Table 6-1. **Classification of Clubfoot Deformity**

I. Congenital
  A. Idiopathic
    1. *Intrinsic:* Also known as type II, rigid, or structural club-foot. The deformity is rigid in nature, with marked fibrosis and abnormally shaped and positioned tarsal bones. This deformity commonly requires surgical correction.
    2. *Extrinsic:* Also known as type I, flexible, pliant, or postural clubfoot. The deformity is flexible in nature and without marked fibrosis. Tarsal bones may be malpositioned but not abnormally shaped. This deformity can respond well to conservative manipulation and serial casting.
  B. Neurogenic: Spinal defects create paralytic musculoskeletal (clubfoot) deformity. Muscle imbalance created by the neurogenic deficit causes contracture, subluxation, possible dislocation, and gross deformity. Growth, development, weight bearing, and progressive paralysis may worsen the deformity.[37]
    1. Open defects
      a. Myelomeningocele (hydromyelia, dysrhaphia, and rachischisis)
      b. Meningocele
      c. Dermal sinus
    2. Closed defects
      a) Spina bifida occulta
        (1) Diastematomyelia
        (2) Intraspinal tumor (lipomas, chondromas, osteomas, angiomas, and dermoids)
      b) Myelodysplasia
        (1) Aplasia or hypoplasia of nerve roots or spinal cord
        (2) Absent anterior horn cells (arthrogryposis)
        (3) Diplomyelia
      c) Errors in skeletal segmentation
        (1) Absent sacrum or lumbar vertebra
        (2) Hemivertebra
        (3) Congenital segmental fusion
  C. Myogenic: abnormal muscle and tendon insertions[38]
    1. Anterior tibial
    2. Triceps surae
    3. Peroneals
    4. Plantaris
    5. Flexor accessorius longus
  D. Osteogenic: absence of tibia or medial malleolus
  E. Collagenous[39]
    1. Amniotic bands
    2. Arthrogryposis multiplex congenita
  F. Cartilaginous (diastrophic dwarfism)[40]
II. Acquired
  A. Neurogenic
    1. Poliomyelitis
    2. Cerebral palsy
    3. Meningitis
    4. Sciatic nerve damage
  B. Vascular
    Volkmann's paralysis of the lower extremity

tures and idiopathic clubfoot has been reported.[52,53] Both conditions have been assumed separately to be due to amniotic leakage and changes in the amount and composition of amniotic fluid.

The clubfoot-producing effects of some diseases such as diabetes[54,55] and maternal hypothermia[56] and of certain drugs such as aminopterin,[57] *d*-tubocurarine,[58] methotrexate,[59] as well and a similar effect of oligohydramnios[60] have been documented clinically and in animal experiments. The human embryo is especially vulnerable to the teratogenic effects of radiation, drugs, and viruses during the first 8 weeks of gestation. Later in fetal development malnutrition, multiple pregnancy, placental errors, and environmental stress predominate as potential clubfoot-creating factors.[59]

In summary, these diverse extrinsic theories do not hold up to critical analysis when one attempts to consistently explain the etiology and pathology of the true congenital idiopathic clubfoot. On the other hand, these extrinsic factors may account for many of the flexible or postural clubfeet that respond well to nonsurgical management by manipulation and serial casting.

## Intrinsic and Anatomic Factors

Arrest in the fetal development of the foot, resulting in malposition of the tarsal bones has been suggested as a cause of idiopathic clubfoot.[49,61] Bohm[61] carefully examined six stillborn fetuses from the early stages of gestation (weeks 5 through 16) and documented four specific stages in the normal maturation process of the developing foot. He believed that the idiopathic clubfoot deformity was indistinguishable from the normal fetal foot at the fifth week of gestation both being characterized by 90 degrees of ankle equinus, calcaneus beneath the talus, supinated foot, adducted forefoot, and medial deviation of the navicular with respect to the talus. Despite the failure of this study to show any structural abnormalities within the tarsal bones, Bohm postulated that idiopathic clubfoot is caused by arrest in the development of the normal fetal foot at approximately 5 weeks of gestation.[61]

In contrast, Irani and Sherman,[62] supported by others,[50,63,64] believe that a germ plasm defect of the anterior cartilaginous anlage of the talus creates the basis for the development of idiopathic clubfoot. They consider all other deformities involving soft tissue and bone to be secondary or adaptive responses to the malposition created by the deformed head and neck of the talus. Shapiro and Glimcher's study,[50] revealing the histiologic differences between the tali of a 9-day-old infant with unilateral idiopathic clubfoot, further supports this theory.

There has been recent interest in the frequency of arterial dysgenesis in fetal limbs with congenital idiopathic clubfoot deformity.[65] In arteriographic studies of such limbs, 63 of 71 limbs (89 percent) exhibited reduction or absence of the anterior tibial (dorsalis pedis) artery and the medial plantar artery,[50,66-71] whereas congenital deficiency of these vessels in otherwise normal populations has a reported incidence of only 2.4 to 7.1 percent.[72] This vascular abnormality in an area of endochondral ossification may disrupt the normal morphogenesis of the talus and thus contribute to the development of the clubfoot deformity.

Theories of anomalous tendon insertions involving the anterior and posterior tibial, Achilles, and peroneal longus tendons have been suggested[73-76] and opposed.[47,62,63,77] Fried[78] believed that the idiopathic clubfoot deformity was due to the hypertrophic and plantarly positioned insertion of the posterior tibial tendon, which he verified in 56 dissected clubfeet. Others[73,74] postulated that idiopathic clubfoot may be caused by the abnormal medial insertion of the Achilles and peroneal longus tendons, which in conjunction with the anterior tibial muscle creates a muscle imbalance capable of producing the equinovarus deformity early in gestation.

Theories regarding abnormalities in the muscle itself have been suggested[75,79,80] and opposed.[47,49,62,63,77,81] Mau[82] and Wiley[47] documented abnormal histologic changes (loss of normal striations and a decrease in muscle fiber size) in the calf musculature of idiopathic clubfoot limbs. Isaacs et al.[83] examined 111 muscle biopsies from the peroneal and gastrocnemius muscle groups and found evidence (increased collagen content) to suggest early denervation, which they claimed could create a subtle muscle imbalance and thus a clubfoot deformity. Other electromicroscopic and electromyographic studies,[84-86] however, have failed to reveal any abnormal findings (such as variable fiber size and increased collagen content or fibrillation, polyphasic potential, or lower motor neuron lesions) that would support this neurogenic theory.

Numerous other unsupported theories persist. Keith[87] thought that the idiopathic clubfoot was a form of Streeter's fetal dysplasia (congenital constriction bands) caused by a local error in circulation, resulting in necrosis and a fibrotic mass. Bechtol and Mossman[80] theorized that the idiopathic clubfoot was due to an uneven rate of bone and muscle growth, which created a structural imbalance and thus produced the deformity. Hirsch[88] felt that an abnormally taut or contracted deltoid ligament was responsible for the varus hindfoot deformity.

In summary, the most consistent evidence supports the theory of a primary defect in the development of the head and neck of the talus. The specific cause of this defect is unknown. It is important to remember that none of these intrinsic or anatomic theories has been shown to be constant and thus they should all be considered to account for part of the pathology rather than the etiology of idiopathic clubfoot.

## Heredity and Intrauterine Environment

Late in the nineteenth century reference was made to the significance of heredity in association with idiopathic clubfoot.[42,44] Since then numerous studies have documented the increased incidence of idiopathic clubfoot among family members and relatives, which greatly exceeds the number expected by chance alone[54,81,89-94] (Table 6-2).

The classic studies of Wynne-Davies,[95-97] Palmer,[98] and Yang et al.[99] show that the incidence of idiopathic clubfoot is strongly influenced by race. In whites the

Table 6-2. **Clubfoot Incidence and Family History**

| Author/Year | Clubfoot Patients | Significant Family History | % |
|---|---|---|---|
| Ehrenfried,[89] 1912 | 185 | 14 | 8 |
| Kite,[90] 1932 | 166 | 37 | 22 |
| Crabbe,[54] 1960 | 164 | 16 | 10 |
| MacEven, et al.,[91] 1961 | 149 | 29 | 19 |
| Kite,[92] 1964 | 1447 | 54 | 4 |
| Steno and Slivka,[93] 1978 | 174 | 45 | 26 |
| Gray and Katz,[81] 1981 | 78 | 22 | 29 |
| Blakeslee and DeValentine,[94] 1992 | 43 | 3 | 7 |
| Total | 2406 | 220 | 9 |

incidence is 1.00 to 1.24 per 1,000 live births, which is approximately twice the 0.57 per 1,000 live births found in Oriental races. In contrast, Polynesians have a much higher incidence, 6.81 per 1,000 live births. Common to all races is the male to female ratio of 2:1. Most studies show no statistically significant relationship between the incidence of idiopathic clubfoot and the patient's birth weight, birth number, or maternal age.

Current well constructed studies investigating idiopathic clubfoot have supported several modes of inheritance, including autosomal recessive, sex-linked recessive, and autosomal dominant patterns.[98-101] None of these recent studies, however, can fully explain the questions raised by Idelberger's[102] classic 1939 research (nearly 50 years earlier) involving 174 pairs of twins (40 identical, or monozygotic and 134 fraternal, or dizygotic) with idiopathic clubfoot. He found the incidence in monozygous twins was 32.5 percent, as compared with only 2.9 percent in dizygous twins. In other words, 67 percent of the identical twins, who shared the same uterine environment, were not affected, but they did exhibit a significant increase as compared with the fraternal twins.

Furthermore, Wynne-Davies documented a 20- to 30-fold increased incidence of idiopathic clubfoot in first-degree relatives and a 6-fold increased incidence in second-degree relatives. The incidence in third-degree relatives was the same as that of the general population, namely, 0.1 percent.

Currently most research supports the theory of polygenic multifactorial inheritance with a sex-linked threshold effect.[103-105] Within this complex mode of inheritance, which takes into account the intrauterine environment, the idiopathic clubfoot deformity cannot occur until the number of abnormal genes exceeds the threshold level. The threshold appears to be sex-related, with a higher tolerance being found in females. This would explain why males are twice as often affected as females. This concept may also help explain the fact that the deformity tends to be less severe in males because fewer abnormal genes are required. Females, in contrast, require a higher number of abnormal genes to produce the deformity and therefore would tend to have a more severe and resistant type. This sex-linked concept also explains why first-degree relatives of affected females are more likely to be affected than those of affected males.

In summary, idiopathic clubfoot deformity probably is the result of complex multifactorial polygenic inheritance intimately influenced by a sex-related threshold effect and obscure intrauterine environmental factors.

## PATHOLOGIC ANATOMY

Prior to reviewing the pathologic anatomy of idiopathic clubfoot one must have a good understanding of normal lower extremity anatomy. Detailed discussion of this lengthy topic, which will not be addressed here, has been provided by Sarrafian.[106] Also, the majority of anatomic dissections investigating clubfoot have not been performed on true idiopathic clubfeet but on specimens available following fetal demise due to multiple birth defects. Thus the reported literature may not represent the pure idiopathic anatomy.

Historically, Scarpa[107] in 1818 and Adams[108] in 1886 presented clear and accurate descriptions of the clubfoot deformity. Both these authors felt that the root of the problem was to be found in the shape and position of the talus and that the other soft tissue and bony abnormalities were adaptive in nature.

Currently there is general agreement regarding the classic deformity, which is due to the abnormal relationship of the tarsal bones, specifically, the medial displacement of the navicular and calcaneus around the talus[109-111] (Fig. 6-3). The severity of this deformity depends upon the degree of articular malalignment, whereas the resistance to anatomic reduction and correction is determined by the rigidity within the surrounding soft tissues. Some of the abnormalities in the bones and soft tissues are acquired as a result of persistent structural deformity. The adaptive osseous changes are acquired in accordance with Wolff's law, whereas the adaptive soft tissue contractures are acquired in accordance with the law of Davis.[111] These adaptive changes, which may progress with the growth and development of the untreated or inadequately treated clubfoot, are discussed in detail in the section on complications.

The following is a concise review of the pathologic anatomy that contributes to the classic deformity characteristic of idiopathic clubfoot, specifically (1) adducted forefoot; (2) inverted hindfoot; (3) ankle equinus; (4) plantar-medial displacement of the navicular on the head of the talus (subluxation or dislocation of the talonavicular joint); and (5) lateral rotation of the longitudinal axis

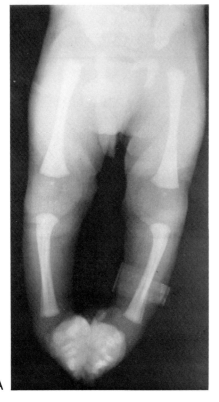
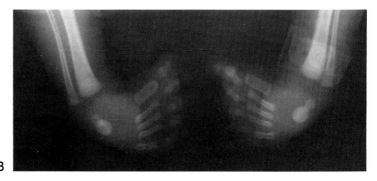

**Fig. 6-3.** **(A)** Anteroposterior radiograph of a newborn's feet and legs illustrate the degree of deformity present in idiopathic clubfoot at birth. **(B)** Lateral radiograph of bilateral clubfeet at birth.

of the talus in the ankle mortise, resulting in posterior displacement of the fibula and medial spin of the entire foot.[112-121]

## Soft Tissue

In general, all soft tissues (muscles, tendons, ligaments, retinaculum, fasciae, vinculi, joint capsules, nerves, arteries, veins, and skin) on the plantar, medial, and posterior aspects of the foot, ankle, and distal leg are hypertrophied, contracted, fibrosed, or shortened[109,122-127] (Table 6-3). Controversy persists as to whether these structures are actually contracted or whether they have simply grown to their shortened length by conforming to the contours of the abnormally shaped and/or positioned tarsal bones.[110,111,128]

Despite complete peritalar release (posterior, medial, and lateral) of all soft tissue contractures contributing to the deformity, frequently the idiopathic clubfoot cannot

be manipulated into a normal anatomic position because of the remaining intrinsic osseous deformities.[129-131]

## Osseous

In two significant 1963 studies Irani and Sherman[129] and Settle[128] independently reported findings from detailed anatomic dissections of 27 fetal clubfoot specimens. Both studies revealed similar abnormal pathology involving the talus, specifically, an essentially normal body with the majority of the deformity located within the head and neck region. This deformity, comprising reduced size, malalignment, and angulation of the talar head and neck, was consistent in all fetal specimens (Fig. 6-4). The navicular and calcaneus were to a lesser degree misshapen and/or malpositioned. The remainder of the bones in the foot and leg were essentially normal in size and configuration, but secondary postional changes were present at this early stage of development, presumably because of

Table 6-3. **Soft Tissue Deformities Commonly Present in Idiopathic Clubfoot**

| Structure | Pathologic Anatomy |
|---|---|
| Skin[111] | Absent posterior heel skin lines or wrinkles |
| | Deep cleft just above heel and/or on medial plantar arch surface |
| Muscle[122,131] | |
| Posterior tibial | Histochemical and electron microscopic studies suggest neurogenic disease resulting in dysplasia (thinned or shortened) in all posterior and lateral leg musculature |
| Gastrocnemius | |
| Soleus | |
| Flexor digitorum longus | |
| Flexor hallucis longus | |
| Peroneals | |
| Abductor hallucis | |
| Tendon insertions[132-135] | |
| Achilles | Contracted medial insertion |
| Posterior tibial | Hypertrophied plantar insertion |
| Anterior tibial | Dorsomedially displaced |
| Peroneals | Stretched or lengthened |
| Long flexors | Contracted or shortened |
| Short flexors | Contracted or shortened |
| Abductor hallucis | Contracted or shortened |
| Abductor digiti minimi | Contracted or shortened |
| Ligaments[136] | |
| Superficial deltoid | Hypertrophied and shortened |
| Calcaneofibular | Hypertrophied and shortened |
| Plantar calcaneonavicular | Contracted or shortened |
| Posterior talofibular | Contracted or shortened |
| Bifurcate | Contracted or shortened |
| Talocalcaneal interosseous | Contracted or shortened |
| Short and long plantar | Contracted or shortened |
| Retinaculum | |
| Superior peroneal | Contracted or shortened |
| Inferior extensor | Contracted or shortened |
| Fascia[126] | |
| Medial | Abnormal contractile properties due to high concentration of myofibroblasts |
| Plantar | Contracted or shortened |
| Vinculi | |
| Master knot of Henry | Thickened and attached to plantar surface of navicular |
| Joint capsule | |
| Calcaneocuboid | Contracted or shortened |
| Naviculocuneiform | Contracted or shortened |
| Talonavicular | Contracted or shortened |
| Subtalar medial and posterior | Contracted or shortened |
| Ankle, posterior | Contracted or shortened |
| Arteries[137] | |
| Anterior tibial/dorsalis pedis | Absent or reduced in size |
| Medial plantar | Absent or reduced in size |
| Calf[138] | Atrophy of posterior and lateral leg musculature leading to decreased circumference |

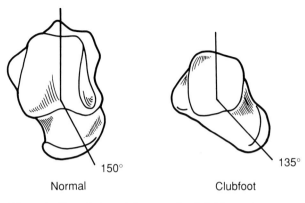

Normal 150°    Clubfoot 135°

**Fig. 6-4.** Dorsal view of the normal and clubfoot talus, revealing the deformity in size, alignment, and angulation of the talus (right). The overall size is reduced, and the head and neck are malaligned and angulated in the plantar-medial direction. The declination angle in the normal talus is 150 degrees, whereas in the clubfoot it is reduced to 135 degrees. (From Turco,[111] with permission.)

the articular malalignments created by the intrinsic abnormalities described above[132-139] and outlined in Tables 6-3 and 6-4.

## Articular Malalignments

### Ankle (Talocrural) Joint

In clubfoot the talus is plantarflexed and anteriorly displaced out of the ankle mortise, exposing 25 to 33 percent of its trochlear surface.[110,117] Also present is lateral rotation of the longitudinal axis of the talus in the ankle mortise, resulting in posterior displacement of the fibula. The lateral malleolus may be posteriorly displaced off its articular talar facet. This is referred to as a *horizontal breach* and leads to a decrease in the bimalleolar axis (the acute angle clinically measured between the longitudinal bisection of the hindfoot and the malleolar plane), the normal value of which is 75 to 90 degrees[109,116-119,138] (Fig. 6-5A).

### Subtalar (Talocalcaneal) Joint

The calcaneus is rotated in all three cardinal planes while pivoting on the talocalcaneal interosseous ligament. Around a vertical axis its anterior aspect is displaced plantar-medially beneath the head and neck of the talus while its posterior aspect is displaced dorsolaterally

Table 6-4. **Osseous Deformities Commonly Present in Idiopathic Clubfoot**

| Structure | Pathologic Anatomy |
|---|---|
| Talus[117,124,128-131,138] | Restricted endochondral growth due to lack of motion and constriction. |
| | Alterations in vascularity and ossification |
| | Progressive plantar-medial deviation of head and neck with associated neck shortening |
| | Declination angle (the angle formed by the long axis of the talar head and neck with the long axis of the talar body) decreased to 115–135 degrees (normal 150–160 degrees) (Fig. 6-4) |
| | Talar neck obliquity (the medial tilting of the anterior part of the talus) increased to 50–65 degrees (normal 12–32 degrees) |
| Calcaneus[110,117,139] | Reduction of the normal three talocalcaneal articular facets to only two by blending of the anterior and middle facets |
| | Plantar medial angulation of the distal calcaneal articular facet |
| | Underdeveloped sustentaculum tali |
| Navicular[110,117,121] | Diminished in overall size with medial tuberosity hypertrophy |
| | If severely subluxed, a pseudoarticulation or accessory joint with the medial malleolus may develop |
| Cuboid[110] | Grossly normal |
| Cuneiforms[110] | Grossly normal |
| Metatarsals[110] | Grossly normal |
| Phalanges[110] | Grossly normal |
| Foot size[138] | Adult length decreased 2.5 cm |
| Tibia[110,111,138] | Mild length inequality (shortened) with no torsional component |
| Fibula[110,111,138] | Mild length inequality (shortened) with no torsional component |
| Femur[110,111,138] | Mild length inequality (shortened) with no torsional component |

toward the lateral malleolus. The longitudinal axes of the calcaneus and talus become increasingly parallel and superimposed. This concept of rotation within the subtalar joint is important in understanding the clinical presentation of the adducted (medially spun) forefoot despite the lateral rotation of the talus within the ankle mortise.[121,140] The calcaneus inverts around a horizontal axis and laterally subluxes into the characteristic varus hindfoot position[117,141,142] (Fig. 6-5B and C).

### Midtarsal (Talonavicular and Calcaneocuboid) Joints

Depending on the severity of the soft tissue and osseous abnormalities described earlier, the navicular is plantarmedially displaced (subluxed or dislocated) off the head of the talus and may abut the medial malleolus.[110,117,120] The cuboid is also displaced in a plantarmedial direction below the navicular and cuneiforms, because (1) the distal calcaneal articular facet is abnormally angulated plantar-medially; and (2) the ligamentous connections between the navicular and cuboid distract the cuboid by ligamentotaxis.[110,117] The equinoadductovarus orientation of the midfoot and forefoot (Lisfranc's and metatarsophalangeal joints) is secondary to the gross abnormalities described above.

These triplane articular malalignments involving a complex system of joints, created by intrinsic and adaptive abnormalities in the soft tissue and osseous structures, produce the five principal deformities characteristic of idiopathic clubfoot: (1) adducted forefoot, (2) inverted hindfoot, (3) ankle equinus, (4) talonavicular subluxation, and (5) lateral rotation of the talus in the ankle mortise.

## CLINICAL EVALUATION
### General Evaluation

The purpose of the examination of the clubfoot patient is twofold: (1) to accurately classify the type of deformity present on the basis of the suspected etiology and the nature of the deformity itself; and (2) to determine and initiate the appropriate treatment regimen to correct the deformity. The patient's history may be obtained from multiple and contradictory sources. Patient cooperation will be variable and influenced by age. Normal findings change with age and development. A systematic evaluation, reviewing all systems, is outlined in Table 6-5.

### Radiographic Evaluation

The purpose of radiographic evaluation of idiopathic clubfoot should be to accurately document the type and degree of all articular malalignments present. However, there has been no commonly accepted comprehensive, practical, and quantitative method for accurately diagnosing and treating idiopathic clubfoot. Although we now realize that five principal deformities may be present in varying degrees at birth, only three of these are easily detectable on clinical or radiologic examination. Talonavicular subluxation is difficult to document in infancy because the navicular does not start to ossify and thus is radiographically silent until the third year of life or

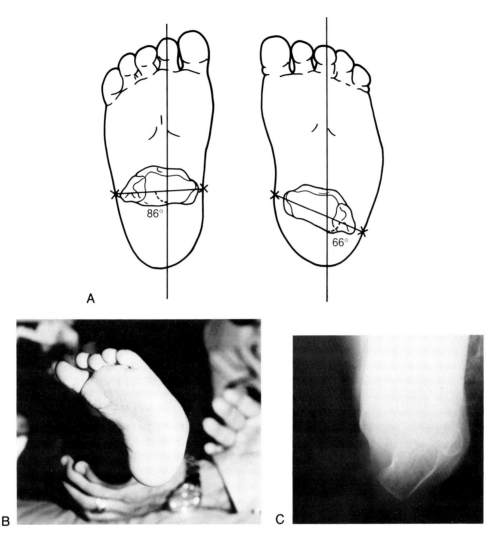

**Fig. 6-5.** **(A)** Bimalleolar axis (the acute angle measured clinically between the longitudinal bisection of the hindfoot and the bimalleolar plane). This angle is 75 to 90 degrees in the normal 12-month-old infant. In clubfoot, owing to the lateral rotation of the talus in the ankle mortise ("horizontal breach") and the resultant posterior displacement of the fibula, this angle decreases to less than 75 degrees. **(B)** Plantar view of an infant clubfoot, illustrating the adducted (medially spun) forefoot. **(C)** Calcaneal axial radiograph, illustrating the calcaneal varus present in a 6-year-old child with untreated idiopathic clubfoot.

later.[143] Also, lateral rotation of the longitudinal axis of the talus in the ankle mortise and calcaneal inversion are difficult to evaluate directly from anteroposterior and lateral radiographs.[144] Furthermore, until recently there was no standard method for quantitatively measuring the extent of the deformities present either before, during, or after conservative or surgical treatment. Thus, the laudable goal of obtaining a foot that is near "normal" in both appearance and function is rarely achieved.

Historically, Barwell in a series of short papers published in 1896 was the first to use radiography as a technique to assist in the evaluation and treatment of clubfoot.[145-147] He described the use of the standard anteroposterior and lateral views in a qualitative manner. Many other authors followed suit, citing the descriptive and diagnostic value of clubfoot radiographs.[148-151] Wisburn[152] in 1932 was the first to make quantitative angular measurements in the evalua-

**Table 6-5. General Clinical Evaluation of the Clubfoot Patient**

I. History
  A. *Chief complaint:* Parents should be able to provide the most accurate history regarding the deformity's presentation, course, current status, and response to previous treatment.
  B. Past medical history
    1. *Prenatal:* The medical history begins with a thorough review of the pregnancy, including the number of weeks of gestation and any illnesses or trauma experienced by the mother. Maternal exposure to prescription, over-the-counter, and recreational drugs must be investigated.
    2. *Perinatal:* Many aspects of the labor and delivery are important, such as duration, type of anesthesia used, neonatal seizures or apnea, and complications.
    3. *Growth and development:* Parents should be able to provide important milestone information, such as age at which patient first lifted head, rolled over, grasped, sat up, and walked. One must remember, however, that there is great variation, in normal development among individuals and families.
II. Examination
  A. *Musculoskeletal:* The characteristic equinoadductorvarus foot deformity with calf atrophy should be carefully evaluated. In general, the severity of the deformity depends on the degree of articular malalignments, whereas the resistance to anatomic reduction and correction is determined by the rigidity within the surrounding soft tissue. In the newborn a single deep skin cleft or furrow may be present just above the heel and in the plantarmedial arch area. The skin quality may be thin, and there may be an absence of posterior heel skin wrinkles. The calcaneus and medial malleolus commonly are difficult to palpate, whereas the medially displaced navicular anlage may be prominent. These clinical deformities are the direct result of the malpositioned talocalcaneonavicular joint complex.

The degree of flexibility of the clubfoot deformity is critically important. A large degree of passive joint motion is normal in the newborn. It is not uncommon to be able to passively dorsiflex the foot onto the anterior aspect of the leg. A flexible clubfoot, one that is easily manipulated into normal anatomic alignment, may be due to extrinsic causes and thus may respond well to conservative manipulation and serial casting. An excessive amount of flexibility or "floppiness," however, is abnormal and may indicate an underlying neuromuscular disorder. In contrast, a rigid clubfoot may portend the failure of conservative therapy.

Thorough examination of the patient's back and hips is essential. Sacral abnormalities, both cutaneous and bony, should be looked for, as should pigmented skin lesions. The incidence of congenital dislocation of the hip is higher in the presence of idiopathic clubfoot and must be ruled out as well.
  B. *Neurophysiologic:* A thorough assessment of the patient's neurophysiologic status is required to accurately classify the type of clubfoot present. This involves evaluation of (1) muscle tone and motor function; (2) sensation and reflex activity; and (3) motion and gait if feasible. This process is discussed in detail in Chapter 3.
  C. *Special diagnostic studies:* It is our experience that some infants who are initially classified as having idiopathic clubfoot seem to have very subtle neurologic abnormalities, which become noticeable only with later development and often are so subtle that a specific diagnosis is never made. In such complicated cases a neurology consultation should be obtained. Currently, sagittal plane magnetic resonance imaging of the lumbar spine has proved useful in detecting previously undiagnosed abnormalities such as cord tethering or lipomatous impingement, which may be the true cause of the clubfoot deformity.

**Table 6-6. Normal Ranges of Radiographic Angular Measurements[a]**

| Author | Anteroposterior | | | Lateral | |
| --- | --- | --- | --- | --- | --- |
| | Talocalcaneal Angle | Talus–First Metatarsal Angle | | Talocalcaneal Angle | Talocalcaneal Index |
| Debrunner[155] | 30–45 | — | | 30–40 | — |
| Ponseti and Smoley[156] | >20 | — | | — | — |
| Heywood[154] | 20–40 | — | | 35–50 | — |
| Templeton et al.[157] | 15–50 | — | | >40 | — |
| Beatson and Pearson[158] | 10–50 | — | | 15–55 | 40–85 |
| Taylor et al.[159] | >30 | — | | >30 | — |
| Lloyd-Roberts[160] | 30 | — | | 30 | — |
| Ponseti and Campos[161] | — | — | | — | 40–85 |
| Debrunner[162] | >30 | — | | 40 | — |
| Denis and Paquot[163] | — | — | | 40–60 | — |
| Simons[171,172] | 20–40 | 0–(−20) | | 35–50 | — |
| Price[164] | 20–40 | — | | 35–50 | — |
| Approximate averages | 20–40 | 0–(−20) | | 35–50 | 40–85 |

[a] Table 6-7 shows the pertinent measurements and their normal ranges for the standard anteroposterior and lateral views at 12 months of age[152,153,167] (Fig. 6-6).

tion of clubfoot.[152] He described the talocalcaneal angle in the anteroposterior view. Kite supported this and other angular measurements and stressed the importance of the normal divergence of the longitudinal axes of the talus and calcaneus.[153] Heywood evaluated changes in the talocalcaneal angle in the lateral view while the foot was placed in forced dorsiflexion and equinus positions.[154] Numerous additional angular measurements involving the talus, calcaneus, and adjacent osseous structures have been proposed. A wide range of normal values[154-164] is presented in Tables 6-6 and 6-7, and Figure 6-6 shows such measurements for a normal foot of a 12-month-old infant.

Many other special views, such as the suroplantar and posterior tangential (both variations of the Harris and Beath or "ski-jump" projections) have been proposed for use in the evaluation of clubfoot.[165,166]

Controversy exists regarding the quantitative use and predictive value of radiographs in the evaluation of infant clubfoot.[167-169] This conflict persists because of (1) the

**Table 6-7. Radiographic Angular Measurements at 12 Months of Age**

| Views | Normal Range (degrees) |
|---|---|
| Anteroposterior | |
| Talocalcaneal angle | 15–50 |
| Talus–first metatarsal angle | 0–(–30) |
| Calcaneus–fifth metatarsal angle | 0 |
| Lateral | |
| Talocalcaneal angle | 25–50 |
| Tibiocalcaneal angle | 25–60 |
| Tibiotalar angle | 70–110 |
| Talus–first metatarsal angle | 0–20 |
| Calcaneus–first metatarsal angle | 130–150 |
| Combination anteroposterior and lateral | |
| Talocalcaneal index | 40–85 |

(Data from Wisburn,[152] Kite,[153] and LeNoir.[167])

complexity of the triplanar articular malalignments; (2) the impaired ossification and consequently diminished size and/or abnormal shape of the tarsal bones; (3) the complete radiographic absence of the navicular until the age of 3 years or later; and (4) the lack of a practical,

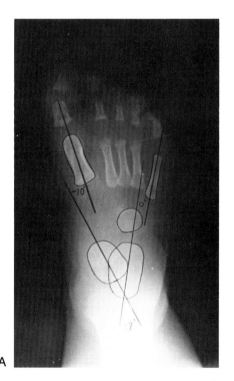
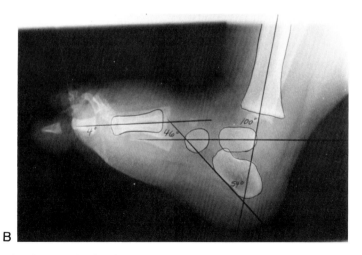

**Fig. 6-6.** Anteroposterior and lateral radiographs of a normal infant foot at 12 months of age. **(A)** Anteroposterior: talocalcaneal angle, 37 degrees; talo-first metatarsal angle, –10 degrees; calcaneal-fifth metatarsal angle, 0 degrees. **(B)** Lateral: talocalcaneal angle, 46 degrees; tibiocalcaneal angle, 54 degrees; tibiotalar angle, 100 degrees; talo-first metatarsal angle, 4 degrees; calcaneal-first metatarsal angle, 135 degrees. Talocalcaneal index, 83.

comprehensive, quantitative, and standardized method of evaluation.

Beatson and Pearson[158] and Simons[170] independently devised two different methods in an attempt to quantitatively analyze the articular malalignments present in clubfoot. These two methods represent the most common techniques currently used in the diagnosis and treatment of clubfoot in infancy.

**Beatson and Pearson Assessment Method**

Beatson and Pearson developed a simple, quantitative radiographic technique to assess the clinical correction of the talocalcaneal articular malalignments using standard anteroposterior and lateral veiws.[158] Patients were positioned in the following manner: for the anteroposterior views, supine with 30 degrees of ankle joint plantar flexion, weight-bearing foot plantigrade, and central x-ray beam 30 degrees from perpendicular; for the lateral views, supine with 30 degrees of ankle joint plantar flexion, weight-bearing foot plantigrade, and central x-ray beam 90 degrees from the perpendicular.

In the anteroposterior view the talus and calcaneus are bisected longitudinally and the subtended angle is

Table 6-8. **Beatson and Pearson Radiographic Clubfoot Criteria**

| Foot Type | Anteroposterior | Lateral | Talocalcaneal Index |
|---|---|---|---|
| Normal | 10–50 | 15–55 | 40–85 |
| Clubfoot | 0–55 | −5–40 | 0–55 |

(Data from Beatson and Pearson.[158])

measured. In the lateral view the talus is bisected longitudinally, a line is drawn to the inferior border of the calcaneus, and the angle subtended is measured (Fig. 6-7). These two angles are added together, and the sum is referred to as the *talocalcaneal index.* Table 6-8 represents a summary of their results.

Comparison of the anteroposterior and lateral angular measurements reveals significant overlap between normal and clubfeet. However, when the talocalcaneal indices are compared, a much smaller overlap is noted. Only 10 of the 147 clubfeet evaluated by Beatson and Pearson had a talocalcaneal index over 40 degrees, and there were no normal feet with a talocalcaneal index under 40 degrees. Thus, Beatson and Pearson concluded that a talocalcaneal index of 40 degrees was the dividing line between the normal foot and the clubfoot. These

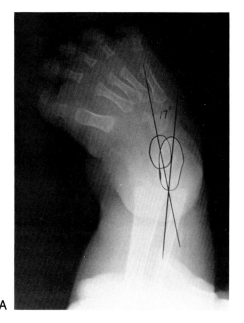
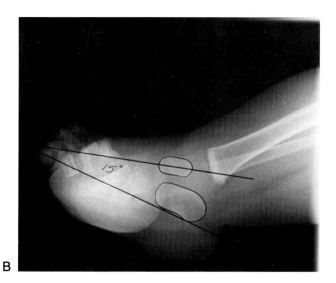

A                                   B

**Fig. 6-7.** Radiographic evaluation of idiopathic clubfoot according to the Beatson and Pearson assessment method.[158] **(A)** Anteroposterior: talocalcaneal angle, 17 degrees. **(B)** Lateral: talocalcaneal angle, 15 degrees. Talocalcaneal index, 32; talonavicular subluxation predicted.

parameters have been shown to predict the subluxation of the talonavicular joint in infancy with 90 percent accuracy.[170] According to Beatson and Pearson, "should the correction be inadequate—that is, should the talocalcaneal index be under 40 degrees even though, clinically, the foot appears corrected—further treatment should immediately be undertaken."[158]

## Simons's Assessment Method

Simons developed an analytical method for the radiographic evaluation (analytical radiography) of four of the principal deformities in idiopathic clubfoot, namely forefoot adductus, hindfoot varus, ankle equinus, and most importantly, talonavicular subluxation.[171,172] This analytical method predicts the presence of talonavicular subluxation before ossification occurs within the navicular with near 100 percent accuracy,[170] while using only standard anteroposterior and lateral radiographic views. Simons' standardized technique is based on positioning the patient's clubfoot in its maximally corrected position in the following manner: for the anteroposterior view, sitting with knees and hips flexed, forefoot maximally abducted and ankle maximally dorsiflexed 15 to 20 degrees or as close as the equinus deformity will allow, weight-bearing foot plantigrade, and x-ray beam 30 degrees from perpendicular; for the lateral view, hindfoot parallel to cassette, ankle maximally dorsiflexed without raising heel, x-ray beam 90 degrees from perpendicular.

Simons advocates the use of three angular measurements obtained from standard anteroposterior and lateral views to assess four potential deformities. On the anteroposterior view the talus, calcaneus, and first metatarsal are longitudinally bisected, and the talocalcaneal and talo-first metatarsal angles are measured (Fig. 6-8). In the clubfoot, as the talus and calcaneus become parallel and superimposed, the talocalcaneal angle (normal 20 to 40 degrees) decreases below 15 degrees; a negative angle may result if the anterior aspect of the calcaneus slides beneath the head and neck of the talus, indicating severe inversion of the rearfoot. The talo-first metatarsal angle (normal 0 to −20 degrees), in contrast, increases in a positive direction as the bisection of the externally rotated talus moves to the lateral side of the first metatarsal. By comparing radiographic angular measurements with intraoperative findings in a retrospective study, Simons[172] showed that talonavicular subluxation was present in every case in which the talo-first

metatarsal angle was greater than 15 degrees and the talocalcaneal angle less than 15 degrees. This relationship is called the *Simons rule of 15.*

The talus and calcaneus are bisected on the lateral view, in the usual manner as described by Beatson and Pearson.[158] The talocalcaneal angle (normal 35 to 50 degrees) decreases to less than 35 degrees and approaches a negative value, indicating severe hindfoot equinus. With forced dorsiflexion in a clubfoot this angle may decrease even further owing to the pull of the already contracted and taut Achilles tendon on its calcaneal insertion.[154,173,174]

According to Simons, four principal deformities may be present to varying degrees in any clubfoot; thus, 16 different deformity combinations are theoretically possible. However, Simons's clinical experience has confirmed the existence of only seven such combinations (Table 6-9). This reduced number is probably due to the following reasons: first, talonavicular subluxation always occurs in conjunction with hindfoot varus, which eliminates combinations 4, 8, 9, and 14. The converse, however, is not true; hindfoot varus may occur without talonavicular subluxation (i.e., combinations 6 and 13). Second, because of the articular relationship between the talus and calcaneus, hindfoot varus is always present in conjunction with ankle equinus, which eliminates combinations 3, 7, 11, and 15. Again, the converse is not true; ankle equinus may occur without hindfoot varus (i.e., combinations 2 and 10).

Table 6-9. **Theoretical and Actual Clubfoot Deformity Combinations**

| Combination | Forefoot Adductus | Hindfoot Varus | Ankle Equinus | Talonavicular Subluxation |
|---|---|---|---|---|
| 1 | − | − | − | − |
| 2[a] | − | − | + | − |
| 3 | − | + | − | − |
| 4 | − | − | − | + |
| 5[a] | + | − | − | − |
| 6[a] | − | + | + | − |
| 7 | − | + | − | + |
| 8 | + | − | − | + |
| 9 | − | − | + | + |
| 10[a] | + | − | + | − |
| 11 | + | + | − | − |
| 12[a] | − | + | + | + |
| 13[a] | + | + | + | − |
| 14 | + | − | + | + |
| 15 | + | + | − | + |
| 16[a] | + | + | + | + |

[a] Clubfoot deformity combinations clinically identified by Simons.[171,172]

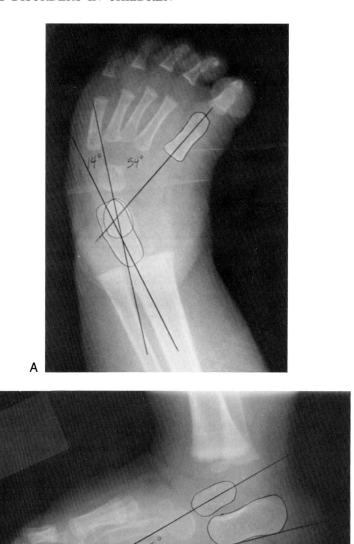

**Fig. 6-8.** Radiographic evaluation of idiopathic clubfoot according to Simons's assessment method.[112,113] **(A)** Antero-posterior: talocalcaneal angle, 14 degrees; talo-first metatarsal angle, 54 degrees. Talonavicular subluxation predicted according to Simons' rule of 15. **(B)** Lateral talocalcaneal angle, 15 degreees. All four principal deformities present; talocalcaneal index, 16.

There are two main sources of error in using any radiographic clubfoot assessment method in infants. First, patients must be properly positioned. More importantly, they must be held in the maximal degree of correction obtained by conservative care, so that only the true remaining articular malalignment (s) will be re-

vealed. Second, once acceptable radiographs have been obtained, the small ossification centers of the talus and calcaneus should be carefully outlined to aid in their bisection before angular measurements are attempted. Unfortunately, lines drawn through the ossific nuclei of these bones do not necessarily determine the axis of the entire bone. Shapiro and Glimcher[175] have clearly shown that the ossific nucleus of the clubfoot talus is positioned eccentrically in the neck of the talus. Therefore, an axis determined by the ossific nucleus does not necessarily coincide with the axis of the entire bone (Fig. 6-9). Moreover, the talus is an irregularly shaped bone even in the normal foot, and to assign a single major axis to the talus is quite difficult. An accurate description of the talus may require separate measurements of both the neck and body axes.

Tomography[176] and arthrography[177] have also been proposed as methods of improving the radiographic evaluation of clubfoot; however, to obtain the "bird's-eye" anteroposterior projection (view) is difficult because the tibia blocks the body of the talus. CT has also been used for evaluating the subtalar joint in clubfoot.[144] Unfortunately, CT does not accurately define the positional relationships of the tarsal bones in three dimensions because any given slice is only a two-dimensional image. In addition, the outline of the cartilage anlage is not well depicted by CT.

Herzenberg et al.[178] utilized three-dimensional CT modeling techniques to investigate the shape and axis placement of the individual tarsal bones, as well as their positional relationship to each other in two neonatal cadaver feet, one a clubfoot and one normal. This study supported the accepted theories regarding the intrinsic morphologic abnormalities commonly present in idio-

pathic clubfoot and clarified the abnormal positional relationships between the hindfoot bones. In the clubfoot the talar neck was shown to be internally rotated relative to the mortise, but the talar body was externally rotated in the ankle mortise.

Theoretically, it is possible to repeat this study by MRI examination of living patients instead of histologic study of pathologic specimens. This technique could provide preoperative three-dimensional models of a patient's clubfoot to help plan the surgical treatment. This approach, developed for use in skeletally mature patients undergoing reconstructive hip joint surgery,[179] currently requires CT data, which are not well suited to the unossified structures of the neonatal foot. We are hopeful that practical three-dimensional MRI modeling will soon be available for clinical use in the pre- and postoperative evaluation of clubfoot.

## TREATMENT

### Nonoperative Treatment

Hippocrates, Kite, and many others have stressed the importance of beginning treatment of clubfoot as soon after birth as possible. Infants with clubfoot should be seen in the newborn nursery soon after delivery, certainly within the first 24 hours after birth. The old tongue-in-cheek axiom that a breech delivery is preferred so that manipulation of the foot can begin before the head is delivered emphasizes the importance of early treatment. It is during the first few days to the first 3 weeks of life that the infant's ligaments and soft tissues are most pliable and most amenable to stretching, partly because of the presence of residual maternal relaxing hormones. All children with congenital clubfoot should be treated by manipulation. Surgeons with considerable experience often feel that they can discriminate very early after birth between those children with the more flexible positional type of clubfoot and those with the more rigid types that will undoubtedly require surgery. Even so, the child with a rigid or teratologic clubfoot should be treated to promote and maintain as much pliability of the soft tissue as possible until such time as the child is old enough and the foot large enough to allow surgical intervention.

In order to reduce the joint subluxation that occurs at the talocalcaneal and midtarsal joints in clubfoot, it is necessary to elongate the involved ligaments, capsule, tendon sheaths, and other tissues that surround these

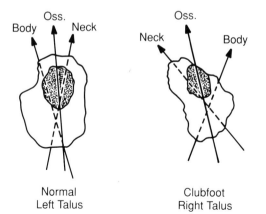

**Fig. 6-9.** Two-dimensional view of normal and clubfoot talus from a histologic section. Axes drawn through the talar neck and body do not coincide with an axis drawn through the ossific nucleus (OSS). This is why drawing axes on standard radiographs of the neonatal clubfoot may be misleading. (Adapted from Shapiro and Glimcher,[124] with permission.)

joints. Coleman described the three ways in which these tissues can be elongated as (1) growth; (2) gradual elongation of the elastic components of connective tissue through constant and repetitive application of force; and (3) traumatic or surgical interruption.[180] The success of nonoperative manipulation and immobilization is based upon the first two principles. Growth is essential for reduction of the deformity, and therefore the rapid growth period of early infancy is the most ideal time for treatment. This is typically illustrated in children with growth-limiting disorders who exhibit minimal or no improvement with prolonged periods of manipulation. It is also important to remember that the strain resistance of infant connective tissue is greater than that of cartilaginous pediatric bone. Excessive force is more likely to crush or sublux bone than to rupture ligaments and often leads to the common findings of dorsally displaced or wedge-shaped navicular, flat-top talus, or avascular necrosis of the navicular, talus, or distal tibial epiphysis. The most conservative and usually least traumatic approach in rigid clubfeet that do not exhibit an adequate clinical and radiographic response to treatment is often soft tissue release, while the most radical and inappropriate choice may be continued nonoperative care.

The ultimate goal of treatment, whether operative or nonoperative, should be to reduce the equinovarus and rotational subluxation of the talocalcaneal and midtarsal articulations to anatomic position, thereby creating a plantigrade foot, while maintaining a functional ankle range of motion (ROM). Although this is the end point that should be striven for in each case, anatomic and functional normality is often not possible. It is important to remember the pathologic anatomy of clubfoot and the abnormal shape of the talus (and often other tarsal bones) and to realistically discuss the prognosis with the parents. In most cases a functional foot can be achieved that will not result in any activity restriction but will not appear cosmetically perfect, and slight over- or undercorrection is frequent. The possibility of recurrent deformity (even after several years) and the potential need for future surgery should also be discussed with parents within the first few weeks of treatment.

### Manipulation and Serial Casting

There are three components to successful nonoperative reduction of clubfoot deformity: (1) gentle stretching of the soft tissue; (2) manipulation of the subluxed talocal-

caneal and midtarsal joints toward a reduced position; and (3) maintenance of the reduced position with plaster of Paris bandages. Stretching and manipulation should be performed with intermittent application of gentle but firm force over a period of 10 to 15 minutes. Manipulation and stretching provides the correction and the plaster cast should be used only to maintain position.

Various techniques for manual stretching and reduction have been recommended.[180-190] In our preferred technique (Fig. 6-10), tincture of benzoin or a skin adherent is placed about the posterior heel, and the right clubfoot is grasped, with the left thumb-index web space firmly gripping the heel and with the thumb tip applying pressure in a medial direction against the lateral aspect of the prominent talar head. The thumb and index finger of the right hand are then used to apply an abduction force together with distal traction to the right forefoot. With the thumb tip of the left hand applying firm counterpressure to the lateral talar head, the thenar crease is used to apply distal traction to the heel and the left index finger to apply an eversion force to the medial heel. This technique can be applied as a unit or one or two components at a time. It is, however, necessary to attempt to reduce all components of the deformity from the start of therapy in order to achieve satisfactory reduction. One cannot afford to allow the equinus component to become rigid while attempting to reduce the adduction and varus components. It is essential to visualize the pathologic anatomy of clubfoot while performing the manipulation. The calcaneocuboid-navicular complex should be visualized as a unit, which must be externally rotated about a vertical axis through the distal tibia and at the same time everted and dorsiflexed at the subtalar joint.

Once stretching and manipulaton have been accomplished, tincture of benzoin or a pediatric skin adherent is applied to the foot and leg. Newborn infants require more padding due to their lack of subcutaneous fat padding. By the second or third cast application, one or two layers of Webril are applied directly to the skin. Three people are necessary for proper cast application. The parent is instructed to occupy the child, who is placed supine on the cast table while a cast technician applies the Webril and plaster. We often instruct the parent to delay one feeding until the manipulation and cast application. This usually relaxes the child and facilitates manipulative correction. The physician should maintain the proper position of the foot. A short leg cast is applied initially by using 2-inch extra fast setting plaster or Gyp-

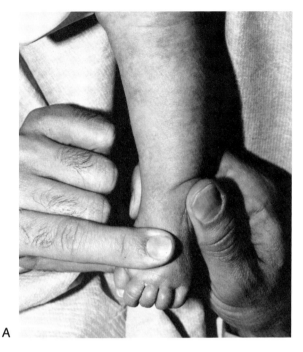

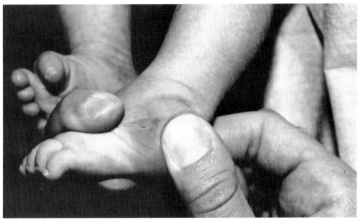

**Fig. 6-10.** Technique of soft tissue stretching and manipulation of infantile clubfoot deformity. **(A)** Manipulation of adduction, varus, and rotational components of deformity. **(B)** Manipulation of equinus by dorsiflexion of rear foot and distal traction of posterior calcaneus. *(Figure continues.)*

sona (Johnson & Johnson). The physician then molds the cast with the foot in the reduced position while the assistant stabilizes the thigh. In infants, the plaster is extended above the knee with the knee flexed 75 to 90 degrees while the physician holds the foot in gentle external rotation. Parents and nurses should always be instructed to check the neurovascular status of the infant's toes and watch for proximal migration of the foot in

the cast. If this occurs, the cast should be changed immediately to provide effective control and prevent neurovascular compromise.

Serial manipulation and casting should be performed at least once a week initially (in newborns) and for at least 1 to 2 months, at which time the frequency is decreased to every 10 to 14 days. Once satisfactory clinical and radiographic reduction is achieved, casting is discontin-

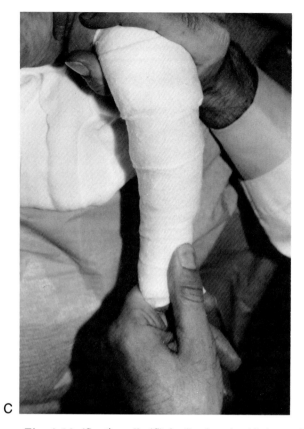
C

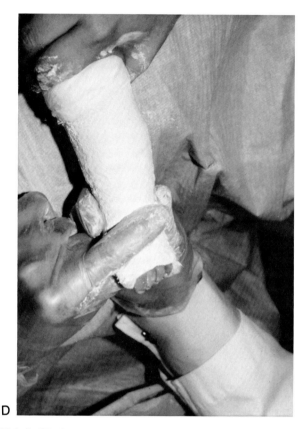
D

**Fig. 6-10** *(Continued).* **(C)** Application of a thin layer of Webril. **(D)** Application of below-knee portion of molded plaster cast, which is then extended above knee.

ued. The last casts are bivalved and used as night splints. Once children begin to walk, they are placed in pre-walker-type straight last shoes. Dennis-Browne bars are not normally used unless a significant rotational abnormality persists. Postoperative splinting should be continued 24 hours per day for a time at least twice as long as the child's age at surgery, or at completion of serial casting.

## Evaluation and Results of Nonoperative Treatment

Manipulation and serial casting should be continued until the foot exhibits satisfactory clinical and radiographic correction or until no further correction can be obtained. Radiographs should be taken at 1- to 2-month intervals after the first 2 to 3 months to assess the patient's progress. Improvement in appearance of the foot alone is

not adequate evidence of satisfactory reduction, since soft tissue compensation can occur at another level while the talocalcaneonaviculocuboid subluxation remains unimproved. Gradual recurrence to some degree is almost certain unless adequate radiographic evidence of reduction can be demonstrated.

In 1933 Kite reported an 88 percent success rate using his technique of manipulation and serial plaster of Paris casting.[181-184] Children were typically treated for several months to several years. Later authors have not been able to reproduce Kite's success rate, and the more recent literature most often quotes success rates of 35 to 45 percent.[189,191-197] (Table 6-10). Although some would argue that the lower success rates of recent years are the result of less diligence or persistence, it is our opinion that this is more a function of adherence to more stringent criteria in recent studies. Many older studies relied only on subjective clinical evaluations, their primary criterion for a good result being a plantigrade foot.

Table 6-10. **Results of Nonoperative Treatment of Clubfoot**

| Author | Method[a] | Year Reported | No. of Feet | Success Rate (%) |
|---|---|---|---|---|
| Brockman[191] | | 1930 | 73 | 54 |
| Kite[184] | M/P | 1933 | 100 | 88 |
| Bertelsen[192] | | 1957 | 114 | 66 |
| Jansen[193] | | 1957 | 150 | 60 |
| Dangelmajor[195] | | 1961 | 200 | 40 |
| Ponseti and Smoley[194] | M/P | 1963 | 94 | 44 |
| Blockey and Smith[196] | M/T | 1966 | 186 | 35 |
| Turco[189] | M/P | 1981 | (Not Reported) | 35 |
| Nather and Bose[197] | M/P | 1987 | 174 | 58 |

[a] Abbreviations: M, manipulation; P, plaster; T, taping.

More recent authors have demonstrated that radiographic correction and function approaching that found in the normal foot are also necessary for long-term good results and have included these factors in their studies. This point was illustrated by Heywood, who found that many of the children who were classified as having "corrected" clubfeet by Kite actually had radiographically uncorrected clubfeet by presentday criteria.[198]

## Operative Treatment of the Infant and Young Child

Surgical soft tissue release should be considered an extension of stretching and manipulation of clubfoot deformity and not an alternative to conservative treatment. The rationale for and goals of surgical release should parallel those of nonoperative treatment; namely, to attempt to restore the bones and joints (primarily the talocalcaneonaviculocuboid complex) to as near anatomic normality as possible through elongation of the periarticular soft tissue contractures. The gradual trend toward more comprehensive surgical soft tissue releases since about 1970 is a function not only of a better understanding of the pathologic anatomy of clubfoot but also of more stringent criteria for an acceptable correction.

### Criteria for Surgical Intervention

Nonoperative treatment should be continued as long as gradual improvement is being realized. One should consider soft tissue release when no further improvement has occurred over a period of 1 month in the face of unsatisfactory clinical and radiographic correction. The hallmarks of inadequate clinical correction are all too familiar to most clinicians who treat clubfoot in infants. Even though the foot may grossly appear plantigrade

without significant adduction, varus, or equinus, the talar head is noticeably prominent laterally and is nonpalpable in its usually prominent medial location at the talonavicular joint. The sinus tarsi is not identifiable, and the dorsolateral skin appears stretched. The heel typically appears very small and foreshortened, and ankle dorsiflexion is limited. McKay also considers inadequate reduction of the relationship between the bimalleolar plane and the longitudinal bisection of the foot as one of his criteria for surgical release.[199] Satisfactory evidence of radiographic correction in the infant is usually limited to normalization of the talocalcaneal angle on standard anteroposterior and lateral radiographs. The talocalcaneal angle in newborn infants is usually very difficult if not impossible to assess because of the very spheroidal to ovoid ossification centers of the talus and calcaneus, and for this reason radiographs are usually not very helpful before the age of 2 to 3 months.

Although the nonoperative and operative treatment of infants and children with nonidiopathic clubfoot is often very similar to that used in idiopathic clubfoot, there are some important differences. The likelihood of recurrent deformity with soft tissue release alone is much higher with nonidiopathic clubfoot (especially the neurogenic and arthrogrypotic varieties). It is often more prudent to delay operation until children are old enough to allow muscle balancing and/or fusion operations (e.g., extraarticular arthrodesis or triple arthrodesis). Repeat procedures are often necessary, and the prognosis for lasting correction is guarded.

### Timing of Operative Treatment

The debate over early versus delayed soft tissue release is not a new one. It is often difficult to compare results of many early authors with the results of more recent studies, since most early surgeons tended to perform what would now be considered incomplete releases. Codvilla[16] in 1906 recommended early soft tissue release, and Attenborough[19] in 1966 recommended an extended posterior release between 2 and 4 months of age.[16,19] However, Attenborough's operation did not involve complete subtalar and midtarsal release and proved inadequate for complete correction. Somppi and Sulamaa[200] reported operations on 54 patients (87 feet) under the age of 2 weeks between 1959 and 1966. Their operation consisted of a modification of Brockman's medial release operation combined with Achilles tenotomy, and they reported 34 percent good and 41 percent fair results. In 1978 the French surgeons Pous and Dimeglio reported neonatal surgical release between 1 and 6 weeks of age.[201] Their procedure included posterior, medial, and plantar releases but did not include complete subtalar joint release. They felt that their results after a short 2-year follow-up in over 100 clubfeet were superior to those in patients treated with delayed surgical procedures; however, they did not provide clinical or radiographic documentation.

The rationale for early soft tissue release for resistant clubfoot within the first few weeks to months of life is based on the sound principle that rigid contractures in the growing child must be reduced as soon as possible to prevent secondary osseous deformation and to allow remodeling of bony abnormalities that may already exist. Disagreements over the benefits of early versus later operation have generally centered around technical considerations. Turco believes that the ideal age for surgical release is between 1 and 2 years of age.[185,199,200] He reported a higher incidence of failures in children who underwent operation between 5 and 8 months of age. Turco and Spinella [202] stated the following reasons (based on technical considerations) for their view that surgical release at less than 1 year of age is not indicated: loss of correction in plaster is more likely to occur following removal of internal fixation owing to the small size of the foot; overcorrection is more likely to occur because a minimal overcorrection is magnified with growth; tarsal remodeling is more apt to be stimulated by weight-bearing in the older child; and there is a greater likelihood of operation on an unrecognized nonidiopathic clubfoot that would be better treated conservatively.

Other more recent authors have disputed Turco's arguments, claiming that the technical complexity of very early release can be satisfactorily managed and the benefits of early contracture release outweigh the potential risks. Most have recommended comprehensive soft tissue release for resistant clubfoot between 3 and 12 months of age.[203-211] DeRosa and Stepro[207] in 1986 reported a retrospective review of 69 children (99 feet) with resistant clubfoot, in which they divided the children into three groups on the basis of their age at surgery: group I under 12 months, group II between 12 and 36 months; and group III over 36 months. Group I had 79 percent good results as opposed to 46 percent in group II. These authors recommended early soft tissue release, although not before 3 months of age. They also believed that the operation is technically difficult and should not be attempted by surgeons who do not regularly treat clubfoot. DePuy and Drennan[208] in 1989 reviewed 30 patients (44 feet), whom they divided into three groups according to average age at surgery: group I averaged 4.4 months, group II 9.1 months, and group III 16.1 months. The early operated group (I) displayed better clinical results (less hindfoot valgus and less tarsal deformity) and better radiographic results after an average follow-up of 4.5 to 6 years.

Our preference is to operate on those children who have demonstrated resistant soft tissue contracture between 3 and 8 months of age. The operation is technically much more difficult before 3 months of age owing to the physically small size of the foot, and 3 months of conservative care usually constitutes the minimum time required to adequately determine clinical and radiographic response to treatment. In addition, the benefit of operating prior to age 3 months has not been clearly established. Depending upon the experience and technical skills of the surgeon, it may be more appropriate to wait until the child is a little older and the foot a little larger. Although soft tissue release alone may be performed in children up to several years of age, our experience has shown that results are not as good when operations are performed in children over 1 year of age.

## Selection of Surgical Incisions

Comprehensive soft tissue release of clubfoot deformity requires extensive surgical exposure of the medial, plantar, posterior, and portions of the lateral aspect of the midfoot and hindfoot. Numerous surgical incision approaches have been described,[196,199,200,204,212-214] including (1) two incisions, medial and posterior; (2) a long posterior medial incision; (3) two incisions, medial and posterolateral; (4) two incisions, posteromedial and lateral; and (5) a transverse Cincinnati incision (Fig. 6-11). The two-incision medial and posterior approach does not provide adequate exposure to the subtalar joint and does not ensure protection of the posterior tibial neurovascular structures; therefore it is not recommended. The other incisional approaches are capable of providing satisfactory exposure in most cases, each having its own advantages and disadvantages.

Beyond adequate exposure, which must be the primary goal of any surgical incision, other considerations include avoiding violation of neurovascular structures, preservation of vascularity of skin flaps, and cosmesis. Taylor and Palmer mapped out five major vascular territories of the lower leg and foot which they termed *angiosomes*[215] (Fig. 6-12). They felt that incisions that

violated these angiosomes would be more likely to cause skin slough. The posteromedial incision described by Turco provides good exposure to the medial, plantar, and posterior structures and does not interrupt the vascular distribution to the skin. The disadvantage of the Turco-type incision alone is that it provides very limited exposure to the lateral structures. Some surgeons, including one of us (S.J.D.), believe that a satisfactory lateral release can often be performed through this incision by "reaching across" the foot through the subtalar and midtarsal joints. If more exposure of the lateral structures is necessary, a lateral incision can be added, as suggested by Carroll et al.,[204] Porat and Kaplan,[206] and Lehman et al.,[213] without violating vascular supply to the skin. The transverse Cincinnati incision was recommended by Crawford et al.[212] in 1982 and has been

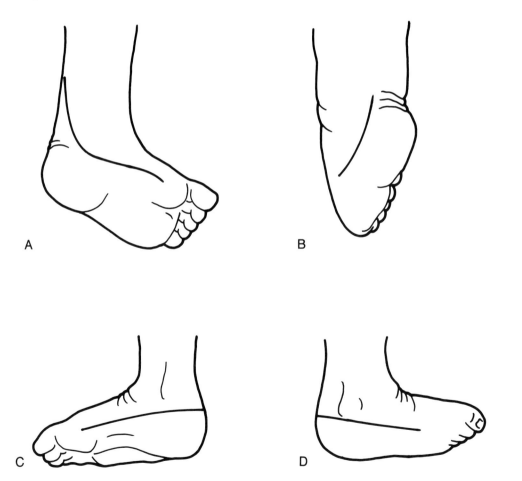

**Fig. 6-11.** Surgical approaches to clubfoot. **(A)** Turco posteromedial incision. **(B)** Posterolateral incision. **(C&D)** Medial and lateral arms of Cincinnati incision.

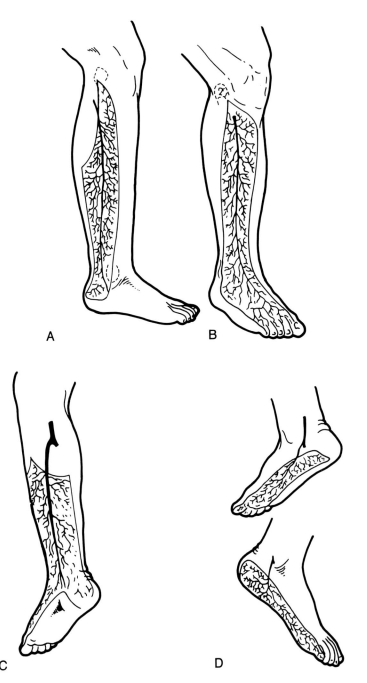

**Fig. 6-12.** The five major angiosomes (vascular territories) of the lower leg and foot as mapped by Taylor and Palmer.[215] Arterial skin distribution of: **(A)** peroneal artery; **(B)** anterior tibial artery; **(C)** posterior tibial artery; and **(D)** medial and plantar arterial branches of posterior tibial artery.

adopted by many as the incision of choice for clubfoot repair. Crawford et al. believed that this approach provides superior exposure and cosmesis and reported using this incision on 99 patients (154 feet) between the ages of 1.5 months and 15 years with only seven superficial skin sloughs, all of which healed uneventfully.[212] Although the Cincinnati incision does provide excellent exposure, it does violate vascular supply to the skin (angiosomes) in two ways: angiosomes are transversely incised, and adjacent angiosomes are interrupted. However, the incidence of skin slough in the experience of most surgeons is surprisingly low. Brougham and Nicol[216] reviewed 16 patients (24 feet) with idiopathic clubfoot who had soft tissue releases utilizing the Cincinnati incision between 3 and 15 months of age (average age 6 months). Only four skin problems occurred (including one pin tract infection and one tourniquet skin "burn"). Long-term results were equivalent to those of most other studies. Additional potential problems with the Cincinnati incision include limited exposure to the superior portion of the Achilles tendon without extensive undermining of the medial and lateral skin flaps and difficulty in obtaining closure when significant equinus is present. The incision should be carried superior to the insertion of the Achilles tendon at ankle joint level posteriorly.[217] It does tend to follow Langer's lines and is often cosmetically superior to linear incisions.

Our preference is to use either a posteromedial incision as described by Turco, with the addition of a lateral incision if necessary, or the Cincinnati incision. We prefer not to use the transverse approach in cases of severe equinus or in older children, in whom vascular compromise is more likely. Of course, skin slough is a potential complication in clubfoot surgery regardless of the incisional approach used. The tourniquet should be released prior to skin closure, and complete hemostasis should be achieved. The posterior tibial pulse should be palpable and skin edges should be well perfused with the foot in the corrected position. If not, it may be necessary to place the foot in slight equinus temporarily to avoid vascular embarrassment.

### Comprehensive Soft Tissue Release

The rationale for use of the comprehensive one-stage soft tissue release is based upon the concept proposed by Turco[218] and expanded upon by Carroll et al.[204] McKay,[219] and Simons,[220] that the equinovarus deformity is a multiplanar deformity characterized by adduction, inversion, internal rotation, and equinus of the calcaneocuboideonavicular complex about the talus. Because of the nature of the talocalcaneonaviculocuboid complex, it is impossible to reduce any one component of the deformity without simultaneously reducing all components. One should visualize this subluxation of the calcaneocuboideonavicular complex (and thus of the foot) about the talus, which is fixed within the ankle mortise, when performing the operation. Reduction is accomplished by circumferential or near circumferential release of all soft tissues that attach the calcaneocuboideonavicular complex to the talus, followed by manual reduction and fixation. The technique is essentially an anatomic dissection of the soft tissues of the hindfoot and midfoot, which is performed in an orderly and sequential manner until satisfactory reduction is achieved (Fig. 6-13). Turco and Spinella stated that there are two prerequisites to attaining a lasting correction: (1) a complete correction must be attained; and (2) normal tarsal relationships must be maintained until stable articular surfaces develop.[202]

The operation is performed under general anesthesia with use of a midthigh pneumatic tourniquet. The child may be positioned prone or supine with a large bump placed under the contralateral hip. Either approach gives adequate exposure, since the limb and/or the child can easily be turned from side to side during the procedure. We prefer the supine approach in most cases simply because it is more consistent with our usual visual and spatial approach to the foot. The skin incision of choice is made, and the skin flaps, along with the entire subcutaneous layer, are extensively reflected from the deep fascia to provide wide exposure to the hindfoot and midfoot. All dissection deep to skin is performed with fine, blunt-tipped dissecting scissors. We prefer to conduct the release in the following sequence: (1) posterior; (2) medial, including subtalar; (3) lateral; and (4) plantar. The deep fascia and laciniate ligament over the tarsal tunnel are divided to expose the posterior tibial neurovascular bundle, which is freely mobilized and retracted with a small Penrose drain.

The origin of the abductor hallucis is then reflected, taking care to avoid the neurovascular bundle as it passes inferior to the muscle belly. A Z-plasty-type lengthening of the Achilles tendon is then performed from its insertion to the myotendinous junction in either the sagittal or coronal plane. The sheath of the flexor hallucis longus

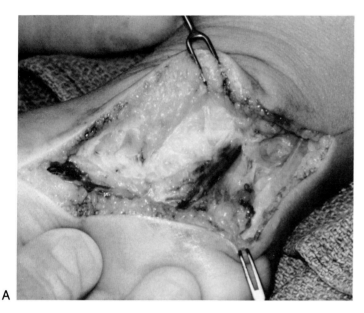
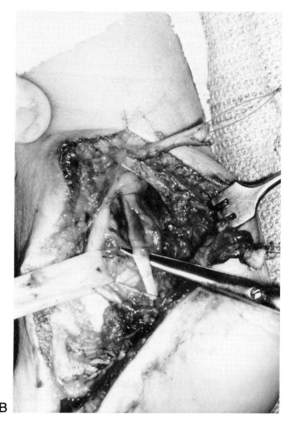

A                                    B

**Fig. 6-13.** Posteromedial portion of comprehensive soft tissue release procedure of the right foot of a 6-month-old child with congenital idiopathic clubfoot. **(A)** Turco-type skin incision with elevation of full thickness skin flaps. **(B)** Mobilization of posterior tibial neurovascular bundle and completion of posterior release. *(Figure continues.)*

tendon is identified posterior to the ankle joint and incised vertically and transversely, and the tendon is retracted medially to expose the posterior ankle and subtalar joint. With the talocalcaneal and ankle joints in marked equinus, the distal tibial physis, talotibial, and subtalar joints are in very close proximity, only millimeters apart. One must be careful not to mistake the distal tibial physis for the ankle joint. A vertical incision is made in the periosteum and joint capsules, which are then sectioned. The capsule of the ankle joint is sectioned from just posterior to the central axis on both the medial and lateral sides, with care taken not to section the anteromedial portion of the deep deltoid ligament so as not to allow valgus subluxation of the talus in the ankle mortise. The peroneal tendon sheaths are incised transversely and circumferentially superior to the ankle joint,

and the inferior portion of the sheath is reflected from the lateral wall of the calcaneus. The posteromedial, posterior, and posterolateral portions of the subtalar joint capsule, as well as the posterior talofibular and calcaneofibular ligaments, are then sectioned.

Attention is next directed to the posterior inferior tip of the medial malleolus, where the posterior tibial and flexor digitorum longus tendons are identified and reflected from their sheaths and the sheaths are divided transversely. A Z-plasty lengthening of the posterior tibial tendon is performed, and the distal stump is used to locate the talonavicular joint. At the medial side of the foot the plane of the talonavicular joint is often parallel to the long axis of the foot, and the medial navicular tuberosity may articulate with the medial malleolus. The talonavicular joint capsule is progressively divided medi-

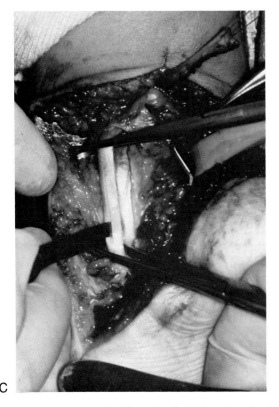
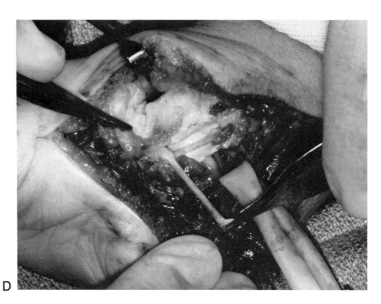

**Fig. 6-13** *(Continued).* **(C)** Z-plasty lengthening of posterior tibial tendon. **(D)** Exposure and release of talonavicular joint using posterior tibial tendon to locate joint. *(Figure continues.)*

ally, dorsally, plantarly, and laterally by using a small bone hook to distract the navicular distally and laterally. The plantar calcaneonavicular (spring) ligament and Henry's knot (the fibrous attachment of the flexor hallucis longus and flexor digitorum longus to the plantar navicular) should also be divided.

The dissection is then carried proximally, following the inferior contour of the talar neck to release the entire medial subtalar joint capsule and superficial deltoid ligament. The subtalar joint can then be opened almost like the pages of a book. The interosseous talocalcaneal ligament can be divided as necessary. Once the subtalar joint is opened, a more extensive release of the lateral talonavicular joint, bifurcate ligament, and lateral subtalar joint can be performed either through the medial side or through the lateral incision if one is used. A plantar, naviculocuneiform, or cuneiform-first metatarsal release can then be performed as deemed necessary. We do not

find these releases necessary in most cases; however, they are more likely to be needed in older children.

Once the surgeon feels that satisfactory reduction of the deformity has been achieved, .062 Kirschner wires or small Steinman pins are used to stabilize the talonavicular and subtalar joints. The talonavicular pin is inserted from the posterior aspect of the talus. A temporary pin placed longitudinally in the posterior calcaneus may aid in reduction of the rotational component of the deformity. Caution must be exerted to avoid excessive lateral displacement or dorsal displacement of the navicular. It is also important to remember that, although the calcaneus must be everted, its posterior aspect must be internally rotated and its anterior aspect must be externally rotated to avoid valgus heel deformity postoperatively.

Once fixation is complete, the tourniquet is released, mild compression is applied for 5 minutes, and intraoperative anteroposterior and lateral radiographs of the foot

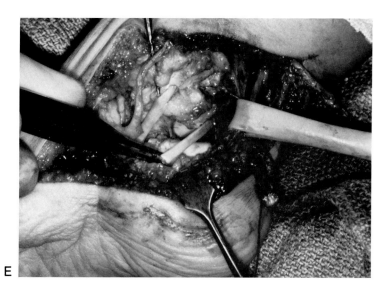

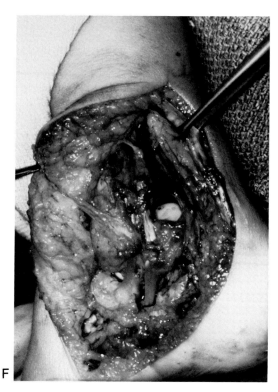

E

F

**Fig. 6-13** *(Continued).* **(E)** Release of medial subtalar joint. **(F)** Repair of Achilles and posterior tibial tendon after pin fixation. *(Figure continues.)*

are obtained to confirm adequate reduction. Complete hemostasis is then obtained, and the posterior tibial and Achilles tendons are repaired with absorbable sutures under physiologic tension with the foot in neutral position. The subcutaneous layer is approximated to reduce skin tension, and the skin is closed with absorbable suture (subcuticular and Steri strips if possible). A posterior tibial pulse should be palpable, and skin flaps should be well vascularized with the foot held in the reduced position. If any vascular impairment is present, the foot should be immobilized in slight equinus and gradually reduced at successive postoperative cast changes. A padded long leg cast is applied and bivalved anteriorly to allow for some swelling. If satisfactory reduction in plaster is achieved intraoperatively, the casts are usually left in place for 3 weeks. Percutaneous pins are removed in the clinic at 6 weeks, and cast immobilization is continued for 3 to 4 months postoperatively. The last casts, made of fiberglass, are bivalved prior to removal and used as

night splints, and the child is allowed to use a prewalker-type straight last shoe during the day.

## Operative Treatment of Recurrent or Residual Equinovarus Deformity

As previously stated, the best results with surgical treatment of resistant clubfoot are achieved when comprehensive one-stage soft tissue release is performed before the age of 1 year. Regardless of the method of treatment, however, clinically significant deformity will recur in some cases. One should always reinvestigate the possibility of some primary underlying cause of nonidiopathic clubfoot.[221] Turco[189,218] reported satisfactory results with soft tissue release alone in children up to 6 to 8 years of age; however, we feel that isolated soft tissue release does not usually produce satisfactory results beyond 3 years of age. By 3 to 4 years of age the neglected or recurrent clubfoot has usually developed a

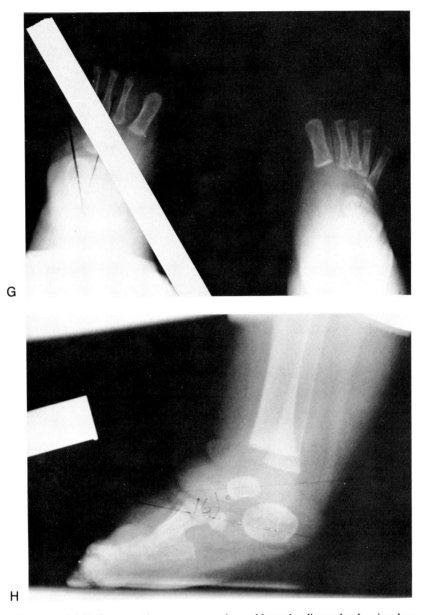

**Fig. 6-13** *(Continued)*. **(G&H)** Preoperative anteroposterior and lateral radiographs showing decreased talocalcaneal angles. *(Figure continues.)*

relatively shorter medial column secondary to the intrinsic deformity of the talus and soft tissue contracture. In his 1961 account of relapsed clubfoot, Dillwyn Evans also expressed the view that a relative "overgrowth" of the lateral column occurs, and he recommended wedge re-

section of the calcaneocuboid joint along with medial release.[222] Lateral column osteotomy together with comprehensive soft tissue release is effective in most children between 2 and 6 years of age in our experience. The upper limit may be extended to age 8 in some in-

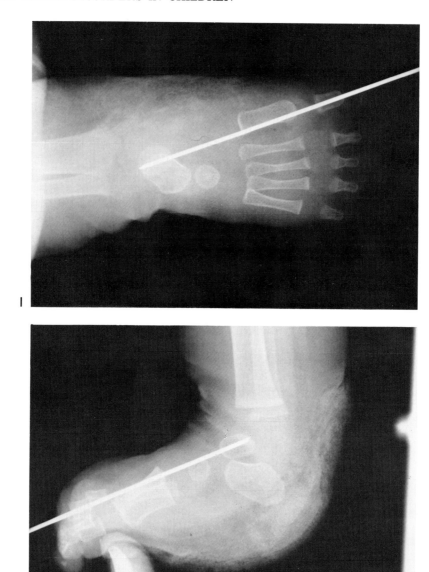

**Fig. 6-13** *(Continued).* **(I&J)** Intraoperative anteroposterior and lateral radiographs showing talonavicular pin fixation and satisfactory improvement of talocalcaneal angles.

stances. Limited procedures may be useful when one component of clubfoot (e.g., metatarsus adductus, heel varus) predominates. Salvage procedures (e.g., triple arthrodesis) are reserved for children with recurrent or neglected deformity that is too severe for lesser procedures.

**Comprehensive Soft Tissue Release Combined with Lateral Column Osteotomy**

Evans recommended calcaneocuboid joint wedge resection and fusion, believing that in addition to equalizing column length, the fusion would further stabilize and retard lateral column growth.[222] This principle is very effective in the older child but should be used with caution in children under 4 years of age for fear of producing overcorrection. Wedge resection of the cuboid (decancellation) is a good alternative to calcaneocuboid fusion in the child under age 4. This technique, originally described in 1902 by Ogston[223] and in 1958 by Johanning,[224] has been used successfully by Lehman[188] and others. Another variation of lateral column shortening in very young children, originally described by Lichtblau in 1973 is resection of the anterior calcaneus.[225] If this procedure is performed while the anterior portion of the calcaneus is largely cartilaginous, regeneration of the articular surface usually occurs.

Lateral column shortening osteotomy is always combined with posteromedial or comprehensive soft tissue release. Soft tissue release is performed first, and if inadequate correction is obtained owing to unequal column lengths, then lateral column osteotomy is performed. A two-incision approach is preferred because of the

greater risk of skin slough in the older child. The extensor digitorum brevis muscle is reflected distally, and a thin wedge of bone is resected from the cuboid or the calcaneocuboid joint (Fig. 6-14). Care should be taken not to resect too large a wedge since overcorrection is easily produced. When cuboid osteotomy is performed in children under age 4, fixation is usually not necessary. Calcaneocuboid fusion is preferred in the older child; it provides greater stability and durability and to some extent limits lateral column growth, thus providing an ongoing corrective force to equalize column length. Fixation is accomplished with staples or Kirschner wires. As with soft tissue release alone, cast immobilization is necessary for 3 to 4 months.

Evans originally reported operating on 30 feet in children between the ages of 3 and 15 years.[222] Most of these patients were between 6 and 8 years old and had severe "recurrent" clubfoot that had not been treated surgically. Long-term results, as reported by Tayton and Thompson, were clinically and radiographically satisfac-

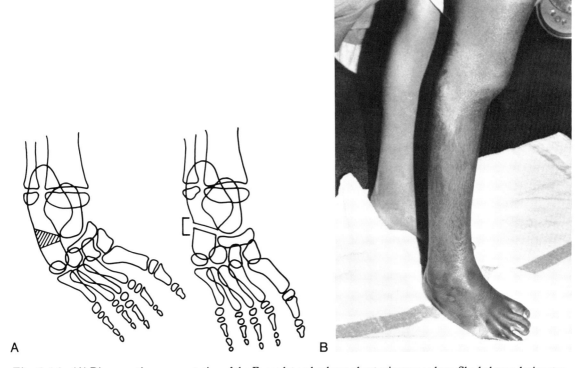

**Fig. 6-14.** (A) Diagramatic representation of the Evans lateral column shortening procedure. Shaded area designates resected wedge of bone at the calcaneocuboid joint. (B) Residual rigid equinovarus deformity in an 8-year-old child. *(Figure continues.)*

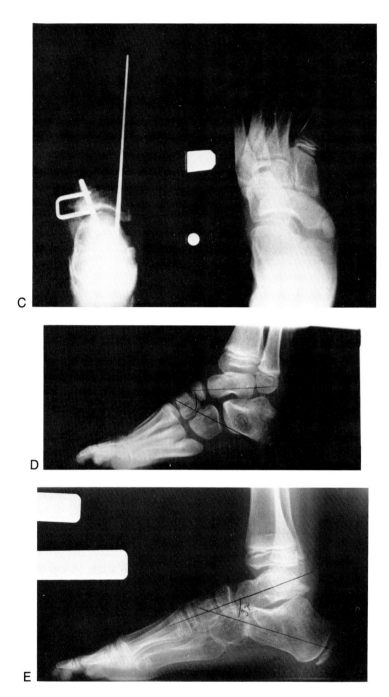

**Fig. 6-14** *(Continued).* **(C)** Immediate pre- and postoperative anteroposterior radiographic appearance of child in Fig. B. **(D&E)** Preoperative and 1-year postoperative radiographic appearance of child in Fig. B.

tory in 66 percent of patients.[226] Addison et al. also reported 66 percent satisfactory results in 45 feet in 4- to 14-year-old patients; 42 of these feet had been subjected to previous operations (multiple procedures in many cases).[227] Of these patients, 92 percent were able to participate in all desired athletic activities. Most feet in both studies exhibited significant stiffness, which is probably as much attributable to long-standing uncorrected deformity prior to operation as to calcaneocuboid fusion.

### Limited Precedures for Correction of Isolated Residual Deformity

*Metatarsus Adductus*

Some degree of residual metatarsus adductus is a common finding in clubfoot, whether treated operatively or nonoperatively. In 1973 Lowe and Hannon found residual metatarsus adductus in 52 percent of 73 feet that had undergone various surgical procedures for clubfoot.[228] Otremski et al. reviewed 28 children (44 feet) who had undergone a one-stage (Turco) posteromedial soft tissue release at 6 months to 2 years of age.[229] In 21 feet (48 percent) residual adduction deformity, mainly caused by metatarsus adductus, was clinically evident. The patients were 8 to 11 years of age at the time of review. Otremski felt that earlier soft tissue release (3 to 10 months) and more attention to abductor and plantar release resulted in less residual metatarsus adductus deformity (9 percent in an early follow-up of 22 feet). Clinically significant metatarsus adductus does not respond well to stretching and manipulation after 12 to 18 months of age. A minimal degree of residual metatarsus adductus which as a common sequela of clubfoot, does not impair function or interfere with normal shoe wear and does not deserve exposure to the potential risks and complications of elective foot surgery. A greater amount of metatarsus adductus in a young child can, however, result in significant problems, which may not become symptomatically apparent until adolescence or early adulthood. Difficulty with normal shoe wear, cosmesis, compensatory hindfoot pronation (skewfoot), hallux valgus, and claw toe formation have all been associated with residual metatarsus adductus deformity.[230]

The tarsometatarsal soft tissue release described by Heyman et al.[231] is very effective if the child is young enough. Most authors have recommended this procedure up to 6 to 8 years of age.[188,231] We have found, however that adequate correction after 4 years of age is

very difficult if not impossible, owing to progressive ossification of the bones that compose the interlocking tarsometatarsal joints. Good results can be obtained if the release is performed between the ages of 18 months and 3 years, with an upper limit of 4 years of age.

A transverse incision distal to the level of the tarsometatarsal joints is preferred in children (Fig. 6-15). This incision provides the wide exposure and clear visualization necessary for successful completion of the procedure. Skin slough has not been a problem because of the marked vascularity of the soft tissues of young children. Full thickness skin flaps, along with the underlying subcutaneous tissues, are mobilized proximally and distally, and the long and short extensor tendons and deep peroneal neurovascular bundle are mobilized, elevated, and retracted with a Penrose drain. The tarsometatarsal joints can then be visualized as a unit by retracting the dorsal tendons and neurovascular structures alternately in a medial and a lateral direction. All tarsometatarsal ligaments except for a few fibers at the plantar lateral aspect of each joint are sectioned. This usually requires two successive releases, starting medially and progressing to the lateral side. A large gap will be present at the medial side of each metatarsocuneiform joint when the forefoot is reduced. Internal fixation with cross Kirschner wires is necessary to hold the reduction and prevent dorsal displacement of the metatarsals. Intraoperative radiographs should be obtained to ensure adequate reduction. Percutaneous pins are removed at 6 weeks, and cast immobilization is continued for 3 to 4 months.

Soft tissue release is the most common technique employed for correction of residual metatarsus adductus deformity in our clinic. Appropriate use of this procedure requires early detection of those cases that will require surgery and adequate prior correction of any hindfoot deformity. Various osteotomy procedures have been described for correction of metatarsus adductus in the older child. Most authors do not recommend metatarsal osteotomy before 8 years of age in order to avoid potential adverse effects on foot growth. The reader is referred to Chapter 8 on metatarsus adductus for a complete discussion of these procedures.

*Residual Heel Varus*

A residual heel varus deformity is never seen as an isolated condition in clubfoot, but it may remain the most significant portion of an incompletely corrected clubfoot

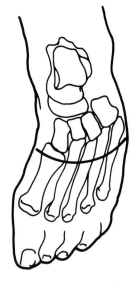 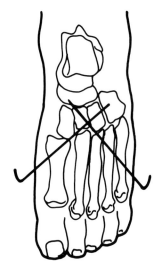

**Fig. 6-15.** Diagramatic representation of surgical incision and fixation recommended for Heyman-Herndon-Strong tarsometatarsal soft tissue release. See Fig. 8-12 A&B for clinical photographs of procedure.

deformity. Calcaneal osteotomy may be of value in a child with this deformity who is too old for soft tissue release and too young for triple arthrodesis or in whom the deformity may not be severe enough to warrant triple arthrodesis. In our experience, however, calcaneal osteotomy is rarely indicated. Most children over 4 years of age who require additional surgery have a compound residual deformity that is more appropriately treated by soft tissue release with lateral column osteotomy or triple arthrodesis. The best indication for calcaneal osteotomy would be a structural deformity of the posterior calcaneus (C-shaped calcaneus); however, this is rarely seen.[221] Although calcaneal osteotomy can be useful in the absence of structural deformity, one must keep in mind that this procedure corrects varus heel and subtalar joint position by creating a compensatory valgus structural deformity of the posterior calcaneus and that it will not alter midfoot or forefoot position. Thus, calcaneal osteotomy for residual heel varus should only be considered when the heel is rigidly inverted with a plantigrade forefoot.

Most authors agree that the operation should not be performed before age 4 because the body of the calcaneus is insufficiently ossified to allow reliable fusion in children aged 3 and under. The object of calcaneal osteotomy should be to wedge or translocate the weight-bearing posterior tuberosity of the calcaneus just lateral

to the central axis of the ipsilateral tibia. This can be accomplished by medial opening wedge osteotomy, lateral closing wedge osteotomy, or lateral translocation of the posterior tuberosity. In 1963 Dwyer recommended medial opening wedge osteotomy for correction of residual heel varus in clubfoot.[232] This opening wedge procedure has the advantage of elongating the usually small, underdeveloped heel found in residual clubfoot deformity. A medial osteotomy is made roughly perpendicular to the long axis of the posterior calcaneus, leaving the lateral cortex intact (Fig. 6-16). The osteotomy site is opened with the aid of a pin inserted in the posterior tuberosity until satisfactory correction is achieved and an appropriate corticocancellous graft is fashioned and inserted. The bone graft can be taken from the iliac crest, upper tibia, or allograft bank bone. Pin or staple fixation can be used to secure the graft.

Dwyer originally performed the operation through a long posteromedial incision (similar to Turco's incision), allowing simultaneous posterior and plantar release.[232] The combination of soft tissue release and structural elongation of the heel results in a very significant gap in the normally taut skin directly over the osteotomy site. Portions of the wound usually must be left open and allowed to heal by secondary intention, often resulting in hypertrophic scar and contracture. Tachdjian recommended placing the incision perpendicular to the plane of

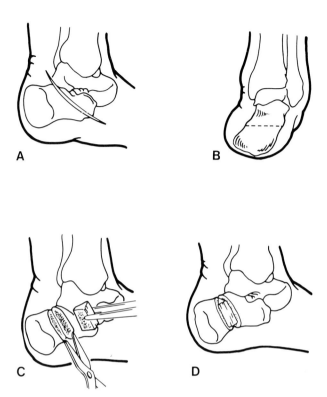

**Fig. 6-16.** Dwyer-type medial opening wedge calcaneal oste-otomy as used for clubfoot repair. **(A)** Skin incision. **(B&C)** Osteotomy cut. **(D)** Insertion of corticocancellous wedge of bone graft.

the osteotomy and delaying soft tissue release (if neces-sary) for about 6 weeks.[186] For cases in which prior posteromedial release has been performed and hyper-trophic scar is already present, Tachdjian recommended a Z-plasty skin incision (Fig. 6-17). Regardless of which technique is used, considerable skin tension is produced by wound closure, and skin slough can occur. Portions of the wound may need to be left open, and split thickness skin graft may be necessary. Dwyer reported 48 percent good and 52 percent fair results in 56 operated feet.[232] Many of the children in his study had had prior failed piecemeal operations, and the rating of results was based primarily on function, not on cosmesis.

Although the medial opening wedge osteotomy is theoretically preferred when the heel is small and not well developed (as it usually is in clubfoot) in order to prevent further reduction in heel size, the lateral closing wedge osteotomy is technically easier to perform, does not require bone graft, and is preferred by some au-

thors.[233,234] The lateral closing wedge osteotomy is also a good choice if the calcaneus is large and prominent enough to allow some shortening (this is more likely in older children). Dekel and Weissman reported the re-sults of lateral closing wedge operations of the calcaneus in 33 children (38 feet) with clubfeet of varying etiol-ogy.[233] Although these authors felt that osteotomy in younger growing children helped prevent progression of the deformity, they did note that corrections performed in older children were less likely to result in recurrence. Dekel and Weissman rated the results of 12 calcaneal osteotomies for clubfoot as good in 11 cases and fair in the other case. About half of the children in this study required additional tarsal reconstructive surgery later. Fisher and Shaffer reported results of 26 calcaneal oste-otomies in 20 patients as good in 13, fair in 7, and poor in 2 cases.[234] A third alternative, the lateral translocation or displacement osteotomy, is preferred by Coleman.[180] Although we have no experience with this procedure in children, it may be of value in some situations.

The medial subtalar stabilization procedure reported by Schneider and Smith may be useful in the manage-ment of progressive or unstable varus heel or equino-varus deformity, particularly when the etiology is para-lytic.[235] This procedure is a variation of subtalar stabilization by lateral extra-articular arthrodesis, as originally proposed by Grice for stabilization of paralytic pes plano valgus or heel valgus deformity in children.[236] These procedures are indicated in children with paralytic muscle imbalance or instability who are too young for triple arthrodesis (approximately ages 6 to 10). A pos-teromedial soft tissue release is almost always needed, and tendon transfer should be performed as necessary to recreate muscle balance equilibrium. An appropriate length graft of iliac bone is then placed across the middle facet of the subtalar joint with the heel in the desired position and is held in place with a Kirschner wire. This procedure is a nonexcision, intra-articular arthrodesis across the middle subtalar facet. Schneider and Smith[235] reported having performed this procedure on 40 pa-tients, most with neglected varus deformity, and dis-cussed short-term results on six patients. In all cases a solid union was obtained; however, two patients required revision because of technical errors in positioning. The unforgiving nature of fusion (or even heel osteotomy) emphasizes the need for exact positioning, which is best accomplished by performing these procedures with the patient prone.

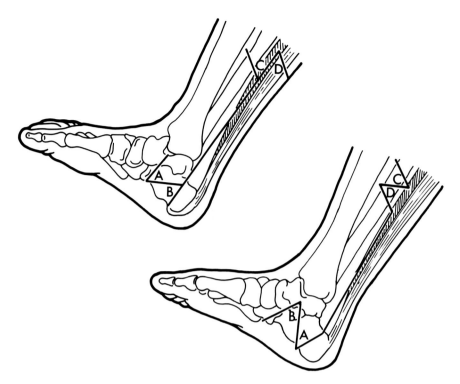

**Fig. 6-17.** Tachdjian's Z-plasty skin incision.

## Salvage Procedures

### Talectomy

Talectomy, originally reported as a treatment for talipes equinovarus deformity in the late 1800s, has been advocated as either a primary or a salvage procedure for severe rigid clubfoot deformity associated with certain neuromuscular diseases (e.g., arthrogryposis multiplex congenita or myelomeningocele) by numerous authors since.[237-240] Although periodic reports have appeared in the literature affirming the value of talectomy, this procedure has been a subject of great controversy among many surgeons. The objections to talectomy are well founded. Removal of the talus shortens the affected limb; lowers the malleoli, making shoes fit less well; creates a potentially unstable pseudarthrosis between the tibia and calcaneus; and renders any further reconstructive procedures (including fusion) extremely difficult if not impossible. The best indication for talectomy as reported by most recent authors is found in the child with severe rigid clubfoot secondary to arthrogryposis or myelomeningocele (especially at the thoracic level).[241] Rigid equinovarus is the most common deformity that is seen in arthrogryposis multiplex congenita and has an incidence of 25 to 36 percent in myelomeningocele.[241-245]

Most authors reporting the results of talectomy for arthrogryposis and myelomeningocele in the recent literature have indicated satisfactory results in 70 to 80 percent of cases.[243,245-249] Segal et al. compared the results of primary talectomy (performed at an average age of 6 to 8 years) in children with arthrogryposis and myelomeningocele with those of posteromedial release (performed at an average age of 1 to 2 years) in a similar group.[241] Poor results occurred in 63 percent of children with arthrogryposis and 27 percent of children with myelomeningocele who had undergone posteromedial release, as opposed to only 7 percent poor results in arthrogrypotic feet and 50 percent poor results (only four feet total) in myelomeningocele feet treated by primary talectomy. Those children who had primary posteromedial releases tended to have more procedures (averaging 2.1 to 2.3 procedures per foot), higher recurrence rates, and less satisfactory results than those children who had primary talectomies. The authors concluded that primary talectomy is a useful procedure in the management of severe rigid equinovarus feet associated with arthrogryposis and that it may be effective in the management of thoracic level myelomeningocele.

Although talectomy has been reported in the treatment of severe idiopathic clubfoot that is not associated with other conditions, reports have been few and follow-up has not been well documented.[240,250-252] Talectomy should be considered a last resort salvage procedure in patients with idiopathic clubfoot who have uncorrected or rigid deformity that is not amenable to soft tissue release and/or column osteotomy and who are too young for triple arthrodesis. Additional indications might include severe rigid deformity associated with extensive medial scar formation or severe talar deformity or avascular necrosis that is not amenable to reconstruction.

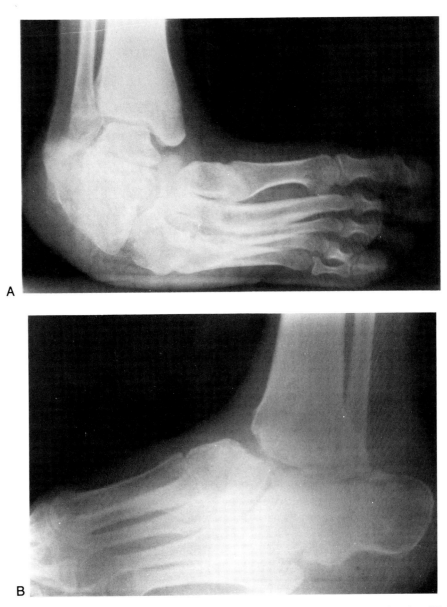

**Fig. 6-18.** (A) Radiograph of an 18-year-old man with severe rigid untreated clubfoot deformity. (B) Three years post-talectomy and wedge osteotomy. The foot is now plantigrade, and the patient is able to ambulate without pain. (Courtesy of Mitchell Pokrassa, D.P.M.)

Talectomy is a relatively simple procedure as compared with other more physiologic reconstructive techniques for clubfoot repair. Most authors recommend that this procedure be performed between the ages of 4 and 8 years, although those limits can be expanded in some cases.[180,252] Soft tissue release is more appropriate for idiopathic clubfoot in children under age 4. Severe neurogenic clubfoot is often better treated by nonoperative care and bracing initially. A more stable correction can generally be achieved in children over age 10 through triple arthrodesis.

Talectomy is usually performed through a straight anterolateral incision. The talus is excised by dividing all ligamentous attachments. It is imperative to position the foot as far posteriorly on the tibia as possible. (Fig. 6-18). The navicular should articulate with the medial malleolus, and the fibula should be in line with the calcaneocuboid joint. The position must be held with a large Steinman pin inserted axially through the calcaneus and into the tibia for 4 to 6 weeks until adequate soft tissue fibrosis has occurred. Cast immobilization is usually recommended for 3 months. Long-term or permanent use of an ankle-foot orthosis-type brace is recommended postoperatively.

### Triple Arthrodesis

Triple arthrodesis is an excellent and time-honored salvage operation for management of symptomatic, recurrent, or inadequately corrected clubfoot deformity in the older child. Loss of subtalar and midtarsal joint motion due to arthrodesis is not a significant concern, since children with residual equinovarus deformity usually have relatively stiff, rigid feet prior to arthrodesis. Triple arthrodesis merely converts a stiff foot that is fixed in a position of poor function to a stiff foot that is placed in a better functional position. The disadvantages of triple fusion are limited to some shortening of the foot and lowering of malleolar height along with the potential risks and complications of a major bone operation. Many children with clubfoot have a mild to moderate amount of residual deformity that results in minimal or no functional impairment. These children should not be considered candidates for fusion since the potential risks of a major operation usually outweigh any marginal improvement in function. Since triple arthrodesis is a salvage procedure that does not improve cosmesis and since it can be performed at any time after skeletal maturity if the deformity progresses, it should only be considered if

a significant improvement in function can be expected. It is just as important that parents and children have realistic expectations. This operation will not make the foot normal; it will simply improve position.

Triple arthrodesis should be reserved for children with a severe, rigid equinovarus deformity that is not correctable with soft tissue release and column osteotomy because osseous adaptation has occurred to such a degree that correction is only possible by osseous wedge resection through the subtalar and midtarsal joints. Fusion is also the preferred method of stabilizing residual clubfoot deformity in the presence of neuromuscular imbalance. When triple arthrodesis is performed on a neurogenic clubfoot, tendon transfer may still be indicated to restore as much muscular balance as possible in order to prevent recurrent deformity at the ankle or distal joints.

Most authors have recommended that triple arthrodesis in children be postponed until skeletal maturity or very near skeletal maturity in order to avoid excision of large wedges of nonossified cartilaginous bone with the subsequent complications of excessive shortening of the foot and potentially increased risk of nonunion.[253-256] Crego and McCarroll also stated that the risk of recurrent deformity is higher if fusion is performed prior to skeletal maturity.[257] Children with severe untreated clubfoot or those with rigid recurrent deformity who are older than 7 to 8 years of age are often required to wait as long as several years before they can undergo operation. Talectomy is an option in some of these children, but fusion can be expected to provide a more stable long-term result and should always be selected over talectomy if possible. If the child is near skeletal maturity and can be braced or accommodated until the foot is near completion of growth (usually at 10 to 12 years of age), then fusion is the regimen that is usually preferred. Triple fusion may also be performed prior to skeletal maturity in select cases.

Galindo et al. reviewed 19 triple arthrodeses in 13 children aged 10 years or younger with neurogenic, arthrogrypotic, or severe idiopathic clubfoot.[258] Their average foot shortening was 0.81 inch, which was not significant when compared with a group of clubfoot control patients who had similar degrees of shortening without fusion. These authors reported 68 percent good and excellent results, with nonunion occurring in 16 percent of feet and 7 percent of joints. They stated that fair and poor results were primarily due to failure to completely correct the deformity in most cases and expressed the view that triple arthrodesis is functionally and cosmetically superior to talectomy. Hill et al. reported similar results in 43 triple arthrodeses in children 8 years of age and under, with a nonunion rate of 12 percent of feet and 6 percent of joints.[259] According to Galindo et al., these statistics compare favorably with a reported nonunion rate in adolescent feet varying from 9.1 to 23 percent.[258,260,261]

Some degree of soft tissue release is almost always necessary in conjunction with triple arthrodesis for equinovarus deformity. This may consist of only percutaneous Achilles tendon lengthening or complete open posterior release in milder degrees of deformity, but complete posteromedial soft tissue release may be necessary in more severe deformity. In most cases soft tissue release can be performed coincidently with fusion, since bone

resection usually provides enough reduction of tension on vascular structures to allow complete correction without vascular compromise. The procedure should be carried out in a sequential manner, with soft tissue release performed first. If the tension on soft tissue and vascular structures is considered to be too great with manipulation of the foot into a more corrected position, then arthrodesis can be postponed until after a period of manipulation, stretching, and casting under general anesthesia. Tachdjian recommends a four-step regimen of correction in cases of severe deformity, which includes (1) manipulation, stretching, and casting of contracted soft tissues; (2) soft tissue release; (3) a second period of manipulation, stretching, and casting; and (4) triple arthrodesis.[186] Primary closure of medial skin incisions

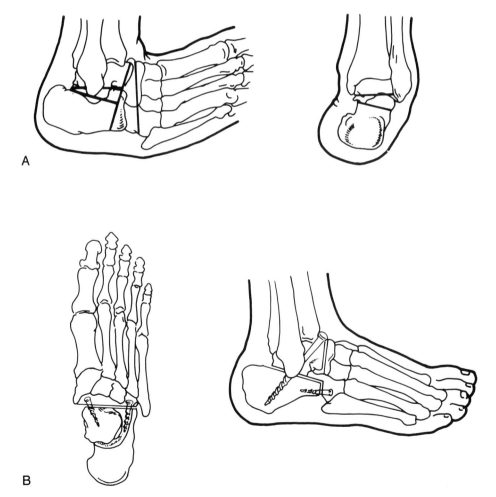

**Fig. 6-19.** Triple arthrodesis. **(A)** Wedge resection of midtarsal and subtalar joint. **(B)** Reduction of deformity with rigid internal fixation.

may not be possible in the older child or adolescent, and one should be prepared to primarily or secondarily apply a split thickness skin graft to the medial wound.

Adequate visualization of the talocalcaneonaviculocuboid skeletal complex is imperative for successful realignment of the tarsal bones. This is best accomplished through lateral and medial incisions. The medial incision begins inferior to the medial malleolus and extends distally over the dorsomedial talonavicular joint just inferior to the insertion of the anterior tibial tendon, following the medial column of the foot. This incision may be modified or extended proximally as the standard Turco-type incision to allow soft tissue release. We prefer a lateral curvilinear incision extending from just posterior and inferior to the tip of the fibula, coursing parallel and dorsal to the peroneal tendons, and then gently curving medially distal to the midtarsal joint. This leaves a bipedicle island of skin between the two incisions, which is elevated along with the superficial nerves, extensor tendons, and anterior tibial neurovascular bundle to provide full visualization of the entire midtarsal joint from the lateral wound. The extensor digitorum brevis muscle belly is reflected distally to expose the calcaneocuboid joint, and the entire soft tissue contents of the sinus tarsi

are excised. The calcaneofibular ligament and talocalcaneal ligaments are sectioned to allow exposure to the subtalar joint. The calcaneofibular ligament should later be repaired to prevent ankle instability. As much correction as possible should be attempted through soft tissue release and repositioning of the tarsal bones. The remainder of the correction is provided by resection of appropriately sized wedges of bone from the subtalar and midtarsal joints (Fig. 6-19).

The cuts are usually started with a sagittal saw and completed with thin, wide osteotomes. The talonavicular and calcaneocuboid joints should be resected as if this were one large joint, and the surfaces should then be matched by reciprocal planing with the power saw. The subtalar joint is resected in a similar manner. The bones are then temporarily held in the reduced position with pins placed axially through the subtalar joint and obliquely from medial and lateral through the midtarsal joint. An intraoperative radiograph should be taken at this point to confirm the adequacy of the reduction (Fig. 6-20). Once the position is judged satisfactory, permanent fixation with interfragmental screws is performed. The use of interfragmental screw fixation in tarsal fusions is greatly facilitated by the use of a cannulated

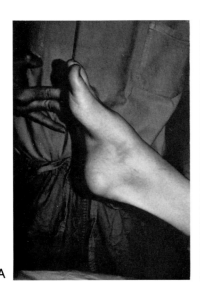 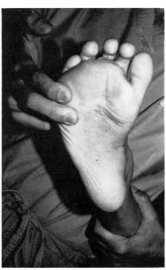 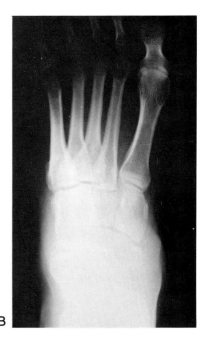

A      B

**Fig. 6-20. (A)** Preoperative clinical appearance of 13-year-old boy with rigid residual and recurrent clubfoot after nonoperative treatment as a child. **(B)** Preoperative anterioposterior radiograph. *(Figure continues.)*

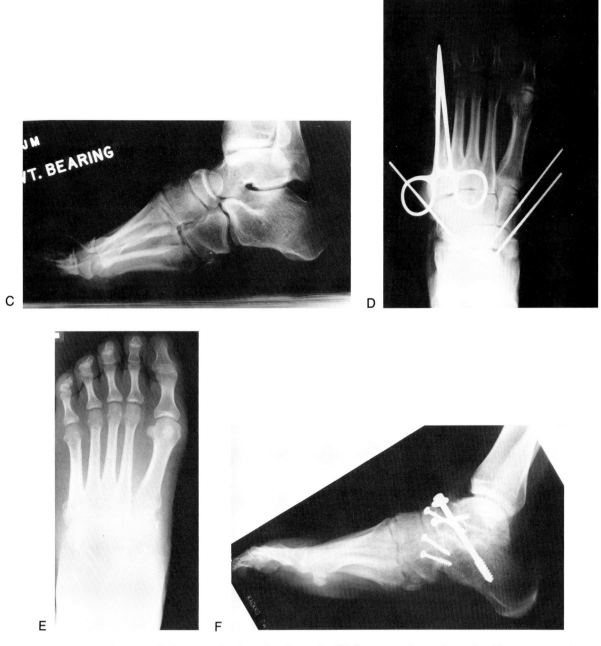

**Fig. 6-20** *(Continued).* **(C)** Preoperative lateral radiograph. **(D)** Intraoperative radiograph with temporary pin fixation. **(E&F)** Postoperative radiographs with rigid internal fixation.

screw system that allows insertion of a screw directly over a guide wire that has been inserted initially for temporary fixation. We usually release the tourniquet prior to closure to obtain maximum hemostasis, and we also use a closed suction drainage tube postoperatively. The patient is kept in a non-weight-bearing short leg cast for 6 weeks postoperatively and then in a short leg walking cast until radiographic evidence of union is obtained (usually about 3 months postsurgery).

## LONG-TERM RESULTS OF CLUBFOOT SURGERY

### Review of the Literature

Comparing the results of clubfoot treatment is not an easy task for the following reasons:

1. No general agreement regarding the classification of clubfoot exists. Many studies have inaccurately combined idiopathic and acquired clubfoot, and few have made efforts to distinguish between the flexible and rigid foot types.
2. Little consistency exists between studies regarding materials and methods, (e.g., initiation and duration of conservative treatment, age at time of surgery, specific type and number of surgical pro-

cedures performed, postoperative bracing regimen, and length of follow-up).
3. There are no uniform model or criteria for reviewing and comparing the results of treatment. Clubfoot has been evaluated on a subjective, clinical, functional, and radiographic basis as well as by multiple combinations of these approaches. The classification of results differs widely from the simple (e.g., satisfactory or unsatisfactory) to the complex (e.g., excellent, good, fair, poor, overcorrected, and failure).
4. There is no general agreement about the definition of treatment failure versus relapse, recurrence, or imcomplete correction.

In general, most physicians agree that the initial management of the newborn clubfoot is closed, gentle manipulation and serial casting. McKay[262] states that 9 out of 10 cases of clubfoot can initially be anatomically reduced by gentle manipulation if treatment is started a few days following birth. However, in only about 15 percent of these cases can the correction be maintained with continued daily manipulations and night splints. Table 6-11 reviews the results of successful long-term treatment, conservative versus operative, in 18 studies involving 3,657 clubfeet.[263-280] In summary, 52 percent of clubfeet attained satisfactory correction with nonoperative treatment alone. Kite,[268] a strong proponent of

Table 6-11. **Conservative versus Operative Treatment Results in 18 Studies Involving 3,657 Clubfeet**

| Author | Conservative Treatment, % | Operative Treatment, % | No. of Feet |
|---|---|---|---|
| Bachmann,[263] 1953 | 37 | 63 | 24 |
| Fredenhagen,[264] 1955 | 69 | 31 | 532 |
| Debrunner,[265] 1956 | 50 | 50 | 87 |
| Jansen,[266] 1957 | 59 | 41 | 150 |
| Solonen & Parkkulainen,[267] 1958 | 38 | 62 | 108 |
| MacEven, et al.,[268] 1961 | 67 | 33 | 237 |
| Seyfarth,[269] 1961 | 30 | 70 | 74 |
| Ponseti & Smoley,[270] 1963 | 21 | 79 | 94 |
| Kite,[271] 1964 | 92 | 8 | 922 |
| Wynne-Davies,[272] 1964 | 30 | 70 | 121 |
| Hersch,[273] 1967 | 56 | 44 | 159 |
| Denham,[274] 1967 | 79 | 21 | 223 |
| Tonnis & Bikadorov,[275] 1968 | 65 | 35 | 263 |
| Preston & Fell,[276] 1976 | 36 | 64 | 33 |
| Richardson & Westin,[277] 1978 | 50 | 50 | 362 |
| Tripathi & Chatuverdi,[278] 1979 | 80 | 20 | 32 |
| Kumar,[279] 1979 | 66 | 34 | 32 |
| Laaveg & Ponseti,[280] 1980 | 12 | 88 | 104 |
| Total | 52% | 48% | 3,657 |

nonoperative treatment, reported a very high (92 percent) success rate, which has never been duplicated. One must assume either that Kite's talents were truly superior or that his criteria for an acceptable result were less stringent than those of other researchers.

Nichols in 1897 expressed the view that failure of nonoperative treatment was due to incomplete or inadequate correction of the subtalar and/or midtarsal joint deviations.[281] Müller,[282] supported by others,[283-285] cited many causes for the failure of conservative and operative care, which included (1) delayed start of treatment; (2) poor technique (e.g., overzealous, forceful manipulation and casting); (3) insufficient initial correction of hindfoot varus deformity; (4) insufficient maintenance of the corrected position; (5) undetected neuromuscular condition; and (6) failure of patient (or parents) to follow the treatment regimen.

Innumerable methods of corrective clubfoot surgery can be found in the literature, but their effectiveness varies considerably. Fripp and Shaw[286] stated, "At least 15 years elapse before any surgeon can assess the merit of the particular method he adopts." Table 6-12 compares the results of four different common methods of corrective surgery performed on 960 infant clubfeet.[263,275,285,289-297] These 14 studies were well constructed and used comparable assessment criteria; thus an excellent to good result was a painless, plantigrade foot with good ROM, propulsive gait, good correction of all components of the deformity, and normal radiographic tarsal relationships. The purpose of this comparison is not to advocate any specific procedure but to show the tremendous variability among similar studies.

Most researchers agree that the fate of the surgically treated idiopathic clubfoot, prior to Turco's preliminary report[292] in 1971, included individual piecemeal proce-

Table 6-12. **Summary of Results of Four Different Corrective Clubfoot Procedures in 960 Cases**

| Author | Percentages | | | | Number of Feet |
| | Excellent/ Good | Fair | Poor | Failure | |
|---|---|---|---|---|---|
| **A. Achilles Tendon Lengthening with Posterior Capsular Release** | | | | | |
| Lindemann,[287] 1934 | 54 | 30 | 16 | 0 | 44 |
| Bachmann,[263] 1953 | 33 | 33 | 33 | 0 | 66 |
| Kuhlman & Bell,[288] 1956 | 73 | 13 | 14 | 0 | 30 |
| Tonnis & Bikadorov,[275] 1968 | 8 | 42 | 44 | 6 | 48 |
| Total | 42% | 30% | 27% | 1.5% | 188 |
| **B. Achilles Tendon Lengthening with Posterior Capsular Release, Partial Medial Release, and Anterior Tibialis Tendon Transfer** | | | | | |
| Critchley et al.,[287] 1952 | 73 | 9 | 18 | 0 | 22 |
| Kuhlman & Bell,[288] 1956 | 86 | 7 | 7 | 0 | 29 |
| Tonnis & Bikadorov,[275] 1968 | 16 | 63 | 21 | 0 | 19 |
| Nyga,[290] 1979 | 58 | 24 | 12 | 6 | 34 |
| Total | 56% | 26% | 15% | 1.5% | 104 |
| **C. Traditional (Turco Method) Posteromedial Soft Tissue Release with Temporary Internal Fixation** | | | | | |
| Bosch,[291] 1953 | 24 | 38 | 38 | 0 | 69 |
| Turco,[292] 1971 | 87 | 10 | 3 | 0 | 58 |
| Herring et al.,[293] 1977 | 55 | 33 | 12 | 0 | 72 |
| Imhauser,[285] 1980 | 72 | 21 | 7 | 0 | 204 |
| Bensahel et al.,[294] 1987 | 88 | 9 | 3 | 0 | 101 |
| Total | 65% | 22% | 13% | 0% | 504 |
| **D. Modified Turco (McKay or Carroll Method) or Posterior Medial Lateral Release with Temporary Internal Fixation** | | | | | |
| McKay,[295] 1983 | 82 | 3 | 15 | 0 | 55 |
| Magone et al.,[296] 1989 | 63 | 13 | 25 | 0 | 17 |
| Magone et al.,[296] 1989 | 46 | 17 | 38 | 0 | 24 |
| Magone et al.,[296] 1989 | 48 | 29 | 23 | 0 | 35 |
| Porat & Kaplan,[297] 1989 | 82 | 0 | 18 | 0 | 33 |
| Total | 64% | 12% | 24% | 0% | 164 |

dures and incomplete corrections, resulting in multiple operations and far less than satisfactory results (Table 6-12A and B). Since then, many "philosophies" regarding the morbid anatomy of clubfoot have evolved, resulting in different procedures that attack the pathology differently[259,292,295-297] (Table 6-12D). In our opinion, these most recent procedures, referred to as *modified Turco* or complete or comprehensive posteromedial and lateral soft tissue release, are much more similar than dissimilar, and all paralled Turco's one-stage posteromedial soft tissue release with temporary internal fixation[292] (Table 6-12C). In general, the data indicate that the best long-term satisfactory results are achieved when all the components of the deformity are released simultaneously. When the releases were limited solely to the apparent cause of the residual deformity, the results were less satisfactory.

Controversy over the timing of a comprehensive soft tissue release for idiopathic clubfoot correction exists throughout the literature. Turco[301] reported 84 percent good or excellent results in 149 feet of patients from 6 months to 8 years of age. He reported the best results and fewest complications especially overcorrection, in children undergoing surgery between the ages of 1 and 2 years. He claimed that this "delayed" surgery is technically less difficult and that toddler ambulation stimulates tarsal remodeling. His extensive study, however, did not separate the results of early (age under 6 months) versus late (age over 36 months) posteromedial releases. In addition, important variables such as flexibility of the initial deformity and specific postoperative management were not addressed.

Main et al.[302] noted 70 percent good results in 77 feet of children undergoing surgery at less than 6 months of age. These results are difficult to assess because two different surgical procedures were used (posterior and posteromedial releases) and additional surgery was performed on feet that did not have an initial satisfactory outcome.

Porat et al.[303] reported 82 percent good results with surgical correction performed on patients whose average age was 3 months versus only 23 percent favorable results in patients averaging 3 years, 7 months of age. However, direct comparisons in this study are difficult because the older patients had more rigid and severe deformities.

Ostremski et al.[304] published results of early and delayed posteromedial releases. Patients whose feet were operated on at over 9 months of age had a 50 percent

incidence of residual forefoot adductus, whereas 91 percent of patients who underwent surgery at an average age of 4 months achieved satisfactory correction of the adducted forefoot component.

In conclusion, treatment of the clubfoot should be directed toward giving the patient a lifelong functional foot with the least amount of deformity and disability. Approximately 52 percent of all clubfeet will respond favorably to nonoperative treatment by gentle manipulation and serial casting; the remaining 48 percent require some type of surgical intervention. The specific procedure performed should depend upon the degree of residual deformity that persists after a conservative treatment plateau has been reached. Each foot is unique, and the procedure, whether a posterior, posteromedial, or complete posteromediolateral release, should be adapted to the specific pathology present. Acceptable (fair, good, and excellent) clinical and radiographic results can be achieved in approximately 75 to 85 percent of cases by use of either an early or delayed soft tissue release, although a truly "normal" foot and leg are never achieved.

## Blakeslee and DeValentine 1990 Idiopathic Clubfoot Study

### Material and Methods

Over a 10-year-period (1978 to 1988) 248 infants with clubfoot deformities were hospitalized for surgical correction at Kaiser Foundation hospitals in northern California. Infants with nonidiopathic clubfoot were excluded from this study, as were patients with inadequate conservative therapy and/or incomplete hospital and outpatient records. Also excluded were children who were over 36 months of age at the time of surgery and/or were treated by procedures other than a single Turco-type posteromedial soft tissue release with internal fixation, as originally outlined by Turco,[289] followed by the appropriate postoperative management. This left a total of 45 patients with 63 idiopathic clubfeet (conservative manipulation and serial casting were unilaterally successful in three patients).

The parents of all patients completed a subjective questionnaire that provided insight relative to foot pain, limitations in activity, and overall satisfaction with the current result. Clinic and hospital records were reviewed to provide information regarding prenatal history, perinatal history, and family history of clubfoot.

**Table 6-13. Clubfoot Functional Rating System**

| Category | Points |
|---|---|
| 1. Hindfoot position | |
|     Neutral to 5 valgus | 5 |
|     >5 valgus | 3 |
|     varus | 0 |
| 2. Forefoot position | |
|     Neutral to 5 adducted | 3 |
|     >5 adducted | 0 |
| 3. Equinus | |
|     Dorsiflexion to 90+ | 5 |
|     <90 dorsiflexion | 0 |
| 4. Cavus | |
|     Absent | 5 |
|     Present | 0 |
| 5. Forefoot varus (supinated) | |
|     Absent | 3 |
|     Present | 0 |
| 6. Total ankle motion by radiographs | |
|     >40 | 25 |
|     31–40 | 20 |
|     21–30 | 15 |
|     11–20 | 8 |
|     <11 | 0 |
| 7. Flexion of hallux (toe purchase) | |
|     Present | 5 |
|     Absent | 0 |
| 8. Bimalleolar axis | |
|     75–85 | 10 |
|     70–74, 86–90 | 8 |
|     65–69, >90 | 4 |
|     <65 | 2 |
| 9. Heel walking | |
|     Present or not applicable[a] | 5 |
|     Absent | 0 |
| 10. Toe walking | |
|     Present or not applicable[a] | 5 |
|     Absent | 0 |
| 11. Pain | |
|     Never | 12 |
|     With heavy activity | 8 |
|     With routine activity | 6 |
|     With walking | 3 |
| 12. Function | |
|     Never limits | 12 |
|     Limits heavy activity | 8 |
|     Limits routine activity | 6 |
|     Limits walking | 3 |
| 13. Satisfaction | |
|     Satisfied | 5 |
|     Neither | 3 |
|     Dissatisfied | 0 |

[a] Child not penalized if too young to cooperate with task.
(From Magone et al.,[296] with permission.)

All 45 patients had a musculoskeletal and neurologic examination performed by an independent examiner who did participate in that patient's surgical cure (T.J.B.). Muscle strength, gait, active and passive ROM, residual deformity, and calf circumference were recorded. In addition, all patients had their feet traced to determine length and width differences as well as their bimalleolar axes (Fig. 6-5A).

Our radiographic evaluation included an anteroposterior and two lateral radiographs as standardized by Simons.[305–308] All patients were positioned by the same examiner (T.J.B.); the lateral radiographs were taken with the feet in maximum dorsiflexion and maximum plantar flexion, a hinged positioning device being used so that total available ankle joint motion was recorded. We also recorded any abnormalities in the position, shape, and nature of the tarsal bones. A functional rating system designed by Magone et al.,[296] with 100 points indicating a normal foot was used. This system intentionally weighs ankle motion and patient subjective responses in reference to pain and function more heavily than radiographic measurements (Table 6-13).

The results are classified according to the following scores: excellent, 90 to 100; good, 80 to 89; fair, 70 to 79; and poor, under 70.

## Results

### Clinical Results

The 45 patients in the study included 35 boys (78 percent) and 10 girls (22 percent); 27 (60 percent) were white, 10 (22 percent) were Hispanic, and 8 (18 percent) were black. The parents of 7 percent of the patients could confirm the incidence of idiopathic clubfoot within their nuclear or extended families.

The average age at operation was 12.4 months, with a range of 5 to 36 months. Average postoperative follow-up was 67.2 months. At the time of this study no patient had a recurrence of deformity significant enough to warrant additional surgery. Of the 63 affected feet, 34 (54 percent) were right and 29 (46 percent) were left feet. Bilateral clubfoot was present in 18 of the 45 patients (40 percent).

In all patients with unilateral clubfoot, the normal foot was longer and wider than the clubfoot and the circumference of the leg was greater on the normal side than on the side with the clubfoot. The mean difference between the lengths of the feet was 1.4 cm, that between the widths of the feet was 0.7 cm, and that between the

Table 6-14. **Results of Idiopathic Clubfoot Study Based on Radiographic Criteria (Mean values)**

| Functional Rating Score | No. and % of Feet | AP[a] | | Lat[a] | Age at Surgery (months) | Follow-up Duration (months) | Talocalcaneal Index | Bimalleolar Axis, Mean (degrees) | Ankle Joint ROM (degrees) |
| | | TC[a] Angle Mean (degrees) | T-1MT[a] Angle Mean (degrees) | TC Angle Mean (degrees) | | | | | |
|---|---|---|---|---|---|---|---|---|---|
| Normal | | 20–40 | 0–(−20) | 35–50 | | | 40–85 | 75–85 | >40 |
| 90–100 | 29 (46%) | 23.1 | −1.1 | 38.8 | 11.1 | 55.5 | 61.9 | 79.0 | 36.1 |
| 80–89 | 15 (24%) | 20.3 | +5.8 | 37.4 | 14.7 | 64.1 | 57.7 | 73.3 | 28.5 |
| 70–79 | 8 (13%) | 21.9 | +3.4 | 41.1 | 7.9 | 74.6 | 63.0 | 72.9 | 17.8 |
| <70 | 11 (17%) | 13.9 | +11.6 | 38.5 | 12.2 | 96.2 | 52.4 | 67.8 | 25.4 |

[a] Abbreviations: AP, anteroposterior; Lat, lateral; TC, talocalcaneal; T-1MT, talo-first metatarsal.

circumferences of the legs was 2.1 cm. Physical examination showed that all patients had well formed sinus tarsi laterally, normal bony prominences medially, and good heel formation; 3.2 percent had residual hindfoot varus, 3.2 percent had residual equinus, 22.2 percent had cavus, 22.2 percent had residual forefoot varus, and 41.3 percent had residual forefoot adductus. Our measured value for the bimalleolar axis in the 63 clubfeet averaged 74.9 degrees.

The mean functional rating score was 84.0 points, with a standard deviation of 11.9 and a range of 52 to 100 points. The results were rated as excellent in 46 percent of the feet, good in 24 percent, fair in 13 percent, and poor in 17 percent. In 95 percent of cases the parents were satisfied with the current result, although 59 percent believed that their child would have physical limitations in the future, and 40 percent of the patients stated that they occasionally experienced pain that caused limping.

### Radiographic Results

Tables 6-14 and 6-15 summarize the pertinent results of our radiographic evaluation as compared with the functional rating subgroups excellent, good, fair, and poor. Both the anteroposterior and lateral talocalcaneal angles

reflect the hindfoot position. The anteroposterior talo-first metatarsal angle used in conjunction with the anteroposterior talocalcaneal angle can provide information regarding the congruity of the talonavicular joint.

Of the 63 clubfeet, 56 (89 percent) had an ossified navicular, and 9 (14.3 percent) revealed signs suggestive of avascular necrosis of the navicular. Only 37 feet (58.7 percent) exhibited normal talonavicular joint congruity, while 22 feet (34.9 percent) revealed dorsal subluxation. Three feet (4.8 percent) were displaced medially (undercorrected) by one-third of the talar head, and one foot (1.6 percent) was laterally displaced (overcorrected) by one-third of the talar head. In 33 feet (52.4 percent) there was some degree of abnormal talar dome flattening.

### Discussion

This study demonstrates the well known and complex interrelationships between the different components of the pathologic anatomy that persist after successful surgical correction of idiopathic clubfeet. However, drawing any specific conclusions from our research is difficult owing to our small number of cases (63 feet) and our short average follow-up period of approximately 6.5 years. Ideally, this study should be repeated when these 45 patients become skeletally mature adults. When results of clubfoot surgery are discussed, one frequently hears the statement: That foot looks good — for a clubfoot. Our goal in clubfoot management, regardless of the method of treatment, is to approach the condition of a normal foot as closely as possible, not only in terms of static deformity but, more importantly, in terms of dynamic functional results. However, especially in unilateral idiopathic clubfoot, the calf and foot will almost always be smaller than the contralateral normal side because of the primary muscle pathology.[272,309,310] Histori-

Table 6-15. **Comparison of Radiographic Results with Functional Rating Subgroups**

| Score | Incidence of Flat-Top Talus, % | Incidence of Navicular Dorsal Subluxation, % |
|---|---|---|
| 90–100 | 37.9 | 34.5 |
| 80–89 | 73.3 | 46.7 |
| 70–79 | 37.5 | 50.0 |
| <70 | 72.7 | 45.5 |

cally, corrective clubfoot assessment studies have given little consideration to dynamic foot function while focusing on correction of the static deformity; i.e., evaluation of traditional radiographic tarsal relationships (talocalcaneal and talo-first metatarsal angles). In our attempt to answer the question of what features constitute a good functional clubfoot, we utilized Magone et al.'s[296] progressive rating system for the assessment of the postoperative clubfoot, which weighs functional results most heavily.

Total ankle joint motion as measured on standardized lateral radiographs is worth up to 25 of the total possible 100 points. A criticism of operatively treated clubfeet is their stiffness and decreased ankle joint motion. Radiographic studies of these children have shown that most plantar flexion and dorsiflexion occurs not in the ankle joint but in the midtarsal joint. Giannestras[311] considers 60 degrees to be the normal ankle motion in children. Stauffer et al.[312] reported that the average ankle ROM during normal walking is 24.4 degrees. Simons[313] in 1990 compared radiographic true ankle motion in clubfeet prospectively, both preoperatively and after posteromedial release. Average preoperative ROM was 31 degrees; postoperatively ROM was 29 degrees, but the arc of motion was directed more toward dorsiflexion by 10 degrees. Our average postoperative ankle ROM was 30.1 degrees, and we found a direct relationship to exist between the ankle joint ROM and the functional rating score: patients with the best functional results had more ankle joint ROM (36.1 degrees), as well as a lower incidence of navicular dorsal subluxation (34.5 percent) and flat-top talar changes (37.9 percent). Morever, a calcaneal gait secondary to possible overlengthening of the Achilles tendon was not seen in any of our 63 cases.

Simons[314] has shown that pinning of the navicular in a dorsally subluxed position at the time of operation causes long-term incongruity and is closely associated with a cavus foot type. He reports that this problem may not become apparent until years after the operation, when the foot enlarges and the patient develops shoe wear trouble because of the high arch. Our findings support this conclusion, indicating a direct correlation between cavus deformity and dorsal navicular subluxation.

Simons[315] and Staheli[316] have documented the high incidence of residual forefoot adductus and persistent in-toeing in clubfeet that have received successful operative treatment, in conjunction with a posteriorly positioned lateral malleolus. This medially spun foot and lat-

erally rotated talus (horizontal breach) may illustrate the persistent intrinsic deformity within the talus as well as reflect the limitations of all soft tissue releases that do not directly address this level of pathology. Residual forefoot adductus was present in 41.3 percent of our patients, although the average bimalleolar axis approached the normal range at 75.9 degrees (standard deviation 7.1). Patients with the best functional results (7 out of 29, or 24 percent) had the highest average bimalleolar axis (79.0 degrees) and the least amount of residual forefoot adductus. Morever, these patients, who were within the excellent subgroup, exhibited no residual hindfoot varus, equinus, or cavus deformities.

In summary, three general conclusions can be drawn from our study. First, our results (83 percent acceptable) are comparable with those of other studies using similar materials, methods, and assessment criteria. Second, an inverse relationship exists between the functional rating score and the length of follow-up (i.e.; acceptable results decrease over time as the patient approaches skeletal maturity). Third, anatomic realignment of the talocalcaneo-navicular joint complex is directly correlated to better functional results.

# COMPLICATIONS

## FLAIR D. GOLDMAN
## PAUL D. DAYTON

The early diagnosis and management of the diverse group of deformities that may occur as the result of the treatment of patients with congenital clubfoot requires considerable experience and insight. Unsatisfactory results are often not obvious until the child is older and the foot is skeletally more mature, by which time the opportunity for less drastic forms of treatment has passed. A thorough knowledge of potential complications will aid the astute clinician in anticipating their occurrence and in early management. It is equally important to keep parents completely informed of the treatment plan and the child's prognosis. All parties need to be aware of the complexity of clubfoot management and accept the reality that treatment may involve multiple nonoperative and/or operative procedures. In fact, a "normal" foot is not likely to be obtainable; the goal of providing a pain-free plantigrade foot is more realistic.

## Complications of Nonoperative Treatment

### Skin Complications

An infant's skin is sensitive to many environmental irritants. Sensitivity to skin adherent used in serial casting is not unusual. A primary irritant dermatitis is uncomfortable for the child and can predispose to secondary bacterial infection. If dermatitis develops, skin adherents should be immediately discontinued. Temporary cessation of cast therapy and topical treatment of dermatitis may occasionally be necessary.

Pressure blisters, ulcerations, and full thickness necrosis are rare complications of serial casting. Poorly padded or molded casts with sharp edges provide the source for these mechanical abrasions. We have also seen mechanically induced paronychia, which has resulted from casts molded around the distal aspect of a digit. The need for adequate padding to avoid pressure on prominent areas must be balanced against the requirement of good plaster contact for transmission of corrective forces. The practitioner must be aware of this potential iatrogenic complication and not hesitate to remove or replace a cast if the baby is unusually fussy. In the majority of cases discontinuation of casting and local wound care constitute adequate therapy to allow healing.

### Rocker Bottom Foot

Rocker bottom foot occurs when external forces designed to produce dorsiflexion at the ankle are resisted by contracted posterior ankle soft tissues, resulting in dorsiflexion at the midfoot. This iatrogenic result of overzealous casting can cause significant foot deformity with functional deficit and pain in the older child and adult. Early rocker bottom deformity may not be readily evident in the small, pudgy infant foot. Initially there is loss of the normal longitudinal arch. The heel remains in fixed equinovarus as the forefoot is dorsiflexed at the midfoot. Plantar prominence and abnormal motion at the midfoot joints may be appreciated.

A similar deformity may develop in the ambulatory child with residual hindfoot equinus as weight-bearing forces transmitted through the forefoot produce a compensatory midfoot dorsiflexion. Additionally, we (Goldman and Dayton) have noted developmental dorsal deviation of the fifth metatarsal bone secondary to residual equinovarus in several patients. This gives the clinical appearance of a rocker bottom foot (Fig. 6-21).

Radiographically the deformity is marked by increased or negative (reversed) angle between the inferior surface of the calcaneus and the fifth metatarsal. Normally this angle measures approximately 140 degrees or more. Stress dorsiflexion radiography will demonstrate the midfoot break as the axis of the talus (as well as the parallel calcaneus) assumes a plantar-flexed position relative to the forefoot (Fig. 6-22).

Kite believed that sequential casting of the triad of deformities in clubfoot, starting with forefoot adductus and ending with reduction of the equinus only when the forefoot is totally corrected, prevents this harmful complication.[317] This has been disputed by other authors. Wesely et al. recognized that in certain cases even though the midfoot and rearfoot may be well aligned, the amount of force necessary to oppose the equinus produces a midfoot break regardless of the care taken.[318] Realistically, in the case of significant firm equinus it is difficult to apply force from plaster to the small, dorsally

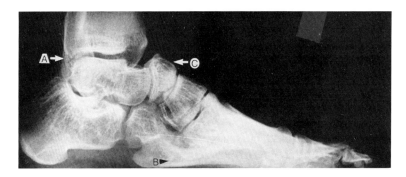

**Fig. 6-21.** Treated clubfoot at skeletal maturity. Arrow A shows flattening of the trochlear surface of the talus; arrow B shows developmental dorsal deviation of the fifth metatarsal. Arrow C shows wedging and dorsal subluxation of the navicular.

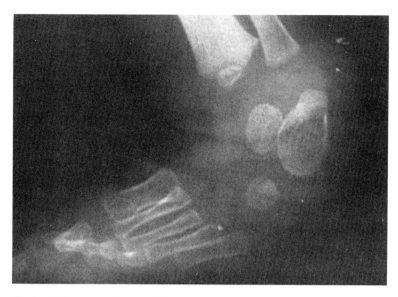

**Fig. 6-22.** Rocker deformity. Note dorsiflexion of the midfoot, while the hindfoot remains in equinus.

recessed heel. Consequently, a great deal of force is applied through the midtarsal joint and forefoot in an attempt to stretch the posterior structures. Our experience has been similar to that of Weseley et al.[318] in that inability to reduce equinus is usually the cause of failure of conservative therapy. Avoidance of exposure to surgical risks is usually the factor that leads many practitioners to continue casting in these patients to a point at which adverse effects may outweigh corrective forces. Soft tissue release should not be delayed when hindfoot equinus persists and is a more conservative approach than overly forcible manipulation! We have successfully treated rocker deformity early in its course by posterior medial release, with or without midfoot release, followed by Kirschner wire fixation and casting. Although satisfactory results were obtained, avoidance of this complication is preferred. When the rocker deformity is not recognized and treated early in its course, it becomes fixed, necessitating osteotomy and/or fusion.

**Flat-Top Talus**

When a dorsiflexion force placed on the forefoot is resisted by contracted posterior soft tissues, the immature cartilaginous talar body can be crushed. Keim and Ritchie compared the talus to a walnut in a nutcracker.[319] The result is an osteochondral compression fracture and flattening of the trochlear surface of the talus (Fig. 6-21).

Keim and Ritchie[319] classified the degree of deformity as follows: (1) mild, in which some convexity of the upper talus is lost but height is retained; (2) moderate, in which superior convexity is lost (may be concave), with minimal height loss; and (3) severe, which involves compression to 50 percent of normal height along with subtalar or tibial changes.

Swann et al. believed that the external rotation of the talus within the ankle mortise in clubfoot deformity can produce the illusion of flat-top talus by the overlapping of the medial and lateral lobes of the talar trochlear surface.[320] Dunn and Samuelson evaluated 12 treated clubfeet with multiple oblique lateral views to prevent an illusion of flattening and showed true flat-top talus deformity to be present in all 12 cases.[321] To avoid the radiographic illusion of flat-top talus, they recommended that lateral radiographs be taken with the foot internally rotated so that the medial and lateral malleoli are superimposed.

The true incidence of flat-top talus deformity is unknown. It has been our experience that a mild degree of flattening occurs in most clubfeet regardless of treatment. This may suggest that changes in the contour of the talar dome occur during early stages of development or with very early treatment. The result of talar dome flattening is decreased total ROM of the ankle joint. Although loss of this important function of gait may preclude certain athletic and occupational activities, pain and disability are rare unless the deformity is marked. Compensation for lost ankle dorsiflexion is seen in several forms: accessory dorsiflexion at the midfoot, adaptation of the forefoot bones, recurvatum of the knee, and abnormal gait. This deformity can be prevented through gentle casting technique, avoidance of manipulation under anesthesia, and early posterior release. Severe disabling pain is managed with tibiotalar fusion.

### Fracture

The delicate bones of the neonate are easily overpowered by the hands of the surgeon. Care must be taken if fracture and epiphyseal injury are to be avoided. Weseley et al. described fracture of the distal tibia and fibula in four cases as a result of forceful casting; they recommend early posterior release in cases resistant to firm manipulation.[318] Miller and Bernstein described wedging of the distal tibial epiphysis following overzealous serial casting and warned that this can lead to disabling valgus ankle deformity.[322] We have noted one case of fracture of the medial cuneiform secondary to casting (Fig. 6-23). We have not seen this described previously.

When bone injury is noted, manipulation should be discontinued and soft tissue release performed to relieve the destructive forces on the bone. An abnormal weight-bearing force at the distal tibial epophysis caused by an overcorrected, laterally displaced hindfoot requires correction by balancing osteotomy and/or tendon transfer. Manipulation under anesthesia holds great potential for fracture and is best avoided.

### Navicular Wedging

Wedging or truncation of the navicular on the lateral radiographic projection as described by Miller and Bernstein is a common occurrence secondary to forceful manipulation.[322] Dorsal dislocation of the navicular on the talus is found with similar frequency. Radiographically, the appearance on the lateral projection is a wedge-shaped navicular, based dorsally (Fig. 6-21). The ossification center may be fragmented, indicating the presence of avascular necrosis (AVN). Wedging may also be

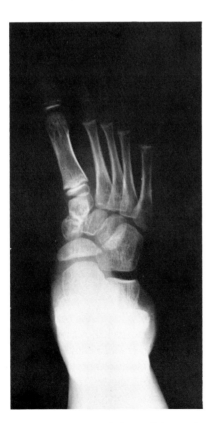

**Fig. 6-23.** Fracture of the medial cuneiform.

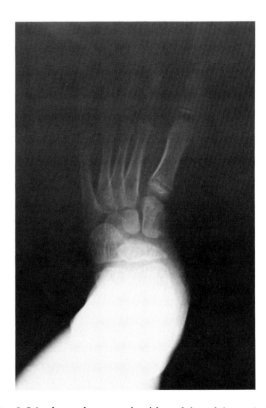

**Fig. 6-24.** Avascular necrosis with wedging of the navicular.

seen in the anteroposterior projection again caused by forceful angulation of the forefoot (Fig. 6-24).

Pain and/or disability have not been specifically associated with this deformity, and operative treatment to improve navicular position is not recommended. Operative treatment of clubfoot is also well known to cause subluxation and deformity of the navicular, as will be discussed below.

## Complications of Operative Treatment

### Wound Complications

Congenital contractures of the lower extremity involve not only tendons, ligaments, and bones but also the overlying skin. Release and lengthening of the deep structures can lead to problems with skin closure. Care should be taken to plan incisions that provide adequate exposure without producing excessive skin tension during closure. Preoperative serial casting can also help by stretching the overlying skin.

Soft tissue wound complications are most often attributed to problems with tissue handling (e.g., crushing of tissues, nonanatomic dissection, wound hematoma, excessive skin tension, and excessive operation time). The skin and subcutaneous tissues should be elevated from the deep fascia as a single layer to preserve maximal vascular supply to the skin and should be gently retracted during operation. The posterior tibial neurovascular bundle should be completely mobilized from surrounding soft tissues and allowed to "float free" during closure to minimize traction ischemia. Excessive tension should be avoided during skin closure. The pneumatic tourniquet should be released prior to closure, complete hemostasis should be obtained, and a posterior tibial pulse and well vascularized skin flaps should be present with the foot in the corrected position. When adequate circulation is not re-established, it may be necessary to cast the foot in an incompletely corrected position of slight equinus (internal fixation is imperative to retain osseous correction). Complete reduction can be achieved by serial cast changes under anesthesia. When postoperative serial casting is necessary, sutures should be left in place for a prolonged period. Turco found that wound dehiscence is much less likely if sutures are left for 6 weeks.[323] In some cases (severe deformity or an older child) it may be necessary to leave a portion of the wound open, allowing healing by granulation or by primary or delayed primary split thickness skin grafting.

### Avascular Necrosis

AVN results when normal periosteal and endosteal bone blood flow is interrupted. Trauma from casting, as well as surgical trauma inflicted on the bones of the foot, has led to this complication. Reports of AVN of the navicular, talus, and calcaneus are found in the literature.[324-326]

Navicular ossification does not normally occur until 3 to 4 years of age. This and the fact that the center of ossification can appear fragmented in the normal foot make the diagnosis of AVN difficult. AVN may result in late appearance of navicular ossification, deformity of the bone, fragmentation, sclerosis, and degenerative arthritis. In view of the amount of dissection usually necessary to relocate the navicular on the talus and the force produced with casting, it is surprising that this finding is not more common. In fact, Magone et al. found the incidence of navicular avascular necrosis to be 1 in 17 to 25 cases, depending on the procedure used.[326]

The talus lacks muscular attachment and therefore receives its entire nutrient blood supply from a series of independent perforating vessels. The anatomy of this vascular network is well known, as are reports of AVN of the talus following trauma, surgery, infection, or steroid therapy and as a result of undetermined causes. Extensive dissection, which is required in clubfoot surgery, poses a significant risk for disturbance of the tenuous talar vascular network. Repeat surgery has also been associated with a higher incidence of AVN. Concomitant subtalar and sinus tarsi dissection should be avoided if possible, and lateral release should be judiciously performed when extensive subtalar dissection has been necessary medially. AVN of the talus may result in limited ankle and subtalar joint motion and degenerative arthritis and may require fusion after skeletal maturity. When AVN is detected in its early stages in children, it should be treated with protected weight-bearing (e.g., ankle-foot orthosis [AFO] or the patellar tendon-bearing type of AFO) until revascularization occurs, which may take up to 3 years.

### Navicular Subluxation

Late ossification of the navicular prevents plain film radiographic evaluation of its pre- and postoperative position in the child under age 3. An eccentric position of the center of ossification in the navicular also increases the difficulty of evaluating its position when ossification has begun. Additionally, AVN secondary to surgical or manipulation trauma may delay the onset of ossification.

The incidence of subluxation of the navicular following conservative as well as surgical treatment is high. Schlafly et al.[325] reported 43 percent dorsal dislocation following posteromedial release. These dislocations included up to 50 percent of the navicular body. Medial and lateral subluxations were also noted but less commonly. Ponseti and Becher[327] noted 34 percent dislocation following Achilles tendon lengthening and casting, although they graded it as mild and noted no disability. Schlafly et al.[325] as well as Magone et al.[326] this subluxation, when marked, to be due to surgical error in placement and fixation of the navicular on the talar head rather than to sequential migration over time. Turco[323] has noted the difficulty in finding the optimal position of the navicular in relation to the deformed head of the clubfoot talus during posteromedial release.

In most cases dorsal navicular subluxation seems to have a lesser effect on the functional success of the procedure than does medial displacement. Medial dislocation carries the highest risk for pain and disability. Dorsal and lateral dislocation produce a cavus appearance of the foot and may present shoe wear difficulties due to dorsal prominence. Pain and disability are rare in dorsal subluxation unless the navicular impinges on the distal tibia, thereby limiting ankle joint motion (Fig. 6-25).

Our experience is consistent with previous authors who find no need for reoperation to improve dorsal or lateral navicular position. In fact, some authors recommend against any attempt at surgical reduction of dorsal or lateral navicular position.[325] On the other hand, medial subluxation, which has a relatively high incidence of adverse sequelae and probably indicates undercorrection of the clubfoot, can be addressed by additional posterior or medial release surgery.

### Persistent Metatarsus Adductus

It has been our experience and that of others that forefoot adduction associated with clubfoot is often persistent following posteromedial release.[328-330] On the other hand, it has been reported that 85 percent or more of neonatal cases of isolated metatarsus adductus resolve spontaneously.[327] This suggests that these two deformities are distinct entities and may require two separate and distinct management approaches. Radiographic evaluation of a group of treated clubfeet showed persistent adductus in 74 percent and clinical evidence in 52 percent.[329]

The cause of persistent metatarsus adductus is usually failure to address the forefoot deformity with a separate and specific procedure when the initial rearfoot release surgery is performed. Tayton and Thompson[331] noted the inability of the posteromedial release operation to effect positional change in forefoot deformity distal to the navicular. Additionally, this deformity may be induced in isolated instances by inadvertent release of the peroneus longus tendon from its plantar medial attachments, allowing the anterior tibial tendon to pull the forefoot into adductus and varus. It has also been suggested, but not universally accepted, that weak peroneal tendons may be an inherent component of the clubfoot and a component factor in the development of the deformity.

Persistent adductus is a troublesome complication, as the child retains a clumsy, intoed gait. Compensation places significant external rotatory forces on the ankle, knee, and hip. Additionally, there are resultant pronatory forces on the midfoot and hindfoot that procduce the difficult to treat serpentine ("Z") foot deformity. In our experience, persistent forefoot adductus has occurred relatively frequently and has necessitated prolonged casting or shoe therapy and in some cases surgical intervention. Procedures that are useful in treating this deformity are dependent on its severity and the age of the child; Approaches that have been advocated for the treatment of metatarsus adductus include release of tarsometatarsal joints,[332] release of the abductor hallucis[327] and osteotomy of the metatarsals[333,334] or of the cuboid[335,336] and/or the cuneiforms.[337] Tarsometatarsal release has been used successfully in our practice in children up to the age of 6 years.

Recently we have used multiple opening wedge osteotomies to correct forefoot adductus in the older child, as described by Rab.[338] The osteotomy is made with the lateral cortex kept intact. The forefoot is then shifted laterally as a unit and pinned through the first and fifth metatarsals. The pins are left for 6 to 8 weeks, and casting is continued for a total of 3 months. Osteotomy, with wedge resection and/or decancellization of the cuboid, can also be used to effectively shorten the lateral column. The Evans[335] closing wedge resection and fusion of the calcaneocuboid joint not only shortens the lateral column, thereby correcting the forefoot, but also provides stability through fusion. We have used a similar approach in which a wedge is resected from the cuboid and inserted into the navicular (Fig. 6-26). When degen-

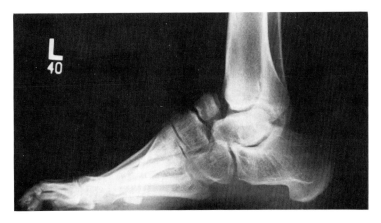

**Fig. 6-25.** Complete dorsal dislocation of the navicular with ankle joint impingement.

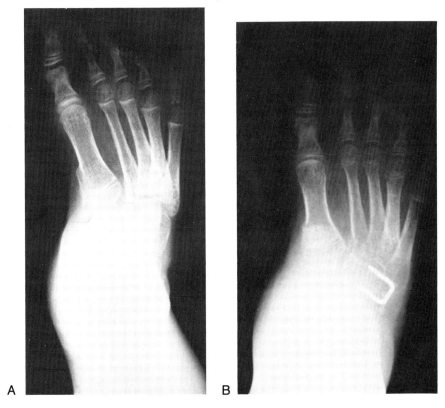

A                    B

**Fig. 6-26.** **(A)** Residual metatarsus adductus. **(B)** After correction by wedge resection from the cuboid with wedge insertion in the navicular.

erative changes in the hindfoot joints are advanced, triple arthrodesis with appropriate wedging may be necessary.

It has been suggested that the adducted forefoot be addressed during the initial posteromedial release operation by adductor muscle release and tenotomy,[328] and/ or tarsometatarsal release.[331] Ostremski et al. specifically addressed this deformity with a plantar fascial and short flexor release and achieved improved results over the standard posteromedial release.[328] Specifically addressing this component of the clubfoot may improve the overall success rate of one-stage correction.

### Persistent Equinovarus

Unless the original equinovarus deformity is due to a progressive neuromuscular imbalance, persistent equinovarus results from failure to obtain adequate correction at the original surgery or failure to maintain correction postoperatively. The approach to management of recurrent clubfoot deformity has been described in connection with operative treatment of recurrent or residual equinovarus deformity.

### Calcaneus Deformity

The *calcaneus foot* can be defined as a foot that has an extremely high calcaneal inclination angle and that in its most severe form lacks plantar flexion and the ability to bear weight on the forefoot (Fig. 6-27A). Calcaneus deformity is one of the most devastating complications of clubfoot surgery and one of the most difficult to manage. Such a foot bears all its weight on the posterior heel, functioning much as does a foot that has had a Symes amputation. Compensation occurs through knee flexion in an attempt to make the foot plantigrade. Calcaneus deformity often develops insidiously and is usually progressive, which adds to the overall morbidity of this condition.

The true incidence of calcaneus after clubfoot repair is difficult to determine. The literature contains only sporadic case reports, and many series do not mention this or other specific complications. Wijesinha and Menelaus[339] reported 3 cases in "approximately 500"; Aronson and Puskarich[340] reported 2 cases in a series of 29; and Simons[341] reported 6 cases in 34. With a high index of suspicion and critical evaluation of postoperative results, this deformity may be recognized as more prevalent than once realized.

The most common cause of calcaneus deformity following clubfoot repair is weakening of the triceps surae muscle group by overlengthening of the Achilles tendon

and overcorrection of the deformity with pin and cast fixation (Fig. 6-28). Simons states that calcaneus deformity can be prevented by pinning the calcaneus and talus with the posterior part of the subtalar joint closed, repairing the Achilles tendon at a maximum of 10 degrees of ankle dorsiflexion, and addressing anterior ankle joint contracture before complete subtalar joint release.[341] The loss of the normal length-tension relationship of the gastrosoleus muscle group, combined with strong intrinsic muscles and the remaining long flexor muscles that insert into the forefoot (peroneals, flexor hallucis longus, flexor digitorum longus, and posterior tibial) results in a progressive calcaneus (vertical) migration of the heel. As the calcaneus becomes more vertical, the triceps surae lever arm is further weakened and the progression of the deformity is perpetuated. Secondary contracture of the plantar fascia reinforces the deformity. The neurogenic calcaneus deformity is usually accompanied by cavus and varus or valgus heel deformity, which results from long flexor muscle contracture. The long flexor muscles are often released or severely weakened in clubfoot surgery, so that forefoot equinus and frontal plane heel deformity may not be present.

Once calcaneus deformity is recognized, early operation may allow the child's remaining growth to aid in correction rather than perpetuate this deformity. A combination of the following surgical techniques may be needed: extensor tendon and ankle capsule release or lengthening; Achilles tendon shortening; posterior transfer of anterior muscles (i.e., the peroneals and anterior tibial); and posterosuperior displacement osteotomy of the calcaneus.[342,343] We have treated two such patients, one with pure calcaneus deformity and the other also having varus rotation and adduction of the forefoot. Both were successfully managed by anterior ankle joint release; lengthening of the extensor hallucis longus, extensor digitorum longus, and anterior tibial muscles; and shortening of the Achilles tendon. The more severe case required a superior displacement osteotomy of the calcaneus, osteotomy with wedge excision of the cuboid, and osteotomy with dorsal medial wedge placement in the navicular.

### Pes Plano Valgus

Overcorrection or excessive lateral shift of the calcaneus on the talus during posteromedial release surgery will result in hindfoot valgus. Although a mild to moderate amount of hindfoot valgus is well tolerated by children

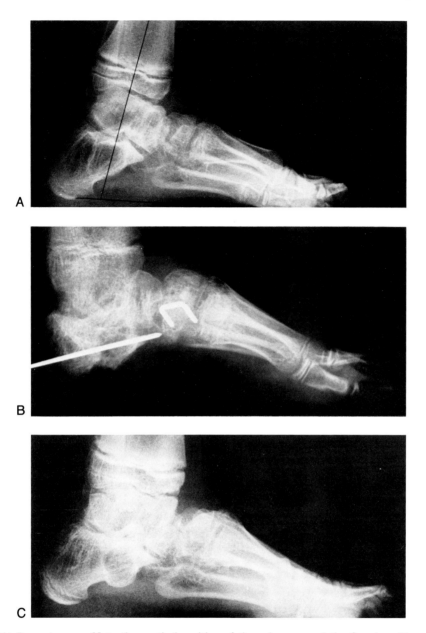

**Fig. 6-27. (A)** Pes calcaneus. Note the vertical position of the calcaneus and the flexed position of the leg on weight-bearing lateral radiograph. **(B)** Postoperative lateral, showing superior displacement osteotomy of the calcaneus and plantar forefoot displacement. **(C)** Three years post surgery, with decreased cavus attitude of the hindfoot and forefoot able to bear weight.

and adults, collapsing pes plano valgus can prove to be a painful and difficult to treat problem. With the subtalar joint axis lateral to the body's center of gravity, growth and increasing body weight contribute to and perpetuate the valgus deformity. The distal tibial epiphysis may be wedged in valgus as well (Fig. 6-29).

The incidence of this deformity has not been adequately determined. Although most practitioners treating clubfoot recognize pes valgus as a potential hazard, few have quantified its incidence. McKay noted lateral calcaneal displacement following clubfoot surgeries that included extensive subtalar release in five cases.[344] He

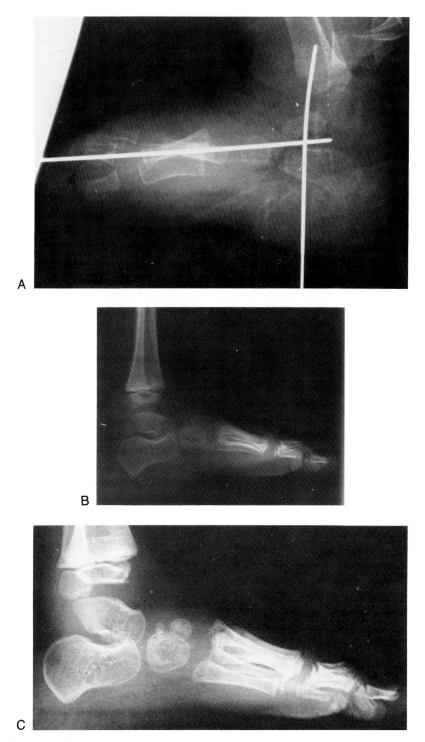

**Fig. 6-28.** (A) Postoperative lateral, showing overcorrection of hindfoot equinus. (B) Appearance of patient in Fig. 6-8, 2 years post surgery. Note lack of ground purchase of the forefoot on this weight-bearing lateral view. (C) Following correction by Achilles tendon shortening.

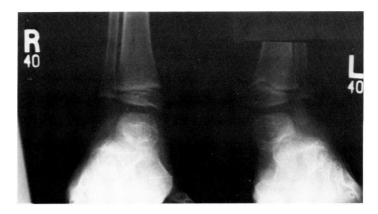

**Fig. 6-29.** Overcorrection, with lateral displacement of the calcaneus on the talus. Note also the wedging of the distal tibial epiphysis in valgus.

found no such complication when this extensive release was not performed. Porat and Kaplan noted a 9 percent incidence of overcorrected hindfoot in 33 surgically treated clubfeet.[345] Many practitioners agree that this deformity is intimately linked to surgical technique and specifically to the adequacy of anatomic reduction of the talus and calcaneus.

The role of the interosseus talocalcaneal ligament release in the overcorrected clubfoot has been discussed by McKay.[344] Since a high incidence of lateral calcaneal shift has followed release of this ligament, he recommends limited release in all cases except those in which correction can not be otherwise obtained. Simons[341] noted that release of this ligament did not make the subtalar joint perceptibly less stable than with the ligament unreleased but that the lateral shift of the calcaneus was secondary to poor surgical reduction. That is, the motion in the subtalar joint was limited to the same degree in cases in which the ligament was released as in those in which it was not. Lateral or valgus shift of the hindfoot therefore results from poor surgical reduction rather than from progressive shift secondary to instability.

Hindfoot valgus is produced by excessive eversion or lateral translocation of the calcaneus, without reduction of the rotational component of the subtalar joint deformity as recommended by McKay[344] and Simons.[341] If the body of the calcaneus is externally rotated about an imaginary vertical axis through the subtalar joint and also everted slightly, the subtalar joint axis is not translocated far medial to the body's center of gravity, and severe collapsing pes plano valgus will not occur.

Mild hindfoot valgus is usually asymptomatic and re-

quires no intervention. Conservative and/or surgical intervention is necessary when the deformity leads to functional disability or pain. The operative treatment of flatfoot is discussed in Chapter 14.

# REFERENCES

## History

1. Bosch J: Operative oder konservative Klumpfussbehandlung. Z Orthop 83:8, 1953
2. McKay DW: New concept of and approach to clubfoot treatment. I. Principles and morbid anatomy. J Pediatr Orthop 2:347, 1982
3. Simons GW, Sarrafian S: The microsurgical dissection of a stillborn fetal clubfoot. Clin Orthop 173:275, 1983
4. Lyons AS, Petrucelli RJ: Medicine. An Illustrated History. Harry N. Abrams, New York, 1978
5. Strach EH: Club-foot through the centuries. p. 215. In Rickham, PP (ed): Progress in Pediatric Surgery. Springer-Verlag, Berlin, 1986
6. Mann RW, Owsley DW: Anatomy of uncorrected talipes equinovarus in a fifteenth-century American Indian. J Am Podiatr Med Assoc 79:436, 1989
7. Hippocrates: The Genuine Works of Hippocrates. Williams & Wilkins, Baltimore, 1939
8. Scarpa A: Memoirs on Congenital Clubfeet. A. Constable, Edinburgh, 1818
9. Stromeyer, L: The classic contribution to operative orthopedics or experiences with subcutaneous section of shortened muscles and their tendons. Clin Orthop 97:2, 1973
10. Little WJ: Preface to A Treatise on the Nature of Club-

Foot and Analogous Distorsions, Including Their Treatment Both with and without Surgical Operation (1839). In The Classic. Clin Orthop 233:3, 1988

11. Kite JH: The treatment of congenital club-feet. Surg Gynecol Obstet:190, 1933

12. Kite JH: Principles involved in treatment of clubfoot. J Bone Joint Surg 2:595, 1939

13. Kite JH: The Clubfoot. Grune & Stratton, Orlando, FL, 1964

14. Kite JH: Non-operative treatment of congenital clubfoot. Clin Orthop 70:79, 1970

15. Phelps AM: International Congress of Medical Science, Copenhagen, 1884

16. Codvilla A: Tendon transplant in orthopaedic practice. The Classic. Clin Orthop 118:2, 1976

17. Brockman FP: Modern methods of treatment of clubfoot. Br Med J 2:572, 1937

18. Bost FC, Schottstaedt ER, Larsen LJ: Plantar dissection. An operation to release the soft tissues in recurrent or recalcitrant talipes equinovarus. JBJS 42:151, 1960

19. Attenborough, CG: Severe congenital talipes equinovarus. J Bone Joint Surg [Br] 48(1):31, 1966

20. Goldner JL: Congenital talipes equinovarus—fifteen years of surgical treatment. Curr Pract Orthop Surg 4:61, 1969

21. Turco VJ: Surgical correction of the resistant club foot. One-stage posteromedial release with internal fixation: a preliminary report. J Bone Joint Surg [Am] 53A:477, 1971

22. McKay DW: New concept of and approach to clubfoot treatment. I. Principles and morbid anatomy. J Pediatr Orthop 2:347, 1982

23. McKay DW: New concept of and approach to clubfoot treatment. II. Correction of the clubfoot. J Pediatr Orthop 3:10, 1983

24. McKay DW: New concept of and approach to clubfoot treatment. III. Evaluation and results. J Pediatr Orthop 3:141, 1983

25. Simons GW: Complete subtalar release in club feet. I. A prelimanary report. J Bone Joint Surg [Am] 67A:1044, 1985

26. Simons GW: Complete subtalar release in club feet. II. Comparison with less extensive procedures. J Bone Joint Surg [Am] 67A:1056, 1985

## Incidence

27. Congenital Malformations Surveillance: Jan-Dec, 1977. U. S. Public Health Service, Atlanta, Georgia

28. Stewart SF: Clubfoot: its incidence, cause, and treatment. J Bone Joint Surg [Am] 33A:577, 1951

29. Chung CS, Menecheck RW, Larsen IJ, Ching GHS: Genetic and epidemiological studies of clubfoot in Hawaii, general and medical considerations. Hum Hered 19:321, 1969

30. Wynne-Davies R: Heritable Disorders in Orthopaedic Practice. Blackwell Scientific Publications, Oxford, 1973

31. Tachdjian MO: The Child's Foot. WB Saunders, Philadelphia, 1985

32. Kite JH: Principles involved in treatment of clubfoot. J Bone Joint Surg 2:595, 1939

33. Turco VJ: Surgical correction of the resistant clubfoot. One-stage posteromedial release with internal fixation: a preliminary report. J Bone Joint Surg [Am] 53A:477, 1971

34. Wynne-Davies R: Family studies and the cause of congenital clubfoot. J Bone Joint Surg [Br] 46:445, 1964

35. Palmer RM: The genetics of talipes equinovarus. J Bone Joint Surg [Am] 46:542, 1964

## Classification

36. Hersh A: The role of surgery in the treatment of club feet. J Bone Joint Surg 49(8):1684, 1967

37. Committee For Care Of Handicapped Child, American Academy of Orthopedic Surgeons. Bull Am Acad Orthop Surg 14:No (2):15, 1966

38. Stewart SF: Club-foot: its incidence, cause, and treatment. An anatomical-physiological study. J Bone Joint Surg [Am] 33:577, 1951

39. Torpin R: Amniochorionic mesoblastic fibrous strings and amniotic bands. Associated constricting fetal Malformations or Fetal Deaths. Am J Obstet Gynecol, 91:65, 1965

40. Stover CH, Hayes JT, Holt JF: Diastrophic dwarfism. AJR 89:914, 1963

## Etiology

41. Little WJ: A Treatise on the Nature of Club-Foot and Analogous Distortions including their Treatment with and without Surgical Operations. W. Jeffs, London, 1839

42. Adams W: Club-Foot: Its Causes, Pathology and Treatment. John Churchill & Sons., London, 1866

43. Hippocrates: 400 B.C., translated by Withington ET William Heinemann, London, Putnam New York, 1927

44. Parker RW, Shattock SG: The pathology and etiology of congenital club-foot. Trans Pathol Soc Lond 35:423, 1884

45. Browne D: Congenital deformities of mechanical origin. Arch Dis Child 30:37, 1955

46. Browne D: The pathology and classification of talipes. Aust J Surg 29:85, 1959

47. Wiley AM: Club foot. An anatomical and experimental study of muscle growth. J Bone Joint Surg [Br] 41:821, 1959

48. Bagg HJ: Hereditary abnormalities of the limbs, their origin and transmission. Am J Anat 43:167, 1929
49. Fripp A, Shaw NE: Club-foot. E & S Livingstone, Edinburgh London, 1967
50. Shapiro F, Glimcher MJ: Gross and histological abnormalities of the talus in congenital club foot. J Bone Joint Surg [Am] 61:522, 1979
51. Critchley JE, Taylor RG: Transfer of the tibialis anterior tendon for relapsed clubfoot. J Bone Joint Surg [Br] 34:49, 1952
52. Baker CJ, Rudolph AJ: Congenital ring constrictions and intrauterine amputations. Am J Dis Child 121:393, 1971
53. Cowell HR, Hensinger RN: The relationship of clubfoot to congenital annular bands. In Bateman J (ed): Foot Science. WB Saunders, Philadelphia, 1976
54. Scrabbe WA: Aetiology of congenital talipes. Br Med J 2:1060, 1960
55. Duraiswami PK: Experimental causation of congenital skeletal defects and its significance in orthopedic surgery. J Bone Joint Surg [Br] 34:646, 1952
56. Edwards MJ: The experimental production of clubfoot in guinea pigs by maternal hyperthermia during gestation. J Pathol 103:49, 1971
57. Shaw EB, Steinbach HL: Aminopterin-induced fetal malformations. Am J Dis Child 115:477, 1968
58. Jago RH: Arthrogryphosis following treatment of maternal tetanus with muscle relaxants. Arch Dis Child 45:277, 1970
59. Melincoff RH, Davis RH: The development of lower extremity deformity. J Am Podiatr Med Assoc 68:631, 1978
60. DeMyer W, Baird I: Mortality and skeletal malformations from amniocentesis and oligohydramnions in rats: cleft palate, clubfoot, microstomia and adactyly. Teratology 2:33, 1969
61. Bohm M: The embryologic origin of club-foot. J Bone Joint Surg 11:229, 1929
62. Irani RN, Sherman MS: The pathological anatomy of clubfoot. J Bone Joint Surg [Am] 45:45, 1963
63. Settle GW: The anatomy of congenital talipes equinovarus: sixteen dissected specimens. J Bone Joint Surg [Am] 45:1341, 1963
64. Kaplan EB: Comparative anatomy of the talus in relation to idiopathic clubfoot. Clin Orthop 85:32, 1972
65. Sodre H, Bruschini S, Mestriner LA et al: Arterial abnormalities in talipes equinovarus as assessed by angiography and the Doppler technique. J Pediatr Orthop 10:101, 1990
66. Ben-Menachem Y, Butler JE: Arteriography of the foot in congenital deformities. J Bone Joint Surg [Am] 56:1625, 1974
67. Greider MD, Siff SJ, Gerson P, Donovan NM: Arteriography in clubfoot. J Bone Joint Surg [Am] 64:837, 1982
68. Hootnick DR, Levinsohn EM, Crider RJ, Packard DS Jr: Congenital arterial malformations associated with clubfoot. Clin Orthop 167:160, 1982
69. Hootnick DR, Packard, DS, Levisohn EM et al: The anatomy of a congenitally short limb with clubfoot and ectrodactyly. Teratology 29:155, 1984
70. Polo GV, Ruiz GP: Reporte preliminar al hallazgo de la ausencia vascular en enfermos con pies equino cavo varo aducto congenito. Rev Ortop Latinoam 8:27, 1968
71. Sodre H, Filho JL, Napoli MMM et al: Estudo arteriografico em pacientes portadores de petorto equinovaro congenito. Rev Bras Ortop 22:43, 1987
72. Sarrafian SK: Anatomy of the foot and ankle. JB Lippincott, Philadelphia, 1983
73. Flinchum D: Pathological anatomy in talipes equinovarus. J Bone Joint Surg [Am] 35:111, 1953
74. Stewart FS: Club-foot: its incidence, cause, and treatment. J Bone Joint Surg [Am] 33:577, 1951
75. Garceau GJ: Congenital talipes equinovarus. In Instr Course Lect 18:178, 1961
76. Inclan A: Anomalous tendinous insertions in the pathogenesis of club foot. J Bone Joint Surg [Br] 40:159, 1958
77. Ippolito E, Ponseti, IV: Congenital clubfoot in the human fetus. J Bone Joint Surg [Am] 62:8, 1980
78. Fried A: Recurrent congenital clubfoot. The role of the m. tibialis posterior in etiology and treatment. J Bone Joint Surg [Am] 41:243, 1959
79. Attenborough CG: Early posterior soft-tissue release in severe congenital talipes equinovarus. Clin Orthop 84:71, 1972
80. Bechtol CO, Mossman HW: Club-foot. An embryological study of associated muscle abnormalities. J Bone Joint Surg [Am] 32:827, 1950
81. Gray DH, Katz JM: A histochemical study of muscle in club foot. J Bone Joint Surg [Br] 63:437, 1981
82. Mau C: Muskelbefunde und ihre Bedeutung beim angeborenen Klumpfussleiden. Arch Orthop Trauma Surg 28:292, 1930
83. Isaacs H, Handelsman JE, Bandenhorst M, Pickering A: The muscles in club foot — a histologic, histochemical and electron-microscopic study. J Bone Joint Surg [Br] 59:465, 1977
84. Orofino CF: The etiology of congenital clubfoot. Acta Orthop Scand 20:59, 1960
85. Takasy S: Electromyographic study of congenital clubfoot. J Jpn Orthop Assoc 36:857, 1980
86. Fearnley ME: cited as personal communication in Attenborough CG: Early posterior soft tissue release in severe congenital talipes equinovarus. Clin Orthop 84:71, 1972
87. Keith A: Concerning the origin and nature of certain malformations of the face, head and foot. Br J Surg 28:173, 1940
88. Hirsch C: Observations on early operative treatment of

congenital clubfoot. Bull Hosp Jt Dis Orthop Inst 21:173, 1960

89. Ehrenfried A: The occurence and etiology of club-foot. JAMA 59:1940, 1912

90. Kite JH: The treatment of congenital clubfoot. A study of the results in two hundred cases. JAMA 99:1156, 1932

91. MacEven GD, Scott DJ Jr, Shands, AR Jr: Follow-up survey of clubfoot. JAMA 175:427, 1961

92. Kite JH: The clubfoot. Grune & Stratton, Orlando, FL, 1964

93. Steno M, Slivka M: Etiological factors in talipes equinovarus. Acta Chir Orthop Traumatol Cech 45:65, 1978

94. Blakeslee TJ, DeValentine SD: To be submitted for publication, 1992 J Foot Surg

95. Wynne-Davies R: Family studies and the cause of congenital clubfoot — talipes equinovarus, talipes calcaneovalgus and metatarsus varus. J Bone Joint Surg [Br] 46:445, 1964

96. Wynne-Davies R: Talipes equinovarus — a review of eighty-four cases after completion of treatment. J Bone Joint Surg [Br] 46:463, 1964

97. Wynne-Davies R: Genetic and environmental factors in the etiology of talipes equinovarus. Clin Orthop 84:9, 1972

98. Palmer RM: The genetics of talipes equinovarus. J Bone Joint Surg [Am] 46:542, 1964

99. Yang H, Chung CS, Nemechek RW: A genetic analysis of clubfoot in Hawaii. Genet Epidemiol 4:299, 1987

100. Carter CO: Progress in Medical Genetics. Vol. 4. Grune & Stratton, Orlando, FL, 1965

101. Chung CS, Nemechek RW, Larsen IJ, Ching GHS: Genetic and epidemiology studies of clubfoot in Hawaii, general and medical considerations. Hum Hered 19:321, 1969

102. Idelberger K: Die Ergebnisse der Zwillingsforschung beim angeborenen Klumpfuss. Verh Dtsch Orthop Ges 33:272, 1939

103. Wynne-Davies R: Heritable disorders in orthopaedic practice. Blackwell Scientific Publications, Oxford, 1973

104. Palmer RW, Conneally PM, Pao LY: Studies on the inheritance of idiopathic talipes equinovarus. Orthop Clin North Am 5:99, 1974

105. Wynne-Davies R, Littlejohn A, Gormley J: Aetiolgy and interrelationship of some common skeletal deformities. J Med Genet 19:321, 1982

## Pathologic Anatomy

106. Sarrafian SK: Anatomy of the Foot and Ankle. JB Lippincott, Philadelphia, 1983

107. Scarpa A: A Memoir on the Congenital Club Foot in Children. Wishart JW (transl): Constable, Edinburgh, 1818

108. Adams W: Clubfoot. Its Causes, Pathology and Treatment. J & A Churchill, London, 1886

109. Carroll NC, McMurtry R, Leete SF: The pathoanatomy of congenital clubfoot. Orthop Clin North Am 9:225, 1978

110. Tachdjian MO: The Child's Foot. WB Saunders, Philadelphia, 1985

111. Turco VJ: Clubfoot. Churchill Livingstone, New York, 1981

112. Simons GW: Analytical radiography of clubfoot. J Bone Joint Surg [Br] 59:485, 1977

113. Simons GW: Analytical radiography and the progressive approach in talipes equinovarus. Orthop Clin North Am 9:187, 1978

114. Simons GW: A standardized method for the radiographic evaluation of clubfeet. Clin Orthop 135:107, 1978

115. Simons GW: The diagnosis and treatment of deformity combinations in clubfeet. Clin Orthop 150:229, 1980

116. Swann M, Lloyd-Roberts GC, Catterall A: The anatomy of uncorrected clubfeet. A study of rotation deformity. J Bone Joint Surg [Br] 51:263, 1969

117. McKay DW: New concept of and approach to clubfoot treatment. I. Principles and morbid anatomy. J Pediatr Orthop 2:347, 1982

118. McKay DW: New concept of and approach to clubfoot treatment. II. Correction of the clubfoot. J Pediatr Orthop 3:10, 1983

119. McKay DW: New concept of and approach to clubfoot treatment. III. Evaluation and results. J Pediatr Orthop, 3:141, 1983

120. Bensahel H, Huouenin P, Themar-Noel C: The functional anatomy of clubfoot. J Pediatr Orthop 3:141, 1983

121. Fagan JP: The four-quadrant approach to clubfoot surgery. Clin Podiatr Med Surg 4:223, 1986

122. Isaacs H, Handelsman JE, Bandenhorst M, Pickering A: The muscles in club foot — a histological, histochemical and electron microscopic study. J Bone Joint Surg [Br] 59:465, 1977

123. Campos da Paz A Jr, DeSouza V: Talipes equinovarus: pathomechanical basis of treatment. Orthop Clin North Am 9:171, 1978

124. Shapiro F, Glimcher JJ: Gross and histological abnormalities of the talus in congenital clubfoot. J Bone Joint Surg [Am] 61:522, 1979

125. Ippolito E, Ponseti IV: Congenital club foot in the human fetus. J Bone Joint Surg [Am] 62:8, 1980

126. Zimny ML, Willig SJ, Roberts JM, D'Ambrosia RD: An electron microscopic study of the fascia from the medial and lateral sides of the clubfoot. J Pediatr Orthop 5:577, 1985

127. Handelsman JE, Bandalamente MA: Neuromuscular studies in clubfoot. J Pediatr Orthop 1:23, 1981

128. Settle GW: The anatomy of congenital talipes equino-

varus: sixteen dissected specimens. J Bone Joint Surg [Am] 45:1341, 1963

129. Irani RN, Sherman MS: The pathological anatomy of clubfoot. J Bone Joint Surg [Am] 45:45, 1963

130. Irani RN, Sherman MJ: The pathological anatomy of idiopathic clubfoot. Clin Orthop 84:14, 1972

131. Waisbrod H: Congenital club foot. An anatomical study. J Bone Joint Surg [Br] 55:796, 1973

132. Stewart FS: Club-foot: its incidence, cause, and treatment. J Bone Joint Surg [Am] 33:577, 1951

133. Garceau G.J: Congenital talipes equinovarus. In: Instr Course Lect 18:178, 1961

134. Incan A: Anomalous tendious insertions in the pathogenesis of club foot. J Bone Joint Surg [Br] 40:159, 1958

135. Wiley A.M: Club foot. An anatomical and experimental study of muscle growth. J Bone Joint Surg [Br] 41:821, 1959

136. Hirsch C: Observations on early operative treatment of congenital clubfoot. Bull Hosp Dis Orthop Inst 21:173, 1960

137. Sodre H, Bruschini S, Mestriner LA et al: Arterial abnormalities in talipes equinovarus as assessed by angiography and the Doppler technique. J Pediatr Orthop 10:101, 1990

138. Wynne-Davies R: Talipes equinovarus. A review of eight-four cases after completion of treatment. J Bone Joint Surg [Br] 46:464, 1964

139. Schlicht D: The pathological anatomy of talipes equinovarus. Aust N Z J Surg 33:2, 1963

140. Bleck EE: Congenital clubfoot. Pathomechanics, radiographic analysis, and results of surgical treatment. Clin Orthop 125:119, 1977

141. Simons GW, Sarrafian S: The microscopic dissection of a stillborn fetal clubfoot. Clin Orthop 173:275, 1983

142. Fahrenbach GJ, Kuehn DN, Tachdjian MO: Occult subluxation of the subtalar joint in clubfoot (using computerized tomography). J Pediatr Orthop 6:334, 1986

## Clinical Evaluation

143. Sarrafian SK: Anatomy of the Foot and Ankle. JB Lippincott, Philadelphia, 1983

144. Fahrenbach GJ, Kuehn DN, Tachdjian MO: Occult subluxation of the subtalar joint in clubfoot (using computerized tomography). J Pediatr Orthop 6:334, 1986

145. Barwell R: On various forms of talipes as depicted by x-rays. Lancet II:160, 1896

146. Barwell R: On various forms of talipes as depicted by x-rays. Lancet II:234, 1896

147. Barwell R: On various forms of talipes as depicted by x-rays. Lancet II:1521, 1896

148. Ogston A: A new principle in curing clubfoot in severe cases in children a few years old. Br Med J 1:1524, 1902

149. Brockman EP: Congenital Clubfoot (Talipes Equinovarus). William Wood, Bristol, England, 1930

150. Browne D: Congenital deformities of mechanical origin. Proc R Soc Med 29:1409, 1936

151. McCauley JC, Krida A: The early treatment of equinus in congenital clubfoot. Am J Surg 22:491, 1933

152. Wisburn W: Neue Gesichtpunkte zum Redressemente des angeborenen Klumpfusses und daraus sich ergebende Schlussfolgerungen bezüglich der Ätiologie. Arch Orthop Unfallchir 31:451, 1932

153. Kite JH: The Clubfoot. Grune & Stratton, Orlando, FL, 1964

154. Heywood AWB: The mechanics of hind foot in club foot as demonstrated radiologically. J Bone Joint Surg [Br] 46:102, 1964

155. Debrunner H: Die Therapie des angeborenen Klumpfusses. Z Orthop 88:1, 1956

156. Ponseti IV, Smoley EN: Congenital clubfoot: the results of treatment. J Bone Joint Surg [Am] 45:261, 1963

157. Templeton AW, McAlister WH, Zim ID: Standardization of terminology and evaluation of osseous relationships in congenitally abnormal feet. AJR 93:374, 1965

158. Beatson TR, Pearson JR: A method of assessing correction in clubfeet. J Bone Joint Surg [Br] 48:40, 1966

159. Taylor JF, Oyemade GAA, Shaw E et al: Primary treatment of rigid congenital talipes equino-varus. Physiotherapy 62:89, 1976

160. Lloyd-Roberts GC: Orthopaedics in Infancy and Childhood. Butterworths, London, 1971

161. Ponseti IV, Campos J: Observations on pathogenesis and treatment of congenital clubfoot. Clin Orthop 84:50, 1972

162. Debrunner H: Orthopädisches Diagnosticum. Georg Thieme Verlag, Stuttgart, 1973

163. Denis X, Paquot JP: Examen radiologique et surveillance du pied bot congenital. Ann Radiol (Paris) 18:339, 1975

164. Price CT: Congenital clubfoot. J Fla Med Assoc 66:104, 1979

165. Kandel B: The suroplantar projection in the congenital clubfoot of the infant. Acta Orthop Scand 22:161, 1952

166. Kleiger B, Mankin HJ: A roentgenographic study of the development of the calcaneus by means of the posterior tangential view. J Bone Joint Surg [Am] 43:961, 1961

167. LeNoir JL: Congenital Idiopathic Talipes. Charles C Thomas, Springfield, IL, 1966

168. Evans D: Relapsed club foot. J Bone Joint Surg [Br] 43:722, 1961

169. McKay DW: New concept of and approach to clubfoot treatment. II: Correction of the clubfoot. J Pediatr Orthop 3:10, 1983

170. Blakeslee TJ: Comparative radiographic analysis of congenital idiopathic talipes equinovarus (clubfoot) in infancy: a retrospective study. J Foot Surg 27:188, 1988

171. Simons GW: Analytical radiography and the progressive approach in talipes equinovarus. Orthop Clin North Am 9:187, 1978
172. Simons GW: A standardized method for the radiographic evaluation of clubfeet. Clin Orthop 135:107, 1978
173. Tachdjian MO: The Child's Foot. WB Saunders, Philadelphia, 1985
174. Fagan JP: The four-quadrant approach to clubfoot surgery. Clin Podiatr Med Surg 4:223, 1986
175. Shapiro F, Glimcher JJ: Gross and histological abnormalities of the talus in congenital clubfoot. J Bone Joint Surg [Am] 61:522, 1979
176. Ono K, Hayashi H: Residual deformity of treated congenital club foot. A clinical study employing frontal tomography of the hind part of the foot. J Bone Joint Surg [Am] 56:1577, 1974
177. Hjelmstedt EA, Sahlstedt B: Arthrography as a guide in the treatment of congenital club foot. Acta Orthop Scand 51:321, 1980
178. Herzenberg JE, Carroll NC, Christofersen MR et al: Clubfoot analysis with three-dimensional computer modeling. J Pediatr Orthop 8:257, 1988
179. Woolson, ST, Dev, P, Fellingham LL, Vassiliadis A: Three-dimensional imaging of bone from computerized tomography. Clin Orthop 202:239, 1986

## Treatment

180. Coleman SS: Complex Foot Deformities in Children. Lea & Febiger, Philadelphia, 1983
181. Kite JH: The treatment of congenital club-feet. Surg Gynecol Obstet :190, 1933
182. Kite JH: Principles involved in treatment of clubfoot. J Bone Joint Surg 2:595, 1939
183. Kite JH: The Clubfoot. Grune & Stratton, Orlando, FL, 1964
184. Kite JH: Non-operative treatment of congenital clubfoot. Clin Orthop 70:79, 1970
185. Lovell WW, Price CT, Meehan PL: The foot. p. 911. In Lovell WW, Winter RB (eds): Pediatric Orthopaedics. JB Lippincott, Philadelphia, 1978
186. Tachdjian MO: The Child's Foot. WB Saunders, Philadelphia, 1985
187. Fixsen J, Lloyd-Roberts G: The Foot in Childhood. Churchill Livingstone, New York, 1988
188. Lehman WB: The Clubfoot. JB Lippincott, Philadelphia, 1980
189. Turco VJ: Clubfoot. Churchill Livingstone, New York, 1981
190. McKay DW: New concept of and approach to clubfoot treatment: II. Correction of the clubfoot. J Pediatr Orthop 3:10, 1983

191. Brockman FP: Modern methods of treatment of clubfoot. Br Med J 2:572, 1937
192. Bertelsen A: Treatment of congenital clubfoot. J Bone Joint Surg [Br] 39:599, 1957
193. Jansen K: Treatment of congenital clubfoot. J Bone Joint Surg [Br] 39:599, 1957
194. Ponseti IV, Smoley EN: Congenital club foot: the results of treatment. J Bone Joint Surg [Am] 45(2):261, 1963
195. Dangelmajor RC: A review of 200 clubfeet. Bull Hosp Special Surg 4:38, 1961
196. Blockey NJ, Smith MGH: The treatment of congenital club foot. J Bone Joint Surg [Br] 48:660, 1966
197. Nather A, Bose K: Conservative and surgical treatment of clubfoot. J Pediatr Orthop 7:42, 1987
198. Heywood AWB: The mechanics of the hindfoot in club foot as demonstrated radiographically. J Bone Joint Surg [Br] 46:102, 1964
199. McKay DW: Surgical correction of clubfoot. Instr Course Lect 37:87, 1988
200. Somppi E, Sulamaa M: Early operative treatment of congenital clubfoot. Acta Orthop Scand 42:513, 1971
201. Pous J, Dimeglio A: Neonatal surgery in clubfoot. Orthop Clin North Am 9:233, 1978
202. Turco VJ, Spinella AJ: Current management of clubfoot. Instr Course Lect 31:218, 1982
203. Carroll NC: Congenital clubfoot: pathoanatomy and treatment. Instr Course Lect 36:117, 1987
204. Carroll NC, McMurtry R, Leete SF: The pathoanatomy of congenital clubfoot. Orthop Clin North Am 9:225, 1978
205. Cummings RJ, Lovell WW: Current concepts review. Operative treatment of congenital idiopathic club foot. J Bone Joint Surg [Am] 70:1108, 1988
206. Porat S, Kaplan L: Critical analysis of results in clubfeet treated surgically along the Norris Carroll approach: seven years' experience. J Pediatr Orthop 9:137, 1989
207. DeRosa GP, Stepro D: Results of posteromedial release for the resistant clubfoot. J Pediatr Orthop 6:590, 1986
208. DePuy J, Drennan J: Correction of idiopathic clubfoot: A comparison of results of early versus delayed posteromedial release. J Pediatr Orthop 9:44, 1989
209. Main BJ, Crider RJ: An analysis of residual deformity in clubfeet submitted to early operation. J Bone Joint Surg [Br] 60:536, 1978
210. Porat S, Milgram C, Bentley G: The history of treatment of congenital clubfoot at the Royal Liverpool Children's Hospital: improvement of results by early extensive posterormedial release. J Pediatr Orthop 4:331, 1984
211. Otremski I, Salamaa R, Khermosh O, Wientroub S: An analysis of the results of a modified one-stage posteromedial release (Turco operation) for the treatment of clubfoot. J Pediatr Orthop 7:149, 1987

212. Crawford AH, Marxen JL, Osterfeld DL: The Cincinnati incision: a comprehensive approach for surgical procedures of the foot and ankle in childhood. J Bone Joint Surg [Am] 64:1355, 1982

213. Lehman WB, Silver L, Grant AD et al: The anatomical basis for incisions around the foot and ankle in clubfoot surgery. Bull Hosp Jt Dis Orthop Inst 47:218, 1987

214. Fagan JP: The four quadrant approach to clubfoot surgery. Clin Podiatr Med Surg 4:233, 1987

215. Taylor GI, Palmer JH: The vascular territories (angiosomes) of the body: experimental study and clinical applications. Br J Plast Surg 40:113, 1987

216. Brougham DI, Nicol RO: Use of the Cincinnati incision in congenital talipes equinovarus. J Pediatr Orthop 8:696, 1988

217. Karlin J: The Cincinnati incision. J Am Podiatr Med Assoc 6:386, 1986

218. Turco VJ: Surgical correction of the resistant club foot. One-stage posteromedial release with internal fixation: preliminary report. J Bone Joint Surg [Am] 53:477, 1971

219. McKay DW: New concept of and approach to clubfoot treatment. I. Principles and morbid anatomy. J Pediatr Orthop 2:347, 1982

220. Simons GW: complete subtalar release in clubfoot. I. A preliminary report. J Bone Joint Surg [Am] 67:1044, 1985

221. Scurran BL, DeValentine SJ: Clubfoot considerations in the older child. Clin Podiatr Med Surg 4:247, 1987

222. Evans D: Relapsed club foot. J Bone Joint Surg [Br] 43:723, 1961

223. Ogston A: A new principle of curing club-foot in severe cases in children a few years old. Br Med J 1:5243, 1902

224. Johanning K: Excochleatio ossis cuboidei in treatment of pes equino-varus. Acta Orthop Scand 27:310, 1958

225. Lichtblau S: A medial and lateral release operation for club foot. A preliminary report. J Bone Joint Surg [Am] 55:1377, 1973

226. Tayton K, Thompson T: Relapsing clubfeet, late results of delayed operation. J Bone Joint Surg [Br] 61:474, 1979

227. Addison A, Fixsen JA, Lloyd-Roberts GC: A review of the Dillwyn Evans type collateral operation in severe clubfeet. J Bone Joint Surg [Br] 65:12, 1983

228. Lowe LW, Hannon MA: Residual adduction of the forefoot in treated congenital club foot. J Bone Joint Surg [Br] 55:809, 1973

229. Otremski I, Salama R, Khermosh O, Wientroub S: Residual adduction of the forefoot. A review of the Turco procedure for congenital club foot. J Bone Joint Surg [Br] 69:832, 1987

230. Yu GV, Wallace GF: Metatarsus adductus. p. 324. In McGlamry ED (ed): Foot Surgery. Williams & Wilkins, Baltimore, 1987

231. Heyman CH, Herndon CH, Strong JM: Mobilization of the tarsometatarsal and intermetatarsal joints for the correction of resistant adduction of the forefoot in congenital metatarsus varus. J Bone Joint Soc [Am] 40:299, 1958

232. Dwyer FC: The treatment of relapsed clubfoot by the insertion of a wedge into the calcaneum. J Bone Joint Surg [Br] 45:67, 1963

233. Dekel S, Weissman SL: Osteotomy of the calcaneus and concomitant plantar stripping in children with talipes cavovarus. J Bone Joint Surg [Br] 55:802, 1973

234. Fisher RL, Shaffer SR: An evaluation of calcaneal osteotomy in congenital clubfoot and other disorders. Clin Orthop 70:141, 1970

235. Schneider DA, Smith CF: Medial subtalar stabilization with posterior medial release in the treatment of varus feet: a preliminary report. Orthop Clin North Am 7:949, 1976

236. Grice DS: An extra-articular arthrodesis of the subastragalar joint for correction of paralytic flat feet in children J Bone Joint Surg [Am] 34:927, 1952

237. Lund (1872), cited by Kite JH: The treatment of congenital clubfoot. JAMA 99:1156, 1932

238. Whitman R: Operative orthopedics as illustrated by a hospital service. Med Rec NY 88:143, 1915

239. Sharrard WJW: The management of deformity and paralysis of the foot in myelomeningocele. J Bone Joint Surg [Br] 50:456, 1968

240. Kilfoyle RM, Broome JS, Hardy JH, Curtis BH: Talectomy. p. 162. In Bateman JE (ed): Foot Science, WB Saunders, Philadelphia, 1976

241. Segal LS, Mann DC, Feiwell E, Hoffer MM: Equinovarus deformity in arthrogryposis and myelomeningocele: evaluation of primary talectomy. Foot Ankle 10:12, 1989

242. Gibson DA, Urs NDK: Arthrogryposis multiplex congenita. J Bone Joint Surg [Br] 60:96, 1978

243. Green ADL, Fixsen JA, Lloyd-Roberts GC: Talectomy for arthrogryposis multiplex congenita. J Bone Joint Surg [Br] 66:697, 1984

244. Guidera KJ, Drennan JC: Foot and ankle deformities in arthrogryposis multiplex congenita. Clin Orthop 194:94, 1985

245. Lloyd-Roberts GC, Lettin AWF: Arthrogryposis multiplex congenita. J Bone Joint Surg [Br] 52:494, 1975

246. Menelaus MB: Talectomy for equinovarus deformity in arthrogryposis and spina bifida. J Bone Joint Surg [Br] 53:468, 1971

247. Sherk HH, Ames MD: Talectomy in the treatment of the myelomeningocele patient. Clin Orthop 110:218, 1975

248. Trumble T, Banta JV, Raycroft JF, Curtis BH: Talectomy for equinovarus deformity in myelodysplasia. J Bone Joint Surg [Am] 67A:21, 1985

249. Dias LS, Stern LS: Talectomy in the treatment of resistant talipes equinovarus deformity in myelomeningocele and arthrogryposis. J Pediatr Orthop 7:39, 1987
250. Young AB: Clubfoot treated by astragalectomy. 50-year follow-up of a case. Lancet I:670, 1962
251. Burkhart SS, Petersen HA: 60-Year follow-up of talectomy for congenital talipes equinovarus: brief report. J Bone Joint Surg [Br] 71B:325, 1989
252. Rodgeveller BN: Clubfoot. p. 354. In McGlamry ED (ed): Comprehensive Textbook of Foot Surgery. Vol I. Williams & Wilkins, Baltimore, 1987
253. Ryerson EW: Arthrodesing operations on the feet. J Bone Joint Surg [Am] 5:453, 1923
254. McCauley JC: Triple arthrodesis for congenital talipes equinovarus deformities. Clin Orthop 34:25, 1964
255. Banks HH: The management of spastic deformities of the foot and ankle. Clin Orthop 122:70, 1977
256. Bernau A: Long term results following Lambrinudi arthrodesis. J Bone Joint Surg [Am] 59:473, 1977
257. Crego CH Jr, McCarroll HR: Recurrent deformities in stabilized paralytic feet. J Bone Joint Surg [Am] 20:609, 1938
258. Galindo MJ Jr, Siff SJ, Butler JE, Cain TE: Triple arthrodesis in young children: a salvage procedure after failed releases in severely affected feet. Foot Ankle 7:319, 1987
259. Hill NA, Wilson HJ, Chevres F, Sweterlitsch PR: Triple arthrodesis in the young child. Clin Orthop 70:187, 1970
260. Seitz DG, Carpenter EB: Triple arthrodesis in children: a ten year review. South Med J 67:1420, 1974
261. Adelaar RS, Dannelly EA, Meunier PA et al: A long term study of triple arthrodesis in children. Orthop Clin North Am 7:895, 1976

## Long-Term Results of Clubfoot Surgery

262. McKay DW: New concept of and approach to clubfoot treatment. II: Correction of the clubfoot. J Pediatr Orthop 3:10, 1983
263. Bachman R: Klinisches und röntgenologisches Behandlungsergebnis angeborener Klumpfusse nach 5 Jahren. Zentralbl Chir 41:1738, 1953
264. Fredenhagen H: Der Klumpfuss. Vorkommen, Anatomie, Behandlung und Spätresultate. Z Orthop 85:305, 1955
265. Debrunner H: Die Therapie des angeborenen Klumpfusses. Z Orthop 88:1, 1956
266. Jansen K: Treatment of congenital clubfoot. J Bone Joint Surg [Br] 39:599, 1957
267. Solonen KA, Parkkulainen KV: Congenital clubfoot. Results of treatment. Ann Chir Gynaecol 48:130, 1958
268. MacEven GD, Scott, DJ Jr, Shands AR Jr: Follow-up survey of clubfoot. JAMA 175:427, 1961
269. Seyfarth H: Derzeitige Gesichtspunkte in der Therapie des angeborenen Klumpfusses. Forsch Fortschr 36:362, 1962
270. Ponseti IV, Smoley, EN: Congenital clubfoot: the results of treatment. J Bone Joint Surg [Am] 45:261, 1963
271. Kite JH: The Clubfoot. Grune & Stratton, Orlando FL, 1964
272. Wynne-Davies R: Talipes equinovarus. A review of eighty-four cases after completion of treatment. J Bone Joint Surg [Br] 46:464, 1964
273. Hersch A: The role of surgery in the treatment of club feet. J Bone Joint Surg [Am] 49:1684, 1967
274. Denham RA: Congenital talipes equinovarus. J Bone Joint Surg [Br] 49:583, 1967
275. Tonnis D, Bikadorov V: Untersuchungen über die Ergebnisse verschiedener Behandlunsmethoden bei angeborenen Klumpfuss. Z Orthop 104:218, 1968
276. Preston E, Fell TW: Congenital idiopathic clubfoot. Clin Orthop 122:102, 1976
277. Richardson AB, Westin WG: The complete vs incomplete surgical release of the congenital clubfoot. Orthop Trans 2:213, 1978
278. Tripathi RP, Chaturvedi SN: Treatment of clubfoot by one-stage medial soft tissue release operation. J Indian Med Assoc 73:33, 1979
279. Kumar K: The role of footprints in the management of clubfeet. Clin Orthop 140:32, 1979
280. Laaveg SJ, Ponseti IV: Long-term results of treatment of congenital club foot. J Bone Joint Surg [Am] 62:23, 1980
281. Nichols EH: Anatomy of congenital equino-varus. Boston Med Surg J 136:150, 1897
282. Müller G: Die morphologischen Ergebnisse der Klumpfuss behandlung aus klinischer und röntgenologischer Sicht. Beitr Orthop Traumatol 179:594, 1970
283. Stein V: Einflussfaktoren bei der Entstehung einer Klumpfussrezidivs. Beitr Orthop Traumatol 27:138, 1979
284. Somppi E, Sulamaa M: Early operative treatment of congenital club foot. Acta Orthop Scand 42:513, 1971
285. Imhauser G: The idiopathic clubfoot and its treatment. Georg Thieme Verlag, New York, 1986
286. Fripp AT, Shaw NE: Clubfoot. E & S Livingstone, Edinburgh, 1967
287. Lindemann K: Die Behandlung des kindlichen Klumpfusses späterer Jahre und des Klumpfussrezidivs. Verh Dtsch Ges Orthop 29:188, 1934
288. Kuhlman RF, Bell JF: A clinical evaluation of operative procedure for congenital talipes equinovarus. J Bone Joint Surg [Br] 38B:929, 1956
289. Critchley, JE, Taylor RG: Transfer of the tibialis anterior tendon for the relapsed clubfoot. J Bone Joint Surg [Br] 34:49, 1952
290. Nyga W: Ergebnisse der Tibialis anterior – Verlagerung

zur Behandlung des kongenitalen Klumpfuss. Beitr Orthop Traumatol 26:44, 1979

291. Bosch J: Operative oder konservative Klumpfuss behandlung. Z Orthop 83:8, 1953

292. Turco VJ: Surgical correction of the resistant club foot. One-stage posteromedial release with internal fixation. A preliminary report. J Bone Joint Surg [Am] 53:477, 1971

293. Herring JA, Aston JW Jr, Schneider RW, Carrel B: The Turco posteromedial release. Orthop Trans 1:107, 1977

294. Bensahel H, Csukonyi Z, Desgrippes Y, Chaumien JP: Surgery in residual clubfoot: one-stage medioposterior release "à la carte." J Pediatr Orthop 7:145, 1987

295. McKay DW: New concept of and approach to clubfoot treatment. III. Evaluation and results. J Pediatr Orthop 3:141, 1983

296. Magone JB, Torch MA, Clark RN, Kean JR: Comparative review of surgical treatment of the idiopathic clubfoot by three different procedures at Columbus Children's Hospital. J Pediatr Orthop 9:49, 1989

297. Porat S, Kaplan L: Critical analysis of results in club feet treated surgically along the Norris Carroll approach: seven years of experience. J Pediatr Orthop 9:137, 1989

298. Carroll NC, McMurty R, Leete SF: The pathoanatomy of congenital clubfoot. Orthop Clin North Am 9:225, 1978

299. McKay DW: New concept of and approach to clubfoot treatment. I: Principles and morbid anatomy. J Pediatr Orthop 2:347, 1982

300. Fagan JP: The four-quadrant approach to clubfoot surgery. Clin Podiatr Med Surg 4:223, 1986

301. Turco VJ: Resistant congenital club foot—one stage posteromedial release with internal fixation. J Bone Joint Surg [Am] 61:805, 1979

302. Main BJ, Crider RJ, Polk, M et al: The results of early operation in talipes equinovarus. J Bone Joint Surg [Br] 59:332, 1977

303. Porat S, Milgrom C, Bentley G: The history of treatment of congenital clubfoot at the Royal Liverpool Children's Hospital: Improvement of results by early extensive posteromedial release. J Pediatr Orthop 4:331, 1984

304. Otremski I, Salama R, Khermosh O, Wientroub S: An analysis of the results of a modified one-stage posteromedial release (Turco operation) for the treatment of clubfoot. J Pediatr Orthop 7:149, 1987

305. Simons GW: Analytical radiography of clubfoot. J Bone Joint Surg [Br] 59:485, 1977

306. Simons GW: Analytical radiography and the progressive approach in talipes equinovarus. Orthop Clin North Am 9:187, 1978

307. Simons GW: A standardized method for the radiographic evaluation of clubfeet. Clin Orthop 135:107, 1978

308. Simons GW: The diagnosis and treatment of deformity combinations in clubfeet. Clin Orthop 150:229, 1980

309. Isaacs H, Handelsman JE, Bandenhorst M, Pickering A: The muscles in club foot—a histological, histochemical and electron microscopic study. J Bone Joint Surg [Br] 59:465, 1977

310. Waisbrod H: Congenital club foot. An anatomical study. J Bone Joint Surg [Br] 55:796, 1973

311. Giannestras NJ: Foot Disorders. Medical and Surgical management. Lea & Febiger, Philadelphia, 1967

312. Stauffer RN, Chao EYS, Brewster RC: Force and motion analysis of the normal diseased, and prosthetic ankle joint. Clin Orthop 127:189, 1977

313. Simons GW: Ankle range of motion in club feet, abstracted. Orthop Trans 1990

314. Simons GW: Complete subtalar release in club feet. II: Comparison with less extensive procedures. J Bone Joint Surg [Am] 67:1056, 1985

315. Simons GW: Complete subtalar release in club feet: I. Preliminary report. J Bone Joint Surg [Am] 67:1044, 1985

316. Staheli LT, Corbett M, Wyss C, King H: Lower-extremity rotational problems in children. J Bone Joint Surg [Am] 67:39, 1985

## Complications

317. Kite JH: Errors and complications in treating foot conditions in children. Clin Orthop 53:31, 1967

318. Weseley MS, Barenfeld PA, Barrett N: Complications of the treatment of clubfoot. Clin Orthop 84:93, 1972

319. Keim HA, Ritchie GW: Nutcracker treatment of clubfoot. JAMA 189:613, 1964

320. Swann M, Lloyd-Roberts GC, Catterall A: The anatomy of uncorrected club feet. J Bone Joint Surg [Br] 51:263, 1969

321. Dunn HK, Samuelson KM: Flat-top talus. J Bone Joint Surg [Am] 56A:57, 1974

322. Miller JH, Bernstein SM: The roentgenographic appearance of the corrected clubfoot. Foot Ankle 6:177, 1986

323. Turco VJ: Surgical correction of the resistant club foot. J Bone Joint Surg [Am] 53:477, 1971

324. Applington JP, Riddle CD: Avascular necrosis of the body of the talus after combined medial and lateral release of congenital clubfoot. South Med J 69:1037, 1976

325. Schlafly B, Butler JE, Siff SJ et al: The appearance of the tarsal navicular after posteromedial release for clubfoot. Foot Ankle 5:222, 1985

326. Magone JB, Torch MA, Clark RN, Kean JR: Comparative review of surgical treatment of the idiopathic clubfoot by three different procedures at Columbus Children's Hospital. J Pediatr Orthop 9:49, 1989

327. Ponseti IV, Becker JR: Congenital metatarsus adductus: the results of treatment. J Bone Joint Surg [Am] 48A:702, 1966

328. Ostremski I, Salama R, Khermosh O, Wientroub S: An analysis of the results of a modified one-stage posteromedial release (Turco operation) for the treatment of clubfoot. J Pediatr Orthop 7:149, 1987

329. Lowe LW, Hannon MA: Residual adduction of the forefoot in treated congenital clubfoot. J Bone Joint Surg [Br] 55:809, 1973

330. Lichtblau S: Section of the abductor hallucis tendon for correction of metatarsus varus deformity. Clin Orthop 110:227, 1975

331. Tayton K, Thompson P: Relapsing club feet. J Bone Joint Surg [Br] 61:474, 1979

332. Heyman CH, Herndon CH, Strong JM: Mobilization of the tarsometatarsal and intermetatarsal joints for the correction of resistant adduction of the forepart of the foot in congenital clubfoot or congenital metatarsus varus. J Bone Joint Surg [Am] 49:299, 1958

333. Berman A, Gartland JJ: Metatarsal osteotomy for the correction of adduction of the fore part of the foot in children. J Bone Joint Surg [Am] 53:498, 1971

334. Yu GV, Wallace GE: Metatarsus adductus. p. III:324. In McGlamary ED (ed): Comprehensive Textbook of Foot Surgery. Vol. 1. William & Wilkins, Baltimore, 1987

335. Evans D: Relapsed club foot. J Bone Joint Surg [Br] 43B:722, 1961

336. Johanning K: Excochleatio ossis cuboidei in the treatment of pes equinovarus. Acta Orthop Scand 27:310, 1958

337. Lincoln CR, Wood KE, Bugg EI: Metatarsus varus corrected by open wedge osteotomy of the first cuneiform bone. Orthop Clin North Am 7:795, 1976

338. Rab GT: Congenital deformities of the foot. In Chapman MW (ed): Operative Orthopaedics. JB Lippincott, New York, 1988

339. Wijesinha SS, Menelaus MB: Operation for calcaneus deformity after surgery for club foot. J Bone Joint Surg [Br] 71:234, 1989

340. Aronson J, Puskarich C: Deformity and disability from treated clubfoot. J Pediatr Orthop 10:109, 1990

341. Simons GW: Complete subtalar release in club feet. J Bone Joint Surg [Am] 67:1044, 1985

342. Herndon CH, Strong JM, Heyman CH: Transposition of the tibialis anterior in the treatment of paralytic talipes calcaneus. J Bone Joint Surg [Am] 38:751, 1956

343. Makin M, Yossipovitch Z: Translocation of the peroneus longus in the treatment of paralytic pes calcaneus. J Bone Joint Surg [Am] 48:1541, 1966

344. McKay DW: New concept of and approach to clubfoot treatment. III. Evaluation and results. J Pediatr Orthop 3:141, 1983

345. Porat S, Kaplan L: Critical analysis of results in club feet treated surgically along the Norris Carroll approach: seven years of experience. J Pediatr Orthop 9:137, 1989

# SUGGESTED READINGS

Adams W: Clubfoot. Its Causes, Pathology and Treatment. J & A Churchill, London, 1886

Barwell R: On various forms of talipes as depicted by x-rays. Lancet II:160, 1896

Barwell R: On various forms of talipes as depicted by x-rays. Lancet II:234, 1896

Barwell R: On various forms of talipes as depicted by x-rays. Lancet II:1521, 1896

Beatson TR, Pearson JR: A method of assessing correction in clubfeet. J Bone Joint Surg [Br] 48:40, 1966

Bensahel H, Huouenin, P, Themar-Noel C. The functional anatomy of clubfoot. J Pediatr Orthop 3:191, 1983

Blakeslee TJ: Comparative radiographic analysis of congenital idiopathic talipes equinovarus (clubfoot) in infancy: a retrospective study. J Foot Surg 27:188, 1988

Bleck EE: Congenital clubfoot. Pathomechanics, radiographic analysis, and results of surgical treatment. Clin Orthop 125:119, 1977

Brockman EP: Congenital Clubfoot (Talipes Equinovarus). William Wood, Bristol, England, 1930

Browne D: Congenital deformities of mechanical origin. Proc R Soc Med 29:1409, 1936

Campos da Paz A Jr, DeSouza V: Talipes equinovarus: pathomechanical basis of treatment. Orthop Clin North Am 9:171, 1978

Debrunner H: Orthopädisches Diagnosticum. Georg Thieme Verlag, Stuttgart, 1973

Denis X, Paquot JP: Examen radiologique et surveillance du pied bot congenital. Ann Radiol (Paris) 18:339, 1975

Evans D: Relapsed club foot. J Bone Joint Surg [Br] 43B:722, 1961

Fahrenbach GJ, Kuehn DN, Tachdjian MO: Occult subluxation of the subtalar joint in clubfoot (using computerized tomography). J Pediatr Orthop 6:334, 1986

Garceau GJ: Congenital talipes equinovarus. Instr Course Lect 18:178, 1961

Handelsman JE, Bandalamente MA: Neuromuscular studies in clubfoot. J Pediatr Orthop 1:23, 1981

Herzenberg JE, Carroll NC, Christofersen MR et al: Clubfoot analysis with three-dimensional computer modeling. J Pediatr Orthop 8:257, 1988

Heywood AWB: The mechanics of hind foot in club foot as demonstrated radiologically. J Bone Joint Surg [Br] 46:102, 1964

Hirsch C: Observations on early operative treatment of congenital clubfoot. Bull Hosp Joint Dis 21:173, 1960

Hjelmstedt EA, Sahlstedt B: Arthrography as a guide in the treatment of congenital club foot. Acta Orthop Scand 51:321, 1980

Incan A: Anomalous tendinous insertions in the pathogenesis of club foot. J Bone Joint Surg [Br] 40:159, 1958

Ippolito E, Ponseti, IV: Congenital club foot in the human fetus. J Bone Joint Surg [Am] 62:8, 1980

Irani RN, Sherman MS: The pathological anatomy of clubfoot. J Bone Joint Surg [Am] 45:45, 1963

Irani RN, Sherman MS: The pathological anatomy of idiopathic clubfoot. Clin Orthop 84:14, 1972

Kandel B: The suroplantar projection in the congenital clubfoot of the infant. Acta Orthop Scand 22:161, 1952

Kleiger B, Mankin HJ: A roentgenographic study of the development of the calcaneus by means of the posterior tangential view. J Bone Joint Surg [Br] 43:961, 1961

LeNoir JL: Congenital Idiopathic Talipes. Charles C Thomas, Springfield, IL, 1966

Lloyd-Roberts GC: Orthopaedics in Infancy and Childhood. Butterworths, London, 1971

McCauley JC, Krida A: The early treatment of equinus in congenital clubfoot. Am J Surg 22:491, 1933

Ogston A: A new principle in curing clubfoot in severe cases in children a few years old. Br Med J 1:1524, 1902

Ono K, Hayashi H: Residual deformity of treated congenital club foot. A clinical study employing frontal tomography of the hind part of the foot. J Bone Joint Surg [Am] 56:1577, 1974

Price CT: Congenital clubfoot. J Fla Med Assoc 66:104, 1979

Ponseti IV, Campos J: Observations on pathogenesis and treatment of congenital clubfoot. Clin Orthop 84:50, 1972

Sarrafian SK: Anatomy of the Foot and Ankle. JB Lippincott, Philadelphia, 1983

Scarpa A: A memoir on the congenital club foot in children. Wishart, JW (transl): Constable, Edinburgh, 1818

Schlicht D: The pathological anatomy of talipes equinovarus. Aust N Z J Surg 33:2, 1963

Settle GW: The anatomy of congenital talipes equinovarus: sixteen dissected specimens. J Bone Joint Surg [Am] 45:1341, 1963

Shapiro F, Glimcher JJ: Gross and histological abnormalities of the talus in congenital clubfoot. J Bone Joint Surg [Am] 61:522, 1979

Simons GW, Sarrafian S: The microscopic dissection of a stillborn fetal clubfoot. Clin Orthop 173:275, 1983

Sodre H, Bruschini S, Mestriner LA et al: Arterial abnormalities in talipes equinovarus as assessed by angiography and the Doppler technique. J Pediatr Orthop 10:101, 1990

Stewart FS: Club-foot: its incidence, cause, and treatment. J Bone Joint Surg [Am] 33:577, 1951

Swann M, Lloyd-Roberts GC, Catterall A: The anatomy of uncorrected clubfeet. A study of rotation deformity. J Bone Joint Surg [Br] 51:263, 1969

Tachdjian MO: The Child's Foot. WB Saunders, Philadelphia, 1985

Taylor JF, Oyemade GAA, Shaw E et al: Primary treatment of rigid congenital talipes equino-varus. Physiotherapy 62:89, 1976

Templeton AW, McAlister WH, Zim ID: Standardization of terminology and evaluation of osseous relationships in congenitally abnormal feet. AJR 93:374, 1965

Turco VJ: Clubfoot. Churchill Livingstone, New York, 1981

Wiley AM: Club foot: an anatomical and experimental study of muscle growth. J Bone Joint Surg [Br] 41:821, 1959

Wishburn W: Neue Gesichtpunkte zum Redressemente des angeborenen Klumpfusses und daraus sich ergebende Schlussfolgerungen desgleich der Ätiologie. Arch Orthop Unfallchir 31:451, 1932

Woolson ST, Dev P, Fellingham LL, Vassiliadis A: Three-dimensional imaging of bone from computerized tomography. Clin Orthop 202:239, 1986

Zimny ML, Willig SJ, Roberts JM, D'Ambrosia RD: An electron microscopic study of the fascia from the medial and lateral sides of the clubfoot. J Pediatr Orthop 5:577, 1985

# 7
# Congenital Pes Valgus

*STEPHEN H. SILVANI*

*Flatfoot* and *pes planus* are rather vague terms used to describe a group of morphologically similar conditions. The descriptive term *flatfoot* provides little information concerning the etiology, prognosis, or disability of a particular deformity. Since the conditions referred to as flatfoot run the gamut from normal variants that are completely asymptomatic to severe deformities that may be truly disabling, it is imperative that the clinician's approach to the management of flatfoot in children be based upon an accurate diagnosis made on the basis of etiology. A simplified classification of flatfoot is presented in Table 7-1.

This chapter will discuss the rigid convex pes valgus and the flexible calcaneovalgus deformities that are usually identified in the neonatal period. Other types of congenital flatfoot, such as that secondary to tarsal coalition and triceps surae contracture, are usually not clinically apparent until after infancy and will be discussed in other chapters dealing with congenital disorders. Congenital and acquired flatfoot secondary to neurologic disease or of the developmental type, which may occur from early childhood to adolescence, will be discussed separately in the sections on neurologic and developmental disorders.

## CONGENITAL CONVEX PES VALGUS

Congenital convex pes valgus is a very rare type of pedal deformity that presents as a rigid, rocker bottom flatfoot. It is composed of a vertical talus and a rigid dislocation of the talocalcaneonavicular joint. It must be differentiated from other types of congenital valgus feet with oblique tali in order to properly direct therapeutic attention. It is difficult to predict the results of treatment owing to the small number of reported cases and the limited follow-up of these cases, as well as to the variety of surgical techniques reported in the literature.

The first complete anatomic, radiographic, and pathologic description of this condition was published in 1914 by Henken.[1,2] He called it *congenital valgus flatfoot*. In 1934 Rocher and Pouyanne[3] called it *congenital flatfoot due to vertical talus* (pied plat congenital par subluxation sous-astragalienne congénitale et orientation verticale de l'astragale). The first report in the English language literature, in 1939 by Lamy and Weissman,[4] proposed the term *congenital convex pes valgus*. This term is used in preference to others. *Teratologic dorsolateral dislocation of the talocalcaneonavicular joint* is the term used by Tachdjian[5,6] to describe the pathologic, anatomic, and therapeutic implications of this rare entity.

It appears that less than 500 cases of congenital convex pes valgus have been reported in the English language literature, including my own cases.[4,7-12] The incidence corresponds to less than 1 percent of live births. In surveying the literature, there seems to be an equal sex distribution, although not all the cases are identified by gender. The majority of reported cases occur bilaterally; of those that do not, the deformity has a predilection for the right side.

## Classification

Several classification schemes for the types of congenital convex pes valgus are presented in the literature.[9,13,14] All pertain to the severity of the deformity and associated neuromuscular and other orthopedic problems. The most complete scheme appears to be that of Hamanishi,[9] who divides these feet into groups with neural tube defects, neuromuscular disorders, malformation

157

Table 7-1. **Types of Flatfoot**

Congenital
    Convex pes valgus
    Calcaneovalgus
    Tarsal coalition
    Triceps surae contracture
Acquired
    Developmental (e.g., idiopathic, familial, ligamentous laxity)
    Paralytic (cerebral palsy, spinal dysraphism, myopathic)
    Traumatic (e.g., posterior tibial tendon rupture, Lisfranc's
        fracture-dislocation)
    Arthritic (e.g., rheumatoid arthritis)

syndromes, chromosomal aberrations, and idiopathic etiology. The Lichtblau[13] classification scheme differentiates between the teratogenic type, the neurogenic type, and the acquired type. Either of these schemes allows investigators to compare groups of different etiologies with varying prognoses. However, classifying a specific case according either of these schemes remains difficult.

## Etiology

The etiology of congenital convex pes valgus is not totally clear. It is generally accepted that an intrauterine or developmental muscular imbalance, consisting of contractures or overactivity of the gastrosoleus complex, the ankle dorsiflexors, and the peronei, may be primarily responsible for the deformity. A contracted triceps surae holds the calcaneus in equinus, with the interosseous ligament-bound talus following. The forefoot is pulled into dorsiflexion and valgus by the shortened foot dorsiflexors and peronei. Because of the tight osseous and ligamentous constraints of the ankle mortise, the talus cannot evert to follow the calcaneus; therefore the talar head protrudes plantarly and medially. The navicular is positioned against its head and neck. The osseous and ligamentous changes occur secondarily to the abnormal muscular contraction and subsequent fibrosis.

This neuromuscular theory is confirmed by the rabbit experiments of Ritsila,[15] who produced a vertical talus deformity by inducing contractures of both the triceps surae and the foot dorsiflexors. Drennan and Sharrad[16] also believed that a dynamic imbalance between strong dorsiflexors and evertors and a weak posterior tibialis leads to this deformity.

In contrast, a developmental delay or alteration in limb embryogenesis was considered causative by Bohm.[17] He believed that if an arrest of development of the first stage of tarsal derotation occurs at the end of the second and the beginning of the third intrauterine month, a vertical talus will be present at birth.

Regardless of the true etiologic process, this deformity may be inherited. Reports of congenital vertical talus occurring in members of the same family — for example, mother and son,[4] mother and daughter,[18] identical twins,[19] and two brothers[4] — are found in the literature.

Genetic defects have been reported to be associated with this deformity. These include trisomy 13-15, trisomy 18,[20] double trisomy,[21] and autosomal trisomy of group 16-18 chromosomes.[20] Congenital vertical talus is also associated with defects of the neuromuscular system and is commonly found with arthrogryposis and myelomeningocele. It is also seen in conjunction with congenital dislocation of the hip, a contralateral talipes equinovarus, neurofibromatosis, congenital absence of the patella, vertebral fusion, congenital ankylosis of the joints, mental retardation, and microcephalia.

## Pathologic Anatomy

The pathologic anatomy of congenital convex pes valgus may be considered as involving bones and joints, ligaments, and muscles and tendons. This information, which is currently confirmed at the time of surgery, was first described by investigators working with stillborn and necropsy specimens.[16,22,23]

### Bone and Joint Changes

The navicular articulates rigidly with the dorsal aspect of the talus, not with the head (Fig. 7-1). The talar head is directed downward and medially and is flattened superiorly. The collum tali is shortened and may have an abnormal facet for the navicular articulation. The calcaneus is rigidly locked in equinus, being in close contact posteriorly with the fibula. The subtalar joint facets are abnormal, being hypoplastic or absent. The sustentaculum tali is often absent, since the normal talocalcaneal contact is missing. The lateral column of the foot is rigidly concave, being subluxed dorsolaterally at the calcaneocuboid joint. The relationship of the navicular and the cuboid to the cuneiform and the metatarsals is normal.

### Ligamentous Changes

The tibionavicular, the lateral portion of the dorsomedial talonavicular, the bifurcate, interosseous talocalcaneal, and calcaneofibular ligaments are all dramatically short-

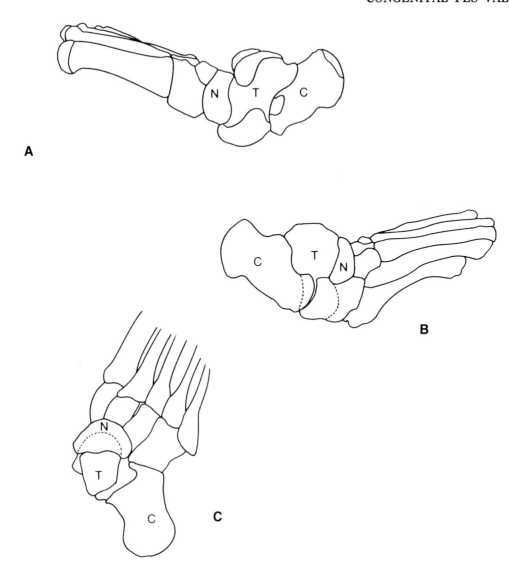

**Fig. 7-1.** Bone and joint changes of congenital convex pes valgus. **(A)** Medial view. **(B)** Lateral view. **(C)** Dorsoplantar view.

ened. The posterior ankle and the subtalar joint capsules are contracted. Conversely, the plantar calcaneonavicular (spring) ligament and the plantar medial capsule of the talonavicular joint are elongated.

### Muscle and Tendon Abnormalities

The tibialis anterior, the extensor hallucis longus, the extensor digitorum longus, the peroneus brevis, and the triceps surae muscles and tendons are contracted. The tibialis posterior and the peroneal tendons act as foot dorsiflexors due to their anterior displacement over the malleoli.

### Clinical Features

The rigid deformity is dramatically present at birth and is so distinctive that a clinical diagnosis is readily made (Fig. 7-2). The sole is rigidly convex, with a severe rocker bottom, and the talar head is palpable plantar-medially. The forefoot is abducted and dorsiflexed at the midtarsal joint, with taut anterior and lateral muscles

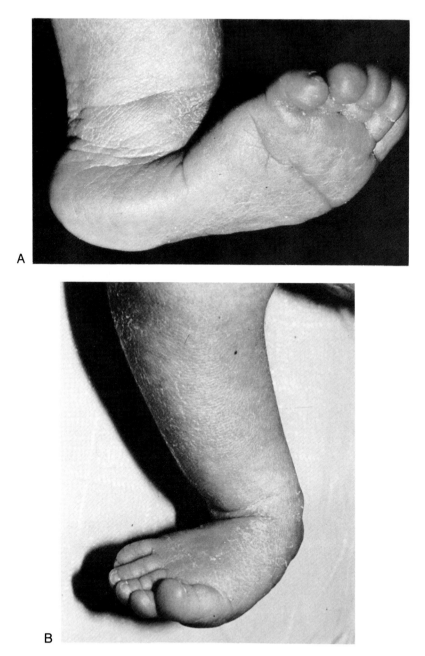

**Fig. 7-2.** Clinical appearance of convex pes valgus at birth. **(A)** Note the rigid convex plantar sole and the dorsiflexed and abducted forefoot. **(B)** Note the prominent plantar talar head.

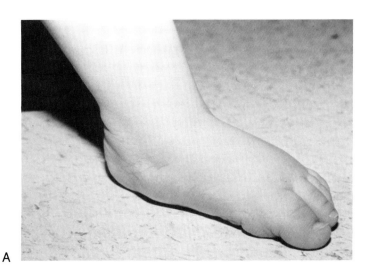
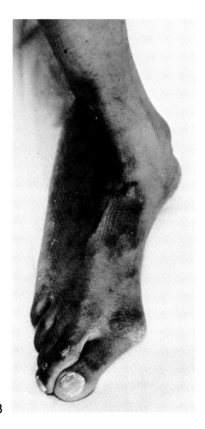

A                                                                    B

**Fig. 7-3.** **(A)** Attempted weight-bearing (maximally dorsiflexed) appearance of convex pes valgus after 8 months of casting. **(B)** An untreated young adult with convex pes valgus with painful subtalar joint and plantar talar head keratosis.

that resist plantar flexion and inversion. Attempted weight-bearing does not change the general appearance of the foot; weight is borne over the medial border of the foot and the talar head, with the rearfoot in equinovalgus. In untreated children, gait is awkward, with external angle and medial sole contact (Fig. 7-3A). These children are asymptomatic until their teenage years, when marked rearfoot joint pain and formation of keratoses occur (Fig. 7-3B).

## Radiographic Findings

The congenital convex pes valgus foot should be evaluated radiographically by anteroposterior and lateral views of attempted weight-bearing, as well as lateral views of stress plantar flexion. The linear bisections of the visible ossification centers of the talus, calcaneus, and the first metatarsal are readily drawn (Fig. 7-4A and B). The lateral standing view shows the talus lying paral-

lel to the tibia, the calcaneus in equinus, and the forefoot dorsiflexed. The talar body bisection projects well below the first metatarsal bisection. The weight-bearing anteroposterior view shows increased talocalcaneal angle and the valgus of the forefoot (Fig. 7-4C).

Until the advent of magnetic resonance imaging (MRI), the dorsal dislocation of the navicular upon the talus could not be visualized. This is because the navicular does not ossify until the age of 3 to 4 years and is therefore radiographically silent in the neonate. Historically, the use of the talo–first metatarsal relationship in the standing and the forced (stress) plantar flexion lateral views was crucial in differentiating the true vertical talus from the flexible oblique (plantar-flexed) talus (Fig. 7-5). In the normal infant the talar and first metatarsal axes are parallel because of normal talonavicular and talocalcaneal joints. In both flexible plantar-flexed and rigid vertical tali, the talar axis passes through the sole of the foot and the first metatarsal axis passes dorsal to the

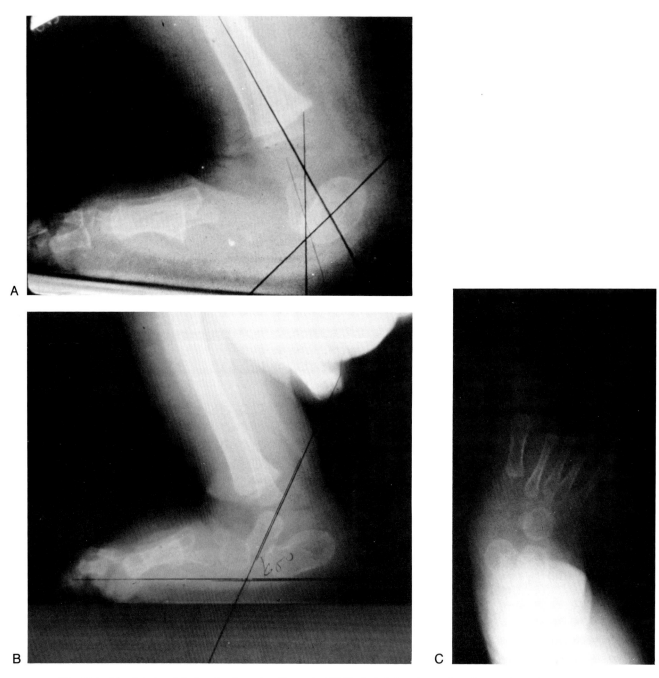

**Fig. 7-4.** Simulated weight-bearing lateral radiograph. **(A)** Birth. **(B)** Age 6 months, after casting. **(C)** Anteroposterior radiograph.

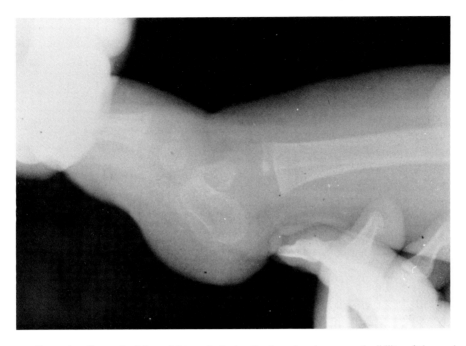

**Fig. 7-5.** Lateral radiograph of forced (stress) plantar flexion, showing nonreducibility of the navicular.

head of the talus. In congenital convex pes valgus, the axes stay misaligned because of the nonreducibility of the navicular on the stress plantar flexion views; this differentiates congenital convex pes valgus from the flexible plantar flexed talus, in which the axes realign in stress plantar flexion views.

The technology of the MRI scan allows direct visualization of the cartilaginous anlage of the navicular and its relationship to the talus (Fig. 7-6). The wedge-shaped navicular is clearly seen articulating with the dorsum of the talar head, and the talonavicular joint dislocation is obvious. Thus, the MRI scan is the definitive diagnostic tool in making the diagnosis of congenital convex pes valgus. When the navicular ossifies in the older uncorrected child, its complete dorsal dislocation is evident and it may appear irregularly ossified or wedge-shaped (Fig. 7-7).

## Differential Diagnosis

In the neonate, talipes calcaneovalgus is commonly mistaken for congenital convex pes valgus. However, the characteristic rigidity and nonreducibility of the vertical talus will differentiate it from talipes calcaneovalgus and pes planovalgus with gastrosoleus equinus. Likewise, paralytic pes planovalgus associated with cerebral palsy,

myelomeningocele, or poliomyelitis is easily distinguished by its suppleness and reducibility. Imaging techniques easily differentiate congenital convex pes valgus from a spastic flatfoot secondary to a tarsal coalition or a prominent medial bulge caused by an accessory navicular.

## Treatment

The object of treatment of congenital convex pes valgus is to restore the normal anatomic relationship of the navicular and calcaneus to the talus as soon as possible. Historically, a variety of therapeutic approaches have been proposed. Common to most of them are the findings that conservative measures usually fail, a posterior release must always be done, the talonavicular joint dislocation must be reduced, and the postoperative bony relationships must be fixated rigidly until complete healing occurs.

Treatment should begin at birth with gentle manipulation to stretch the contracted soft tissues. Reduction of the talocalcaneonavicular joint is possible, although rarely performed, by the method reported by Becker-Anderson and Reimann.[24] When it is evident after 4 to 6 months that the deformity is not being adequately re-

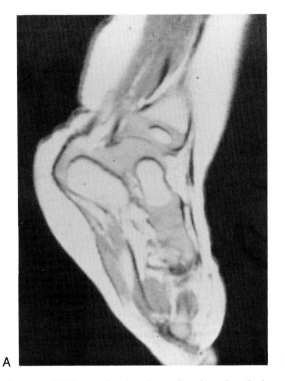
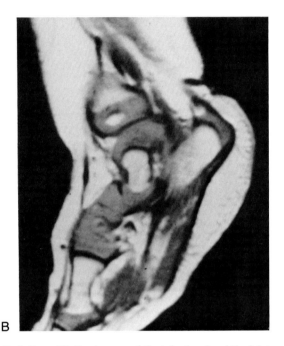

A            B

**Fig. 7-6.** MRI scan showing the wedge-shaped navicular articulating with the dorsum of the talar head and the joint dislocation. **(A)** Normal foot. **(B)** Involved foot.

duced by closed manipulation, open reduction should be performed immediately. The longer the talocalcaneonavicular joint dislocation persists, the more the soft tissues become contracted and the more the osseous adaptive changes become severe and irreversible. The lateral column growth is slowed, and alterations occur at the calcaneocuboid joint.

Early manipulation is performed as follows. Gentle stretching of the triceps surae and the calcaneofibular ligaments is achieved by distal and medial traction with one hand and pressure on the anterior calcaneus with the other. The forefoot is then pulled into plantar flexion, inversion, and adduction to stretch the ankle dorsiflexors and evertors. Distal traction on the forefoot and the navicular and manipulation into adductus and varus stretches the tibionavicular and talonavicular ligaments. These positions are held for 10 to 15 seconds and then released. The whole process is continued for 15 to 20 minutes before a well molded, padded long leg cast of extra fast setting plaster is applied.

Ideally, these casts should be changed twice a week for 6 to 8 weeks, at which time closed reduction of the talocalcaneonavicular dislocation is attempted. Distal traction on the forefoot and the navicular is first applied to increase the deformity (dorsiflexion and eversion). Then the forefoot is brought into plantar flexion as the talar head is pushed into dorsiflexion and the calcaneus is pulled beneath the talus. It is hoped that this will restore the talocalcaneonavicular relationship, as confirmed by postreduction radiographs. MRI or computed tomography (CT) scans may be necessary for absolute confirmation. In the very rare, successful instance of closed reduction, percutaneous pinning under image intensification is necessary to hold the talonavicular joint for 8 weeks.

In most cases when conservative treatment by appropriate manipulation for 4 to 6 months has failed, open reduction should be performed. Many surgical procedures and approaches have been reported in the literature.[5,6,18,25,26] The following surgical procedure is the most direct and effective method for infants and is the one that I favor.

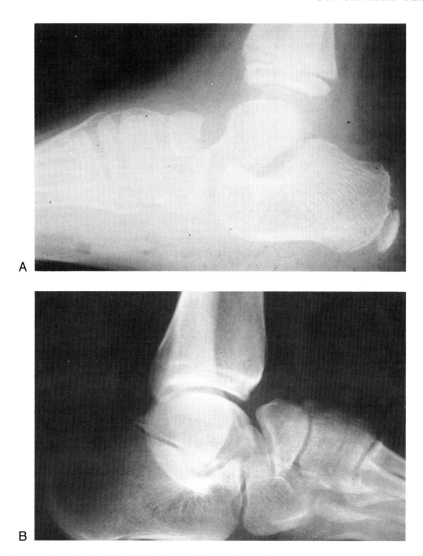

**Fig. 7-7.** Persistent talonavicular joint dislocation and irregular navicular seen in the untreated patient. **(A)** Age 9 years. **(B)** Age 18 years.

The skin incision is made medially, extending from the first metatarsocuneiform joint proximally to the inferior tip of the medial malleolus and curving superiorly to overlie the tendo Achillis. The deep fascia is incised with meticulous care to visualize, mobilize, and retract the medial neurovascular bundle. Systematically, the tendons are lengthened and the contracted ligaments are released. The muscles to be lengthened by Z-plasty are the triceps surae (Fig. 7-8A), the tibialis anterior, the digital extensors, and the peronei. The ligaments to be released are the dorsal and lateral parts of the talonavic-ular, the tibionavicular, the bifurcate (both calcaneona-vicular and calcaneocuboid), the dorsal and lateral aspects of the calcaneocuboid joint capsule, and the cal-caneofibular and the interosseus talocalcaneal ligaments (Fig. 7-8B and C).

After the plantar release, the talar head is manipulated dorsally, and the navicular, with the forefoot, is plantar-flexed and inverted (Fig. 7-8D). A large (0.062-inch) Kirschner wire is driven from the posterior aspect of the talar body anteriorly through the navicular and the cu-neiforms and into the first intermetatarsal space (Fig.

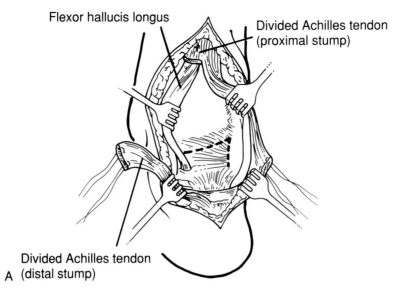

Flexor hallucis longus

Divided Achilles tendon (proximal stump)

Divided Achilles tendon (distal stump)

A

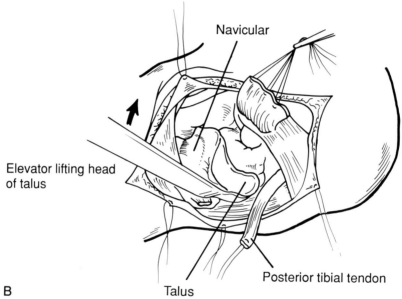

Navicular

Elevator lifting head of talus

Posterior tibial tendon

Talus

B

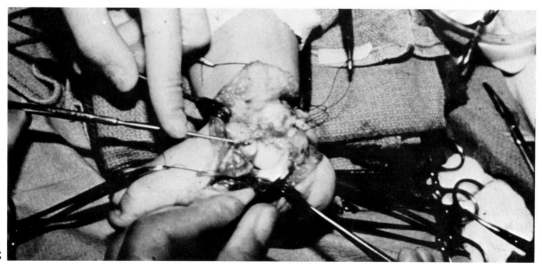

C

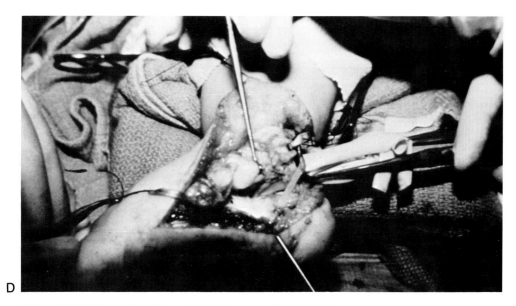

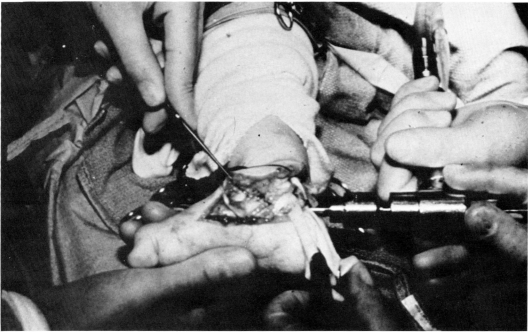

**Fig. 7-8.** Open reduction of congenital convex pes valgus. **(A)** Posterior approach showing tendo achillis Z-plasty lengthening and ankle and subtalar joint release. **(B)** Medial approach showing ligament and tendon division and dorsal rotation of the talus. **(C)** The ligaments have been incised, revealing the navicular (under the upper left skin hook) dorsally located on the talar neck. The talar head is seen protruding plantarward. **(D)** Talar head (skin hook) elevation and plantarward relocation of the navicular. **(E)** The talonavicular joint reduction is held by a Kirschner wire driven from the posterior aspect of the talar body. *(Figure continues.)*

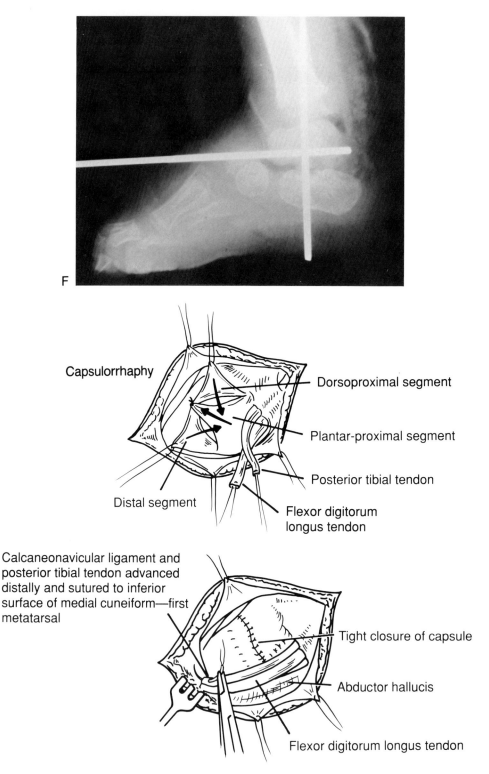

Capsulorrhaphy

Dorsoproximal segment

Plantar-proximal segment

Posterior tibial tendon

Distal segment

Flexor digitorum
longus tendon

Calcaneonavicular ligament and
posterior tibial tendon advanced
distally and sutured to inferior
surface of medial cuneiform—first
metatarsal

Tight closure of capsule

Abductor hallucis

Flexor digitorum longus tendon

F

G

**Fig. 7-8** *(Continued).* **(F)** Kirschner wires are shown holding the corrected talonavicular and talocalcaneal joint relationship in this intraoperative radiograph. **(G)** Capsular plication, reefing of the spring ligament, and tibialis posterior tendon advancement completes the closure.

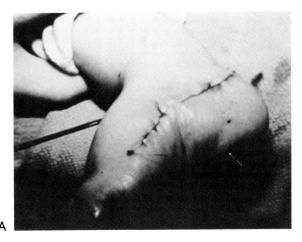

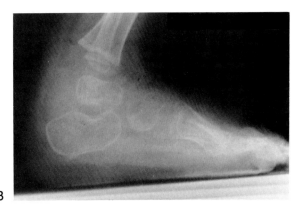

**Fig. 7-9.** **(A)** Postoperative view demonstrating reduction of the rocker bottom deformity absence of the protruding talar head, and formation of an arch. **(B)** Two-year postoperative weight-bearing radiographs showing plantigrade foot and normal talocalcaneal relationships.

7-8E). A second Kirschner wire may be driven from the plantar aspect through the calcaneus into the talus to hold the corrected subtalar joint relationship (Fig. 7-8F). Capsular plication and reefing of the spring ligament, as well as distal transfer of the tibialis posterior tendon under the talar head, may be performed (Fig. 7-8G). Grice[25] and Tachdjian[6] advocate placing the tibialis anterior tendon through the talar neck so that its dynamic force is utilized to prevent recurrence. After skin closure with absorbable suture, an above-knee plaster cast (reinforced with a fiberglass surface roll) is applied for a total of 16 weeks. The cast is changed and the Kirschner wires are removed under general anesthesia 6 to 8 weeks postsurgery (Fig. 7-9A). A nighttime posterior splint is used to hold the ankle at 90 degrees for 1 to 2 years postoperatively (Fig. 7-9B).

Incomplete or lost reduction of the talocalcaneonavicular joint complex will lead to future problems (Fig. 7-10A and B) of stiff, painful feet and degenerative arthritis. Occasionally avascular necrosis of the talus or the navicular may occur (Fig. 7-10C and D). It is therefore important not to disturb the soft tissues close to the neck of the talus during the release. The incidence of avascular necrosis seems to be lower if the patients are older at the time of operation.[27] However, the favorable result of the operation diminishes with increasing age of the child. If the child is first treated at 3 to 6 years of age or if a very rigid deformity persists (as seen in arthrogryposis), an excision of the navicular is the procedure of choice.[18]

This reduces the length of the medial column, allowing the talus to be dorsiflexed, and a somewhat functional joint develops between the talar head and the cuneiforms.

Coleman et al.[26] proposed an alternative two-stage surgery for the child in this age group. The first operation, on the forefoot only, lengthens the contracted tendons, capsulotomizes the talonavicular and calcaneocuboid joints, releases the talocalcaneal interosseus ligament, and fixes the talonavicular joint with a Kirschner wire with the foot in plantar flexion. Occasionally, a talocalcaneal extra-articular bone block is used to stabilize the subtalar joint. After 6 weeks, Achilles tendon lengthening, posterior capsulotomy, and tibialis posterior advancement are performed. Although good results have been reported with this two-stage procedure[7,12,26] in this age group (3 to 6 years), better long-term results are seen with navicular excision,[28] which spares the patient two separate surgical procedures with their inherent risks and complications.

If the child is over 6 years of age, a pantalar release usually fails owing to the deleterious consequences of osseous adaptation of the talus, navicular, and calcaneus. It the patient is symptomatic, a delayed triple arthrodesis with resection of large osseus wedges to correct the deformity may be performed at 10 to 13 years of age[5] (Fig. 7-11). The best overall long-term results occur in those patients who underwent an early (at less than 1 year of age) one-stage pantalar release.[10,11,29]

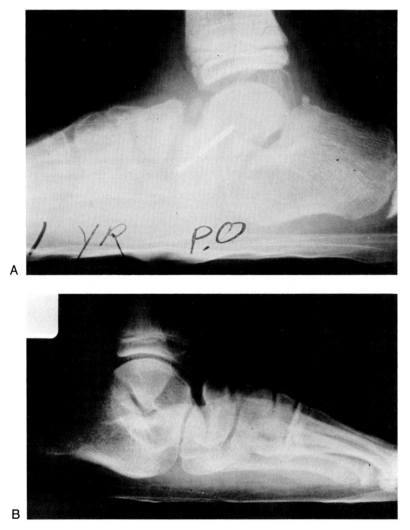

**Fig. 7-10.** Postoperative complications. **(A)** One-year postoperative radiograph showing lost reduction of the talonavicular joint and abnormally shaped navicular. **(B)** Ten-year postoperative radiograph in a patient with painful subtalar and talonavicular joints. *(Figure continues).*

## THE CALCANEOVALGUS FOOT

In contrast to the congenital convex pes valgus foot, the calcaneovalgus foot is a common, relatively benign flexible deformity. It is referred to as the "up and out" deformity since there is marked dorsiflexion and eversion of the foot, with a valgus of the heel. The dorsum of the foot may actually lie against the anterior aspect of the tibia, but soft tissue contractures are not generally severe. The prognosis is good for a functional and pain-free foot as a child matures[30] (Fig. 7-12).

## Incidence and Etiology

The calcaneovalgus foot occurs in 1 to 2 percent of live births,[31] but is probably under-reported owing to the fact that many of these feet spontaneously relax in the first few weeks of life and are therefore not referred to a specialist. My personal experience indicates a 3 percent occurrence rate[32] as seen in a busy (325 births per month) neonatal nursery.

The etiology is unclear but probably involves an abnormal intrauterine position with excessive internal limb

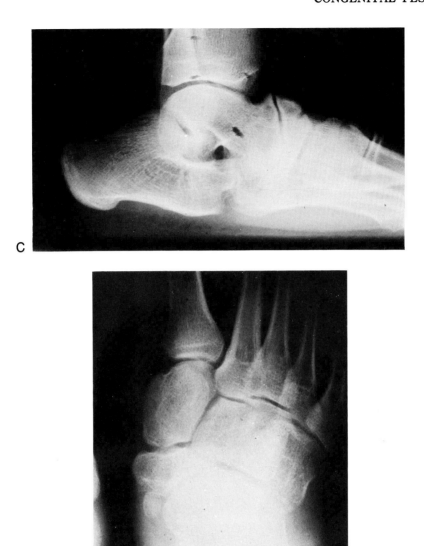

C

D

**Fig. 7-10** *(Continued).* **(C & D)** Avascular necrosis of the navicular, causing talonavicular joint arthritis.

rotation, especially in later fetal life. Oligohydramnios is frequently an associated condition. Calcaneovalgus foot does not usually occur with other congenital neuromuscular abnormalities,[33] but rare reports of associations are found in the literature. Congenital dislocation of the peroneal tendons has been reported to be associated with

calcaneovalgus feet;[34] such feet proved more resistant to correction and needed prolonged treatment as compared with isolated calcaneovalgus deformities. This foot type has also been reported in a patient with multiple chromosomal abnormalities.[35] As with any other pedal birth defect, a thorough general, neurologic, and orthopedic

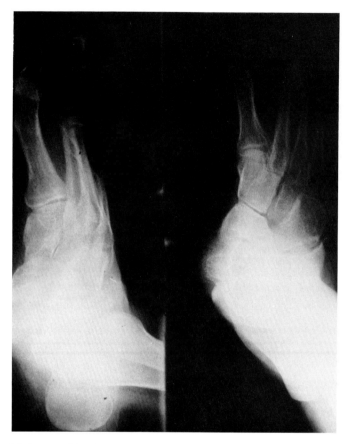

**Fig. 7-11.** A painful adult foot resulting from uncorrected congenital pes valgus. A triple arthrodesis was required to stabilize the foot and to reduce symptoms.

examination is necessary, with consultations as appropriate.

## Pathologic Anatomy and Clinical Features

All the osseous structures are normal in morphology and in their interrelationship with one another, except that the navicular is displaced laterally to the talus. The talus is severely plantar-flexed and adducted, and the distal aspect of the calcaneus is laterally displaced. The forefoot is dorsiflexed and everted, with a prominent plantar-medial talar head. The anterior and lateral musculature is taut and sometimes contracted; the Achilles tendon is not contracted. The talocalcaneal and plantar calcaneonavicular ligaments are relaxed. Redundant folds of skin are usually seen dorsolaterally; however in some cases the skin may be taut, preventing reduction.

All these changes are flexible and easily reduced with plantar flexion and adduction of the forefoot. The hallmarks of *lack* of rigidity and calcaneoequinus clinically distinguish the calcaneovalgus foot from the congenital convex pes valgus foot.

## Radiographic Findings

Simulated weight-bearing radiographs of the calcaneovalgus foot reveal normally shaped ossification centers, a severely plantar-flexed talus, and a lack of calcaneal inclination on the lateral view. The forefoot may appear relatively dorsiflexed. On the anteroposterior view an increased talocalcaneal angle is noted.

As discussed in the previous section, the axes of the talus and the first metatarsal realign on the stress plantar flexion view. This differentiates talipes calcaneovalgus

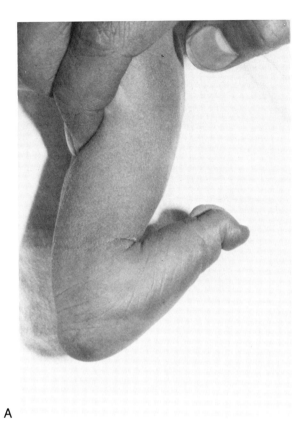
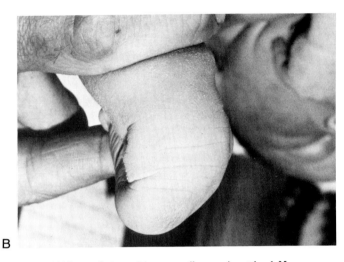

A                                                              B

**Fig. 7-12.** Clinical appearance of a neonatal calcaneovalgus foot. **(A)** Lateral view with a normally prominent heel. No equinus is present. **(B)** Posterior view demonstrating valgus heel position.

from congenital convex pes valgus. In questionable cases, MRI is the definitive diagnostic tool.

## Treatment

The goal of treatment is to reduce the rearfoot valgus and the forefoot dorsiflexion as quickly as possible to prevent deleterious osseous adaptation. Gentle manipulation should be instituted in the neonatal unit by the staff, to be continued postdischarge by the parents. Podiatric supervision with staff in-service and parental demonstration of the manipulation technique are mandatory. The heel should be held parallel to the tibia with one hand while the other hand gently manipulates the forefoot into plantar flexion and adduction. This position is held for 30 seconds and then released. This maneuver should be repeated 15 times per session for 3 or 4 sessions per day. In many cases manipulation alone will

stretch the contracted soft tissue and restore alignment in the first few weeks of life. In the relaxed state, the foot should be perpendicular to the leg with no forefoot valgus or dorsiflexion. If this is not achieved in the first 3 to 4 weeks of proper manipulation, serial casting is appropriate. If the foot appears more rigid and resistant to manipulation, casting should be initiated earlier.

A well padded, short leg cast of a fast-setting plaster is used after a session of manipulation (an above-knee cast may be used if the short leg cast tends to slide off). All the components of the deformity are simultaneously corrected in the cast. The calcaneus is held in slight varus, the foot in slight equinus, and the forefoot in neutral. It is mandatory that the forefoot not be used as a lever arm to bring the rearfoot into varus. The cast is changed at weekly intervals until the foot assumes a normal clinical alignment at rest. Usually the casting period is short, from several weeks to 3 to 4 months in more rigid cases.

The long-term prognosis for a true calcaneovalgus foot is good with appropriate treatment. Most feet mature without further problems. Unfortunately, no good long-term studies have been made. Some of these feet remain flat and if symptomatic may need further treatment, including corrective shoe modifications, orthoses, or possibly surgical repair. Prompt recognition and institution of conservative care will hopefully help limit the need for more aggressive later treatment.

# REFERENCES

## Convex Pes Valgus

1. Henken R: Contribution á l'Étude des Formes Osseuses du Pied Plat Valgus Congénital. Thesis, Univ Lyon, 1914
2. Nove-Josserand L: Formes anatomiques de pied plat. Rev Orthop 10:117, 1923
3. Rocher HL, Pouyanne L: Pied plat congénital par subluxation sous-astragalienne congénitale et orientation verticale de l'astragale. Bordeaux Chir 5:249, 1934
4. Lamy L, Weissman L: Cóngenital convex pes valgus. J Bone Joint Surg [Br] 21:79, 1939
5. Tachdjian MD: Congenital convex pes valgus. Orthop Clin North Am 3:131, 1972
6. Tachdjian MD: The Child's Foot. WB Saunders, Philadelphia, 1985
7. Jacobson S, Crawford A: Congenital vertical talus. J Pediatr Orthop 3:306, 1983
8. Dodge L, Ashley R, Gilbert R: Treatment of congenital vertical talus: a retrospective review of 36 feet with long-term followup. Foot Ankle 7:326, 1987
9. Hamanishi C: Congenital vertical talus: classification with 69 cases and new measurement system. J Pediatr Orthop 4:318, 1984
10. DeRosa G, Ahlfeld S: Congenital vertical talus: the Riley experience. Foot Ankle 5:118, 1984
11. Oppenheim W, Smith C, Christie W: Congenital vertical talus. Foot Ankle 5:198, 1985
12. Walker A, Ghali N, Silk F: Congenital vertical talus. J Bone Joint Surg [Br] 67:117, 1985
13. Lichtblau S: Congenital vertical talus. Bull Hosp Jt Dis Orthop Inst 39:165, 1978
14. Kumar S, Cowell H, Ramsey P: Vertical and oblique talus. Instr Course Lect 31:235, 1982
15. Ritsila VA: Talipes equinovarus and vertical talus produced experimentally in newborn rabbits. Acta Orthop Scand 121:1, 1969
16. Drennan JC, Sharrad WJ: The pathological anatomy of convex pes valgus. J Bone Joint Surg [Br] 53:455, 1971

17. Bohm M: Der Fötale Fuss. Beitrag zur Entstehung des Pes Planus, des Pes Valgus und des Pes Planovalgus. Z Orthop 57:562, 1932
18. Robbins M: Naviculectomy for congenital vertical talus. Bull Hosp Jt Dis Orthop Inst 37:77, 1976
19. Armknecht P: Orthopädische Leiden bei Zwillingen. Verh Dtsch Orthop Ges 26:82, 1932
20. Towns PL, Dettart GK, Hecht F, Manning JA: Trisomy 13-15 in male infant. J Pediatr 60:528, 1962
21. Uchida IA, Lewis AJ, Bowman JM, Wang NC: A case study of double trisomy: no 18 and triple X. J Pediatr 60:498, 1962
22. Campos de Paz A, DeSouza V, DeSouza DC: Congenital convex pes valgus. Orth Clin North Am 9:207, 1978
23. Patterson WR, Fitz DA, Smith WS: The pathological anatomy of congenital convex pes valgus. J Bone Joint Surg [Am] 50:458, 1968
24. Becker-Anderson N, Reimann I: Congenital vertical talus —re-evaluation of early manipulative treatment. Acta Orthop Scand 45:130, 1974
25. Grice DS: The role of subtalar fusion in the valgus deformities of the feet. Instr Course Lect 16:127, 1967
26. Coleman S, Stelling F, Jarrett J: Pathomechanics and treatment of congenital vertical talus. Clin Orthop 70:62, 1970
27. Ellis J, Scheer G: Congenital convex pes valgus. Clin Orthop 99:168, 1974
28. Clark M, D'Ambrosia R, Ferguson A: Congenital vertical talus. J Bone Joint Surg [Am] 59:816, 1977
29. Adelaar R, Williams R, Gould J: Congenital convex pes valgus. Foot Ankle 2:62, 1980

## Calcaneovalgus

30. Wetzenstin H: Prognosis of pes calcaneovalgus congenitus. Acta Orthop Scand 41:122, 1970
31. Widhe T, Aaro S, Elmstedt E: Foot deformities in the newborn—incidence and prognosis. Acta Orthop Scand 59:176, 1988
32. Silvani S: Survey of neonatal feet in the Kaiser Foundation Hospital at Hayward Nursery. Unpublished report, 1984
33. Larsen B, Reimann I, Becker-Anderson H: Congenital calcaneovalgus with special reference to treatment and its relation to other congenital foot deformities. Acta Orthop Scand 45:145, 1974
34. Purnell M, Drummond D, Engber A: Congenital dislocation of the peroneal tendons in the calcaneovalgus foot. J Bone Joint Surg [Br] 65:316, 1983
35. Mankinen C, Sears J, Alvarez V: Terminal long-arm deletion of chromosomes in a 3 year old female. Birth Defects 22 (5):131, 1976

# 8

# Metatarsus Adductus

## JAMES P. FAGAN

*Metatarsus adductus* is a common term used to describe a broad spectrum of deformities in the pediatric foot. It consists of three separate entities—true metatarsus adductus, metatarsus varus, and skewfoot. True metatarsus adductus is characterized by adduction of all five metatarsals in the transverse plane, resulting in a foot that appears C-shaped (Fig. 8-1A). The deformity is restricted to Lisfranc's joint, and the severity of adduction of the metatarsals is greatest medially, progressively decreasing in severity from medial to lateral. *Metatarsus varus* is defined as a frontal plane inversion and adduction of all of the metatarsals at Lisfranc's joint (Fig. 8-1B). Both the inversion and adduction components of the deformity are more pronounced medially. The heel is usually neutral but may assume either a mild varus or, more commonly, a valgus position. *Skewfoot* is characterized by forefoot adduction and inversion, as with metatarsus varus, along with rearfoot eversion at the midtarsal and subtalar joints (Fig. 8-1C). The rearfoot is usually flexible but can be a rigid deformity. The foot appears to have a Z-configuration.

Both metatarsus adductus and metatarsus varus are usually congenital, whereas skewfoot is usually an acquired deformity, resulting from gradual compensation of metatarsus varus that occurs with weight-bearing and shoe wear or occurs iatrogenically as the result of excessive or improper manipulation and casting. There are also some reported cases of true congenital skewfoot.[1,2] Unlike clubfoot, skewfoot involves no sagittal plane deformity or rotational spin of the hindfoot.[3]

Variation in the degree of contracture, flexibility, and the extent of hindfoot involvement has led to the use of multiple descriptions and confusing terms; these terms include metatarsus varus, metatarsus adductus, metatarsus supinatus, metatarsus adductovarus, skewfoot,

hooked forefoot, Z-foot, third of a clubfoot, and serpentine foot. When one reviews the literature, it is important to understand that there is no consistency in the terminology used. For example, different authors have applied the term *metatarsus varus* both to a rigid, nonflexible foot and to a flexible foot with mild pathology. It is preferable to consider metatarsus adductus as a single entity with a broad spectrum of severity.

The deformity was first described in 1863 by Henke and was first acknowledged in the English literature in 1921 by Bankart,[4] who believed that the problem was due to a congenital absence of the internal cuneiform and recommended that the problem be dealt with by excision of the cuboid. In comparison with clubfoot, very little attention has been devoted to this entity in the literature, probably because, unlike clubfoot, metatarsus adductus does not impose major disability. Initial studies of clubfooted children demonstrated that some of them exhibited forefoot contracture without hindfoot involvement. These children seemed to respond more easily to treatment and were in most instances not left with major residual disability.

Historically, there has been great debate regarding treatment. Some authors have stated that the deformity resolves spontaneously.[5-7] Whereas others feel that significant residual deformity often occurs and that treatment should be started as early as possible because of the unpredictable nature of the disorder.[2,8] This issue is clouded even further because of the lack of common terminology used for reference.

Since World War II, the reported incidence of metatarsus adductus has gradually increased while clubfoot has become less common.[2] It is likely that this relative increase in the incidence of metatarsus adductus has resulted primarily from improved recognition of the de-

175

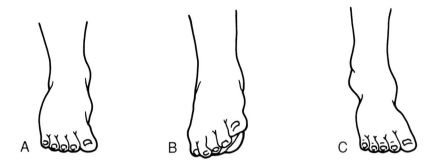

**Fig. 8-1.** The three primary subtypes of metatarsus adductus. **(A)** True metatarsus adductus, with transverse plane adduction of the forefoot only, which is the most common entity. **(B)** Metatarsus varus, in which the deformity consists of transverse plane adduction and frontal plane inversion of the forefoot and, less commonly, rearfoot inversion. **(C)** Skewfoot, in which the deformity consists of forefoot adduction and frontal plane inversion and eversion of the rearfoot.

formity rather than from a real increase in frequency. Wynn-Davies[9] found the incidence of metatarsus adductus to be 1 in 1,000 with a male to female ratio of 0.76 : 1. Other authors have felt that the male to female ratio was essentially equal. Bilateral involvement does not appear to be more common than unilateral involvement.

## CLASSIFICATION

Metatarsus adductus and metatarsus varus can be positional or structural and can vary from flexible and mild to severe and rigid. Dynamic contracture of the foot with weight-bearing is regarded as a separate clinical entity. Positional metatarsus adductus (referred to by Tachdjian as postural metatarsus adductus) is the most common clinical entity and is thought to be caused by abnormal position of the foot in utero.[10] It is quite common for the infant's foot to be slightly adducted. In addition, the foot and great toe of a child under 1 year of age will adduct with plantar stimulation (including simulated weight-bearing) owing to the residual plantar grasp reflex. These mild positional forms of metatarsus adductus will generally resolve without treatment. Treatment may be necessary, however, in the infant who is unable to spontaneously abduct the foot or in whom the forefoot cannot be easily reduced with manual pressure. Unlike the positional deformity, structural metatarsus adductus will usually show increasing or more rigid deformity with age.

Congenital skewfoot is rare. Kite termed this combination of fixed hindfoot valgus and severe, rigid metatarsus adductus *serpentine foot.*[2] Bleck reported only one such case in 21 years among 503 feet reviewed.[8] Peterson, in a review of the entire English literature, noted only 50 cases of skewfoot reported.[1] These children inevitably come to surgery at an early age because of the significance of the deformity.

Residual structural metatarsus adductus deformity is also common in children who have been treated for clubfoot. The residual adduction deformity may be at any level — tarsometatarsal, midtarsal, or talocalcaneonavicular. Simulated weight-bearing radiographs are essential to establish the true level of the contracture.

Metatarsus adductus is most commonly congenital and idiopathic, but rarely, it may have a neurogenic etiology and in some cases may develop slowly in response to muscle imbalance. Neuromuscular conditions such as Charcot-Marie-Tooth disease, Friedreich's ataxia, and arthrogryposis multiplex congenita have been associated with metatarsus adductus.

## ETIOLOGY AND PATHOLOGY

The etiology of metatarsus adductus is unknown; both genetic and environmental theories have been advocated. Wynn-Davies reported a 1 : 20 chance of younger siblings of a child with metatarsus adductus being born with the condition.[9] Kite reported a single family in which the mother and all the children had the severe and rigid form of metatarsus adductus or skewfoot.[2] However, no exact genetic pattern has been identified. The incidence of additional siblings with metatarsus adductus, in my experience, seems to be much higher than the 1 in 20 reported by Wynn-Davies. Various environmental theories have also been proposed. Different authors have implicated abnormalities of the abductor hallucis muscle, anterior and posterior tibial tendons, peroneal tendons, ligaments, and joint capsules. Arrested fetal development is thought by some investigators also to play a role. Just as with clubfoot, there is probably no one specific etiology of metatarsus adductus; it is likely that various etiologic factors can result in a common clinical presentation.

Contracture of the abductor hallucis was reported by Thompson as a possible etiology of hallux varus and metatarsus varus.[11] He reported finding an anomalous insertion of the abductor hallucis into the medial portion of the base of the proximal phalanx in all of his surgical releases for metatarsus adductus. In contrast, Basmajian found only a 5 percent incidence (1 of 22 feet) of anomalous insertion in his dissection of 22 normal adult feet.[12] Furthermore, Thompson stated that when the feet of children with metatarsus adductus were placed in neutral position, forefoot motion was 100 percent in adduction; this may be compared with Basmajian's reports of flexion alone occurring 83 percent of the time when the abductor of normal feet was stimulated. Thompson also believed that the flexor hallucis brevis in children with metatarsus adductus contributed to adduction. Lichtblau reported good or excellent results in 22 of 29 feet of children age 7 months to 11 years who had undergone isolated abductor hallucis tenotomy.[13]

Ponsetti and Becker described an anomalous insertion of the anterior tibial tendon entirely into the base of the first ray, rather than into the first metatarsal base and the first cuneiform equally as in normal feet.[14] They believed that this produced an inversion and elevating force on the first ray, which contributed to development of metatarsus adductus and varus. Reimann and Werner, however, were unable to produce an adductus deformity in a stillborn fetus by merely pulling on the anterior tibial tendon, and in a later study on a stillborn infant with metatarsus adductus they were unable to achieve correction by releasing the anterior tibial tendon alone.[15-17] Correction could not be obtained until the tarsometatarsal capsules and intermetatarsal ligaments were released. These authors therefore concluded that a primary contracture of the joint capsule and ligaments caused metatarsus adductus rather than a muscle imbalance.

Kite speculated that anterior tibial contracture could occur secondary to weakening of the opposing peroneal muscles caused by a mechanical disadvantage imposed by the adductus position.[2] When the foot is manipulated and casted in a neutral position or when the child begins to stand, normal muscle balance is again achieved. Kite's mechanical disadvantage theory of muscle imbalance could explain why metatarsus adductus often improves once the child begins weight-bearing. An abnormal insertion of the posterior tibial tendon distally into the first cuneiform has been described in 14 feet by Browne and Paton,[18] who noticed an increased dynamic contracture in such feet with weight-bearing. They believed that the abnormal insertion contributed to the high arch varus component of the foot, while the lateral insertion of the tendon into the second cuneiform and the bases of the second, third, and fourth metatarsals caused the adduction component of the deformity.

Reimann and Werner postulated the primary etiology of metatarsus adductus to be a congenital subluxation of Lisfranc's joint.[16,17] They noted an anatomic abnormality of the first cuneiform bone, as well as subluxations of the second and third cuneiform metatarsal articulations and slight twisting to the bases of the metatarsals.

Arrested development of the foot in utero has been suggested by Diaz and Diaz.[19] The normal fetal position of the foot is an adducted equinovarus position. If normal development does not take place, the foot will remain locked in that deformed position. Exposure to various toxic substances can result in arrest of normal fetal development at any stage. If arrest occurs during the fibular stage (21 to 30 mm length, 6 to 7 weeks of gestation), clubfoot may result. If arrest occurs during the tibial phase (31 to 50 mm length, 8 to 9 weeks of gestation), metatarsus adductus may occur.

## CLINICAL FEATURES

Examination of the infant with metatarsus adductus should include a complete history of prenatal and perinatal development and a familial history of lower extremity problems. A complete musculoskeletal examination of the spine, hips, and extremities should be performed at the initial visit. Particular attention should be devoted to the stability of the hips, as a 10 percent incidence of associated hip dislocation has been reported with metatarsus adductus.[20,21] Repeat examinations and frog-leg lateral radiographs of the hips should be obtained when any clinical signs of dysplasia are noted. Lack of tibial torsion is also associated with metatarsus adductus; some authors even state that there is always a relationship between the two.[14] I have noted an increased incidence of lack of tibial torsion in children with a familial history of metatarsus adductus.

Examination of the foot should include observation of its appearance, including the presence of adduction and/or varus components of the deformity and heel position. The presence of a vertical cleft along the medial border of the foot may indicate a more rigid deformity. Passive and active motion of the forefoot (abduction and peroneal function) and ankle should be evaluated, and any contracture of the anterior tibial tendon should be noted. Bleck has described a simple, clinically reproducible method that can be used to quantitatively record the degree of deformity.[8] The heel is bisected, with the line of bisection extending through the forefoot. Normally, this line should extend between the second and third toes. If the line of bisection falls through the third toe, between the third and fourth toes, or between the fourth

and fifth toes, mild, moderate, or severe deformity, respectively, is indicated (Fig. 8-2).

To determine the flexibility of the forefoot, the lateral and medial border of the foot should be stimulated by simply stroking the foot. If the child does not spontaneously straighten the foot, proper technique should be used to evaluate true abduction of Lisfranc's joint. The rearfoot must be stabilized in varus and slight plantar flexion in order to prevent rearfoot motion. Pressure should be applied at the level of the first metatarsal head, not beyond. The heel can usually be cradled between the second and third fingers of the opposing hand, while the thumb of the opposing hand projects distally along the base of the cuboid (Fig. 8-3). The amount of correction and the degree of force required to obtain partial or complete correction should be recorded. The tautness of the abductor hallucis muscle should also be evaluated in a relaxed and a simulated weight-bearing position.

The lesser digits of an infant with metatarsus adductus will be aligned in varus and adduction according to metatarsal position. The great toe is usually even more adducted, which creates a cleft between the great and second toes. A dynamic hallux varus will frequently be seen when the forefoot is placed in a simulated weight-bearing position as a result of increased tension of the abductor hallucis and flexor hallucis brevis tendons. In the older

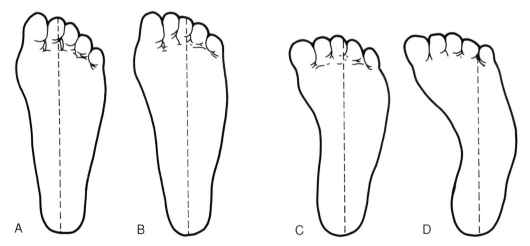

**Fig. 8-2.** Bleck's clinical method of recording the severity of metatarsus adductus deformity. **(A)** Normal child's foot. Bisection of the footprint heel falls between the second and third toes. **(B)** Mild metatarsus adductus. **(C)** Moderate metatarsus adductus. **(D)** Severe metatarsus adductus.

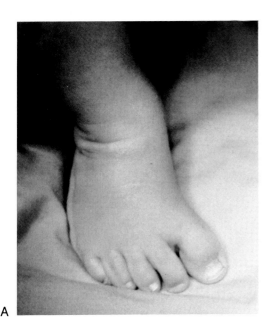
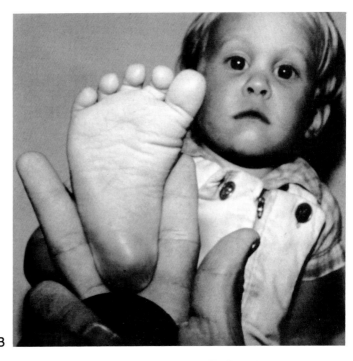

A                                                        B

**Fig. 8-3.** (A) Dorsal view of a 6-month-old child with typical moderate metatarsus adductus. (B) Clinical examination method for determining severity and flexibility of metatarsus adductus. Normally the lateral border of the forefoot should be parallel to the examiner's long finger. The degree of correction that can be obtained with abduction of the forefoot allows the examiner to label the deformity as mild, moderate, or severe. The force required to obtain correction allows the examiner to describe the deformity as flexible, semirigid, or rigid. (Courtesy of S.J. DeValentine, D.P.M.)

child, the degree of deformity may be masked by abduction of the digits at the metatarsophalangeal joints, which gives the illusion of a foot straighter than it actually is.

## RADIOGRAPHIC EVALUATION

Radiographs are not needed to establish a diagnosis in the infant with metatarsus adductus, and response to treatment is usually so rapid that radiographs are academic. However, if the infant does not respond readily to treatment after 4 to 6 weeks or if there is a question of an equinus contracture, radiographs will help differentiate between a clubfoot and metatarsus varus and will establish a baseline parameter (Fig. 8-4). In the toddler who presents for initial evaluation, radiographs will be important to evaluate whether secondary adaptive changes are present in the midfoot and rearfoot and to establish the degree of skeletal ossification. As in clubfoot, all radio-

graphs should be taken in a simulated weight-bearing position. In the infant, the foot should be held by the clinician to ensure proper position and consistency of technique.

Radiographs are also of limited benefit in the infant, because most of the midfoot is cartilaginous until age 2 to 3 years. The traditional reference points for obtaining the bisection of the forefoot are not yet present. Lepow et al.[22] have developed a pediatric metatarsus adductus angle with which they obtained reliable measurements in 15 children before midfoot ossification. The measurement is obtained as follows: one arm of the angle is constructed of the longitudinal bisector of the second metatarsal shaft; and the second arm of the angle is constructed, with the use of a compass and straightedge, by drawing the perpendicular bisector to the line connecting the proximal medial side of the first metatarsal and the proximal lateral side of the base of the fifth metatarsal (Fig. 8-5). The values established for the pe-

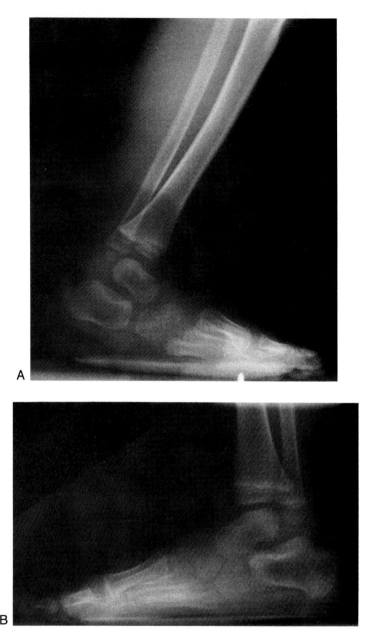

**Fig. 8-4. (A)** Lateral radiograph of residual clubfoot. Note the equinus posture of the os calcis and the low talocalcaneal angle. **(B)** Lateral radiograph of a child with metatarsus adductus. The os calcis is well seated in the heel, and the talocalcaneal angle lies in a normal relationship. *(Figure continues.)*

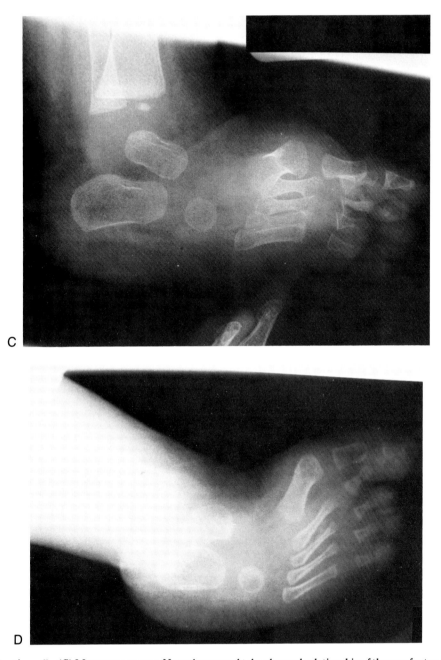

**Fig. 8-4** *(Continued).* **(C)** Metatarsus varus. Note the normal talocalcaneal relationship of the rearfoot and the frontal plane elevation of the first ray. **(D)** Metatarsus adductus. The talocalcaneal angle lies in a normal relationship, as opposed to the reversed talocalcaneal angle in a clubfoot. There is a positive talar first metatarsal angle.

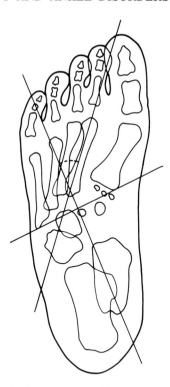

**Fig. 8-5.** Pediatric metatarsus adductus angle as described by Lepow et al.[22] Prior to ossification of the midfoot, this angle measurement is the most accurate way of determining the degree of forefoot angulation. Values obtained are consistent with traditional measurements of 22 to 25 degrees at birth, 15 to 20 degrees by 18 months, and 10 degrees by adulthood. See text for details.

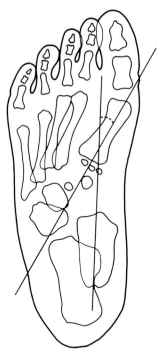

**Fig. 8-6.** Talo-first metatarsal angle. This measurement is used primarily to evaluate true metatarsus adductus. It will be affected by the talocalcaneal angle; it is erroneously increased in clubfoot and decreased in skewfoot.

diatric metatarsus adductus angle as described by Lepow et al. do not vary significantly from those obtained by the traditional method. Normal values for the metatarsus adductus angle are 22 to 25 degrees at birth, 15 to 20 degrees in the toddler, and 10 degrees in the adult.[22] In addition to the metatarsus adductus angle, the talo-first metatarsal, talocalcaneal, lateral talocalcaneal, and calcaneocuboid angles may be helpful parameters in the radiographic evaluation of metatarsus adductus.

The talo-first metatarsal angle on the anteroposterior view is obtained by drawing a bisector through the talus and the first metatarsal (Fig. 8-6). If the bisection of the first metatarsal lies medial to the talar bisector, the angle is assigned a positive value and the foot is considered adducted. The normal angle is 0 to − 20 degrees.[23] This angle is not specific for Lisfranc's joint and will be affected by abnormal movement at Chopart's joint. Therefore it depends upon a normal talocalcaneal angle.

The talocalcaneal angle on the anteroposterior view is formed by the longitudinal bisection of the talus and calcaneus. This can be helpful in differentiating a metatarsus adductus from a clubfoot. The angle would be normal with metatarsus varus; decreased or, more commonly, reversed with clubfoot; and increased with skewfoot. Its normal range is 20 to 40 degrees.[23,24] The talocalcaneal angle does not give information about forefoot adduction, but when combined with the talo-first metatarsal angle, it can be used to evaluate skewfoot, which is defined radiographically by an increased talocalcaneal angle in addition to a positive talo-first metatarsal angle.

The lateral talocalcaneal angle is formed by a bisector of the talus and a line along the inferior aspect of the calcaneus. It helps to differentiate the equinus contracture of clubfoot from metatarsus varus. This angle would be normal in metatarsus adductus and metatarsus varus but decreased in skewfoot. Its normal range is 35 to 55 degrees.[23,24]

The calcaneocuboid angle is formed by a line along the lateral aspect of the calcaneus and a line along the lateral

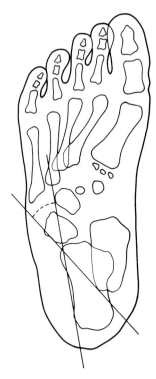

**Fig. 8-7.** Calcaneocuboid angle, which is increased with lateral movement of the rearfoot from Chopart's joint pronation as in skewfoot. This angle should be normal in metatarsus adductus.

aspect of the cuboid (Fig. 8-7) and has a normal value of 0 to 5 degrees. An increase in this angle is expected with Chopart's lateral translational movement, as in skewfoot.[25]

Berg's radiographic classification system for evaluation of metatarsus adductus allows identification of various subtypes of the deformity.[26] The foot is divided into three segments: the forefoot, extending from the digits to Lisfranc's joint; the midfoot, extending to Chopart's joint; and the hindfoot. The forefoot is represented by the talo-first metatarsal angle. The midfoot is evaluated by a bisector through the calcaneus, which should extend through the middle of the cuboid or the base of the fourth metatarsal. If the line lies medially, the midfoot is said to be laterally translated. The hindfoot is evaluated by the talocalcaneal angle on both the anteroposterior and lateral views.

Berg proposed four radiographic subtypes: simple metatarsus adductus (in which the talo-first metatarsal angle is increased but the midfoot and hindfoot are nor-

mally aligned); complex metatarsus adductus or metatarsus varus (in which, in addition to the increase in the talo-first metatarsal angle, the hindfoot is laterally translated); simple skewfoot (in which the talo-first metatarsal angle is increased, the midfoot is normally aligned, and the hindfoot is everted); and complex skewfoot (in which the talo-first metatarsal angle is increased, the midfoot is laterally translated, and the hindfoot is everted).

In the older child, radiographs can be helpful in determining true movement at Lisfranc's joint. An abduction stress test, in which force is applied in the same fashion as when the foot is manipulated for correction, will determine if clinical movement is available at Lisfranc's joint or if the foot is compensating by lateral midfoot or rearfoot translation in hindfoot eversion. This test is also useful in the older child (aged 3 to 4 years) to determine if further casting will be of benefit or if a surgical procedure will be required.

## TREATMENT

The infant with metatarsus adductus and/or varus should be referred for evaluation as early as possible, and treatment should be provided by someone knowledgeable about children's foot problems.[2,6,8,16,27-29] As with clubfoot, overly aggressive manipulation can very clearly lead to rearfoot or midfoot breakdown, creating a skewfoot. Bleck, in a study of 160 children, observed a direct correlation between good results and the age of initiation of treatment.[8] Children who began treatment prior to the age of 8 months did better statistically. Bleck did not find a statistically significant correlation between the severity or flexibility of the deformity and the outcome of treatment. Less favorable results are related to a slower growth curve beyond the age of 8 to 9 months.

It is a commonly held belief among clinicians that most cases of metatarsus adductus resolve spontaneously and that only those children with severe deformity or varus contracture require treatment. Rushford reported an 86 percent spontaneous resolution rate in 130 feet.[5] Ponsetti and Becker noted that only 11 percent of 379 children studied required treatment.[14] These observations were based upon clinical appearance only.

On the basis of the amount of residual forefoot adduction seen clinically and of radiographs in older children and adults, it is obvious that not all deformities resolve spontaneously. Partial reduction may occur in many cases, and the foot may appear to look straighter clini-

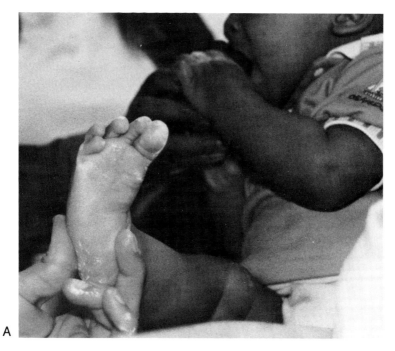

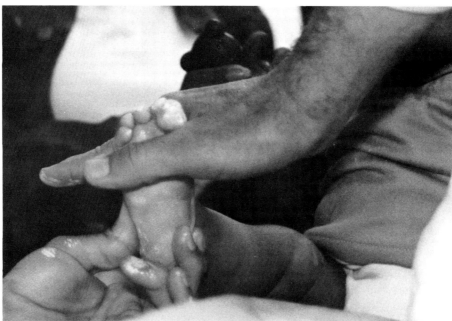

**Fig. 8-8.** Proper manipulation technique used to reduce metatarsus adductus. **(A)** Note the position of the clinician's thumb along the lateral cuboid. The rearfoot should be stabilized in slight varus and plantar flexion by cradling the heel between the second and third fingers with the thumb extended along the cuboid. **(B)** The forefoot is abducted while the rearfoot is stabilized to prevent pronation.

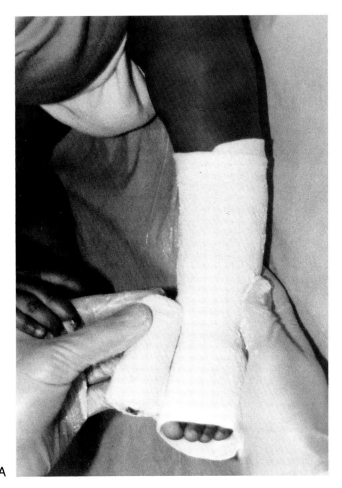
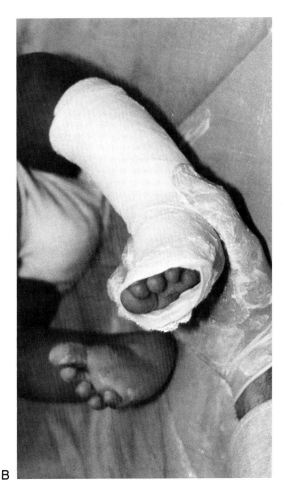

**Fig. 8-9.** Cast application. **(A)** Plaster should be rolled on "against" the deformity with the foot held in the corrected position and externally spun on the lower leg. **(B)** The foot should be held in the same position used for manipulation; the heel should be inverted and slightly plantar-flexed. *(Figure continues.)*

cally because the increased bulk of the foot obliterates bony prominences in the area of the styloid process. Midtarsal and hindfoot pronation creates the illusion of a more rectus foot; however, the osseous structures remain deviated. As the child starts wearing shoes, the digits abduct at the metatarsophalangeal joints, which also creates the illusion of a more rectus foot.

In current practice, in view of the unpredictable outcome of nontreatment it seems reasonable to treat children early rather than to allow the deformity to become more rigid with cartilaginous and bony adaptation. It should be remembered that, unlike the femur and tibia,

no further osseous torsion occurs in the foot after birth. Therefore, unless one completely relies on the theory that muscular action with weight-bearing will realign the foot in all cases, spontaneous resolution is not a valid argument for not treating a child.

## Nonoperative Treatment

Passive stretching and manipulation in infants at diaper changes can be effective in mild cases of flexible deformity if the maneuvers are performed properly and frequently and if parents are adequately instructed in the

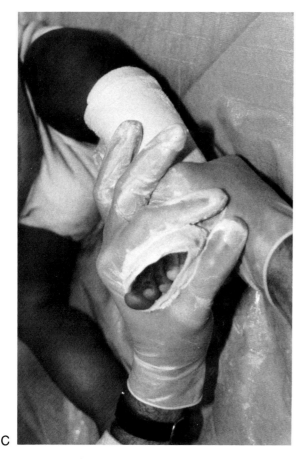

C

**Fig. 8-9** *(Continued)*. **(C)** The forefoot should have lateral pressure directed proximally to the first toe. If there is a varus component to the deformity, the forefoot only should be pronated.

technique (Fig. 8-8). The foot should be stabilized with the hindfoot in slight varus and plantar flexion, with the opposing thumb extending along the lateral rearfoot to the styloid process. Pure transverse plane pressure is then applied to the first ray just behind the first toe. The forefoot should be brought into a neutral to gently abducted position and held there for 1 to 2 minutes. This should be repeated two or three times, with slightly more force applied each time.

If the foot is too rigid to reduce to neutral or if severe deformity exists, it is unlikely that passive stretching alone will be effective. I feel that manipulation should be reserved only for those infants less than 4 months of age who have a flexible deformity and for whom parental

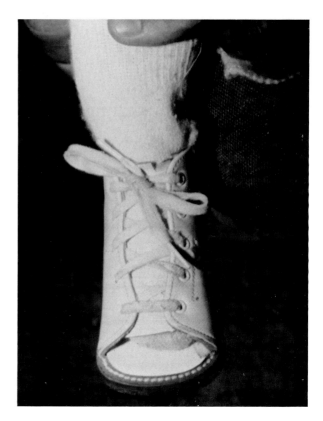

**Fig. 8-10.** A prewalker straight last shoe used to maintain correction after manipulation and reduction of deformity. (Courtesy of S.J. DeValentine, D.P.M.)

compliance is likely to be high. However, nowadays both parents often work, and the day care center staff cannot be relied upon to perform these tasks adequately. These factors must be considered when attempting to select appropriate care.

The prewalker straight last shoe or reverse last shoe, alone or in combination with a Denis Browne bar or Ganley Splint, can also be used for a more flexible deformity. The shoe should be worn 18 to 24 hours a day. The bracing effect of the shoe takes advantage of growth, with gradual adaptation of the cartilaginous structures. The bar is used to produce an external force on the foot and to prevent the child from sleeping in a fetal position. Both the reverse last shoe and the bar have been criticized as tending to produce pronation of the foot. Berg reported a 20 percent rate of residual hindfoot pronation in children treated with a Denis Browne bar.[26] To prevent this, a slight varus bend in the bar as well as a varus

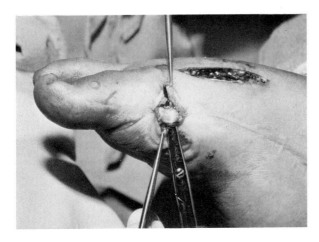

**Fig. 8-11.** Lichtblau tenotomy, shown here combined with a Heyman-Herndon-Strong release, also can be beneficial as an isolated procedure when the abductor hallucis appears taut. Additionally, it is beneficial for a persistent metatarsus primus adductus.

wedge in the heel of the shoe is used to supinate the rearfoot. The Ganley splint is similar to the Denis Browne bar but allows the forefoot and rearfoot relationship to be changed. Various other types of ankle and/or foot orthoses such as the Wheaton Brace, have been designed to place an abduction force on the forefoot. Such braces can be used alone or following a period of casting to help maintain correction.

Manipulation and serial plaster of Paris casting constitute the standard treatment in children with moderate to severe deformity. Those presenting with rigid deformities should be casted from the initiation of treatment. A 12- to 18-month-old infant with even mild residual deformity should be casted because of the progressive increase in rigidity of the deformity with age. Casts should be changed on a weekly basis in infants under 3 months of age; beyond 3 months, casts are usually changed every 2 weeks. As in manipulation and casting of clubfoot, stretching of the soft tissues followed by reduction of deformity is most important. The cast merely holds the foot in the corrected position.

Both padding and plaster should be rolled on "against" the direction of the deformity, and minimal cast padding should be used for maximum retention of position (Fig. 8-9). A short leg cast is usually adequate since there is no need for control of hindfoot rotation in metatarsus adductus. Casting should be continued until the foot is straight. The lateral convexity should be completely eliminated, the styloid process should not be prominent, and the child should be able to spontaneously abduct the foot. The length of time required for casting usually averages 6 to 8 weeks; however, in some children the time is considerably longer. There does not seem to be any direct correlation between the rigidity of the foot and the length of treatment required.

Once correction has been achieved, the foot should be held in the corrected position for one and one-half to two times the length of time required to obtain correction. The child should be closely followed after casting. Recurrent deformity has been reported to occur as much as 11 percent of the time, particularly in younger children.[27] After completion of cast correction, the child is kept in a straight last shoe until the foot has grown by at least two shoe sizes (Fig. 8-10). Thereafter, the parents should be instructed to look for regular shoes built upon a straight last rather than an adducted last.

As in clubfoot, manipulation and serial casting should be continued until correction is achieved or no further progress is observed. It is extremely rare for an infant with metatarsus adductus not to respond to nonoperative treatment. Even in 3- to 5-year-olds, an attempt at cast correction should be made prior to any consideration of surgical treatment. An abduction stress test can be helpful in determining if casting is warranted.

## Operative Treatment

The majority of children with deformity severe enough to require surgical treatment will be those with the residual deformity of clubfoot. A smaller number of children with idiopathic metatarsus adductus will need surgical repair. There are a number of soft tissue and osseous procedures that may be useful in the management of resistant metatarsus adductus, with the appropriateness of each procedure being determined primarily by the severity and rigidity of the deformity and the patient's age. Soft tissue procedures alone may be effective in young children; osseous procedures are required once skeletal adaptation has occurred.

### Limited Soft Tissue Release and Casting

Lichtblau originally described and recommended abductor hallucis tenotomy for persistent bowstringing of the abductor hallucis tendon.[13] A small longitudinal incision

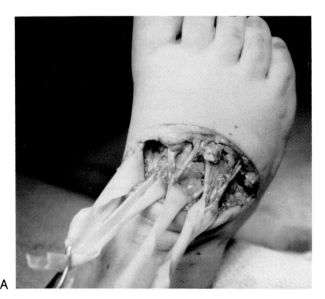
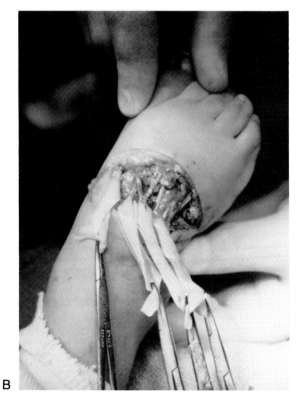

A

B

**Fig. 8-12.** The tarsometatarsal soft tissue release procedure is very reliable if performed properly prior to 4 to 5 years of age. **(A)** Tendons and neurovascular structures are first identified and immobilized through a transverse incision just distal to metatarsocuneiform joint level. **(B)** A progressive soft tissue release of all metatarsocuneiform joints is performed and the forefoot is manipulated into neutral position and fixed with medial and lateral crossed Kirschner wires.

is made medially, just proximal to the first metatarsal head, through which the tendon is sectioned (Fig. 8-11). I have found this procedure, when used in conjunction with dorsal, medial, and plantar release of the first meta-tarsocuneiform joint and followed by additional manipulations and cast correction, to be very effective in milder cases or in younger children who do not require a complete tarsometatarsal soft tissue release. This procedure is also incorporated into my standard medial soft tissue release for clubfoot.

## Complete Tarsometatarsal Soft Tissue Release

The complete tarsometatarsal soft tissue release was originally described by Heyman et al. for treatment of resistant metatarsus adductus in children between the ages of 2 and 7 years.[30] The procedure was described as a complete circumferential release of the capsule and ligaments about the tarsometatarsal, intermetatarsal, and intercuneiform joints. Kendrick et al. modified the original procedure by leaving intact the plantar lateral aspect of the capsules as well as the lateral capsule of the fifth metatarsocuboid joint.[31] This modification was advocated as a stabilizing factor to prevent dorsal drift at the bases of the metatarsals and to allow the metatarsals to be reduced on a stable soft tissue hinge. No fixation was used by either group of authors in their procedures. Both procedures were followed by 3 to 4 months of casting to allow the joint surfaces to remodel to their new positions. Kendrick et al. reported a 92 percent success rate with their modification.[31]

Others have criticized the procedure as producing a stiff and fibrotic foot. Stark et al. reported a 41 percent failure rate and 50 percent incidence of pain in a late follow-up of 48 patients studied over 18 years.[32] Complications such as growth arrest of both the metatarsal bases and avascular necrosis of cuneiforms have also been reported. The procedure was abandoned in children over 8 years of age because of decreased ability for joint surfaces to remodel. Most of the complications of stiffness and arthrosis can be avoided by not performing the procedure in children over 4 to 5 years of age. I have found the tarsometatarsal soft tissue release to be very effective with minimal complications when performed properly in children less than 4 to 5 years old (Fig. 8-12). The technique is described in detail in Chapter 6.

## Osseous Procedures

Johnson[33] described a technique of chondrotomy of the lesser metatarsal bases in which a 2.5-mm wedge of cartilaginous tissue is removed just anterior to the proxi-

mal articular cartilage of the base of the metatarsals and a laterally based wedge osteotomy of the first metatarsal is performed just distal to the epiphysis. The foot is immobilized for 8 to 10 weeks to allow for adaptation. The procedure was originally designed for children ages 6 to 8. I have no personal experience with this procedure and cannot comment on the long-term results.

Children over 8 years of age with significant residual metatarsus adductus deformity generally require corrective osteotomy owing to the degree of ossification, osseous adaptation, and lack of tarsometatarsal joint mobility. The classic procedure described by Berman and Gartland has become the standard. This technique consists of crescentic osteotomies at the bases of the lesser metatarsals, combined with osteotomy of the first metatarsal at least 6 mm beyond the physis, with fixation by crossed pins through the first and fifth metatarsals[34] (Fig. 8-13). Berman and Gartland reported only 4 poor results out of 115 operated feet in a 15-year follow-up.

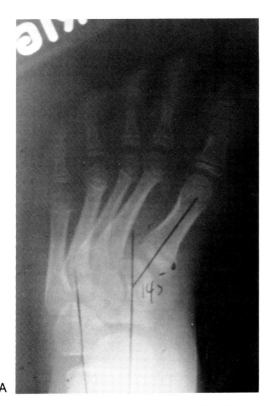 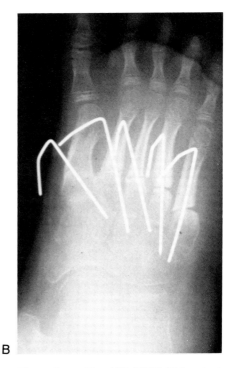

**Fig. 8-13.** (A) persistent right (image reversed) rigid metatarsus adductus in an older child. (B) Multiple osteotomies with Kirschner wire fixation provide satisfactory reduction of the deformity. (Courtesy of B. Scurran, D.P.M.)

Other authors have modified the orientation, location, and fixation of metatarsal osteotomies in an attempt to decrease the likelihood of malunion or nonunion.[35]

Lepird described an oblique osteotomy technique, which allows for rotation of the metatarsals about a common axis without wedge resection of bone.[36] A single oblique osteotomy is performed from dorsal distal obliquely to plantar proximal in the proximal diaphyseal bone of the lesser metatarsals. The cut is made parallel to the plantar surface. Initially, the cut is not made through and through. A 2.7-mm or 3.5-mm hole is drilled perpendicular to the plantar surface using AO technique. After the fixation is ready to be placed, the proximal

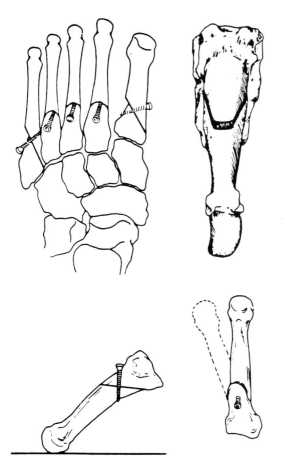

**Fig. 8-14.** Lepird procedure. With the advent of AO principles being utilized in foot surgery, this procedure, although technically more demanding than the Berman-Gartland tarsometatarsal release, provides superior frontal plane stability to the midfoot. (From DiNapoli and Corey,[25] with permission.)

cortex is released and the lag screw inserted. The bone is rotated into correct alignment and the screw secured (Fig. 8-14). By modifying the cut from parallel to the plantar surface to a more vertical orientation, additional frontal plane correction can be obtained. An oblique laterally based closing wedge osteotomy of the first metatarsal is performed. Postoperative care consists of a nonweight-bearing short leg cast for 6 to 8 weeks.

An opening wedge osteotomy of the medial cuneiform can also be used in children over 6 to 8 years of age. Fowler et al. originally described this procedure for treatment of residual forefoot adduction in clubfoot deformity.[37] Adequate ossification of the medial cuneiform is required. A biplanar osteotomy of the medial cuneiform may be performed by making the plantar cut wider than the dorsal in order to correct any forefoot equinus that may be present in residual clubfoot deformity. A corticocancellous wedge of autograft or allograft bone is used to maintain the increased medial column length. Hoffman et al. combined the Fowler procedure with a radical plantar release for correction of residual forefoot adduction secondary to clubfoot and reported good results in 15 of 18 operated feet.[39] A medial cuneiform opening wedge osteotomy should be considered when increased obliquity of the medial cuneiform articulating surface is present. In cases of severe residual adductus deformity in older children with secondary medial and lateral column length discrepancies (especially residual clubfoot), a lateral column shortening osteotomy (Evans procedure) may be combined with medial column lengthening.[40]

## Skewfoot Treatment

Treatment of skewfoot is very difficult because of the complexity of the deformity (Fig. 8-15). Casting and conservative treatment are used exactly as in metatarsus adductus or metatarsus varus. By the time the rearfoot has broken down, conservative therapy is of little expected value. The decision to operate should be based upon increasing deformity, pain, and marked restriction of the child's activities. Historically, most authors have indicated that surgery is necessary at some point in severe skewfoot deformity.

Many procedures have been advocated for correction of the adduction component of the deformity, including all of the previously mentioned procedures, for forefoot correction. In addition, the midfoot and hindfoot defor-

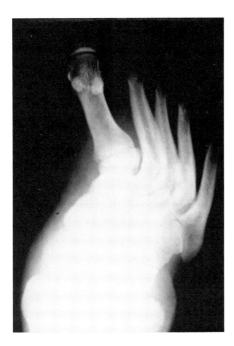

**Fig. 8-15.** Radiograph of skeletally mature child with skewfoot deformity.

mity must be addressed prior to any type of forefoot corrective surgery. If the hindfoot is not fixed rigidly in valgus and shows no sign of degenerative changes, an Evans opening wedge osteotomy of the os calcis is probably the best means of lengthening the lateral column. If substantial adaptation has occurred, a triple arthrodesis or Grice subtalar fusion procedure may be required.

Correction of the midfoot deformity usually requires either a modified Kidner-Young procedure or talonavicular fusion. In the older, heavier child, the talonavicular fusion results in better structural stability of the medial column, although at the expense of some flexibility. The Kidner-Young procedure is performed by advancing the dorsal insertion of the posterior tibial tendon distally and plantarly attaching it to the plantar surface of the navicular. The spring ligament is routinely advanced, which puts an additional sagittal plane pull on the medial column. The anterior tibial tendon is split at its insertion, and the portion of the tendon that inserts onto the first cuneiform is drawn through a notch proximally in the navicular, as classically described in the Young procedure. Surgical management of skewfoot is also discussed in Chapter 14 in connection with the operative management of non-neurogenic pes valgus deformity.

# REFERENCES

1. Peterson H: Skewfoot forefoot adduction with heel valgus. J Pediatr Orthop 6:24, 1986
2. Kite J: Errors and complications in treating foot conditions in children. Clin Orthop 53:31, 1967
3. Fagan J: The four quadrant approach to clubfoot surgery. Clin Podiatr Med Surg 4:233, 1987
4. Bankart B: Metatarsus varus. Br Med J 2:685, 1921
5. Rushford G: The natural history of hooked forefoot. J Bone Joint Surg [Br] 60:530, 1949
6. McCormick D, Blount W: Metatarsus adductovarus. JAMA 141:449, 1949
7. Smith C, Stoltz M, Head K: Dynamic metatarsus adductus. J Bone Joint Surg [Am] 57:1035, 1975
8. Bleck E: Metatarsus adductus: classification and relationship to outcome of treatment. J Pediatr Orthop 3:2, 1983
9. Wynn-Davies R: Family studies and the cause of congenital clubfoot talipes equinovarus, talipes calcaneovalgus and metatarsus varus. J Bone Joint Surg [Br] 46:445, 1964
10. Tachdjian M: The child's Foot. 1st Ed. WB Saunders, Philadelphia, 1985
11. Thompson S: Hallux varus and metatarsus varus. Clin Orthop 16:109, 1960
12. Basmajian J: Muscles Alive, Their Function Revealed by Electromyelography. 2nd Ed. Williams & Wilkins, Baltimore, 1967
13. Lichtblau S: Section of the abductor hallucis tendon for correction of metatarsus varus deformity. Clin Orthop 110:229, 1975
14. Ponsetti I, Becker J: Congenital metatarsus adductus: the results of treatment. J Bone Joint Surg [Am] 48:702, 1966
15. Reimann I, Werner H: Congenital metatarsus varus: a suggestion for a possible mechanism in relation to other foot deformities. Clin Orthop 110:223, 1975
16. Reimann I, Werner H: The pathology of congenital metatarsus varus and its relationship to other congenital deformities of the foot. Acta Orthop Scand 54:847, 1983
17. Reimann I, Werner H: The pathology of congenital metatarsus varus: postmortem study of a newborn infant. Acta Orthop Scand 54:847, 1979
18. Browne R, Paton D: Anomalous insertion of the posterior tibial tendon in congenital metatarsus varus. J Bone Joint Surg [Br] 61:74, 1979
19. Diaz A, Diaz J: Pathogenesis of idiopathic clubfoot. Clin Orthop 185:14, 1984
20. Kumar S, MacEwen D: The incidence of hip dysplasia with metatarsus adductus. Clin Orthop 164:235, 1982
21. Jacobs J: Metatarsus varus in hip dysplasia. Clin Orthop 16:203, 1960
22. Lepow G, Lepow R, Lyson R et al: Pediatric metatarsus adductus angle. J Am Podiatr Med Assoc 77:529, 1987

23. Simons G: Analytical radiography in the progressive approach in talipes equinovarus. Orthop Clin North Am 9:187, 1978
24. Templeton A, McAlister W, Zim I: Standardization of terminology and evaluation of osseous relationships in congenitally abnormal feet. AJR 93:374, 1965
25. DiNapoli R, Corey S: Metatarsal Osteotomy for the Correction of Metatarsus Adductus. In McGlamery, ED (ed): Reconstructive Surgery of the Foot and Leg. Update 89. Podiatry Institute Publishing Co., Tucker, GA, 1989
26. Berg E: A reappraisal of metatarsus adductus in skewfoot. J Bone Joint Surg [Am] 68:1185, 1986
27. McCauley J, Lusskin R, Bromley J: Recurrence in congenital metatarsus varus. J Bone Joint Surg [Am] 46:525, 1964
28. Galuzzo A, Hugar D: Congenital metatarsus adductus: clinical evaluation and treatment. J Foot Surg 18:16, 1979
29. Tax H, Albright T: Metatarsus adductovarus, a simplified approach to treatment. J Am Podiatr Med Assoc 68:331, 1978
30. Heyman C, Herndon C, Strong J: Mobilization of the tarsometatarsal and intermetatarsal joints for the correction of resistant adduction of the forepart of the foot in congenital clubfoot or congenital metatarsus varus. J Bone Joint Surg [Am] 44:299, 1958
31. Kendrick R, Sharma N, Hassler W: Tarsometatarsal mobilization for resistant adduction of the forepart of the foot: a follow-up study. J Bone Joint Surg [Am] 52:61, 1970
32. Stark J, Johanson J, Winter R: The Heyman-Herndon tarsometatarsal capsulotomy for metatarsus adductus: results in 48 feet. J Pediatr Orthop 7:305, 1987
33. Johnson J: A preliminary report on chondrotomies. J Am Podiatr Med Assoc 68:808, 1978
34. Berman A, Gartland J: Metatarsal osteotomy for the correction of adduction of the forepart of the foot in children. J Bone Joint Surg [Am] 53:498, 1971
35. Yu G, Johng B, Freireich R: Surgical management of metatarsus adductus deformity. Clin Podiatr Med Surg 4:207, 1987
36. Yu G, Wallace G: Metatarsus adductus. p. 324. In McGlamry ED (ed): Comprehensive Textbook of Foot Surgery. Vol. 1. Williams & Wilkins, Baltimore, 1987
37. Fowler B, Brooks A, Parrish T: The cavovarus foot. J Bone Joint Surg [Am] 41:757, 1959
38. Lincoln R, Wood K, Bugg E: Metatarsus varus corrected by open wedge osteotomy of the first cuneiform bone. Orthop Clin North Am 7:795, 1976
39. Hoffman A, Constine R, McBride G: Osteotomy of the first cuneiform as treatment of residual adduction of the forepart of the foot in clubfoot. J Bone Joint Surg [Am] 66:985, 1984
40. Evans D: Relapsed clubfoot. J Bone Joint Surg [Br] 43:722, 1961

# 9

# Tarsal Coalitions

*LAWRENCE M. OLOFF*
*GEOFFREY S. HEARD*

Although the initial recognition of tarsal coalition can be attributed to anatomists, who noted abnormal unions between adjoining tarsal bones in cadavers, almost all subsequent advances in diagnosis and treatment have been direct results of new techniques and advancing technologies in the field of radiology.

Buffon in 1769 is credited with the first description of tarsal coalition, and over the next 110 years anatomists described virtually all the types of tarsal coalition.[1] Cruveilhier in 1829 described the existence of calcaneonavicular coalition, Zuckerandl in 1877 described talocalcaneal coalition and Anderson in 1879 described talonavicular coalition.[2-4] While the anatomic presence of these coalitions was well documented, their clinical significance remained unclear until 1880, when Holl proposed a possible relationship between intertarsal bars and flatfoot deformity.[5]

The first step toward proving Holl's hypothesis came with the ability to recognize the presence of tarsal coalition in living as well as postmortem patients. Jones in 1897 provided the first clinical description of peroneal spastic flatfoot, and Kirmissin in 1898 was the first to make a radiographic diagnosis of a tarsal coalition, a mere 3 years after Roentgen's discovery of x-rays.[7] This provided the necessary link allowing correlation of symptoms with the presence of tarsal coalition. Sloman in 1921 was the first to associate peroneal spastic flatfoot with a calcaneonavicular coalition,[8] and Wagoner in 1928 described bilateral congenital calcaneocuboid coalitions.[9] Despite the rapidly growing body of information, little attention was paid to these early contributors until 1948, when Harris and Beath[10] stimulated new interest by using the axial calcaneal projection described in 1934 by

Korvin[11] to show the relationship between peroneal spastic flatfoot and middle facet talocalcaneal coalition. It would be another 21 years before Conway and Cowell, utilizing tomography, were able to demonstrate the association between peroneal spastic flatfoot and anterior facet talocalcaneal coalition.[12]

Owing to the complex anatomy of the mid- and hindfoot articulations, it has previously been difficult to definitively visualize these areas. Visualization of anterior facet coalitions was not possible until the advent of tomography. More recently, computed cross-sectional imaging has played an expanding role in the diagnosis of tarsal coalition. The advent of tomography has allowed for earlier and more accurate diagnoses, as well as quantification of both the amount of joint involvement and the size of the coalition present. Obtaining such precise data was, until only recently, unimaginable, and in the near future computed tomography (CT) may come to dictate treatment of tarsal coalition.

## ASSOCIATION WITH RIGID FLATFOOT

In the majority of cases, tarsal coalitions are associated with rigid flatfoot deformity. Since the deformity may also present with secondary spasm or contracture of the peroneal musculature, any patient presenting with a rigid flatfoot deformity and peroneal spasm or contracture is assumed to have tarsal coalition until proven otherwise. At the same time, it is important to note that although *peroneal spastic flatfoot* has become synonymous with tarsal coalition in much of the literature, this association is not constant. Not all tarsal coalitions present as peroneal spastic flatfoot, and not all cases of peroneal spastic flatfoot are due to tarsal coalition. Some tarsal coalitions may involve spasm of the tibialis anterior or long extensors of the toes and may result in a cavus or even normal-appearing foot.[13] Conversely, other causes, although less common than tarsal coalition, may be responsible for peroneal spastic flatfoot; these include osteoarthritis, rheumatoid arthritis, trauma, infection, neoplasm, osteochondral fractures of the undersurface of the talar head, and tuberculosis.[14-16] There are also iatrogenic causes of peroneal spastic flatfoot, including overzealous casting of clubfoot, postoperative subtalar arthrodesis, and possible sequelae of the Grice extra-articular subtalar fusion procedure.[16]

Variability in the clinical presentation of any pathology demands the utmost of the practitioner's diagnostic acumen, and making correct diagnosis is especially crucial in the management of tarsal coalition, where delay in treatment can lead to significant morbidity. In those cases in which surgical management is deemed necessary and appropriate, the time lost in a delayed or missed diagnosis may result in secondary degenerative changes in surrounding joints, which then demand more drastic surgery.

At this point a few introductory remarks would seem appropriate with regard to emerging concepts in the treatment of tarsal coalitions. As with many musculoskeletal conditions, treatment alternatives can be conveniently divided into nonsurgical and surgical options. Patients with symptomatic tarsal coalition have traditionally been treated by nonoperative methods as long as these methods have been effective in alleviating symptoms. If nonoperative treatment failed to provide relief, arthrodesis was usually performed for talocalcaneal coalitions and resection or arthrodesis for calcaneonavicular coalitions. However, recent studies advocating surgical resection of certain coalitions over arthrodesis in the absence of secondary degenerative changes, offer the prospect of obtaining a foot with close to normal function. This has been made possible to a large degree by new and improved imaging techniques. At the same time, these new imaging modalities raise questions that will have to be addressed regarding criteria for differentiating a candidate for resection from a candidate for fusion.

## ETIOLOGY AND INCIDENCE

Tarsal coalitions may be either congenital or acquired, with those of congenital origin being more frequent. There has been much controversy concerning the etiology of congenital tarsal coalition, and the exact cause is unknown. Pfitzner in 1896 was the first to suggest that tarsal coalitions resulted from the incorporation of accessory intertarsal ossicles into adjacent tarsal bones.[17] It was hypothesized that the os calcaneus secundarius fuses either with the calcaneus and navicular to form the calcaneonavicular coalition or with the calcaneus and cuboid to form the calcaneocuboid coalition. Similarly, the os trigonum was believed to fuse with the talus and calcaneus to form a posterior talocalcaneal coalition, with the os tibiale externum forming the talonavicular coalition.[8,18,19] This theory was supported by many of the earlier investigators and until only recently was the most popular explanation for tarsal coalitions.

A second theory, ascribing tarsal coalitions to the failure of mesenchymal differentiation, was first proposed in 1896 by Leboucq[20] and later advocated by Jack.[21] This etiology seems to have been validated by Harris's discovery of coalitions in fetal feet[22] and is the theory currently most in vogue. If the theory is correct, the question remains as to whether the lack of differentiation is due to an insult in utero or to a hereditary component.

The existence of a hereditary component is supported by numerous reports in the literature of tarsal coalitions occurring in several members of the same family. Rothberg et al. reported bilateral talonavicular coalitions in one family,[23] and Boyd reported a family with three generations of bilateral talonavicular bars.[24] Webster and Roberts found talocalcaneal coalitions in two sisters,[25] and Bersani and Samilson reported a familial incidence of fusion of several tarsal bones.[26] In 1963, Wray and Herndon reported the occurrence of calcaneonavicular coalitions in three generations of one family and theorized that some and perhaps all cases of calcaneonavicular bars are caused by an autosomal dominant gene mutation with variable penetrance.[27] The case for a genetic etiology was further strengthened in 1966 by Glessner and Davis, who reported a set of monozygotic twins both presenting with peroneal spastic flatfoot and tarsal coalition.[28]

The most significant study to date concerning hereditary transmission was that of Leonard, who in 1974

studied 98 first-degree relatives of 31 index patients treated over a 30-year period for symptomatic coalitions[29] and found 39 percent of these relatives to have asymptomatic coalitions themselves. Among first-degree relatives of the 27 index patients with calcaneonavicular coalitions, 25 percent also had calcaneonavicular coalitions, but 14 percent had talocalcaneal or some other type of coalition. From these findings Leonard concluded that (1) tarsal coalitions are most likely inherited as unifactorial disorders of autosomal dominant inheritance of nearly full penetrance; and (2) there does not appear to be any genetic difference in the inheritance of the different coalitions.

Tarsal coalition has also been reported to occur in association with other congenital disorders. Nievergelt described a syndrome consisting of elbow dysplasia, subluxation of the radial heads, fibular overgrowth, carpal coalition, and tarsal coalition in association with clubfoot deformity.[30] This so-called Nievergelt's syndrome has a hereditary transmission. O'Rahilly et al. described phocomelia and hemimelia in patients also displaying talocalcaneal coalition.[31] Many other genetically determined syndromes have been described that include some form of tarsal coalition. An autosomal dominant inheritance was cited by Christian et al. in patients displaying tarsal coalition, multiple osseous dysplasia of long bones of the hands and feet, and platyspondylia.[32] A dominant polyautosomal inheritance pattern is described by Spoendlin in over five generations of one family displaying tarsal coalition, carpal coalition, and congenital stapes ankylosis.[33]

While the majority of tarsal coalitions are congenital, many causes of acquired coalition need to be considered. Although Pfitzner's theory of ossicle incorporation may have fallen into disfavor for explaining congenital coalition, there have been cases of acquired coalition of the posterior facet of the talocalcaneal joint due to fusion of the os trigonum with the talus and calcaneus.[19,34,35] A hypertrophic ossicle may not result in the fusion of two adjacent tarsal bones, but yet it may still restrict motion enough to cause a rudimentary coalition (described in more detail in the section on classification). Acquired coalition is not uncommon in advanced rheumatoid arthritis, juvenile rheumatoid arthritis, and juvenile ankylosing spondylitis, and may also result from neurotrophic joint disease, major tarsal infection, or fractures of the subtalar joint. There have even been reports of acquired

talonavicular coalition following cases of Kohler's disease or tuberculosis infection.[36,37]

When one attempts to determine the incidence of tarsal coalition in the general population by reviewing previously published clinical studies, it is important to realize that any number arrived at is only the incidence of *symptomatic* coalitions. Almost all these studies were of selected populations, in which those patients who were examined complained of pain or presented with obvious deformity, such as peroneal spastic flatfoot. Leonard's study of symptomatic patients and their first-degree relatives showed that of a total of 69 radiographically demonstrable coalitions, only 31 (45 percent) were ever symptomatic. This means that 55 percent of the people with coalitions in his study were asymptomatic and suggests that any study to determine incidence by using pain and deformity as criteria for examination would severely underestimate the true incidence. The difficulty in predicting an average incidence of tarsal coalition by comparing different studies is further compounded by the variable clinical and radiographic techniques used by different investigators, their ability to interpret these tests, and the intensity with which they pursued their studies. For instance, Harris and Beath found 74 cases of peroneal spastic flatfoot among 3,600 army enlistees.[10] This has been incorrectly cited by many subsequent authors as indicating a 2 percent incidence of tarsal coalition. Since only one calcaneonavicular bar was found among the 3,600 enlistees, the actual incidence of tarsal coalition is only 0.03 percent. It is not clear from Harris and Beath's original paper in 1948 whether they were using the so-called coalition view to examine the subtalar joint for coalition, and even if they were, it is likely that they still underestimated the true number of coalitions. A 1955 paper by Harris describes the discovery of incomplete talocalcaneal coalitions that could not be demonstrated by radiography but only by operative exposure.[18]

Another widely cited study is that of Rankin and Baker, in which 24 cases of rigid flatfoot were diagnosed in 60,000 army enlistees.[38] From this they stated the incidence of rigid flatfoot to be 0.4%; however, 24 in 60,000 would be 0.04 percent, not 0.4 percent. Not only have subsequent authors quoted this incorrect 0.4 percent figure as the incidence of tarsal coalition, but Rankin and Baker found that only 16 of the 24 patients demonstrated radiographic evidence of a coalition. This would have produced an incidence of tarsal coalition of 0.03

percent (16 of 60,000), the same as in Harris and Beath's study. Since both these studies involved army recruits and patients who were already symptomatic might not have enlisted in the armed forces, their absence would lead to an artificially low incidence of coalition as compared with that in the general population.

A third study, by Vaughn and Segal, examined approximately 2,000 painful feet among army recruits and found 21 cases of talocalcaneal and calcaneonavicular coalition, which were confirmed by radiography.[39] Thus, 1 percent of the patients with painful feet whom they examined had coalitions, but this figure has no correlation with the incidence of coalition in the general population, as it was conducted on a military population and only painful feet were examined radiographically.

Another commonly cited value for incidence is 0.9 percent, based on a study by Shands and Wentz.[40] In their study, radiographic findings in the feet of 850 children under 17 years of age were evaluated. Initially 4,230 patients were examined, and 1,232 of them were diagnosed as having a primary foot disorder. Out of these 1,232 patients, 850 children were judged by the physicians to be " . . . sufficiently abnormal as to require roentgenograms. . . . ". Shands and Wentz then reported finding spastic or rigid flatfoot in 11 of the 1,232 patients, an incidence of 0.9 percent. Subsequent authors have erroneously stated this 0.9 percent as the incidence of tarsal coalition. Although radiographic findings in these 11 patients did demonstrate definite coalitions in 9 and secondary signs of coalition in the other 2, Shands and Wentz reported five additional definite coalitions and a probable sixth in patients presenting without rigid flatfoot. On the basis of a total of 17 coalitions out of 850 patients radiographed, the incidence of radiographically demonstrable coalitions would be 2.0 percent. However, even this adjusted number has no bearing on what the incidence may be in the general population. The original 4,230 patients from whom these 850 patients were culled did not represent a random sampling of the population but had presented with orthopedic complaints. Furthermore, if all 4,230 patients had been radiographed rather than just those who had sufficient abnormalities in the judgment of the attending physicians to warrant such examination, it is safe to assume that additional asymptomatic coalitions would have been detected. Finally, all patients examined were less than 17 years of age, the average age of the 850 children examined radiographically being 5 years and 3 months. Any estimate arrived at from this population would probably be low, since not all coalitions that eventually become symptomatic manifest themselves during childhood.

It becomes apparent that any calculated incidence derived from these studies would represent the incidence of symptomatic tarsal coalition only and would be an approximation at best. On the basis of present data, the calculated incidence of tarsal coalition would seem to be

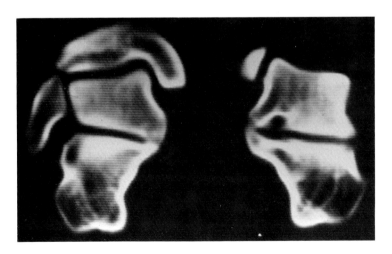

**Fig. 9-1.** Coronal image CT scan demonstrating talocalcaneal coalitions bilaterally. The image on the left demonstrates a posterior facet coalition, while the image on the right displays a middle facet coalition. Talocalcaneal coalitions are the most common type of coalition.

less than 1 percent, but the true incidence is probably much higher.

Conway and Cowell have reported a male to female ratio of 1 : 1 for calcaneonavicular coalitions and 4 : 1 for talocalcaneal coalitions.[12] Beckley et al. reported a male/female ratio of 12 : 5 for all coalitions and 10 : 3 for middle facet talocalcaneal coalitions[34]; Leonard reported close to a 1 : 1 ratio[29]; and Stormont and Peterson reported a ratio of 4 : 1 for all types of coalition.[41] The apparent predominance of males over females seems to refute the present theory of autosomal dominant transmission and may be an artifact of the study parameters.

There has always been a great deal of confusion over which type of coalition is the most common. It appears that talocalcaneal coalitions occur most commonly (Fig. 9-1), followed closely by calcaneonavicular coali-

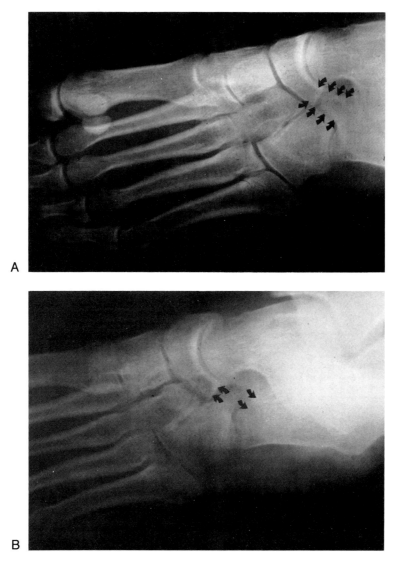

**Fig. 9-2.** (A) A calcaneonavicular coalition is seen on this 45-degree medial oblique view, as outlined by the arrows. These coalitions are second only to the talocalcaneal coalition in frequency of occurrence. (B) Postoperative radiographs of the same patient after resection of the coalition. (Courtesy of Surgery Department, California College of Podiatric Medicine, San Francisco, CA.)

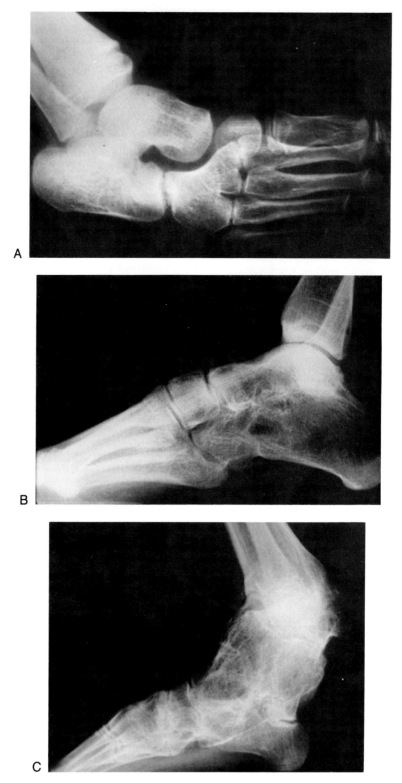

**Fig. 9-3. (A)** An oblique view of a patient with numerous coalitions. Notice the calcaneocuboid, talonavicular, cuboideocuneiform, and intercuneiform coalitions. **(B)** Multiple coalitions in a skeletally mature patient. **(C)** Severe tarsal dysplasia combined with multiple rearfoot coalitions. (Courtesy of S.J. DeValentine, D.P.M.)

tions[10,39,41,42] (Fig. 9-2). Approximately 50 percent of talocalcaneal coalitions and somewhat more than 60 percent of calcaneonavicular, calcaneocuboid, and talonavicular coalitions are bilateral.[15] Talocalcaneal coalitions most commonly occur at the middle facet, followed in frequency by the posterior and anterior facets. Together, talocalcaneal and calcaneonavicular coalitions account for approximately 90 percent of all coalitions encountered.[43] The remainder of coalitions are described as unusual to rare and are accounted for by isolated case reports in the literature (Fig. 9-3). Since Anderson first described talonavicular coalitions in 1879, there have been some 40 more cases reported.[4,24] There are only approximately 10 reported cases of calcaneocuboid and naviculocuneiform coalitions, and even fewer reported cases of cuboideocuneiform coalitions.[9,12,19,44-46] The only coalition not reported is talocuboid. The rarity of some of the less common coalitions may reflect a problem with recognition, since not all coalitions cause sufficient symptoms to warrant medical attention.

## CLASSIFICATION

There are a variety of ways to classify tarsal coalition (Table 9-1). One is by tissue type,[43,47,48] the distinction depending upon whether the intervening tissue is fibrous, cartilaginous, or osseous; these three types of unions are referred to as *syndesmosis, synchondrosis,* and *synostosis,* respectively. However, coalitions may be composed of a combination of tissue types, and the distinction between tissue types may be transient and reflect the stage of maturation of the tissue. The tissue may be fibrous at birth, progress to cartilaginous with growth, and eventually become ossified. The type of tissue potentially determines the clinical features and degree of symptoms.

Syndesmotic and synchondrotic coalitions are gener-

ally more difficult to visualize on radiographs and are less likely to totally limit motion than are synostotic coalitions. Plastic deformation of cartilage and fibrous tissue seems not only to allow greater motion but also to be more forgiving in terms of symptoms. With eventual ossification of the fibrous and cartilaginous tissues, usually in adolescence, motion becomes severely restricted. Lack of joint motion is often associated with the onset of symptoms and may herald the eventual development of osteoarthritic compensatory changes as well. While this series of events represents a common scenario for tarsal coalition, some coalitions persist in their immature tissue type. For example, calcaneonavicular coalitions are occasionally synchondrotic into adult life and were referred to by Sloman[8] as *amphiarthrodial joints.*

The term *tarsal coalition* is usually used in a generic sense to describe varying degrees of tissue types and anatomic characteristics. More exact terminology can be applied that also helps to categorize this anomaly. A distinction may be made between a true coalition and a bar or bridge[49]: a true coalition is represented by an intra-articular fusion of two bones, as seen with a talonavicular or talocalcaneal coalition; a bar or bridge occurs when two bones are fused outside an anatomic joint, as in a calcaneonavicular coalition.

A distinction may also be made according to the completeness of the coalition. Thus coalitions are described as *complete, incomplete,* and *rudimentary.*[18,42] A complete coalition, as the name implies, is due to fused tarsal bones and completely limits joint motion. An incomplete coalition is formed by projections from each of the involved tarsal bones that do not actually unite but are separated by fibrous and/or cartilaginous tissue, while in a rudimentary coalition an osseous projection from one bone inhibits joint motion (e.g., an enlargement or elongation of Steida's process can interfere with subtalar joint motion).

Tachdjian's anatomic classification has gained the most universal acceptance.[48] Coalitions are named according to the specific bones that are abnormally joined. While not totally descriptive, this classification is straightforward. One can expand it by combining it with other classifications. For example, a talocalcaneal coalition might also be described as a complete talocalcaneal synostosis. The majority of accumulated statistical information concerning incidence and prognosis of the various types of tarsal coalitions has been reported in terms of this anatomically descriptive classification.

Table 9-1. **Classification of Tarsal Coalitions**

| Tissue Type | Anatomic Type | Completeness |
|---|---|---|
| Syndesmosis | Talocalcaneal | Complete |
| Synchondrosis | Calcaneonavicular | Incomplete |
| Synostosis | Talonavicular | Rudimentary |
| | Calcaneocuboid | |
| | Cuboideonavicular | |

# CLINICAL FEATURES

Symptoms of tarsal coalition vary with the site of coalition, but pain is the most common symptom. Before the infant begins to walk, signs of a coalition are rare and pain is seldom present. The onset of symptoms and signs depends upon the time of ossification of the tarsal bones involved.

According to Jakayamur and Cowell, ossification of the talonavicular coalition usually occurs between the ages of 3 and 5 years, and symptoms may present as early as the age of 2 to 3 years.[50] While it is hard to make generalizations about talonavicular coalitions, since fewer than 40 have been described in the literature, neither peroneal spasm nor pain seems to be a common presentation.[24,51,52] Sanghi and Roby reported peroneal spastic flatfoot associated with talonavicular coalition, but the most common complaint was usually a tender mass over the navicular.[52]

The more common talocalcaneal and calcaneonavicular coalitions do not usually become symptomatic until the second decade of life. Prior to adolescence the coalitions are cartilaginous, and movement is not severely restricted. It is mostly during the second decade that the coalitions begin to ossify, with the calcaneonavicular coalitions ossifying by the age of 8 to 12 years and the talocalcaneal coalitions by the age of 12 to 16 years.[50] As the coalitions begin to ossify, the restriction of normal tarsal motion, coupled with the greater demand placed upon the tarsal bones by increased weight and activity level and participation in strenuous activities such as sports, results in pain. The onset of pain can be insidious but is more commonly acute after precipitation by trauma. The traumatic incident can vary in intensity from an ankle sprain that fails to resolve to various types of overuse such as running, jumping, walking on uneven terrain, or even standing for long periods. This pain is normally relieved by rest.

During normal gait the tibia rotates around its long axis in the transverse plane by an average of 19 degrees.[53] This transverse motion is then compensated by motion at the ankle joint–subtalar joint complex, to which the subtalar joint is the major contributor. With loss of subtalar joint motion the talus and calcaneus function as a single unit thereby placing more demand upon the ankle joint, especially the lateral collateral ligaments. This may lead to repeated ankle sprains, with ligamentous laxity developing secondarily. Morgan and Crawford advocate a diagnosis of tarsal coalition until proven

otherwise in any active adolescent with recurrent ankle sprains or strains.[54] Admittedly such a sweeping generality may seem unwarranted, but a retrospective study by Snider et al. in which the radiographs of all patients were examined with sprained ankles as the only criterion revealed a 63 percent incidence of calcaneonavicular abnormalities.[55] Granted these abnormalities may not all have been coalitions, but certainly an adolescent complaining of chronic ankle pain and/or instability should fall under a high index of suspicion for coalition.

While pain is the most common symptom, its location can be quite variable. In cases of post-traumatic onset, particularly in calcaneonavicular coalitions, the pain can be localized to the area over the coalition. In talocalcaneal coalitions the pain is often localized to the sinus tarsi or just anterior to the medial malleolus at the middle facet. In other cases the pain can be diffuse and difficult for the patient to localize. Pain in the sinus tarsi, also known as sinus tarsi syndrome, is not diagnostic of coalition; however, it may be the result of excessive pronation, severe ankle sprain, malunion of intra-articular calcaneal fractures, or rheumatoid arthritis. The pain may also be radiating in nature and may mimic tarsal tunnel syndrome if a medial talocalcaneal coalition is impinging on a nerve.[50]

The most consistent sign of tarsal coalition is decreased range of motion of the subtalar and midtarsal joints. Motion at these two joints may be markedly decreased by a fibrous or cartilaginous talocalcaneal coalition, and subtalar motion may be completely lost if the bar is osseous. When examining for inversion or eversion, it is important to dorsiflex the ankle joint so that the talar dome is "locked" into the ankle mortise in order to avoid mistaking ankle joint motion for subtalar joint motion. The amount of subtalar and midtarsal joint motion lost with a calcaneonavicular coalition will characteristically be less than that seen with a talocalcaneal coalition, but the loss may still be quite conspicuous.

The patient may also present with varying degrees of calcaneal valgus, loss of the medial longitudinal arch, and abduction of the forefoot on the rearfoot. This syndrome, most common in talocalcaneal coalitions, has often been erroneously referred to as *peroneal spastic flatfoot;* a more accurate description would be *rigid pes valgus,* since the peroneal tendons are not actually in true spasm. The visibly taut peroneal tendons observed in a long-standing rigid valgus deformity are due to an adaptive state of contracture and not to true spasm, as was demonstrated electromyographically by Blockley when he examined two patients with peroneal spastic flatfoot intraoperatively. He found increased tension but no motor unit activity and was also able to obtain full inversion without force. Blockley speculated that if the increase in muscle-tendon unit tension was not due to organic shortening or to a volley of nerve impulses, then it might be due to changes in local muscle chemistry that are independent of the unit's nerve supply.[56]

All the above is not meant to imply that peroneal spasm is never seen with tarsal coalition. Harris has stated that most patients with tarsal coalition, especially a talocalcaneal or calcaneonavicular coalition, will develop a true spasm at some time during the course of their deformity.[42] Most frequently this spasm is seen in the acutely painful coalition following fracture of the coalition site or a sudden increase in physical activity. Attempts to invert the subtalar joint during physical examination of the patient may also result in reflex peroneal spasm due to pain upon manipulation.

The etiology of true peroneal spasm is still in dispute. Kyne and Mankin discovered that subtalar joint intraarticular pressure is least when the joint is in eversion.[57] They then hypothesized that peroneal spasm might be a guarding reflex to protect the joint against painful inversion. Outland and Murphy observed that spasm can exist even in the presence of a complete bar that prevents any motion at the subtalar joint and reasoned that the subtalar joint was not the cause of peroneal spasm.[16] They then suggested that the superficial branch of the peroneal nerve may supply some innervation to the talonavicular joint. Painful stimuli from degenerative changes at the talonavicular joint may trigger peroneal spasm. Cowell and Elener have postulated that the peroneal muscles shorten to adapt to limited subtalar joint motion.[58] When inversion is attempted, these shortened peroneal muscles contract to protect a painful subtalar joint. At this point it should be reiterated that a rigid pes valgus that presents with peroneal spasm is not pathognomonic for tarsal coalition. Although coalition is the most common etiology, other pathologies (listed above) must also be kept in mind.

## RADIOGRAPHIC EVALUATION

### Standard Radiographic Examination

Once a thorough history has been obtained and a physical examination performed and tarsal coalition is suspected, radiographic examination should proceed in a systematic manner, starting with a few basic plain film views. The presence of tarsal coalition is usually confirmed by plain film interpretation, whereas more sophisticated imaging techniques provide more detailed information. Initial views should include anteroposterior, lateral, and 45-degree medial oblique views. Bilateral views should be obtained even if subjective complaints and objective findings suggest a unilateral deformity. This will enable comparison of any abnormal findings between the two feet and may also detect a presently asymptomatic coalition in the opposite foot.

The diagnosis of calcaneocuboid, talonavicular, and naviculocuneiform coalitions is relatively straightforward as these coalitions are usually identifiable on anteroposterior views. The talonavicular coalition is often apparent on the lateral view, with an altered cyma line and what appears to be an elongated talar neck articulating directly with the medial cuneiform. Exceptions to these statements may be found in the case of smaller coalitions, particularly those that evade direct visualization because of bony superimposition.

Calcaneonavicular coalitions are likewise usually easy to identify on the 45-degree medial oblique views. The calcaneonavicular coalition will usually appear as a 1-cm wide bar bridging the gap normally found between the calcaneus and navicular. A "pseudocoalition" due to bony overlap can give the false impression of a calcaneonavicular bar, and it is often necessary to obtain several medial oblique views at different angles to differentiate between positional artifact and true coalition.[39] A fibrous or cartilaginous calcaneonavicular coalition will not be directly visible on radiography, and the diagnosis will be more difficult. An elongated anterosuperior process of the calcaneus, referred to by some as the "anteater sign," may be seen on the lateral view. The calcaneus and navicular will be closer in proximity than normal on the medial oblique view, and the bones will appear flattened at their junction with dense irregular and indistinct cortical surfaces.[50,58] Hypoplasia of the talar head may also be evident.[50,59] If the results of all these views are still equivocal, further tests may be necessary, as will be discussed later.

Talocalcaneal coalitions are usually difficult to visualize on standard plain film projections. Care must be taken when interpreting the middle facet of the subtalar joint, as both faulty alignment and a valgus position of the calcaneus can obscure a normal subtalar joint and give the false impression of coalition. However, a high index of suspicion exists when there is evidence of secondary changes (discussed below) that are normally suggestive of the presence of a tarsal coalition.

A variety of special plain film imaging techniques are advised in visualizing the talocalcaneal articulations. Harris and Beath were the first to popularize Korvin's 45-degree axial calcaneal projection to visualize the posterior and middle talocalcaneal facets.[10,11] In a later paper Harris suggested taking two or three radiographs with projection angles of 35, 40, and 45 degrees to account for natural variations in the angles of the two facets.[42] We are in agreement with other investigators who recommend measuring the angle of the middle facets in relation to the weight-bearing surface on a lateral view. One view is then taken at this angle and two additional views are taken, one at an angle 5 degrees greater and one at an angle 5 degrees smaller than the original. (In the severely pronated foot the posterior and middle facets are not in the same plane and therefore will have to be examined separately.) An osseous coalition of either of these facets will appear as an obliteration of the joint space.

The diagnosis may not be obvious in a young patient or when the coalition is cartilaginous or fibrous. A coalition should be considered if the two facets of the subtalar joint are found to be oblique to each other; however, long-standing severe pronation can produce a similar appearance. Narrowing and irregularity of the joint space offer further confirmation of a probable subtalar coalition.

Other specific views besides those recommended by Harris and Beath can be used to visualize the subtalar joint. The anterior facet of the subtalar joint is not readily visible on a standing lateral view because of its downward and medial obliquity or on Harris and Beath views because it is obscured by the talar head. A 60-degree medial oblique view will help to visualize the anterior portion of the subtalar joint.

Isherwood has described three views for visualizing the subtalar joint, including the oblique dorsoplantar (oblique lateral) view to visualize the anterior facet.[60] In this view the medial aspect of the foot is placed on the film, and the sole is inclined 45 degrees to the film. The tube is centered 1 inch below and 1 inch distal to the lateral malleolus.

Isherwood's medial oblique axial view is used to visualize the middle facet and also gives a tangential view of the convexity of the posterior facet. The foot is dorsiflexed and when possible, inverted, with this position maintained by the patient with a wide bandage. The limb is medially rotated 60 degrees and the foot is rested on a 30-degree wedge. The tube is directed axially, tilted 10 degrees toward the head and 1 inch below and 1 inch anterior to the lateral malleolus. This projection gives an "end on" view of the sinus tarsi and places the sustentaculum tali close to the film for maximum radiographic detail.

The third Isherwood view, the lateral oblique axial, demonstrates the posterior facet in profile. The foot is dorsiflexed and when possible, everted, with this position also maintained by asymmetric pull on a broad bandage by the patient. The limb is laterally rotated 60 degrees, the knee flexed if necessary, and the foot rested on a 30-degree wedge. The tube is directed axially and tilted 10 degrees cephalad, with the central ray directed 1 inch below the medial malleolus. The tube direction and tilt may be fixed for both oblique axial views. Since it is difficult to situate patients properly and have them maintain the correct position, multiple views are often necessary. Even under optimal conditions these views can fail to yield conclusive results. The advent of newer techniques such as CT, as well as the increased radiation exposure imposed by plain film radiography, makes the use of the Isherwood views less practical.

## Secondary Radiographic Signs of Tarsal Coalition

Plain film techniques are not only used for identification of coalitions; they are also used to identify the secondary signs of coalitions. These signs include talar beaking; broadening of the lateral process of the talus; narrowing of the posterior talocalcaneal facet; failure to visualize the middle facet; a sclerotic ring surrounding the subtalar joint, referred to as the "halo effect"; and a ball-and-socket ankle joint.[34] These secondary signs usually present to varying degrees in adolescence, when the coalitions become ossified. They serve as a reminder that the foot can no longer adjust to what was previously passive restraint of normal motion and now has become more rigid with maturation of the coalition.

### Talar Beaking

Talar beaking is known to result from the alteration of normal subtalar joint motion, but its exact etiology in tarsal coalition remains a subject of debate. Loss of motion at the subtalar joint affects those joints proximal and distal to it, particularly the talonavicular joint. Cinefluoroscopy of a normal foot reveals that dorsiflexion causes the calcaneus to glide anteriorly on the talus until it is stopped, presumably by the capsular ligament. Near the end of dorsiflexion there is an upward gliding motion at the talonavicular and calcaneocuboid joints.[16] Although the calcaneus and navicular do not articulate, they are held in a constant relationship by the plantar calcaneonavicular ligament and the calcaneonavicular portion of the bifurcate ligament. In the foot with a fused subtalar joint, the calcaneus is incapable of gliding forward, and this in turn restricts movement of the navicular. Cinefluoroscopy of a foot that has had a subtalar fusion reveals that the gliding motion of the midtarsal joint is replaced by a hinge motion, with the upper edge of the navicular impinging on the talar head at the end of the dorsiflexion range of motion.[16]

Outland and Murphy have suggested that if one thinks of the talar head as having a plastic consistency prior to ossification, it is easy to visualize the remodeling effect that the navicular will have on the talar head.[16] Conway and Cowell suggest a slightly different etiology for talar beaking.[12] While they agree that the navicular overrides the lateral aspect of the talar head, they believe that the elevation of the talonavicular ligament and repeated minute elevations of the periosteum on the head of the talus cause a periosteal avulsion. Osseous repair of this avulsion results in talar beaking.

Early investigators interpreted this talar beaking, also known as "lipping" or "spurring," as a sign of osteoarthritis occurring at the talonavicular joint[8,10,18] (Fig. 9-4). Osteophyte formation is indeed one of the radiographic signs of osteoarthritis, but it is usually circumferential and occurs on both sides of the joint. In contrast, the talar beaking seen in some coalitions is confined to only the talar side of the talonavicular articulation; even more specifically, it is localized to the dorsolateral aspect of the talar head.[12] Furthermore, other radiographic signs of osteoarthritis such as joint space narrowing, subchondral sclerosis, and cystic bone changes are missing.[16,34] In such cases, in which no other signs of osteoarthritis are present, the existence of a talar beak does not signify arthritic changes. In cases of long-standing coalitions, however, some of these other radiographic signs may be present and herald the presence of true osteoarthritis at the talonavicular joint.

The questions of whether or not talar beaking is indicative of degenerative joint disease and of how to differentiate between a degenerative and nondegenerative talonavicular joint on a case-by-case basis are not just of academic interest. Accurate determination is of critical importance when surgical alternatives are being considered (as will be further discussed in the section on treatment). The absence of a talar beak does not necessarily rule out the diagnosis of talocalcaneal coalition. The beak is less apt to appear in those cases in which the coalition has not completely ossified. Talar beaking may also be

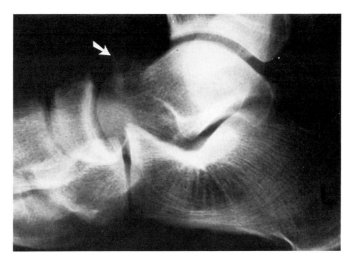

**Fig. 9-4.** Lateral radiograph demonstrating talar beaking. Notice the predominance on the talar side of the joint. (Courtesy of Surgery Department, California College of Podiatric Medicine, San Francisco, CA.)

seen with calcaneonavicular bars (although far less commonly than with talocalcaneal coalitions), rheumatoid arthritis, acromegaly, hypermobile flatfoot, and overzealous cast correction of clubfoot, as well as in long-term follow-up after a Grice procedure.[12,21,34]

### Other Secondary Signs

Broadening of the lateral process of the talus is the result of increased compressive forces exerted on the lateral talar surface by the calcaneus sulcus owing to severe valgus. These same increased compressive forces are responsible for the altered trabecular patterns around the subtalar joint that cause the halo effect.[47]

## Conventional Tomography

The unique capabilities of conventional tomography to diagnose tarsal coalition were first demonstrated in 1969 by Conway and Cowell, with their discovery of the previously undescribed coalition of the anterior facet of the subtalar joint.[12] When examining complex anatomic areas such as the hindfoot, tomography has advantages over conventional radiography by virtue of its ability to bring one section of interest into focus at a time while blurring out structures above and below it. Sections are made at 1, 1.5, and 2 cm less than the measured width of the foot, and an additional section is then made at half the measured distance. The first section bisects the sustentaculum tali, and the second and third sections will usually bisect the anterior facet if it is present. The fourth section at the midplane will bisect the posterior facet. Caution must be exercised, however, when interpreting plain tomograms, as the anterior joint may give the false impression of a coalition owing to its obliquity.[34] Conway and Cowell also noted that it was difficult to differentiate between a cartilaginous coalition and changes in the cartilage occurring secondary to trauma.

## Arthrography

Arthrography of the talocalcaneonavicular joint can be useful for detecting the presence of a talocalcaneal coalition when plain film and tomography findings are equivocal. With a 20- or 22-gauge needle 3 to 4 ml of positive contrast material is injected into the dorsal aspect of the talonavicular joint. Dorsoplantar, lateral, oblique, and Harris and Beath radiographic views are then obtained.

Failure to see contrast material above the sustentaculum tali in the lateral view, as well as failure to visualize contrast filling the middle facet on the Harris and Beath views, indicate a fibrous, cartilaginous, or osseous coalition. An irregular outline of the articular cartilage is indicative of degenerative joint disease.

If a coalition of the posterior facet is suspected, a separate arthrogram must be obtained, as the joint containing the posterior facet is anatomically separate from the talocalcaneonavicular joint containing the anterior and middle facets. Two techniques, both of which use 3 to 4 ml of contrast material, can be used to examine the posterior facet. More contrast medium is required if there is communication between the posterior subtalar joint and the ankle joint, which is seen in approximately 10 percent of the normal population. The first technique uses fluoroscopy to make a posterolateral approach, whereas the second technique involves angling the needle in a posterior direction after making an approach through the sinus tarsi. After injection of contrast material by either of these methods, lateral, lateral oblique, and Harris and Beath views are obtained. In the normal foot there will be a pouching at the posterior aspect of the joint, synovial folds in the area of the interosseous ligament, and a smooth contour over the articular cartilage. Inability to inject the dye is indicative of a posterior facet coalition, and irregular articular margins with thinning of the joint space are indicative of degenerative joint disease.

## Technetium 99 Bone Scanning

Bone scanning with technetium 99 (99 m medronate methylene diphosphonate) has been utilized successfully by some authors, who report a focally augmented uptake in the area of the coalition.[61,62] Deutsch et al. claim that such a finding is nonspecific but may provide localizing information in cases without a clear clinical or radiographic presentation.[61] Goldman et al. claimed a high degree of specificity and sensitivity.[62] In six patients with coalitions later substantiated by surgery or talonavicular arthrography, five coalitions (two osseous and three fibrous) had unique patterns of uptake both at the subtalar joint and at either the superior aspect of the talus or the talonavicular joint. The sixth patient had uptake in only the subtalar region and was later found via arthrography to have a fibrous coalition. None of the scans of 35 other feet without coalition but with an uptake in the hindfoot showed the characteristic pattern exhibited by the five feet with coalitions. Despite their claims that this characteristic pattern is unique to coalitions, Goldman et al. still recommended this technique only as a screening procedure, with the results subject to verification by Harris views, tomography, or arthrography.

## Computed Tomography

All the above-mentioned views and the techniques of conventional tomography, arthrography, and technetium bone scanning have limitations and caveats concerning their interpretation. Each technique represents a stage in the development of increasingly more sophisticated methods, and each has served a purpose in further delineating those coalitions that have evaded visualization by conventional radiographs. At present, CT is considered the gold standard in the diagnosis of tarsal coalition. Plain film radiographs still represent the initial evaluation technique, but ultimately CT scanning represents the definitive diagnostic technique. CT is unsurpassed in its ability to detect coalitions missed by plain films (including Harris and Beath views) or other special techniques, including arthrography, plain tomography, and Tc-99 bone scanning.[61,63–67] Although CT scanning was first conceptualized as a detection tool for tarsal coalitions, the wealth of information that it provides has expanded its role far beyond simple detection. CT displays the exact size of a coalition and its relationships to surrounding structures and often facilitates selection of the most appropriate surgical procedure. Moreover, its usefulness is not limited to preoperative planning; because it offers unparalleled visualization of hindfoot articulations, it allows the surgeon to follow and document postoperative changes. If there is a clinical suspicion that a resected coalition has begun to re-form, CT will allow the surgeon to objectively determine this regrowth almost immediately.[68]

Historically, coalition resection was principally reserved for the adolescent or younger patient with an isolated calcaneonavicular bar and without concurrent arthrosis of the hindfoot articulations. This select group has been expanded over the years, and selected resection of talocalcaneal coalitions in younger patients without adaptive changes is gradually becoming more accepted. Because of CT's ability to determine the size of these coalitions and the presence or absence of degenerative articular changes, it has played a vital role in the development of parameters that will ultimately define which patients are acceptable candidates for resection. For example, although there are some isolated claims of successful resections of coalitions involving the entire middle talocalcaneal facet, it is our experience and that of others that such a coalition is likely to fuse spontaneously some time in the postresection period. This is presumably the result of large areas of raw bone surface in contact with one another. However, if the coalition is limited and has not replaced the entire middle facet and it is feasible to maintain a portion of the middle facet's articular surfaces postresection, a higher success rate would be anticipated. CT can answer questions such as these and will help to further define the relevant parameters in future years.

Optimal visualization of the subtalar joint is obtained by imaging in the coronal plane. The patient lies supine on the CT table, with the knees and thighs flexed in order to place the feet flat on the scanner table. It has been suggested that an ankle in moderate flexion has the same

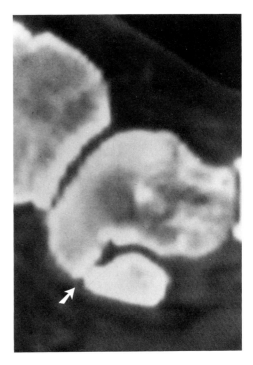

**Fig. 9-5.** Computer-generated sagittal image of the left foot of patient imaged in Fig. 9-1. The posterior facet (arrow) is mostly obliterated by a tarsal coalition. The middle facet is normal.

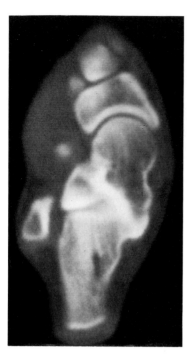

**Fig. 9-6.** Transverse image displaying a middle facet coalition. Notice the obliteration of the middle facet and the sclerosis at this site.

talocalcaneal relationship as a foot in neutral position, so that exact positioning is not critical as long as the two feet are lined up evenly.[69] Direct imaging can then proceed in either the frontal or transverse planes. Direct sagittal imaging is not feasible but can be computer-generated and thus helps to substantiate what is directly imaged (Fig. 9-5). Two-millimeter cuts will optimize visualization of the subtlest of irregularities and also allow for higher-quality computer re-formations in the sagittal plane.

Subtalar middle facet coalitions can theoretically be visualized on either frontal or axial images because the middle facet is typically tilted approximately 45 degrees, which makes it equidistant from both these planes (Fig. 9-6). However, anatomic relationships are better appreciated on the frontal plane images. Coalitions involving joints in the coronal plane such as the talonavicular and calcaneocuboid, as well as calcaneonavicular bars, are best visualized in the axial images.[69] This is accomplished by again placing the patient supine, but with the knees extended and the toes pointed straight up. Since coali-

tions may be fibrous or osseous, it is recommended that imaging be done with both soft tissue and bone windows.

An osseous talocalcaneal coalition will appear as an obvious fusion between the talus and calcaneus, with a continuity in the marrow cavity of the two bones and/or complete cortical bridging.[70] Fibrous or cartilaginous coalitions will present with joint space narrowing, but this will be accompanied by spur formation and cystic or lucent changes in the subchondral bone. We are in agreement with Bower et al.'s contention that markedly angled, enlarged, and deformed midsubtalar joints are congenital variations that will most likely result in tarsal coalition.[70] Stoskopf et al. have shown that in the normal axial views at the longest anterior to posterior dimension of the calcaneus there is a triangle of soft tissue directly anterior to the calcaneus.[63] An osseous calcaneonavicular coalition will show continuity of marrow between the two bones and/or cortical bridging with a loss of the soft tissue triangle. A loss of that soft tissue triangle, but without continuity of marrow or cortical bridging, indicates a fibrous or cartilaginous coalition.

## TREATMENT

Appropriate treatment of tarsal coalition is determined by numerous factors, including the severity of the deformity, the severity of symptoms, the extent of related arthritic changes, and the amount of the joint actually involved in the coalition. While asymptomatic coalitions do not necessarily require treatment, it must be considered that not all asymptomatic coalitions will necessarily remain so. Nonoperative care is usually directed at amelioration of acute symptoms. Surgical treatment can ultimately have one of two purposes; relief of pain or restoration of function. While the two purposes are not necessarily exclusive of one another, this is often the case. For example, restoration of function is best achieved by coalition resection; however, in many cases relief of pain may be most effectively achieved by arthrodesis.

### Nonsurgical Treatment

Nonsurgical treatment is aimed at decreasing the amount of pain and the degree of muscle spasm by limiting motion at the subtalar and midtarsal joints and thereby reducing the stress placed on these joints. Non-operative treatment may include physical therapy, use of accommodative and functional orthoses, injections, and immobilization. Shoe therapy and/or orthotic recommendations are varied and include medial heel wedges, University of California, Berkeley, Laboratory, (UCBL) devices, Thomas heels, Whitman plates, ankle/foot orthoses, and pronated orthoses. The subtalar joint should be gently placed in the closest position to neutral that can be attained without forcibly maintaining this position against spasm or pain when taking cast impressions for orthoses. The height of the rearfoot post can be increased to put the rearfoot in slight equinus and thus allow for greater movement at the ankle joint. The rearfoot post should be flat, not biplanar, as is usual to allow for subtalar joint motion. This will limit rearfoot motion to a minimum. A course of oral nonsteroidal anti-inflammatory medication and physical therapy can be helpful. Peroneal nerve blocks may decrease pain, either temporarily or long-term. Injection of a local anesthetic and corticosteroids into the sinus tarsi not only can serve as a diagnostic aid to determine the location of pain but also can provide long-term relief from spasm and pain in select cases.

Those patients with severe acute onset of symptoms and those who are recalcitrant to other nonoperative forms of treatment can be treated by cast immobilization for 3 to 4 weeks. The foot should be placed as close to the neutral position as possible without forcing the foot into an unnatural or painful varus position. If the results with the first cast are limited, a second period of immobilization may be tried. Failure of two 3- to 4-week periods of cast immobilization suggests the need for surgical intervention.

## Surgical Treatment

### Surgical Treatment of Calcaneonavicular Coalitions

The surgical treatment of tarsal coalition may include resection, arthrodesis, and osseous realignment. Resection is the procedure of choice in calcaneonavicular coalitions in young children without any signs or symptoms of advanced degenerative changes within the subtalar joint complex. In the presence of severe degenerative changes, most commonly seen in older patients, a triple

arthrodesis is usually performed. The presence and degree of adaptive joint symptoms therefore becomes a critical distinguishing factor.

Resection of calcaneonavicular bars was first suggested in 1927 by Badgley.[71] In 1929 Bentzon described essentially the same technique that is used today, which includes interposition of a portion of the extensor digitorum brevis muscle belly into the cavity left after resection of the calcaneonavicular bar.[72] Andreasen in 1968 reported the results of a long-term study of 25 feet which were followed for 10 to 22 years after resection, and reported that 14 patients were asymptomatic, 9 had mild symptoms, and 2 had severe pain requiring triple arthrodesis.[73] In spite of these findings, Andreasen recommended a triple arthrodesis as the procedure of choice, stating that it yielded better long-term results. Mitchell and Gibson in 1967 reported 41 calcaneonavicular bars treated by resection and followed for 4 to 13 years, with an average of 6 years.[74] At follow-up the bar had recurred to a large extent in one-third of the feet and to a lesser extent in another third. Complete relief was achieved in 68 percent of the feet, and over 25 degrees of subtalar inversion was restored in 58 percent of the feet. The procedure of these authors differs from that used today in that they resected a wedge of bone, not a rectangle, and they did not interpose the extensor digitorum brevis muscle into the area of resection.

Current thoughts on surgical treatment of calcaneonavicular bars are summarized by two studies. Cowell reported on 26 bars in 15 patients, which were resected with interposition of the extensor digitorum brevis muscle.[75] Muscle interposition was used in an attempt to achieve two basic goals, namely, to hinder bone reformation and to obliterate the dead space created by bar resection. Of the 26 feet, 23 were asymptomatic after surgery, and the patients were able to resume full activity, including participation in sports. Cowell stated that satisfactory results can be obtained 90 percent of the time in the symptomatic patient who has limitation of motion provided that the patient is less than 14 years old. He also stated that degenerative changes in the talonavicular joint, a completely ossified bar, or a second coalition between the talus and calcaneus contraindicated resection.

Similar findings were reported by Gonzalez and Kumar,[76] who treated 75 feet in 48 patients by resection with interposition of the extensor digitorum brevis mus-

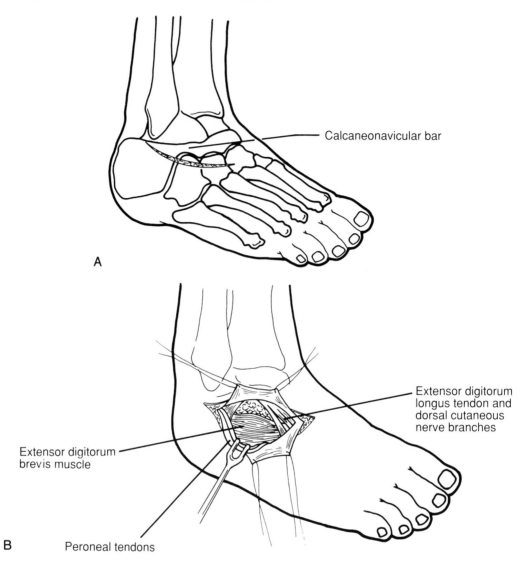

**Fig. 9-7.** Resection of calcaneonavicular coalition with soft tissue interposition. **(A)** A curvilinear lateral Ollier incision is made, extending from just inferior to the tip of the fibular malleolus toward the anteromedial tarsal joints slightly inferior to the calcaneonavicular bar in order to allow proximal retraction of the convex proximal skin flap. **(B)** The deep fascia is divided and reflected, and the long extensor tendons and dorsal cutaneous branch of the superficial peroneal nerve are mobilized and retracted medially. The peroneal tendons, which are visualized along the lateral calcaneal wall at the inferior portion of the wound, are gently retracted inferiorly. The proximal origin of the extensor digitorum muscle is identified, incised sharply to bone, and reflected distally to expose the calcaneonavicular bar. *(Figure continues.)*

cle. The length of follow-up ranged from 2 to 23 years. Results were graded as excellent in 77 percent of the feet, with the best results obtained in the 11- to 15-year-old group. These authors found that the best results were obtained in those patients under the age of 16 years who had a cartilaginous coalition. The age limitation supported by these two studies reinforces the premise that secondary changes and arthrosis are generally observed in the patient in postadolescent years. Once these changes occur, increases in tarsal motion are not well

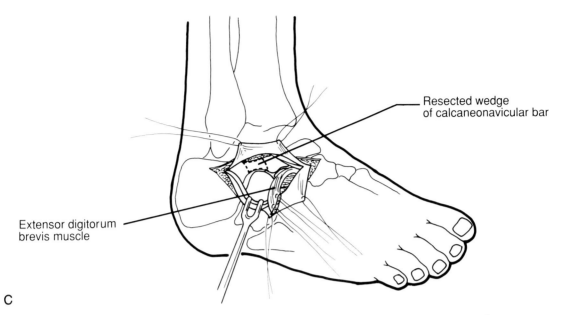

Resected wedge
of calcaneonavicular bar

Extensor digitorum
brevis muscle

C

**Fig. 9-7** *(Continued).* **(C)** A generous rectangular cube-shaped portion of bone is resected from the bar. Care is taken to make the wedge as wide inferiorly as superiorly and also to avoid resecting a portion of the talar head. Bone wax may be applied to the denuded bone surfaces to attempt to prevent recurrent fusion. A heavy absorbable suture is then applied to the free end of the extensor digitorum brevis muscle, which is drawn into the defect via two long, straight needles. The suture is tied over a buttress at the medial arch area. Alternatively, the defect may be packed with autogenous gluteal fat.

tolerated and in fact can exacerbate the problem. Arthrodesis is best advised in such cases.

*Technique of Resection*

Calcaneonavicular bar resection is performed through an anterolateral approach over the area of the sinus tarsi (Figs. 9-7 and 9-8). Dissection is carried down to the level of the extensor digitorum muscle, which is then detached from its origin in order to reflect the muscle belly distally. The coalition and the talonavicular, talocalcaneal, and calcaneocuboid joints are then identified. Care must be exercised to avoid cutting the lateral and dorsal aspects of the talonavicular joint capsule when the bar is excised. After all soft tissues have been reflected from the bar, the bar is resected as a rectangle, either by osteotomes or power instrumentation. After removal of at least 1.0 cm of bone, a rongeur is used to clear any residual bone from the base of the wound. All cartilage needs to be carefully removed from neighboring navicular and calcaneal bone to prevent re-formation of the bar.

A heavy absorbable suture is then threaded onto straight needles and passed first through the extensor digitorum muscle belly and then through the plantar aspect of the medial side of the foot. When the suture is pulled taut, the muscle belly is forced to occupy the space created by the generous resection of the bar. The suture is tied over a button at the plantar medial aspect of the foot. A thin layer of polyurethane foam can then be interposed between the button and the skin to prevent skin necrosis.[76]

Postoperative management consists of immobilization in a short leg non-weight-bearing cast or splint, with the foot in neutral position, for approximately 10 days. Following this, physical therapy is initiated to encourage passive subtalar joint range of motion. Full weight-bearing is generally postponed until subtalar motion is restored or markedly improved.[75]

## Surgical Treatment of Talocalcaneal Coalitions

### Choice of Procedure

The surgical treatment of talocalcaneal coalitions remains somewhat controversial. Acceptable methods of surgical treatment include isolated subtalar joint ar-

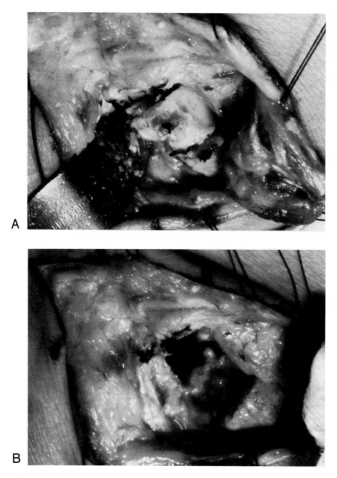

**Fig. 9-8.** Intraoperative photograph demonstrating a calcaneonavicular bar. The extensor digitorum brevis muscle is reflected distally. **(B)** The same patient after resection of the bar. The muscle belly is transposed to the defect to discourage re-formation of the bar. To be a candidate for bar resection, the tarsal articulations need to be normal and free of arthrosis or secondary changes. (Courtesy of Surgery Department, California College of Podiatric Medicine, San Francisco, CA.)

throdesis, arthrodesis of the subtalar and talonavicular joints, triple arthrodesis, calcaneal osteotomy, and resection of the coalition with or without insertion of a fat graft or implant. Until recently, either double or triple arthrodesis was considered by many to be the only reliable and appropriate surgical treatment for talocalcaneal coalitions.

Harris and Beath stated their own preference for either combined arthrodesis of the subtalar and talonavicular joints or arthrodesis of the talonavicular joint alone,[42] the latter option being reserved for those cases in which the talocalcaneal bridge was solid and totally restrictive to any motion and the position of the hindfoot was felt to be satisfactory. When a significant adaptive valgus deformity of the hindfoot was present, appropriate wedge removal and fusion of the subtalar joint was advised regardless of the status of the coalition. Harris and Beath did not advise arthrodesis during early childhood suggesting instead repeated manipulations under anesthesia with cast immobilization in the corrected position until adolescence, at which time arthrodesis could be performed.

While repeated manipulations may no longer be generally accepted, it remains a basic tenet of pediatric foot surgery to avoid the various types of pedal fusions in childhood. Major rearfoot fusions in children are ill-advised in most cases since they usually require resection of large amounts of nonossified bone in order to obtain union, which results in interference with foot growth, markedly abnormal appearance, and increased potential for recurrent deformity. Tachdjian recommended talonavicular fusion alone when rearfoot valgus amounted to less than 15 degrees.[48] If the valgus exceeded 15 degrees, appropriate wedges were resected and a triple arthrodesis was performed. In cases of incomplete coalition, he advised a tri-tarsal arthrodesis. Mann reported good results after performing isolated subtalar joint fusions in patients with talocalcaneal coalitions and no signs of calcaneocuboid or talonavicular joint degeneration.[77] He proposed isolated subtalar fusion as an alternative to more traditional approaches and suggested it as a salvage procedure when resection of the coalition failed.[78]

While fusions certainly can be successful in alleviating the discomfort of tarsal coalition, especially when there are associated degenerative articular changes, the need for exact alignment, the potential morbidity of a major operation (including nonunion), and the potential for eventual arthrosis of surrounding joints argue favorably for an alternate approach. Some authors have reported success in relieving pain by calcaneal osteotomies, performed by three methods, namely, a lateral opening wedge, a medial closing wedge, or crescentic osteotomy with medial displacement of the posterior fragment.[79-81] The opening or closing wedge procedure allows for frontal plane correction, while crescentic osteotomy is more versatile in that it allows for correction in three planes. It has been theorized that calcaneal osteotomy relieves hindfoot pain by alleviating the strain on the tarsal joints imposed by the valgus position usually associated with tarsal coalition. Calcaneal osteotomies may be used alone or as an adjunctive procedure following resection of a tarsal coalition in order to reduce the adaptive valgus deformity resulting from a long-standing coalition.

The newest and certainly most controversial surgical treatment for talocalcaneal coalition is resection. Numerous authors have advised against resection of symptomatic talocalcaneal coalitions if the intent is to restore normal biomechanics to the foot and subtalar joint.[12,15,18,50] Their main argument is based on the assumption that degenerative changes are usually present by the time the diagnosis is arrived at. Furthermore,

some authors feel that resection of middle facet coalitions would place too great a demand upon the remaining subtalar facets. The rationale for coalition resection is less controversial when resection is considered for alleviation of secondary symptoms. For instance, Jakayamur and Cowell[50] resected coalitions in two patients, one with neuroma-like pain from impingement of the medial plantar nerve and the other with mechanical irritation of the ankle joint. The pain was relieved in both instances, but very little subtalar joint motion was actually gained in the final analysis, and these authors recommended triple arthrodesis if more conservative measures fail.

Since about 1980 however, scattered reports have been appearing with greater frequency on the validity of resection to restore more normal foot function.[54,66,82-88] The number of cases in each study is small, and the combined total of reported cases of resection of talocalcaneal coalition is about 50. Owing to the small number of cases as well as the varying preoperative criteria used by the different authors for selecting surgical candidates, the parameters required for a successful outcome are not yet clearly defined. Some surgeons operated in the presence of talar beaking[82,87] and others without regard to the presence of broadening of the lateral process of the talus or narrowing of the posterior facet.[54,84] Scranton arbitrarily decided to operate only on those patients with less than 50 percent of the joint surface between the talus and the calcaneus involved,[87] but some investigators have resected coalitions in which the entire middle facet was involved.[66]

The findings of these different investigators, although still considered preliminary and controversial, seem to warrant attempted resection of talocalcaneal coalition in selected cases. The talonavicular and calcaneocuboid joints should be free of degenerative arthrosis. The presence of talar beaking itself does not appear to be a contradiction to resection.[82,84,87,88] However, other signs of degenerative joint disease at the talonavicular joint, such as sclerosis, joint space narrowing, and osteophytic growths on the navicular, appear to decrease the chances of obtaining optimal results. These changes can be best visualized on the appropriate CT scans. The presence of other secondary signs such as broadening of the lateral process of the talus and narrowing of the posterior facet may not necessarily be contraindications to resection.[85]

Furthermore, Olney and Asher claim their study shows no correlation between results and the type of coalition (e.g., osseous of fibrous), sex of the patient, or age of the patient.[85] However, the oldest patient in their study was only 22 years old, and his results were less than excellent. Although they attributed these results to inadequate resection at their first surgery and a postoperative course complicated by an active Reiter's syndrome, age would certainly have to be considered a factor in most cases, as there is a greater likelihood of degenerative changes in surrounding joints in the older patient. Finally, if the coalition involves a large percentage of the total joint surface between the talus and calcaneus, the advisability of resection is questionable. The exact amount of joint surface that can be successfully resected has yet to be determined, and further studies correlating postoperative results with preoperative quantification of joint involvement via CT are needed. All

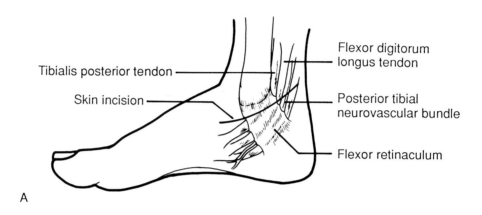

A

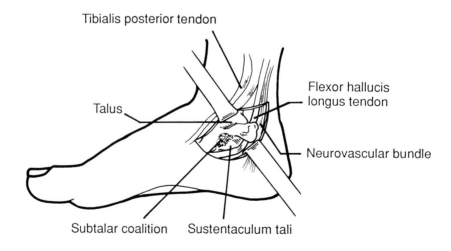

B

**Fig. 9-9.** Surgical resection of middle facet talocalcaneal coalition. **(A)** A medial skin incision is made parallel to the course of the posterior tibial tendon. **(B)** Exposure of the middle facet coalition after division of the flexor retinaculum and mobilization and posterior retraction of the posterior tibial neurovascular bundle. *(Figure continues.)*

the above-mentioned authors are in agreement that arthrodesis should be reserved for patients in whom conservative therapy has failed and who have an unresectable coalition or advanced degenerative changes.

*Technique of Resection*

Although there are minor variations in the techniques used by different surgeons to excise middle facet talocalcaneal coalitions, the basic procedure is as follows. A curvilinear incision beginning posterior to the medial malleolus is carried anteriorly, inferior and parallel to the posterior tibial tendon (Fig. 9-9A). The flexor retinaculum is then incised, care being taken to avoid damaging the underlying tendons and neurovascular structures. The tibialis posterior, flexor digitorum longus, flexor halluces longus, and neurovascular bundle are identified and mobilized. The posterior tibial tendon will be found superior to the middle facet, and the middle facet itself will be found in the interval between the flexor digitorum

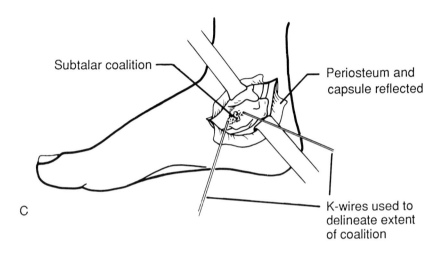

Subtalar coalition

Periosteum and capsule reflected

K-wires used to delineate extent of coalition

C

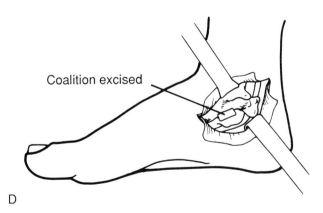

Coalition excised

D

**Fig. 9-9** *(Continued).* **(C)** The location of the subtalar joint and the extent of the coalition are identified by inserting Kirschner wires anterior and posterior to the coalition into the subtalar joint. **(D)** Resection of the coalition. The resected surfaces are covered with bone wax, and a free autogenous fat graft is interposed between the resected surfaces.

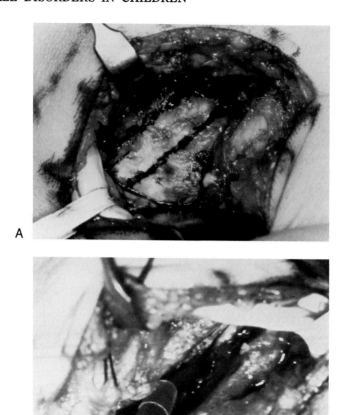

**Fig. 9-10.** **(A)** Intraoperative photograph demonstrating a middle facet coalition in a pediatric patient. The parallel lines represent the sites for proposed bar resection. A preoperative CT scan displayed no other coalitions and no evidence of arthrosis of the subtalar or midtarsal joints. **(B)** The same patient postresection. The resection should be generous. Interposition of soft tissue can be considered, and a sinus tarsi implant may temporarily help to prevent bony contact during the postoperative period.

longus and the neurovascular bundle. Plantar to the middle facet, passing under the sustentaculum tali, will be the flexor hallucis longus.

Once the middle facet has been identified, the periosteum over the coalition is incised and reflected (Fig. 9-9B). The extent of the coalition is then identified by inserting either a Keith needle or a Kirschner wire into normal parts of the subtalar joint anterior and posterior to the coalition (Fig. 9-9C). The coalition is then resected with a rongeur or osteotome. Care must be taken to avoid excessive resection of the sustentaculum tali. The coalition is resected until normal cartilage is visible and no subtalar impingement remains when the subtalar joint

is placed through its range of motion (Fig. 9-10). If limited subtalar joint motion or crepitus remains, further resection is required. Once adequate motion is obtained, the resected surfaces are covered with bone wax. A free autogenous fat graft from either the buttock or pronator quadratus may also be interposed between the resected surfaces (Fig. 9-9D). The flexor retinaculum is then repaired and the subcutaneous tissues and skin closed.

The patient is immobilized in a short leg non-weight-bearing cast for 2 to 4 weeks. After removal of the cast, the patient starts partial weight-bearing and passive range of motion exercises two to three times per day but does not resume full weight-bearing until the motion attained in the joint postoperatively is equal to that seen on the operating table after resection.

The use of subtalar joint implants after coalition resection has not yet been defined. Collins reported good results in five patients who had a condylar implant placed in the talus after resection of a middle facet talocalcaneal coalition.[89] He theorized that implant interposition would improve postoperative subtalar joint motion and prevent undue stress on the anterior and posterior facets.

There are a number of concerns with this approach. The implant used was not designed for this application nor for the location at which it was implanted. Therefore, a high failure rate might be expected. Some implant design concerns might be addressed by using one of the new type of subtalar implants, which is placed in the sinus tarsi and not the sustentaculum tali. The implant is not intended for joint replacement but merely to prevent bone-to-bone apposition. If bone separation is maintained and motion is encouraged postoperatively, then fibrocartilage could potentially form at the site of coalition resection.

One last concern regarding the treatment of talocalcaneal and calcaneonavicular coalitions should be addressed at this point. The incidence of dual calcaneonavicular and talocalcaneal coalitions is probably not rare.[90] Given the high probability of failed resection for either coalition if a second coalition in the foot goes undetected, it is necessary to carefully rule out the presence of other coalitions when contemplating surgical resection.

## Surgical Treatment of Talonavicular Coalitions

Talonavicular coalitions are rarely painful. When a patient does present with pain, the chief complaint is usually bump pain due to shoe irritation over the medial prominence of the talonavicular joint.[24,52] This can often be treated conservatively by shoe modifications and/or with orthoses. When surgical intervention is required, resection of the medial eminence by the Kidner approach is usually successful. Plantar transposition of the tibialis posterior tendon is recommended at the same time as the exostectomy in children with pronated types of feet.[47]

Treatment of other, less commonly occurring coalitions should be determined on an individual basis, with conservative treatment attempted first and surgical intervention undertaken only after all conservative methods have failed.

# REFERENCES

1. Buffon GL: Histoire Naturelle, Générale et Particulière. Vol. 3. Panckouke, Paris, 1769, p. 47
2. Cruveilhier J: Anatomie Pathologique du Corps Humain. Vol. 1. J.B. Ballière, Paris, 1829
3. Zuckerandl E: Ueber einen Fall von synostose chen Talus and Calcaneus. Allgem Wien Med Ztg 22:293, 1877
4. Anderson RJ: The presence of an astragalo-scaphoid bone in man. J Anat 14:452, 1879–1880
5. Holl M: Beiträge zur chirurgischen Osteologie des Fusses. Arch Klin Chir 25:211, 1880
6. Jones R: Peroneal spasm and its treatment. Report of meeting of Liverpool Medical Institution held 22 April, 1897, Liverpool. Med Chir J 17:442, 1897
7. Kirmisson E: Double pied bot varus par malformation osseuse primitive associée à des ankyloses congénitales des doigts et des orteils chez quatre membres d'une même famille. Rev Orthop 9:32, 1898
8. Sloman HC: On coalitio calcaneonavicularis. J Orthop Surg 3:586, 1921
9. Wagoner GW: A case of bilateral congenital fusion of the calcanei and cuboids. J Bone Joint Surg 10:220, 1928
10. Harris RI, Beath T: Etiology of peroneal spastic flatfoot. J Bone Joint Surg [Br] 30:624, 1948
11. Korvin H: Coalitio talocalcanea. Z Orthop 60:105, 1934
12. Conway JJ, Cowell HR: Tarsal coalition: clinical significance and roentgenographic demonstration. Radiology 92:799, 1969
13. Simmons EH: Spastic tibialis varus with tarsal coalition. J Bone Joint Surg [Br] 47:533, 1965
14. Cowell HR: Talocalcaneal coalition and new causes of peroneal spastic flatfoot. Clin Orthop 85:16, 1972
15. Cowell HR: Diagnosis and management of peroneal spastic flatfoot. Instr Course Lect 24:94, 1975
16. Outland T, Murphy ID: The pathomechanics of peroneal spastic flatfoot. Clin Orthop 16:64, 1960
17. Pfitzner W: Die Variationen im Aufbar des Fussskelets. Beiträge zur Kenntnis des menschlichen Extremitätenskelets. VII. Morphol Arbeit 6:245, 1896
18. Harris RI: Rigid valgus foot due to talocalcaneal bridge. J Bone Joint Surg [AM] 37:169, 1955
19. Outland T, Murphy, ID: Relation of tarsal anomalies to spastic and rigid flatfoot. Clin Orthop 1:217, 1953
20. Leboucq H: De la soudure congénitale de certains os du tarse. Bull Acad R Med Belg 4:103, 1896
21. Jack EA: Bone anomalies of the tarsus in relation to peroneal spastic flatfoot. J Bone Joint Surg [Br] 36:530, 1954
22. Harris BJ: Anomalous structures in the developing human foot, abstracted. Anat Rec 121:399, 1955
23. Rothberg AS, Feldman JW, Schuster OF: Congenital fusion of astragalus and scaphoid: bilateral; inherited. NY State J Med 35:29, 1935

24. Boyd HB: Congenital talonavicular synostosis. J Bone Joint Surg [Br] 37:191, 1955
25. Webster FC, Roberts WM: Tarsal anomalies and peroneal spastic flatfoot. JAMA 146:1099, 1951
26. Bersani FA, Samilson RL: Massive familial tarsal synostosis. J Bone Joint Surg [Am] 39:1187, 1957
27. Wray JB, Herndon CN: Hereditary transmission of congenital coalition of the calcaneus and navicular. J Bone Joint Surg [Am] 45:365, 1963
28. Glessner JR Jr, Davis GL: Bilateral calcaneonavicular coalition occurring in twin boys. A case report. Clin Orthop 47:173, 1966
29. Leonard MA: Inheritance of tarsal coalition and its relationship to spastic flatfoot. J Bone Joint Surg [Br] 56B:520, 1974
30. Nievergelt K: Positiver Vaterschaftsnachweis auf Grund erblicher Missbildungen der Extremitäten. Arch Klaus Stift Vererbungsforsch 19:157, 1944
31. O'Rahilly R, Gardner E, Gray DJ: The skeletal development of the foot. Clin Orthop 16:7, 1960
32. Christian JC: A dominant syndrome of metacarpal and metatarsal asymmetry with tarsal and carpal fusions, syndactyly, articular dysplasia and platyspondyly. Clin Genet 8:75, 1975
33. Spoendlin H: Congenital stapes ankylosis and fusion of tarsal and carpal bones as a dominant hereditary syndrome. Arch Otorhinolaryngol 206:173, 1974
34. Beckley DE, et al: Radiology of the subtalar joint with special reference to talocalcaneal coalition. Clin Radiol 26:333, 1975
35. Bentzon PGK: Bilateral congenital deformity of the astragalocalcanean joint: bony coalescence between os trigonum and the calcaneus? Acta Orthop Scand 1:359, 1930
36. Ertel AN, O'Connell FD: Talonavicular coalition following avascular necrosis of the tarsal navicular. J Pediatr Orthop 4:482, 1984
37. Lapidus PW: Bilateral congenital talonavicular fusion. Report of a case. J Bone Joint Surg 20:775, 1938
38. Rankin EA, Baker GI: Rigid flatfoot in the young adult. Clin Orthop 104:244, 1974
39. Vaughn WH, Segal GI: Tarsal coalition with special reference to roentgenographic interpretation. Radiology 60:855, 1953
40. Shands AR, Wentz IJ: Congenital anomalies, accessory bones, and osteochondritis in the feet of 850 children. Surg Clin North Am 33:1643, 1953
41. Stormont DM, Peterson HA: Relative incidence of tarsal coalition. Clin Orthop 181: 28, 1983
42. Harris RI: Retrospect: peroneal spastic flatfoot (rigid valgus foot). J Bone Joint Surg [Am] 47:1657, 1965
43. Perlman MD, Wertheimer SJ: Tarsal coalitions. J Foot Surg 25:1986

44. Wiles S, Palladino SJ, Stavosky JW: Naviculocuneiform coalition. J Am Podiatr Med Assoc 78(7): 1988
45. Gregerson NH: Naviculocuneiform coalition. J Bone Joint Surg [Am] 59:128, 1977
46. Rosen JS: Tarsal coalition: rare or not. J Am Podiatr Med Assoc 74(11):572, 1984
47. Jacobs AM, Sollecito V, Oloff LM, Klein N: Tarsal Coalitions: an instructional review. J Foot Surg 20(4):, 1981
48. Tachdjian M: Pediatric Orthopedics, WB Saunders, Philadelphia, 1972, p. 1346
49. Buckholz J: Tarsal coalitions. Paper presented at Northlake Surgical Seminar, 1975
50. Jayakumar S, Cowell HR: Rigid flatfoot. Clin Orthop 122:77, 1977
51. Sanghi JK, Roby HR: Bilateral peroneal spastic flat feet associated with congenital fusion of the navicular and talus. A case report. J Bone Joint Surg [Am] 43:1237, 1961
52. Lahey MD, Zindrick MR, Harris EJ: A comparative study of the clinical presentation of tarsal coalitions. Clin Podiatr Med Surg 5(2):341, 1988
53. Levens AS, Inman VT, Blosser JA: Transverse rotation of the segments of the lower extremity in locomotion. J Bone Joint Surg [Am] 30:859, 1948
54. Morgan RC, Crawford AH: Surgical management of tarsal coalition in adolescent athletes. Foot Ankle 7(3):183, 1986
55. Snider RB, Lipscomb AB, Johnston RK: The relationship of tarsal coalition to ankle sprains in athletes. Am J Sports Med 9:313, 1981
56. Blockley NJ: Peroneal spastic flat foot. J Bone Joint Surg [Br] 37:191, 1955
57. Kyne PJ, Mankin HJ: Changes in intra-articular pressure with subtalar joint motion with special reference to the etiology of peroneal spastic flatfoot. Bull Hosp Jt Dis Orthop Inst 26:181, 1965
58. Cowell HR, Elener V: Rigid painful flatfoot secondary to tarsal coalition. Clin Orthop 177:54, 1983
59. Braddock GTF: A prolonged follow-up of peroneal spastic flatfoot. J Bone Joint Surg [Br] 43:734, 1961
60. Isherwood I: A radiological approach to the subtalar joint. J Bone Joint Surg [Br] 43:566, 1961
61. Deutsch AL, Resnik D, Campbell G: CT and bone scintigraphy in the evaluation of tarsal coalition. Radiology 144:137, 1982
62. Goldman AB, Pavlov H, Schneider R: Radionuclide bone scanning in subtalar joint coalitions: differential considerations. AJR 38:427, 1982
63. Stoskopf CA, Hernandez RJ, Kelikian A: Evaluation of tarsal coalition by computed tomography. J Pediat Orthop 4:365, 1984
64. Sarno RC, Carter BL, Bankoft MS et al: Computed tomog-

raphy in tarsal coalition. J Comput Assist Tomogr 8:1155, 1984

65. Pineda C, Resnick D, Greenway G: Diagnosis of tarsal coalition with computed tomography. Clin Orthop 208:282, 1986

66. Herzenberg JE, Goldner L, Martinez S: Computed tomography of talocalcaneal coalition: a clinical and anatomic study. Foot Ankle 6:273, 1986

67. Migliori V, Pupp J, Kanat IO: Computed tomography as a diagnostic aid in a middle facet talocalcaneal coalition. J Am Podiatr Med Assoc 75:490, 1985

68. Marchisello PJ: Use of a computerized axial tomography for evaluation of talocalcaneal coalition: a case report. J Bone Joint Surg [Am] 69:609, 1987

69. Smith RW, Staple TW: Computerized tomography scanning technique for the hindfoot. Clin Orthop 177:34, 1983

70. Bower BL, Keyser CK, Gilula LA: Rigid subtalar joint: a radiographic spectrum. Skeletal Radiol 17:583, 1989

71. Badgley CE: Coalition of the calcaneus and navicular. Arch Surg 15:75, 1927

72. Bentzon PGK: Coalitio calcaneo-navicularis, mit besondere-Bezugnahme auf die operative Behandlung des durch diese Anomalie bedingten Platfusses. Verh Detsch Ortho Ges 23:424, 1929

73. Andreasen E: Calcaneo-navicular coalition, late results of resection. Acta Orthop Scand 39:424, 1968

74. Mitchell GP, Gibson JML; Excision of calcaneonavicular bar for painful spasmodic flatfoot. J Bone Joint Surg [Br] 49:281, 1967

75. Cowell HR: Extensor brevis arthroplasty. J Bone Joint Surg [Am] 52:820, 1970

76. Gonzalez P, Kumar SJ: Calcaneonavicular coalition treated by resection and interposition of the extensor digitorum brevis muscle. J Bone Joint Surg [Am] 72:71, 1990

77. Mann RA, Baumgarten M: Subtalar joint fusion for isolated subtalar disorders. Clin Orthop 226:260, 1988

78. Mann RA: Resection as a method of treatment of tarsal coalitions. J Bone Joint Surg [Am] 70:791, 1988

79. Dwyer FC: Causes, significance, and treatment of stiffness of the subtaloid joint. Proc R Soc Med 69:1, 1976

80. Cain TJ, Hyman S: Peroneal spastic flatfoot—its treatment by osteotomy of the os calcis. J Bone Joint Surg [Br] 60:527, 1978

81. Jacobs AM, Oloff LM, Visser HJ: Calcaneal osteotomy in the management of flexible and non-flexible flatfoot—a preliminary report. J Foot Surg 20:57, 1981

82. Swiontkowski MF, Scranton PE, Hansen S: Tarsal coalitions: long term results of surgical treatment. J Pediatr Orthop 3:287, 1983

83. Asher M, Mosiee K: Coalition of the talocalcaneal middle facet: treatment by surgical excision and fat graft interposition. Orthop Trans 7:149, 1983

84. Elkins RA: Tarsal coalition in the young athlete. Am Sports Med 14:477, 1986

85. Olney BW, Asher MA: Excision of symptomatic coalition of the middle facet of the talocalcaneal joint. J Bone Joint Surg [Am] 69:539, 1987

86. Danielsson LG: Talocalcaneal coalition treated with resection. J Pediatr Orthop 7:513, 1987

87. Scranton PE: Treatment of symptomatic talocalcaneal coalition. J Bone Joint Surg [Am] 69(4):533, 1987

88. O'Neill DB, Michel LJ: Tarsal coalition. A follow-up of adolescent athletes. Am J Sports Med 17:544, 1989

89. Collins B: Tarsal coalitions—a new surgical procedure. Clin Podiatr Med Surg 4:475, 1987

90. Wiles S, Palladino SJ, Stavosky JW: Concurrent calcaneo-navicular and talocalcaneal coalition. J Foot Surg 28(5):449, 1989

# 10

# Miscellaneous Congenital Deformities

*STEVEN J. DeVALENTINE*

## POLYDACTYLY

The term *polydactyly* is derived from a combination of Greek and Latin roots, the literal translation of which is "many digits," and is currently used to describe a heterogeneous group of anatomic congenital anomalies characterized by the presence of one or more supernumerary toes or fingers. Polydactyly most commonly occurs as an isolated congenital deformity in which a single supernumerary finger or toe is present, but cases of as many as 13 fingers on one hand and 12 toes on one foot have been reported.[1] References to polydactyly or to individuals with supernumerary digits can be found even in ancient literature. Gould described an ancient Arabian tribe in which polydactyly was so common that children with only five fingers or toes were considered abnormal and were thought to be the product of adultery.[1]

Polydactyly occurs with approximately equal frequency in males and females and is about twice as common in the hand as it is in the foot.[2] The incidence varies with racial type and geographic location. In the white population it has been reported to be between 0.3 and 1.3 per 1,000 live births.[3,4] The incidence in blacks is much higher, with the reported frequency in the United States varying between 3.6 and 13.9 per 1,000 live births.[3,4] Kromberg found the incidence in South African blacks to be 10.4 per 1,000 live births, making polydactyly the most common congenital deformity in the South African black population.[5] The geographic variation of polydactyly is thought to be the result of racial differences in that the incidence is highest in countries in which a higher percentage of the population has black

ancestry. Polydactyly is thought to be slightly more common among Orientals than among whites.[6] In an analysis of 120,000 live births in Baltimore between 1954 and 1958, Frazier found the overall incidence (without respect to race) to be 1.7 per 1,000 live births (white 0.3, black 3.6), which would make polydactyly one of the most common congenital musculoskeletal deformities, along with congenital dislocated hip and congenital talipes equinovarus.[3]

## Classification

Classification systems are generally based on etiology and/or morphology. Since the specific etiology of any individual case of polydactyly is usually not known and since the etiology of this condition does not generally affect prognosis, classification systems that have been described for polydactyly are universally based on morphology. Tetamy and McKusick originally described polydactyly by location of the supernumary digits as preaxial, central, or postaxial.[7] Preaxial polydactyly involves duplication of the first digit and/or ray (Fig. 10-1), postaxial polydactyly duplication of the fifth digit and/or ray (Fig. 10-2), and central polydactyly duplication of the second, third, or fourth digit and/or ray. Postaxial polydactyly is by far the most common type occurring in the foot. In a retrospective review of 125 patients with 194 duplicated toes, Phelps and Grogan found postaxial polydactyly to account for 79 percent of duplications.[8] Preaxial duplication accounted for 15 percent, and central ray duplication was least frequent, accounting for only 6 percent. A combination of preaxial and postaxial polydactyly in the same individual has been referred to by

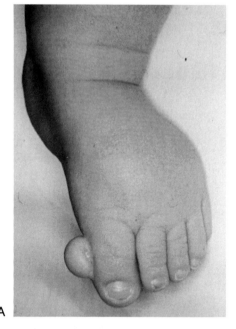

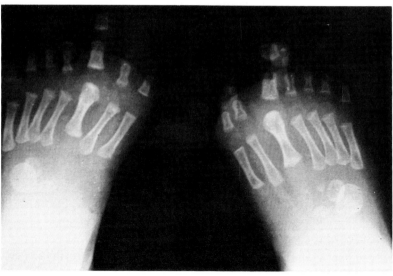

**Fig. 10-1.** Preaxial polydactyly. **(A)** Partial duplication of hallux. **(B)** An unusual complete ray duplication with two supernumerary preaxial digits.

some authors as *mixed polydactyly*.[9] Likewise, a combination of preaxial duplication in the upper extremity with postaxial duplication in the lower extremity or vice versa has been labeled *crossed polydactyly*. Tetamy and McKusick further subdivided postaxial polydactyly into types A and B.[7] Type A digits are well formed, with articulating skeletal components, while type B digits are rudimentary, vestigial digits, often without skeletal components. Type B polydactyly is much rarer than type A and is almost never seen in preaxial involvement.

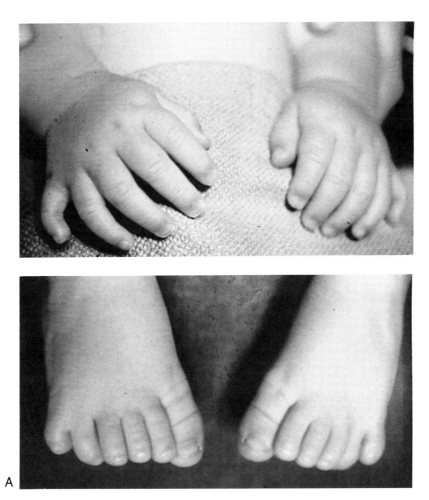

**Fig. 10-2. (A)** Postaxial polydactyly of the hands (top) and feet (bottom) of a young child. *(Figure continues.)*

Venn-Watson provided a useful classification based on the morphologic configuration of the corresponding metatarsal.[10] He divided the six most common metatarsal/digital patterns into lesser metatarsal and first metatarsal types. The lesser patterns are (1) Y-shaped metatarsal, (2) T-shaped metatarsal, (3) normal metatarsal with wide head, and (4) complete ray duplication; the first metatarsal patterns are (1) short block first metatarsal and (2) wide metatarsal head (Fig. 10-3).

Postaxial type A polydactyly has repeatedly been shown to be the most common type of polydactyly, accounting for 84 percent of 153 cases of postaxial polydactyly in Phelps and Grogan's review.[8] They found the following distribution of Venn-Watson metatarsal pat-

terns in that group: normal shaft with wide metatarsal head (45 percent), Y-shaped metatarsal (27 percent), T-shaped metatarsal (13 percent), ray duplication (9 percent), and normal metatarsal with distal duplication (6 percent). Syndactyly frequently occurs in association with postaxial type A polydactyly and may complicate surgical correction. Nogami found syndactyly of the duplicated fifth toes present in 28 percent of 46 cases reviewed in Japan.[11] Even more surprisingly, he found syndactylization of the duplicated fifth toes with the fourth toe in 45 percent of cases (Fig. 10-4). Polydactyly alone without syndactyly was present only 26 percent of the time.

Preaxial polydactyly, although much rarer than post-

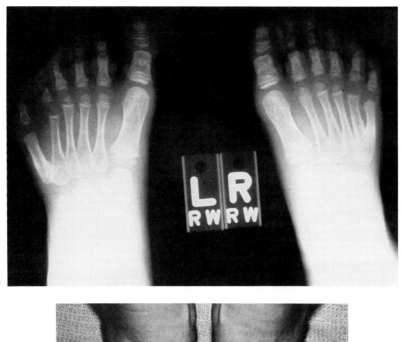

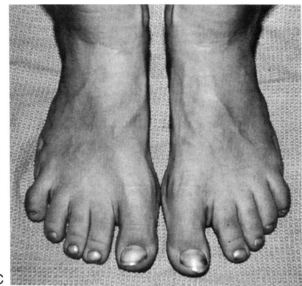

**Fig. 10-2** *(Continued).* **(B)** Postaxial polydactyly, with complete duplication of the fifth ray. **(C)** Same subject as in Fig. B, postrepair.

axial polydactyly, accounts for approximately 15 percent of all cases of polydactyly.[2,8] Preaxial polydactyly is almost always type A. Jahss and Nelson[12] reported 16 cases in 1984, Masada et al.[2] reported 18 cases in 1987, and Phelps and Grogan[8] reported 29 cases in 1985. Both Jahss and Nelson and Phelps and Grogan found block first metatarsals in about 50 percent of their cases. Jahss and

Nelson referred to the block first metatarsal as a transitional ray indicating partial but incomplete duplication of the metatarsal. Almost one-half of Masada et al.'s cases had bifid or incompletely duplicated hallux phalanges, another common finding in preaxial polydactyly. Polydactyly of the hands was more frequently associated with preaxial than with postaxial polydactyly of the feet in

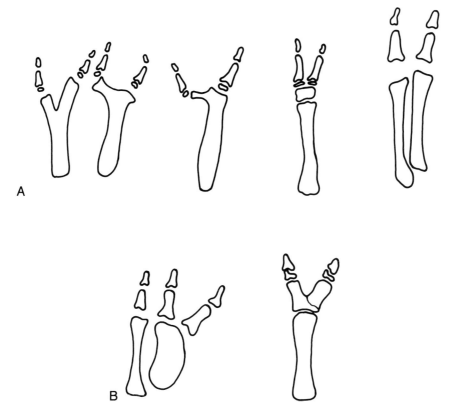

**Fig. 10-3.** Venn-Watson types of metatarsal patterns commonly seen in polydactyly. **(A)** Lesser metatarsal patterns. **(B)** first metatarsal patterns. (From Venn-Watson,[10] with permission.)

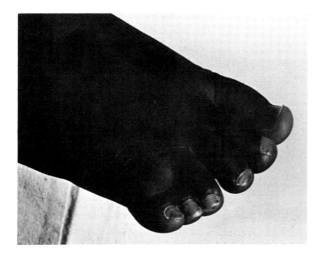

**Fig. 10-4.** Typical polysyndactyly of the fourth and fifth toes.

Masada et al.'s review. Congenital hallux varus was also frequently associated with preaxial polydactyly, and the incidence of recurrent hallux varus was also high after surgery (Fig. 10-5).

## Etiology

Polydactyly is thought to be a genetically transmitted condition. An autosomal dominant pattern with variable penetrance is by far the most common mode of transmission, but autosomal recessive patterns of inheritance have also been described.[7,13,14] Sporadic cases may occur as the result of new gene mutations. In a retrospective chart review of 72 patients with 109 duplicated toes, Venn-Watson found 30 percent of patients to have a positive family history of polydactyly.[10] A wide variation in gene expression was noted. The location of digital

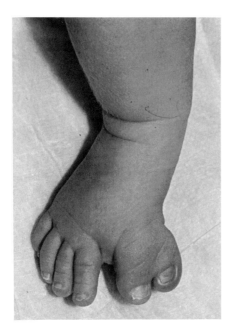

**Fig. 10-5.** Preaxial polydactyly with associated mild hallux varus.

involvement tended to be the same in related individuals, but a wide variation in skeletal and digital structure was present.[10]

Although pedal polydactyly is usually an isolated congenital deformity, it may occur in conjunction with other congenital anomalies or in association with some syndromes or chromosomal nondisjunction disorders. Polydactyly of the hands is the most common associated condition, with a frequency varying between 22 and 33 percent.[8,10] Masada et al. found a slightly higher frequency of polydactyly of the hands associated with preaxial polydactyly of the foot (36 percent).[2] Syndactyly is also fairly common, occurring in about 15 percent of cases.[8] Pedal polydactyly has rarely been reported in association with congenital hip dysplasia, clubfoot, congenital heart disease, or various other isolated conditions. It is unlikely that any etiologic association exists in these cases. Polydactyly has also been reported by several authors in association with Down syndrome (trisomy 21), Lawrence-Moon-Biedl syndrome, chondroectodermal dysplasia, and trisomies 13 and 18.

The exact physiologic mechanism that produces extra digits is unknown. Polydactyly has been produced experimentally in laboratory animals by various teratogens, including exposure to radiation, injection of 6-mercapto-

purine and other cytotoxic agents, and deprivation of folic acid in rats.[15,16] Scott et al. proposed the following mechanism as a result of those experimental studies: cellular death occurs in the limb bud mesoderm, followed by necrosis in the apical ectodermal ridge, which results in a disturbance of the digitation process and the development of excess apical tissue, which develops into the extra digit(s).[16]

## Treatment

Infants with type B vestigial digits are usually recognized and treated in the newborn nursery by ligation or excision of the skin tag-like soft tissue appendage. Radiography is recommended before attempting removal of type B digits to rule out osseous components. Ossification centers for phalanges should be present at birth. If no bone is present, immediate ligation or excision is adequate. If skeletal components are present, it is preferable to wait until the child is a few months old and to excise the digit under anesthesia to ensure complete excision of all accessory bone. The remaining infants with type A digits are usually referred by pediatricians for consultation concerning removal of extra toes when just a few months old. Parents express concern about cosmesis, function, and the stigma of a congenital aberration and usually want the extra toe immediately removed. It is important for the physician to explain to parents that the best cosmetic and functional results are obtained by waiting until the pattern of skeletal involvement becomes clear enough to plan an appropriate surgical approach. Surgery should generally be avoided before 1 year of age, when the child will better tolerate anesthesia, osseous development will be complete enough for adequate surgical planning, and surgical dissection will be facilitated by the larger size. In some cases phalangeal and metatarsal ossification may not be adequate to permit determination of which toe should be removed until age 2 or 3. Surgical excision before the child starts school is preferable to prevent problems with shoewear. Children can be examined radiographically every 6 months to 1 year from age 1 until excision can be performed.

### Postaxial Polydactyly

Each case requires an individual evaluation and surgical approach. The most important decision one has to make is which toe to remove. The most developed and cosmetically normal digit with the most normal metatarsophalangeal joint articulation should be saved. In most cases

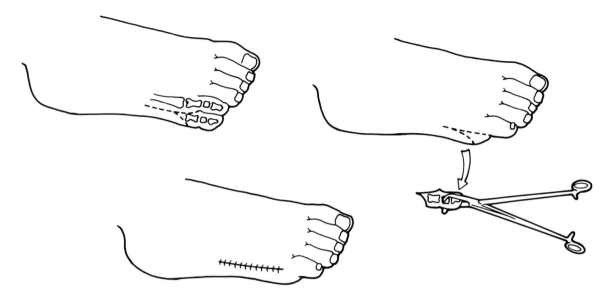

**Fig. 10-6.** Racquet-shaped incision for removal of an outer duplicated toe.

the most lateral digit will be removed. Excision of the most lateral toe is performed through a racquet-shaped incision, which is started at the web space and carried around the base of the toe and proximally along the dorsal lateral fifth metatarsal shaft (Fig. 10-6). The racquet-shaped incision is preferred as it allows maximum conservation of skin flap. Redundant skin can always be removed at the time of closure. The initial incision is made through the skin and subcutaneous layer, and the proximal flaps are reflected enough to expose tendon and bone. Tendons may be duplicated or absent in the extra toe. In most cases the tendon to the extra digit branches in a Y shape from the normal extensor and flexor tendon to the fifth ray and should be resected flush with the main portion of tendon. The toe may then be disarticulated and removed. A block metatarsal or wide metatarsal head should be narrowed with an osteotome to approximate normal size. Long-term follow-up has not shown early physeal closure, and reduction of the metatarsal to normal size contributes to a better cosmetic result.[8] When a T- or Y-shaped fifth metatarsal is present, the extra metatarsal head should be removed flush with the remaining bone, and when a complete duplication of the metatarsal occurs, the entire ray should be excised.

Excision of the most lateral digit has the advantage of simplicity and very effectively narrows the forefoot. In some situations, however, the innermost toe may be more hypoplastic or may not articulate as normally with the metatarsal head as the lateral digit; in such cases the inner toe should be excised (Fig. 10-7). An elliptical incision about the base of the digit may be carried proximally dorsally and plantarly in the same manner as in ray amputation if further exposure or more narrowing by wedge resection is needed. The transverse intermetatarsal ligament should be repaired to maintain narrowing of the forefoot when the more medial toe is excised.

When syndactyly of the duplicated fifth toe is present, the surgical correction is slightly more complex. The nail plate and matrix are excised to bone, and the incision is carried proximally along the nonsyndactylized border of the toe, creating skin flaps out of the remaining digital skin. The bone is "filleted" from the digit, and the skin flaps are remodeled for closure (Fig. 10-7).

Polysyndactyly of the duplicated fifth toe with the normal fifth or fourth toe is also not uncommon. When polysyndactyly of the fourth and duplicated fifth toes is present and the most lateral toe is removed, the fourth and fifth remaining toes should usually be left syndactylized; however, if desyndactyly is performed, it should be staged to prevent vascular compromise. When the innermost of the duplicated fifth toes is abnormal or can be excised, the skin flap that remains can be used to re-create a web space without the need for skin graft or Z-plasty techniques.

Long-term results of surgical treatment of postaxial polydactyly have been generally very good. Phelps and Grogan noted 95 percent good or excellent results in 61 patients with 97 duplications and an average 15.1-year

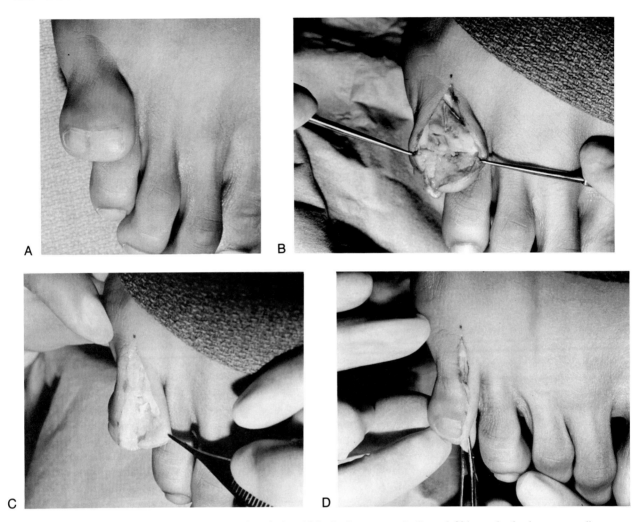

**Fig. 10-7.** (A) Postaxial polydactyly/syndactyly in which the innermost duplicated fifth toe is the least normally articulating digit. (B) Skin incision showing duplicated phalanges and tendon apparatus. (C) All skin is preserved. Accessory inner skeletal and tendon structures are "filleted" and removed. (D) Skin flap is measured for remodeling. *(Figure continues.)*

follow-up.[8] Most of the good (as opposed to excellent) results were due to residual widening of the foot or "abnormal" toe shape, which made some shoe styles more difficult to wear but did not impair function. Residual callus was also assigned a good result.

**Central Ray Duplication**

Central ray duplications can be excised through a racquet-shaped incision with the arm of the racquet carried proximally along the dorsum of the corresponding meta-

tarsal. In complete metatarsal duplication, the entire ray should be removed. The transverse intermetatarsal ligament should be tightly repaired to prevent widening of the forefoot, if possible. In spite of attempts to secure a tight ligament repair and the use of postoperative casts or splints, forefoot widening often occurs, and parents should be warned of this before the operation. Wedge-type ray amputation with removal of dorsal and plantar triangular sections of skin and soft tissue might be more effective in narrowing the foot, but one may have to contend with a potentially problematic plantar scar.

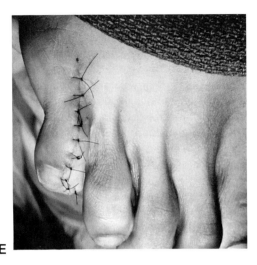

**Fig. 10-7** *(Continued).* **(E)** Skin closure. (Courtesy of B. Scurran, D.P.M.)

## Preaxial Polydactyly

Preaxial polydactyly is a relatively rare condition. Several types have been described, but they occur so rarely that the frequency of occurrence of any particular type has not been established. The following types have been described most often: (1) complete phalangeal duplication with normal first metatarsal; (2) incomplete phalangeal duplication (bifid great toe), with or without wide first metatarsal head; (3) complete ray duplication; and (4) block first metatarsal with complete hallux duplication.[2,8,11]

Jahss and Nelson found block first metatarsals in 50 percent of cases,[12] while Phelps and Grogan found them in 80 percent of their cases of preaxial polydactyly.[8] Masada et al.,[2] in a review of 14 patients with 21 duplicated great toes, found block first metatarsals to be very infrequent. A true congenital hallux varus similar to the isolated deformity that is seen without polydactyly was usually associated with a block first metatarsal.

The same techniques are used in the surgical repair of the first three types of preaxial polydactyly as are used in repair of postaxial polydactyly, but the surgical correction is somewhat more complex, and long-term results are not quite as good. The most frequent long-term problems are recurrent hallux varus deformity and residual splaying of the first ray. One should attempt to evaluate the function of each great toe. It may be necessary to postpone surgical repair until age 1 to 3 to accurately assess clinical function and radiographic development. Complete duplication of tendons, muscle, and ligament attachments may not be present. The most hypoplastic and least functional digit should be removed, whether it is the medial or the lateral one. With all other factors being equal, one should remove the more medial digit. When the most lateral toe is removed, a tight repair of the transverse metatarsal ligament and adductor hallucis tendon to the base of the proximal phalanx should be performed to prevent forefoot widening and hallux varus deformity. I recommend pin fixation for 3 weeks to allow adequate time for soft tissue healing.

Preaxial polydactyly associated with broad short first metatarsal and congenital hallux varus is much more difficult to correct, and long-term results are not as good as with the first three types. Recurrent hallux varus and angular deformity are frequent, and the prognosis for normal first metatarsal development is guarded. The first metatarsal frequently is short and does not adequately bear weight at maturity. The contracture of the medial skin and soft tissue along the first ray presents a problem in surgical correction. When the more medial great toe is removed, the entire digital skin flap can sometimes be used to repair the medial soft tissue deficit that is created. Farmer's procedure, described in the section on congenital hallux varus, may also be useful in this type of preaxial polydactyly.

# SYNDACTYLY

Syndactyly is a relatively common congenital condition affecting the fingers and toes, which is best described as a failure of the separation of the digits during normal fetal development. Syndactylized digits are often referred to as *webbed* fingers or toes. Two or more digits may be involved and are always completely interconnected from proximal to distal through part of or their entire length (Fig. 10-8).

Most authors recommend the following descriptive anatomic classification of syndactyly: (1) complete or incomplete; (2) simple or complex; and (3) complicated complex.[17-19] Incomplete syndactyly is characterized by joining of the digits only along a portion of their length, while complete syndactyly implies interconnection extending to the tips of the fingers or toes. Simple deformity involves only a soft tissue interconnection, while complex deformity may involve shared neurovascular,

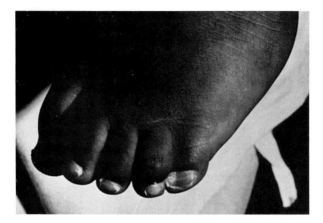

**Fig. 10-8.** Congenital syndactyly of the fourth and fifth toes.

tendinous, or osseous structures. Complex syndactyly affecting three or more digits with interposed incomplete structures is described as complicated complex deformity. Digital syndactylization is most often congenital but can also be acquired through traumatic loss or surgical excision of interdigital skin and subsequent granulation and cicatrix formation. Traumatic syndactylization frequently occurs as a result of burn injury.

Bunnell stated that syndactyly of the fingers occurs once in every 1,000 births.[20] MacCollum placed the incidence of syndactyly of the fingers and toes between 1 in 2,000 and 1 in 2,500 live births.[21] Thus, syndactyly is one of the more common congenital musculoskeletal conditions and is slightly less common than polydactyly. Most authors indicate that boys are affected between one and one-half and three times as often as girls.[17,22,23] Some authors feel that syndactyly occurs in the hands about twice as often as it does in the feet; however the data are questionable, since most reports do not specifically mention whether feet were inspected for syndactyly. Davis and German found syndactyly of the toes without associated syndactyly of the fingers in 11 of 50 patients studied.[17] The second and third toes are most frequently involved in the foot, and the middle and ring finger are most frequently involved in the hand.[17,22,23] Bilateral involvement occurs in approximately one-third to one-half of cases.[20,24]

## Etiology and Pathology

The limb bud appears at about the fourth week of fetal development. The grooves that will eventually allow differentiation of individual digits from the undifferentiated mesenchymal limb bud tissue form during the fifth to eighth week. It is during this crucial period of fetal limb development that normal differentiation and separation of the digits may be prevented. Congenital syndactyly is the result of a failure of separation of the digital mesenchymal limb bud tissue and thus is always manifested by complete joining of the digits from proximal to the distal limit of the webbing. In contrast, acrosyndactyly (partial joining of digits with a proximal opening) is thought to result from a rejoining of the digits after separation, which is most likely due to intrauterine environmental factors (e.g., congenital constriction bands). Although syndactyly has been produced in laboratory animals through nutritional deficiencies or exposure to toxic substances, these mechanisms probably do not play a significant role in the etiology of syndactyly in humans.[25,26]

Genetic factors have been implicated in most studies. Most authors feel that syndactyly is transmitted through an autosomal dominant pattern of inheritance, although other mechanisms have been reported.[27-29] Tetamy and McKusick, in a review of the literature combined with their own experience, found at least five phenotypically different types of syndactyly involving the hands.[27] All were inherited as autosomal dominant traits, with uniformity of the type of syndactyly within any individual family pedigree. Three of the five types were associated with syndactylization of the toes: simple syndactyly of the middle and ring fingers was usually associated with simple syndactyly of the second and third toes, and complex syndactyly of the middle and ring fingers with partial or complete duplication of components of the ring finger was usually associated with syndactyly of the fourth and fifth toes with polydactyly of the fifth toe. Nogami also found this type of complex polysyndactyly of the fourth and fifth toes to be quite common (46 percent of 46 feet with polydactyly of the fifth toe).[28] The third type of complex syndactyly described by Tetamy and McCusick involved syndactyly of the third and fourth fingers and the second and third toes, with an associated fusion of the third and fourth or fourth and fifth metacarpals or metatarsals.

Congenital syndactyly of the hands has been described in combination with many other conditions. The most commonly associated conditions include syndactyly of the toes, polydactyly, and cleft palate.[26] Other conditions, including Apert syndrome (acrocephalosyndactyly), Poland syndrome, dysplasia of long bones, clubfoot, and oculodentodigital dysplasia have been reported.[27] The more complex types of syndactyly tend to be associated with syndromes or multiple congenital problems, whereas the more common simple syndactyly is usually an isolated deformity in a healthy child.

## Treatment

Syndactylization of the fingers is cosmetically unappealing and can significantly impair dexterity and function of the hand. Surgical separation of syndactylized fingers at an early age (1 to 5 years) is generally recommended in order to promote the most functional possible result and prevent contracture. Simple syndactylization of the lesser toes, however, never causes any functional impairment and in most cases provides a stabilizing effect that may help prevent digital deformities such as claw toes or hammer toes. Elective syndactylization is, in fact, a popular reconstructive salvage procedure for unstable or recalcitrant hammer toe deformity. The usual case of syndactylization of two lesser toes is also not unsightly and in my opinion is usually more cosmetically acceptable than the scarring or potential complications associated with the surgical desyndactylization procedure. In most cases parents and adolescents can be easily convinced that this relatively common condition does not need surgical treatment.

In rare cases surgical separation of simple syndactyly deformity may be justified on the basis of psychological and/or cosmetic concerns.[30-32] In these situations it is probably best to postpone the surgical procedure until adolescence, when the child can participate in the decision to operate as well as the postoperative care that is essential to a successful result. Earlier surgical treatment may be necessary in more complex types of syndactyly, including polydactyly, extraosseous structures, or syndactyly of the great toe. In these cases I prefer to operate between the ages of 1 and 5, usually erring toward the upper age limit, to allow more complete preoperative radiographic evaluation and better intraoperative visualization of anatomic structures.

An excellent review of the historical surgical treatment of syndactyly is provided by Coleman et al.[26] The earliest attempts at surgical separation of syndactylized fingers involved simple division or division with limited local skin flaps. The failure rate with these procedures was extremely high because there is never enough skin to cover the defect that is created after separation of the digits and any open area in or near the web space causes troublesome scar formation or resyndactylization. The current principles of desyndactylization surgery, which were developed in the mid-twentieth century, include the following: (1) creation of an adequate web space of the same depth and width as the adjacent digits through the formation of local skin flaps; (2) use of zigzag incisions along the dorsal and plantar aspects of the length of the digits to prevent constriction and reduce scarring; and (3) use of skin grafts to cover all remaining defects, since complete coverage is never possible with local flaps alone.[18,26]

Numerous procedures have been described for desyndactylization of the fingers that fulfill the above requirements. The web space can be constructed with a combination of dorsal and plantar triangular flaps or with a long rectangular dorsal or plantar flap.[18,24,33,34] Weinstock et al.[32] described the use of an elliptical full thickness skin

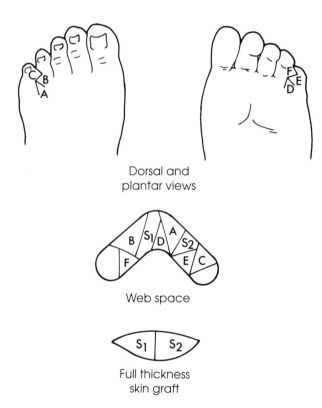

Dorsal and
plantar views

Web space

Full thickness
skin graft

**Fig. 10-9.** Diagramatic representation of desyndactylization incisions and skin flap placement. Dorsal (A) and plantar (D) triangular skin flaps created from the area of syndactylized skin are used to construct a new web space. The remaining triangular skin flaps created from syndactylized skin (B, C, E, F) are interposed to cover defects at the inner and outer edges of the fifth and fourth toes, respectively. Small triangular defects (S1, S2) are covered with a full thickness, defatted skin graft or a split thickness graft from the thigh.

graft placed in the web space after simple sagittal division of the web, but this can only be used in an incomplete, simple syndactyly deformity.

My preferred technique involves the use of dorsal and plantar triangular skin flaps, which are sewn together to create a web space, combined with dorsal and plantar zigzag incisions and a small skin graft to fill any residual defect (Figs. 10-9 and 10-10). The apex of the proximal V-flap should extend to about the midportion of the proximal phalanx. The apices of the transverse V-shaped flaps should extend to at least the midportion of the adjacent toe, and plantar and dorsal flaps should be based

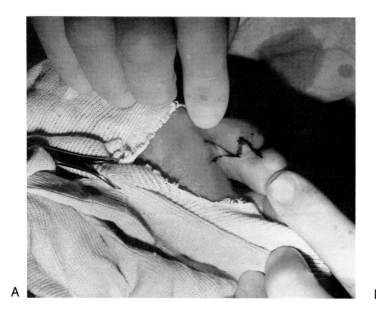

A

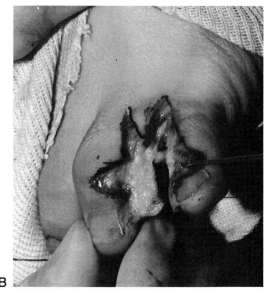

B

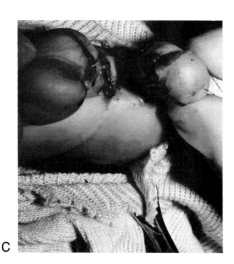

C

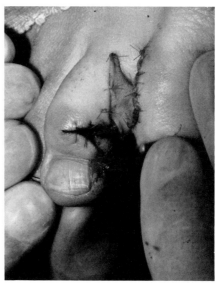

D

**Fig. 10-10.** Desyndactylization procedure. **(A)** Skin incision. Apices of dorsal skin flaps are placed opposite plantar flaps. **(B)** Elevation and mobilization of skin flaps. **(C)** Reconstruction of web space with triangular flaps. **(D)** Closure with skin graft visible at proximal portion of fourth toe.

on opposite toes and placed proximal or distal to one another rather than at the same level. A small needle placed from dorsal to plantar at the apex of the proximal V-flap facilitates incision design. The full thickness triangular skin flaps are undermined and mobilized, with care taken to avoid injury to digital vessels and nerves. Little or no subcutaneous tissue should be left attached to the apex of the flap, but a progressively thicker layer of subcutaneous tissue should be dissected toward the base of the flap in order to preserve its blood supply.

There may be some interdigital connective tissue and fat that can be discarded. This usually leaves a proximal triangular defect on each toe, which is covered with a small skin graft. A full thickness, elliptically shaped, defatted skin graft taken from the thigh is preferred in young children. It may be more prudent to use a split thickness skin graft in adults or adolescents owing to the greater vascular supply that is required for survival of a full thickness skin graft.

The tourniquet should be released prior to closure, and complete hemostasis must be achieved. Skin flaps should be pink after closure. If not, skin tension should be reduced by removing or loosening sutures. A nonadherent dressing should be applied over the incision, followed by a slightly moist gauze sponge, which will conform to the irregular surfaces while applying slight compression. A posterior splint should be applied for complete immobilization, and the patient should be kept non-weight-bearing for a minimum of 2 to 3 weeks.

The most frequent complication of desyndactylization surgery is skin graft or flap slough, which leaves an open granulating interdigital wound. This frequently leads either to resyndactylization or to cosmetically and functionally unappealing scar formation. If skin slough does occur, the toes must be kept separated, and moist to dry dressings should be applied until adequate granulation allows regrafting.

# MACRODACTYLY

Macrodactyly, a specific, relatively rare congenital anomaly affecting the hands and feet, is characterized by localized digital gigantism and common pathologic findings. All structural components of the digits are typically enlarged with the exception of tendons and blood vessels. The term *macrodactyly* should not be used to describe other conditions that may result in digital or extremity enlargement, such as hemangioma, lymphangioma, arteriovenous fistula, lipomatosis, or neurofibromatosis, but these conditions should be kept in mind as part of the differential diagnosis of unexplained digital hypertrophy. Macrodactyly has in the past been referred to in the literature as megalodactyly, macrodystrophia lipomatosa, dactylomegaly, and local gigantism.

Barsky was the first author to publish a comprehensive review of the modern literature concerning macrodactyly.[35] In 1967 he reported finding 64 reported cases of macrodactyly involving the hands and feet in the literature dating back to 1840. All these cases involved only the hands, with the exception of one case of bilateral foot involvement. In 1981 my colleagues and I were able to find an additional 74 cases of macrodactyly involving the feet reported in the English language literature.[36] I have compiled a table of 62 cases (67 feet) reported in the world literature between 1865 and 1988 (Table 10-1). Only cases that contained adequate data concerning distribution and type of involvement were included in this review.

## Classification

Barsky originally classified macrodactyly into two types, static and progressive.[35] In the static type, which is the most common form, the growth rate of the enlarged fingers or toes is proportional to the growth rate of the

Table 10-1. **Review of 62 Cases of Macrodactyly (67 Feet) Reported in 1865 to 1988 World Literature**

|  | Sex | | Side | | | Involvement | | | | Metatarsal and/or Forefoot Involvement | Associated Syndactyly (of 38 Cases) |
|  | F | M | R | L | B/L | Preaxial (1+2 and/or 3) | Central (2,3,4) | Postaxial (3,4,5) | All (4 or more) | | |
|---|---|---|---|---|---|---|---|---|---|---|---|
| No. | 27 | 35 | 33 | 24 | 5 | 30 | 24 | 6 | 7 | 22 | 8 |
| % | 44 | 56 | 49 | 36 | 15 | 45 | 36 | 9 | 10 | 33 | 21 |

Abbreviations: R, right; L, left; B/L, bilateral.

individual. The increase in size of the affected digit is usually most rapid during the first few years of life and tends to stop at maturity. In the much less common progressive type, the growth rate of the enlarged part is disproportionately faster than the growth rate of the child. Swanson expressed the view that all tissues enlarge proportionately in the static type, whereas a disproportionate enlargement of fibrolipomatous and lymphatic tissue is present in the progressive type.[37] He also believed that the progressive type was more likely to be associated with neurofibromas, lymphangiofibromas, and hemangiomas in the distribution of the median nerve of the hand and the medial plantar nerve of the foot.

## Etiology and Pathology

The etiology of macrodactyly is uncertain. No evidence of genetic transmission has been identified. I have not been able to find in the literature any reported cases of true macrodactyly that were associated with a positive family history of the deformity. Barsky reported finding normal chromosomal patterns in his patients with macrodactyly.[35]

Several theories have been proposed to attempt to explain the root cause of this deformity. Barsky believed that a local lack of inhibition of some growth-limiting factor was responsible for digital enlargement but presented no evidence to directly support this theory. Inglis proposed three possibilities: (1) abnormal nerve supply; (2) abnormal blood supply; (3) abnormal hormonal control.[38] Edgerton and Tuerk[39] and numerous other authors believe that macrodactyly is a localized form of neurofibromatosis.

The histopathology of macrodactyly has been well established and agreed upon by most authors.[39-43] The skin is thickened by infiltration of the dermal layer by fibrous bands and flattening of rete pegs. There is an increased volume of fibrofatty subcutaneous tissue that appears similar to adult adipose tissue but with more thickened fibrous bands (Fig. 10-11). The arterial walls are normal in size, but the luminal diameter is decreased by fibrous infiltration. Because the luminal diameter of vessels is small and because the ratio of tissue volume to circulatory capacity is smaller than in normal tissue, digital circulation is less than normal. Capillary skin clearance of iodine 131 is markedly reduced.[39] Tendons are also of normal size but are surrounded by thickened fibrous tissue. One of the most striking and characteristic findings is marked periosteal thickening and fibrosis. Fi-

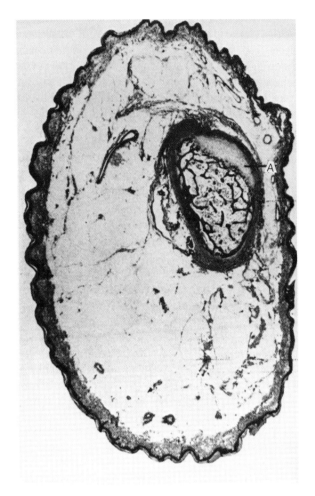

**Fig. 10-11.** Low-power view of cross section of finger with macrodactyly. Most of the enlargement is due to a neurofibrolipomatous mass. **(A)** Some neoenchondromatosis is evident. (From Inglis,[38] with permission.)

broblastic activity is increased near the periosteum, and increased chondroblastic, osteoblastic, and osteoclastic activity associated with new bone formation is characteristic.[40] Small (1mm) subperiosteal nodular areas of chondroblasts contain perineural tissue, which is considered by many investigators to be associated with neurofibromas.[43] Fibrous bands radiate from the periosteum, involved nerve fibers, and blood vessels infiltrating the adipose tissue, which results in an increased thickening and induration of that tissue. The nerves are larger in diameter owing to endoneural and perineural thickening with fibrous tissue infiltration (Fig. 10-12). The axonal fibers are of normal size. The hypesthesia and paresthe-

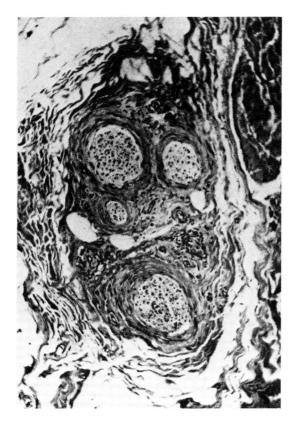

**Fig. 10-12.** Section of enlarged digital nerve in patient with macrodactyly shows relatively normal-appearing axons surrounded by dense fibrous tissue. Cells in this tissue are indistinguishable from those of neurofibromatosis. Thickening of these nerve appears to increase during first few years of life. (From Inglis,[38] with permission.)

sias that occur in a large number of patients may be due to perineural fibrosis or to extrinsic pressure from tissue hypertrophy.

Substantial evidence has been gathered to indicate that at least some cases of macrodactyly represent a localized form of von Recklinghausen's neurofibromatosis.[38,42,45-48] Both conditions show a similar neurogenic pattern of tissue involvement. The distal portions of digits tend to be most significantly affected, and nerve involvement also seems to be progressive from proximal to distal. In fact, thickening and fibrosis of the median nerve in the forearm and the medial plantar nerve in the foot, with associated neurofibromatosis proximal to the area of gigantism, has been noticed at the time of surgical dissection in patients with macrodactyly.[39,47] Adipose

and fibrous tissue proliferation occurs in both conditions, and some macrodactyly patients have lipomas, plexiform neurofibromas, and café-au-lait spots commonly seen in neurofibromatosis.[46] In addition, some experimental evidence exists that macrodactyly may have a neurogenic origin. Brachial plexus trauma in fetal amphibia has been shown to result in digital gigantism, and neurofibromatosis of splachnic nerves in horses has been associated with gigantism of the correspondingly innervated portion of the gut.[39]

## Clinical Features

Although macrodactyly is a congenital deformity, it may not become clinically apparent until early infancy or childhood. Macrodactyly is slightly more common in males than in females. The upper extremity is more frequently affected than the lower extremity, and involvement is usually unilateral; both hands or both feet are affected in less than 10 percent of patients.[39] Hemicorporal involvement of the ipsilateral upper and lower extremities is, to my knowledge, unreported. The distribution of digital involvement is almost always preaxial, with the radial digits of the hand and the great, second, and third toes of the foot affected most often. Although gigantism may be isolated to a single digit, involvement of two or three adjacent digits is a much more common presentation. In cases of multiple digital involvement, all the digits do not usually enlarge at a uniform rate. It is not uncommon to see an infant who has a single enlarged toe that appears to be an isolated deformity gradually develop enlargement of the adjacent toes during early childhood.

The digits enlarge symmetrically in macrodactyly, in contrast to conditions such as hemangioma or lipomatosis, which are identified by their asymmetric pattern. Enlargement is most pronounced distally, with the proximal portion of the digit noticeably less enlarged in most cases (Fig. 10-13). This results in a splayed, almost pear-shaped appearance of the digit. The skin, subcutaneous tissues, nail, and periungual tissues appear thickened even in the young child. A fibrolipomatous thickening of the plantar aspect of the forefoot may also occur in more severe or long-standing cases. The dorsum of the foot other than the digits is usually spared. The enlargement of the digital phalanges gradually become radiographically apparent. The metacarpal and metatarsal bones are not involved in the less severe cases. In more

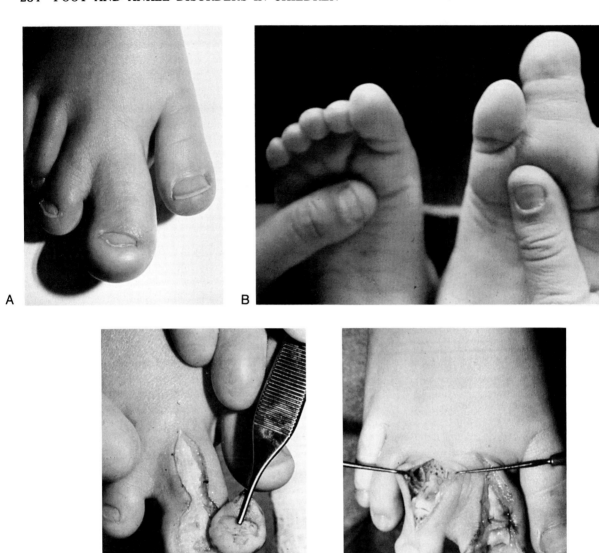

**Fig. 10-13.** (A & B) Typical preaxial macrodactyly in a 4-year-old child. Note that the second digit is already substantially larger than the great toe or a normal adult second toe. The third toe is involved to a lesser degree. (C) Excision of nail bed of second toe prior to shortening. (D) Epiphysiodesis of second and third toes is performed by excising or drilling the physes. *(Figure continues.)*

severe cases the metacarpals and metatarsals may become enlarged over time, but usually to a lesser degree than the more distal portions of the digit.

As the digits enlarge, lateral deviation of the adjacent affected digits away from one another may occur. This may result from a differential increase in epiphyseal growth of the more severely affected side of the digit. Clinodactyly, or curvature of the enlarged fingers or toes, has been less commonly reported and may also be the result of differential epiphyseal growth or may possibly be a mechanically induced deformity due to crowding of the adjacent digits. The tubular bones of the digits

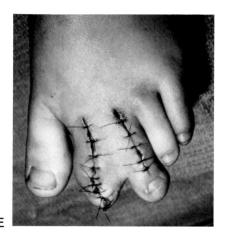

E

**Fig. 10-13** *(Continued).* **(E)** Skin closure. Further debulking can be performed at a later time.

increase in both length and diameter. Continued bone production in mature individuals may result in large osteophytes and calcification of ligaments and tendons. As the digits enlarge, they gradually become stiff and functionless. Sensation is usually normal to examination; however, hypesthesia and paresthesia may be present in long-standing cases. Adult patients also sometimes report paresthesia-type symptoms.

Children are often not seen for macrodactyly until 4 or 5 years of age or older even though the deformity is usually noticeable at birth or within the first few years of life. This is particularly true if the deformity is isolated to the foot. By the time the patient is seen, the enlarged toe or toes are often markedly longer and larger in girth than adjacent more normal digits. Parents usually bring children for consultation because of difficulty in finding shoewear. Adolescents may be extremely self-conscious about foot appearance and present primarily due to cosmetic concerns. Pain other than from shoe pressure is unusual in children or young people. Adults or individuals with more aggressive forms of macrodactyly (i.e., the progressive type) may develop pressure-related symptoms at the plantar aspect of the foot as a result of fibrolipomatous masses, neurofibromas, or osseous exostoses.

Most authors feel that macrodactyly is an isolated deformity not associated with any other congenital deformities.[40,49] However, there are rare reports of macrodactyly occurring in association with syndactyly, polydactyly, hemangiomas, neurofibromas, café-au-lait spots, nevi, and arteriovenous fistula.[39,50–52]

## Treatment

The treatment of macrodactyly is surgical and can be divided into growth-arresting procedures and reduction procedures. The ideal time to begin treatment is during early childhood, before the affected toe is significantly greater in size than the adjacent normal digits or larger than the expected size at skeletal maturity. If surgical treatment is begun early enough, partial or complete growth-arresting procedures along with debulking procedures may be all that are necessary. Primary digital or ray amputations should almost never be performed in children or in adults with the progressive form of the disease. The extent of gigantism is not usually uniformly apparent in the young child. In the progressive disease sequential involvement of adjacent toes may occur after toe or ray amputation, resulting in no functional or cosmetic improvement or in piecemeal additional amputations that leave a poor cosmetic and functional result (Fig. 10-14). Partial amputation or ray resection procedures may be useful in adults with the static form of the disease. If partial amputation or digital shortening is selected, tissue removal should be from the distal aspect of the toe, where enlargement is most pronounced. If debulking procedures are utilized in combination with shortening, multistage procedures are usually necessary to avoid vascular embarrassment. One should keep in mind that the circulation is already compromised by the histopathologic nature of the deformity and that surgical dissection is not as well tolerated as in a normal digit.

Epiphysiodesis, a growth-arresting procedure, can be used in the management of macrodactyly in children (Fig. 10-13D). Although the bone may continue to enlarge in girth and even slightly in length through intramembranous bone formation after epiphysiodesis, this procedure should be considered in any growing child under 10 years of age. Since foot growth only averages about 0.9 cm per year or about half the rate of distal tibial growth after age 5, epiphysiodesis is most effectively performed in younger children.[53] If the toe has not reached expected adult length, only intermediate and distal phalangeal physes should be destroyed. As soon as the affected digit achieves expected adult length, all phalangeal physes should be destroyed. In the older child epiphysiodesis of the corresponding metatarsal should

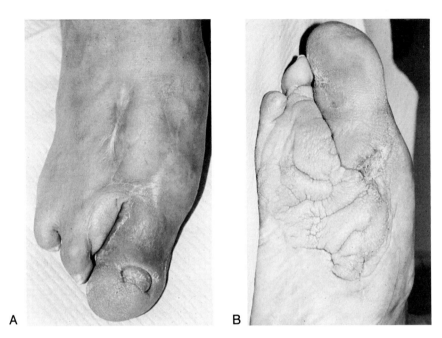

A          B

**Fig. 10-14. (A & B)** A young woman in her twenties who had second and third ray amputation for macrodactyly as a child. The great toe and plantar aspect of the foot have continued to hypertrophy, resulting in a poor cosmetic and functional result.

also be performed. The soft cartilage of the physis can be resected with a knife, or destruction can be accomplished by multiple drillings as recommended by Wilson.[54]

Reduction procedures can be divided into two types, debulking and shortening. Both Barsky and Tsuge described debulking procedures performed through midline medial and lateral digital incisions.[35,41] This approach provides the best exposure, but medial and lateral incisions should be staged not less than 6 weeks apart to avoid digital ischemia. The deep fibrolipomatous tissue should be excised, with care taken to avoid resecting the immediately subdermal fat, which contains the blood supply to the skin. Tsuge in 1967 also recommended excision of the digital nerve branches in the hope that this would slow "neurogenically" stimulated growth.[41] Edgerton and Tuerk recommended longitudinal resection of the main digital nerve trunks.[39] Others have even recommended complete excision of all digital nerve elements. However, in Tsuge's 1985 follow-up paper on the treatment of macrodactyly, he reports that partial or total digital nerve excision has not proved to be a very effective procedure.[55] Extreme care must be taken to avoid digital artery injury during nerve excision.

Various types of shortening procedures have been described. Barsky and Tsuge have described "inch worm"-type plastic shortening procedures that preserve the nail bed (Fig. 10-15). Tsuge's modification is preferred in that the most hypertrophic distal pulp portion of the digit can be resected at the time of shortening. These techniques can be combined with debulking procedures in a series of staged operations about 6 to 8 weeks apart. In situations in which the nail plate is grossly abnormal or nail plate preservation is unimportant to cosmesis, my associates and I recommend a simple dorsal linear incision combined with nail bed and distal pulp excision[36] (Fig. 10-16). Limited debulking of the dorsomedial and dorsolateral skin flaps can be performed at the same time, but care must be taken to avoid digital vessel injury. The nail bed is excised and the distal portion of the toe amputated. This technique has the advantage of being performed as a one-stage procedure and is usually more useful in adults.

Toe amputation or ray resection should be a procedure of last resort and should be reserved for adults with the static form of the disease. Isolated toe amputation often results in an undesirable lateral deviation of adja-

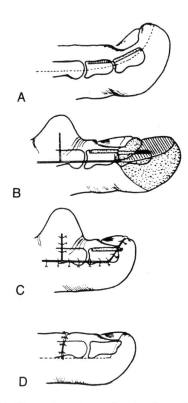

**Fig. 10-15.** Shortening of macrodactyly of toe. **(A)** Incision is made at midlateral line. One-third of dorsal side of terminal phalanx together with the nail is left attached to flap. Next, one-third of dorsal side of middle phalanx is excised. **(B)** Dorsal flap is retracted in measuring worm-like fashion, and a portion of terminal phalanx is placed upon the excised area of middle phalanx. **(C)** Tip of toe is excised, and if nail is enlarged, a partial excision may be performed. **(D)** Secondary surgery is performed to remove surplus skin. (From Tsuge,[41] with permission.)

cent digits and does not narrow the foot. If amputation is necessary, ray amputation is probably more appropriately used to reduce foot width. Diamond described a hemi-ray amputation procedure for treatment of macrodactyly of two adjacent toes.[55a] The medial half of the more lateral toe and metatarsal and the lateral half of the more medial toe and metatarsal are resected along with all intervening soft tissue in a wedge-shaped manner with the apex of the wedge proximal. The wound is repaired in a manner similar to that used in syndactylization. This technique has the advantage of significantly narrowing the foot but still leaves a single abnormally large toe in place of two enlarged toes.

# HALLUX VARUS

*Hallux varus* is a descriptive anatomic term for a condition in which the great toe is deviated medially at the first metatarsophalangeal joint. Foot surgeons usually encounter this problem as an iatrogenic complication of bunion surgery. In contrast, congenital hallux varus is a true congenital deformity, having only the direction of deviation of the great toe in common with the former condition. This usually isolated deformity is very rare and may never be seen by many foot surgeons. McElvenny in 1941 reported finding fewer than 30 cases in the literature.[56] I have been able to find an additional 12 cases reported in the English-language literature. The majority of these cases have the following in common: (1) the first metatarsal is short and broad and is usually in normal alignment with respect to the lesser metatarsals rather than in an adducted position; (2) metatarsus adductus is commonly associated; (3) preaxial polydactyly or polydactyly/syndactyly or partial duplication of medial column bones (phalanges, metatarsal, cuneiform, navicular) is often present; (4) the condition is usually unilateral (Fig. 10-17).

Tachdjian presented a descriptive classification based on associated clinical conditions.[57] He divided congenital hallux varus into three categories: (1) primary hallux varus; (2) hallux varus associated with other forefoot deformities; and (3) hallux varus associated with extensive developmental skeletal disorders. The foot and digits usually appear normal in primary hallux varus except for the medial deviation of the great toe at the metatarsophalangeal joint. This should not be confused with metatarsus primus adductus, in which the medial deviation occurs at the first metatarsal cuneiform joint. The second type is characterized by the short, broad first metatarsal. Partial duplication of phalanges or complete duplication with syndactyly is common as is metatarsus adductus. The third type may be similar to the second type but is usually associated with more extensive congenital abnormalities, such as diastrophic dwarfism.

## Etiology and Pathology

Congenital hallux varus is usually an isolated deformity and is most often unilateral. Preaxial polydactyly has frequently been associated with congenital hallux varus (Fig. 10-5). In some cases complete duplication of the hallux has been described, but more often duplication of

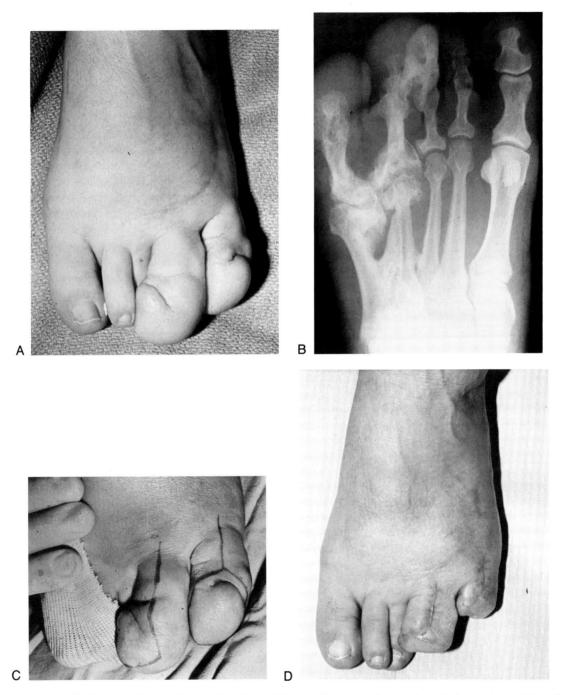

**Fig. 10-16.** **(A)** An unusual postaxial macrodactyly in a 40-year-old woman; the dorsal scar is from prior excision of fibrolipomatous masses. **(B)** Extensive skeletal involvement. **(C)** DeValentine's recommended procedure of distal nail bed and toe amputation with debulking through dorsal incision. **(D)** Postoperative photograph. Further debulking and alignment procedure may be performed at a later time if necessary.

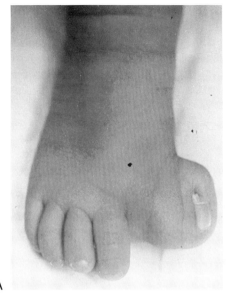 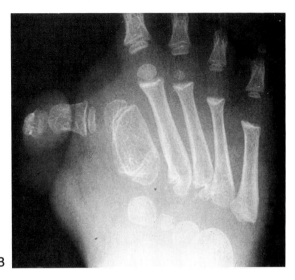

A                                          B

**Fig. 10-17.** **(A)** Congenital hallux varus in 4-year-old child with medial soft tissue contracture. **(B)** Note characteristic broad, short first metatarsal and associated metatarsus adductus.

hallux phalanges with syndactyly occurs.[56–62] The first metatarsal is not usually duplicated but is often broad and short; it is often described at the time of surgery as having the appearance of incomplete duplication. Incomplete formation of medial column accessory bones, including phalanges, metatarsals, cuneiform, and navicular, has also been reported. The first metatarsal head may have an abnormal shape (oblique or flattened), making it difficult to reconstruct a normal articulating surface. A dense mass of contracted scar tissue is generally found along the medial aspect of the first ray. The entire first metatarsophalangeal joint apparatus, including the plantar pad and sesamoid bones, is displaced medially. The tendons and muscles are not abnormal, but duplication may occur and contracture (especially of the abductor hallucis) is the rule.

Many authors have quite logically proposed that congenital hallux varus occurs as the result of incomplete medial column or first ray duplication. The predominant theory is that the first metatarsal portion of the normal duplication fails to develop, resulting in growth arrest and progressive medial deviation of the hallux due to contracture. Most authors have not reported affected family members, but emphasis has been on treatment, and little or no effort has been devoted to investigation of extended family history in most cases. Most isolated

congenital foot deformities, including polydactyly, are thought to be the result of an autosomal dominant form of inheritance, but this pattern has not been demonstrated in congenital hallux varus. Kleiner and Holmes did report two siblings with congenital hallux varus.[61] Both had the typical broad, short first metatarsal, and one had associated polydactyly of the great toe. No relatives were identified with similar problems. These authors concluded that an autosomal recessive, X-linked recessive, or multifactorial inheritance pattern could not be excluded.

### Treatment

Congenital hallux varus is easily recognized at birth, but the growth arrest and partial ray duplication characteristics of this deformity are often not recognized by the inexperienced surgeon. This may lead to a superficial and inadequate attempt to correct the deformity through simple releases or excision of an accessory hallux. Surgical reconstruction should be delayed long enough to adequately assess the skeletal components of the medial column but as early as possible to avoid worsening of the contracture. I prefer to operate on children between 1 and 2 years of age if possible. If left untreated, congenital hallux varus is cosmetically undesirable and makes normal shoe wear almost impossible. The function and propulsive capability of the great toe are usually reduced, and partial growth arrest often occurs with or without surgical treatment, but shoe fit is greatly enhanced with treatment.

Early attempts at surgical correction usually involved medial soft tissue release and lateral capsular plication or tenodesis of the great toe to the second ray but did not adequately address the medial contracture.[56,58,59] Con-

sequently, recurrence and repeat operation were frequently reported. Farmer reported a technique for correction of hallux varus that allows lengthening of contracted medial soft tissues[60] (Fig. 10-18). Farmer's procedure involves transposing a dorsal or plantar flap of skin from the area of the first intermetatarsal space to the area of medial contracture. A partial syndactyly of the great to the second toe may also be performed. In addition, any accessory bones or structures are excised.

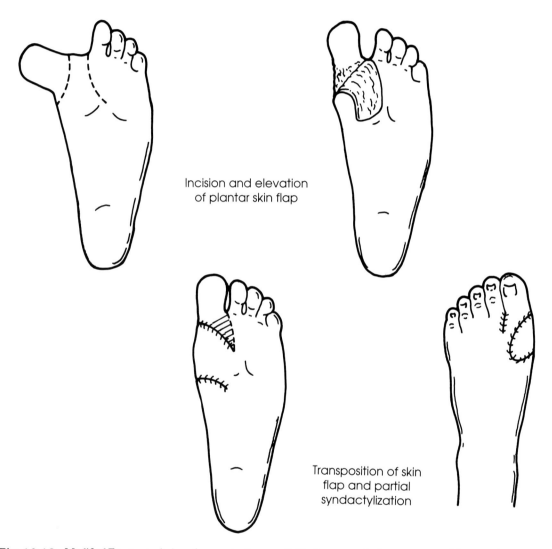

Incision and elevation
of plantar skin flap

Transposition of skin
flap and partial
syndactylization

**Fig. 10-18.** Modified Farmer technique for repair of congenital hallux varus. A plantar transposition skin flap is raised and moved to the areas of medial soft tissue contracture. Excision of accessory bone and medial soft tissue release are also performed. Partial or complete syndactyly of great and second toes may also be performed. (Adapted from Farmer,[60] with permission.)

Longitudinal narrowing of the broad first metatarsal may be necessary to reduce bulk and create an appropriate articulating surface. Sectioning of the abductor hallucis and medial capsule and complete circumferential release of capsular structures about the first metatarsal head are always necessary. Other soft tissue structures are released or sectioned as necessary. A split thickness skin graft may be necessary to fill small residual defects.

Occasionally, when surgical correction is performed early and tissues are very supple or when deformity is mild, transposition flaps and skin grafts may not be necessary. In cases of polydactyly/syndactyly of the great toe, the extra skin that is left after filleting skeletal components can sometimes be used to reconstruct the medial soft tissue defect. I prefer longitudinal Kirschner wire fixation of the great toe and a plaster splint or cast for a minimum of 3 to 4 weeks after surgery.

## HALLUX ABDUCTUS INTERPHALANGEUS

A slight lateral deviation of the distal phalanx of the great toe is a normal finding. This condition has been variably referred to as hallux valgus interphalangeus, ungual phalanx valgus, valgus deviation of the distal phalanx of the great toe, and hallux abductus interphalangeus.[63-67] Barnet found an average of 13 to 14 degrees of hallux abductus interphalangeus in a study of 173 normal British adults (346 feet), as compared with an average of 8 to 10 degrees in a smaller non-shoe-wearing New Guinea native population found in a study by Hardy and Clapham.[65,68] Barnett also found that the average hallux interphalangeal angle in children and in 25 stillborn fetuses of different racial background was similar to that in the adult population. In contrast, several species of nonhuman primates were noted to have little or no interphalangeal hallux abduction. Barnett concluded that interphalangeal hallux abduction is a genetically transmitted characteristic unique to the human species, which has probably evolved through natural selection as a structural trait conducive to upright bipedal locomotion. Sorto et al., in a retrospective review of radiographs, found the incidence of hallux abductus interphalangeus to be slightly higher in patients without hallux valgus.[66] They found that the abduction occurred almost without exception within the distal phalanx and not at the interphalangeal joint. They also theorized that developmental hallux

abductus interphalangeus would more likely occur in shoe-wearing children with stable first rays, who were unlikely to develop hallux valgus owing to medial shoe pressure over the distal great toe. An abduction force exerted by shoe pressure would selectively influence the growth of the physis of the distal phalanx. Those children with less stable first rays would be more likely to develop mild hallux valgus as adults. Tachdjian and Gillett also suggested that shoe wear may be an exacerbating factor in the production of developmental hallux abductus interphalangeus in children with a predisposition toward that condition.[64,69,70]

### Clinical Features

True congenital hallux abductus interphalangeus is a rare disorder, which is distinguished from normal or mild developmental hallux abductus interphalangeus primarily by degree (Fig. 10-19). Gillett established in a study of 389 newborn infants that less than 10 percent had hallux abductus of 10 degrees or more.[64] An interphalangeal angulation greater than 25 degrees should be considered indicative of pathologic congenital hallux ab-

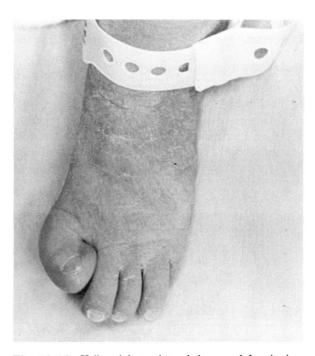

**Fig. 10-19.** Hallux abductus interphalangeus deformity in a newborn infant.

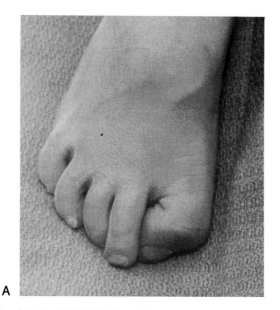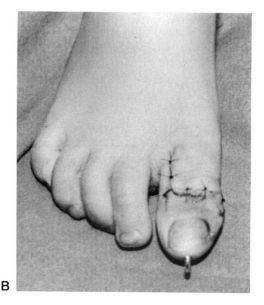

**Fig. 10-20. (A)** Rigid hallux abductus interphalangeus deformity in a 2-year-old boy. **(B)** Soft tissue release through serpentine incision with intramedullary Kirschner-wire fixation. No osteotomy is required as long as the child is young enough to allow for sufficient articular adaptation.

ductus interphalangeus, which in many infants or young children is associated with interphalangeal angles of up to 45 to 90 degrees. The metatarsophalangeal joint in these children is in normal alignment, and there is usually no evidence of congenital bowing or epiphyseal abnormality. In children less than 3 to 5 years of age the deformity appears radiographically as a lateral subluxation of the interphalangeal joint rather than as an angular deviation of the distal phalanx, which is more characteristic in the older child or adult with developmental hallux abductus interphalangeus. The distal tip of the great toe usually abuts or, more often, underlaps the second toe. Although pressure irritation or even blisters may develop at the pressure interface between the digits once the child begins walking, it is more common to see children under age 5 brought for consultation by parents who are concerned about the abnormal appearance of the toe.

## Treatment

As previously mentioned, a mild degree of hallux abductus interphalangeus in a young child is not abnormal or symptomatic and does not require treatment. Surgical correction can always be performed during adulthood if necessary. Moderate to severe deformity should preferably be surgically corrected between the ages of 1 and 5

years. At this age soft tissue release of the collateral ligaments through a transverse or serpentine incision is usually all that is necessary (Fig. 10-20). The distal phalanx should be held in anatomic reduction for 3 to 4 weeks with a small, smooth intramedullary Kirschner wire and a short leg walking cast. In the child over 5 years of age who has developed some degree of osseous adaptation deformity at the interphalangeal joint, a distal wedge osteotomy of the proximal phalanx (Akin procedure) may be necessary. Tachdjian has also recommended epiphysiodesis of the medial half of the distal phalangeal physis if medial overgrowth appears to have occurred.[70] Moderate to severe deformity in the skeletally mature patient, in whom reconstruction of congruent, normally aligned joint surfaces is not possible through osteotomy, can be treated with interphalangeal joint fusion. Intramedullary lag screw fixation, followed by a short leg walking cast for 6 to 8 weeks, is preferred.

## BRACHYMETATARSIA

The term *brachymetatarsia* is used to describe shortening of one or more metatarsals relative to their normally expected length. The condition is not uncommon if all variations are taken into account. Brachymetatarsia may be congenital or acquired, and it may be idiopathic or may occur in association with various syndromes or endocrine disorders. The congenital idiopathic type most often affects the first and fourth metatarsal bones.[71] Short metacarpal bones are often present on examination of the hands. The idiopathic type may be unilateral or bilateral and usually affects only one or two metatarsals. Acquired brachymetatarsia has been reported in association with poliomyelitis and secondary to trauma or surgery.[72-74] Cases associated with polio are thought to be the result of premature epiphyseal closure and only affect the paralytic side.

Congenitally short metatarsals have been described in association with Down, Albright, and Turner syndromes and with multiple epiphyseal dysplasia, diastrophic dwarfism, and myositis ossificans.[72] Shortened metacarpals and metatarsals may also be seen in pseudohypoparathyroidism and pseudopseudohypoparathyroidism, conditions that are genetic and may mimic hypoparathyroidism in clinical and radiographic appearance. The infant appears normal at birth in the latter two conditions, with skeletal changes becoming apparent between 2 and 4 years of age. Multiple exostoses, dwarfism, and subcutaneous calcifications may be present. The first, fourth, and fifth metacarpals and the third and fourth metatarsals are most commonly affected. Parathyroid glands are normal to hyperplastic in pseudohypoparathyroidism, but there is a failure of end organ receptors to respond to parathyroid hormone, resulting in serum hypocalcemia and hyperphosphatemia. Short metacarpals and metatarsals and subcutaneous calcifications are present in pseudopseudohypoparathyroidism as in pseudohypoparathyroidism, but serum calcium and phosphorus are normal.

## Idiopathic Brachymetatarsia

The etiology of idiopathic brachymetatarsia is unclear. Most authors have felt that metatarsal shortening occurs as the result of premature physeal closure, the cause of which is undetermined. A family history of brachymetatarsia may be present, and in some cases identical patterns are noted in related individuals. The relative shortening of affected metatarsals is usually not apparent until after 4 years of age.

Tachdjian states that the incidence of brachymetatarsia is highest in the first metatarsal bone.[71] It is true that a minor degree of shortening of the first metatarsal is not unusual. Harris and Beath found the first metatarsal to be shorter than the second metatarsal by at least 1 mm in 40 percent of 7,167 feet surveyed.[75] In the same study the first metatarsal was found to be longer than the second metatarsal by at least 1 mm in 22 percent of the feet. They did not find a significant difference in the incidence of metatarsalgia or of callus formation beneath the second metatarsal in individuals with slightly shorter first metatarsals. Metatarsalgia associated with a slightly short first metatarsal is probably more a result of elevation of the first metatarsal secondary to a functional unlocking of the midfoot in pronation. This relatively common slightly shortened first metatarsal should not be confused with the much rarer truly pathologic metatarsus primus atavicus and should not be considered a form of brachymetatarsia.

The incidence of idiopathic brachymetatarsia involving lesser metatarsals was found to be between 0.022 and 0.055 percent in a larger sample of Japanese schoolchildren between the ages of 13 and 17 years.[73] Females are affected about 25 times as often as males.[73,76] Congenital shortening of the fourth metatarsal is the most common type of idiopathic brachymetatarsia involving lesser metatarsals. Urano and Kobayashi found isolated shortening of fourth metatarsals in 90 percent of 102 patients with congenital brachymetatarsia.[73] Of these children 10 percent had short first or third metatarsals as well, while 7 percent had associated short metacarpals, usually of the ring or small finger. Both feet were involved in 72 percent of patients. A hereditary pattern was discovered in 5 percent of cases.

## Clinical Features

Brachymetatarsia is rarely noticeable before age 4. Urano and Kobayashi found that brachymetatarsia first became evident to patients or parents between the ages of 4 and 15, with an average of age 9 years.[73] The involved toe or toes appear shorter and dorsally displaced as compared with the surrounding digits. Although the toe and its phalangeal components are of normal length, the patient or parent usually perceives the problem to be isolated to the digit. The toe articulates normally with the corresponding metatarsal head, but because the ray is shortened along an inclining plane from distal to proximal, the digit will often be elevated above the level of the adjacent digits by an entire toe thickness. The flexor and extensor tendon apparatus is usually normal, but the toe is functionless owing to the relative lack of mechanical advantage imposed by shortening. Restoration of long flexor function often occurs with metatarsal lengthening procedures. A skin cleft may develop plantar to the involved metatarsophalangeal joint, and transfer callus may develop plantar to the adjacent metatarsophalangeal joints.

Brachymetatarsia is often completely asymptomatic and is almost never symptomatic before the second or third decade. Transfer metatarsalgia of the adjacent metatarsophalangeal joints may occur, but in my experience a more common complaint is dorsal irritation resulting from the high-riding toe abutting against the toe box of the shoe. Cosmesis may be the patient's primary concern. Surgical correction is not usually recommended if no symptoms are present. An open or extra depth shoe or orthosis is often all that is necessary to alleviate symptoms.

## Classification and Surgical Treatment

Although most authors have reported satisfactory results with metatarsal lengthening and/or shortening procedures in the treatment of brachymetatarsia, one should not recommend or perform this procedure without a certain amount of hesitation. Patients must be made aware that the complexity of the surgical correction is great as compared with the usual minimal symptomatology and that significant potential complications, including digital ischemia, may occur. Surgical correction should not be attempted until after skeletal maturity in order to accurately assess the disparity in metatarsal length and avoid physeal injury.

Brachymetatarsia may be classified into four types by the pattern of metatarsal involvement (Fig. 10-21). Type 1 involves shortening of only the first metatarsal; type 2 involves shortening of one or two lesser metatarsals, usually the fourth and/or third; type 3 is characterized by shortening of the first metatarsal and one or more but not all of the lesser metatarsals; and type 4 involves all metatarsals (Fig. 10-22). Surgical treatment is not recommended for types 1 and 4. Type 4 is asymptomatic. Lengthening of a short first metatarsal is not possible without significantly interfering with first ray function, and type 1 brachymetatarsia, if symptomatic, can be treated mechanically with orthoses. Types 2 and 3 are generally best treated by metatarsal lengthening or a combination of metatarsal shortening and lengthening procedures.

Type 3 brachymetatarsia with short first metatarsal and one to three short lesser metatarsals is best treated by shortening of the normal longer metatarsals together with lengthening of the shorter lesser metatarsals if necessary, the first metatarsal length being used as a guide to reconstruct a more normal metatarsal parabola (Fig. 10-23). Cylindrical portions of bone removed from the longer metatarsals can be used as a bone graft and inserted within the distal third of the short metatarsal(s).[77,78]

Type 2 brachymetatarsia most commonly affects one or two lesser metatarsals. As previously mentioned, the fourth metatarsal is most often affected; when two lesser metatarsals are involved, the third and fourth are the most common combination. Lengthening of the affected lesser metatarsal(s) with an autogenous corticocancellous bone graft is the preferred treatment. Shortening of normal length metatarsals in type 2 brachymetatarsia is not recommended unless minimal differential length is present.

Various lengthening techniques have been described. In 1978 Urano and Kobayashi reported the results of 26 operations using the Jinnaka method of inserting a strut of iliac bone across the involved metatarsophalangeal joint after denuding the articular cartilage.[73] No fixation was applied, and patients were allowed early weight-bearing at 2 weeks. In 63 percent of patients a pseudarthrosis developed at either the proximal or distal end of the graft. Satisfactory results were reported in 74 percent of cases. McGlamry and Cooper in 1969 described the use of an autogenous calcaneal graft inserted in the distal third of the metatarsal.[79] Jimenez[80] and McGlamry and Fenton[81] later recommended modification of this technique by using autogenous tibial or iliac graft. They reported successful metatarsal lengthening of up to 1.5 cm.

I prefer the McGlamry technique of metatarsal lengthening using an autogenous corticocancellous bone graft taken from the proximal or distal tibial metaphysis or the iliac crest (Fig. 10-24). The desired amount of lengthening is calculated from preoperative radiographs. I have found that up to 1 cm of lengthening is frequently possible but attempted lengthenings of greater than 1 cm frequently result in compromise of digital circulation.

The distal segment of the short metatarsal is exposed through a dorsal linear incision. A V-Y-type lengthening of the distal portion of the skin incision overlying the

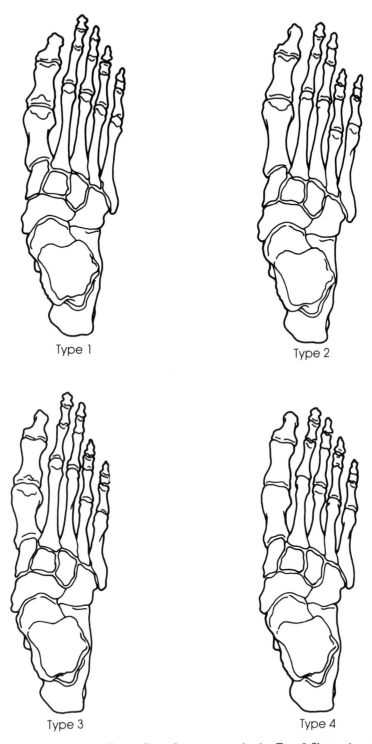

Type 1

Type 2

Type 3

Type 4

**Fig. 10-21.** Types of brachymetatarsia. *Type 1:* Short first metatarsal only. *Type 2:* Shortening of one or two lesser metatarsals. *Type 3:* Short first metatarsal combined with up to three short lesser metatarsals. *Type 4:* All metatarsals short.

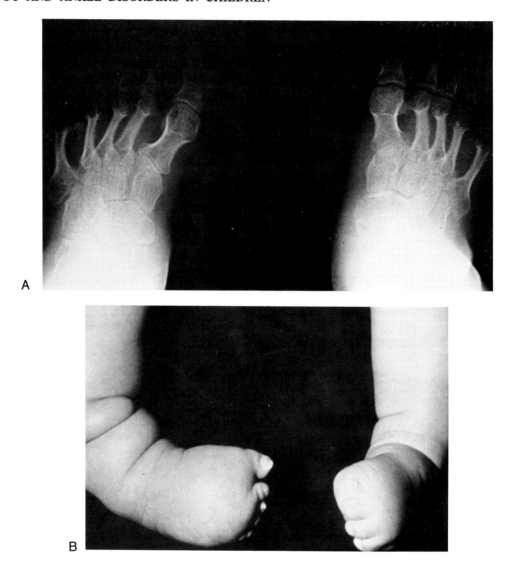

**Fig. 10-22. (A)** Type 4 brachymetatarsia. **(B)** Type 4 brachymetatarsia with brachyphalangia. This condition is sometimes referred to as *microdactyly*.

metatarsophalangeal joint may be necessary. Z-plasty lengthening of the long extensor tendon is performed; the short extensor and interossei are sectioned; a transverse osteotomy of the distal metatarsal is performed from dorsal to plantar; and the periosteum and surrounding soft tissue are sectioned or mobilized. Lengthening of the flexor digitorum longus is usually not necessary and should be avoided in order to provide best toe purchase.

An intramedullary 0.062 Kirschner wire is then passed through the distal fragment, exiting from the distal tip of the toe. The premeasured corticocancellous graft, which may be predrilled, is then inserted, and the pneumatic tourniquet is released. If adequate digital circulation is not present within 5 minutes, the graft is shortened and reinserted until digital circulation is restored. The pin is then passed from distal to proximal through the graft and into the base of the metatarsal, and the long extensor tendon and skin are repaired. Digital circulation should be monitored carefully for the first 24 hours. Postoperative treatment consists of a short leg

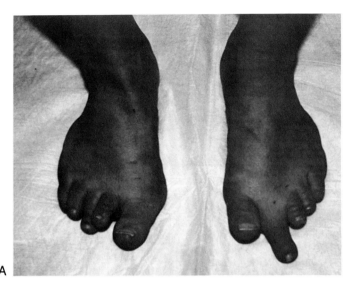

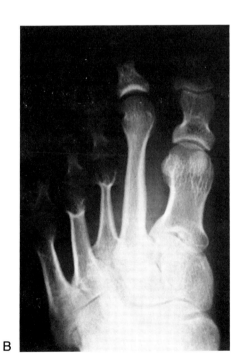

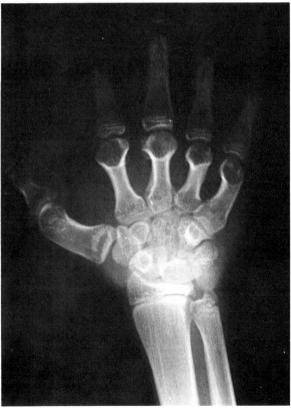

**Fig. 10-23.** **(A)** Type 3 brachymetatarsia in a 12-year-old patient with involvement of both hands and feet. At first glance, this could be confused with macrodactyly. **(B & C)** Radiographs demonstrate stated brachymetatarsia deformity and brachymetacarpia of all metatarsals and metacarpals, except for the second metatarsal of the left foot, which is of normal length. This patient had significant problems with shoewear and second metatarsophalangeal joint metatarsalgia. *(Figure continues.)*

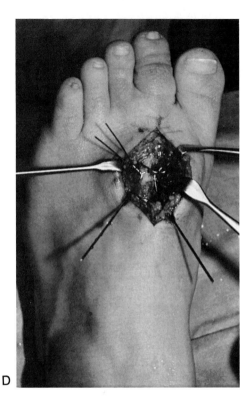
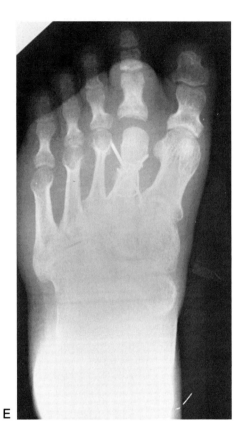

**Fig. 10-23** *(Continued).* **(D & E)** Metatarsal shortening osteotomy with crossed Kirschner wire and tension band fixation.

non-weight-bearing cast for a minimum of 2 months. Cast immobilization should be continued until 3 months postsurgery or until radiographic evidence of graft incorporation is obtained.

## CLEFT FOOT

Cleft foot, often associated with cleft hand deformity, has received significant attention in the literature since about 1890 in view of the relative rarity of this congenital deformity. Its notoriety is probably due to its striking and rather obvious appearance. Cleft foot is a localized form of ectrodactyly (the congenital absence of part or all of one or more fingers or toes) characterized by the congenital absence of two or three of the central digital rays.[82] (Figs. 10-25 and 10-26). This anomaly has also

been commonly referred to as split foot, crab claw, or lobster-claw deformity.

Although cleft hand and foot deformity was described several centuries ago, written reference to this condition prior to 1770 existed only in unscientific reports concerning "monsters."[83] In 1770 Jan Jacob Hartsinck, a director of the East India Company, first reported true cleft hand and foot deformity in a small group of transplanted Africans living in Dutch Guiana in South America.[84] He was the first to use the term "claw" and to suggest a possible hereditary cause. The first description of a case involving cleft hands and feet associated with cleft palate and lip was reported in 1804 by Martens.[85] Béchet in 1829 described a family pedigree with three generations of individuals with both cleft hands and feet,[86] and Geoffroy Saint-Hilaire, a French physician and zoologist, introduced the term *ectrodactyly* in a text

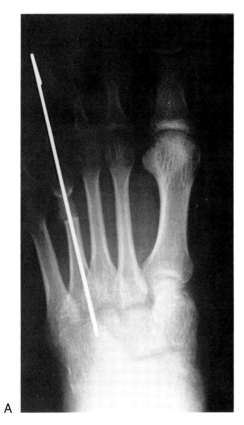 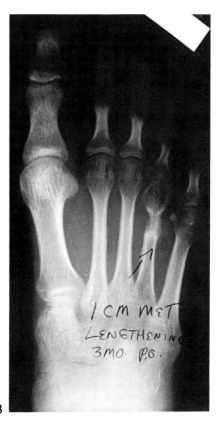

**Fig. 10-24.** **(A)** Lengthening of fourth metatarsal by 1 cm with a corticocancellous bone graft from the distal tibia in a 17-year-old girl with type 2 branchymetatarsia resulting in a "high riding" fourth toe and metatarsalgia of the third metatarsophalangeal joint. **(B)** Three months postsurgery. Full incorporation of autogenous graft.

on congenital anomalies.[87] Numerous reports of cleft hand and foot deformity appeared in the European literature over the next 50 years, documenting cases of cleft hands and feet in various family trees. In 1887 two British surgeons, R.W. Parker and H.B. Robinson, were apparently the first physicians to describe an operation for correction of claw foot.[88] Classic articles concerning the history, etiology, classification, and surgical treatment of this deformity were published between 1949 and 1964 by Birch-Jensen, Walker and Clodius, and Barsky.[83,89,90]

## Classification

Barsky in 1964 was the first to describe a classification system for cleft hand in the English literature.[83] He adapted this classification from descriptions published by

Lange in the German literature in 1936. He discussed two types of cleft hand, typical and atypical. In the typical form, which is frequently familial, usually bilateral, and often accompanied by bilateral cleft foot, a deep cleft is present in the midportion of the hand or foot, with its apex located proximally. In the mildest cases the phalanges of the middle digit are missing, but the corresponding metacarpals or metatarsals may be present and there is only a shallow cleft. In more severe cases two or three of the central digits and corresponding metacarpals and metatarsals are missing, and a deep cleft is present. In the typical form of cleft hand or foot, each component of the "claw" may contain one or two rays. When two sets of phalanges are present, syndactylization usually exists. Considerable variation in the anatomic patterns may occur between families. The typical

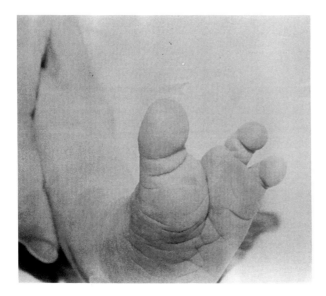

**Fig. 10-25.** A newborn infant with congenital cleft foot. (Courtesy of Stephen Silvani, D.P.M.)

form of cleft hand is not infrequently associated with other congenital anomalies, the most common of which are cleft foot, cleft palate, cleft lip, syndactyly, polydactyly, triphalangeal thumb, tibial aplasia, and deafness.[90-92]

The atypical form of cleft hand, as described by Barsky,[83] is much less common and usually occurs as an isolated deformity with a negative family history. Barsky stated that cleft foot is usually not associated with the atypical cleft hand, which is presumably an isolated congenital anomaly, unrelated to the typical inherited type other than by similarity of appearance. Barsky did not mention the existence of atypical cleft foot as an isolated deformity. However, two cases of isolated cleft foot deformity with negative family history, which may represent atypical cleft foot, have been reported in the podiatric literature.[93,94] The atypical type of deformity is often more severe than the typical type.

## Etiology and Pathology

An autosomal dominant pattern of inheritance with variable penetrance has been documented by numerous investigators in various family pedigrees for the typical type of cleft hand and foot deformity. Males and females are affected approximately equally, and there is no evi-

dence of sex-linked inheritance. Birch-Jensen reviewed 625 patients with hand anomalies and found 36 patients with cleft hands, half of whom also had cleft feet.[89] Barsky found 19 patients with cleft hand, 9 of whom also had cleft feet, in a review of 400 patients with congenital hand anomalies.[83] He calculated the incidence of typical cleft hand deformity as 1 in 90,000 and that of atypical cleft hand deformity as 1 in 150,000. Cleft foot occurred in approximately 42 percent of cases. If one assumes that the number of cases of atypical cleft foot is negligible, then the incidence of cleft foot would be approximately 1 in 180,000.

Various authors have speculated about the embryologic mechanism that results in cleft foot deformity. All feel that something occurs to disturb the normally genetically controlled limb bud differentiation at some time during the first 8 to 12 weeks of gestation. In typical cleft hand and foot, there is presumably a defect in the genetic message that controls the development of the apical portion of the limb bud, resulting in apical dysplasia. Walker and Clodius stated that although the matrix substance is deficient, the tendency toward bone formation remains undisturbed, which results in secondary displacement of bones, extra bone formation, and incomplete separation of osseous structures.[90] This produces the partial fusions that are often seen among metatarsals, phalanges, and tarsal bones in cleft foot deformity. Atypical cleft hand or foot is presumably due to either a new mutation or to the teratogenic effect of some external substance during the vulnerable period of limb bud development.

## Clinical Features

The clinical appearance of cleft foot can vary significantly from one case to another. Central digits may be missing, with portions of or entire metatarsals still present together with only a shallow cleft. More often, only a single first or fifth ray is present, with absence of the middle three rays, which creates a very deep cone-shaped cleft. When two medial or lateral rays are present, syndactyly of the corresponding digits often occurs, resulting in a single large claw at each side of the foot. In these cases division of the first and second metatarsals may fail leaving a single large metatarsal that articulates with the first and second cuneiform bones. Synostosis of the cuboid and lateral cuneiform is often reported. Similar partial fusions of other tarsal bones may occur, but the rear foot is always spared. Occasionally, aplasia of all rays except

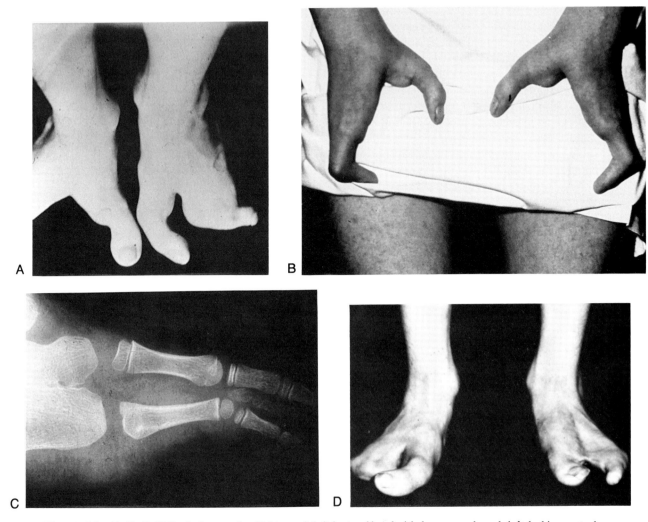

**Fig. 10-26.** **(A, B, & C)** Typical severe familial type of cleft foot and hand with deep cone-shaped cleft, lacking central ray formation. **(D)** After cleft excision and repair.

one or two on the medial or lateral side will produce a "hook" foot or hand. The medial and lateral "claws" tend to curve inward toward the cleft, so that in some cases the distal aspect of the digit will be directed proximally toward the cleft.

Patients with cleft hand and foot deformity have little impairment of function. Cosmesis is a primary concern for most people. In fact, genetic studies of family pedigrees have frequently been complicated by the unwillingness of affected family members to show their deformities to physicians. Accommodation to shoe wear is probably the most significant problem for most people. The splaying of the forefoot that accompanies cleft foot makes it difficult to wear even the most accommodative type of shoe.

## Treatment

Surgical treatment of congenital cleft foot should accomplish three objectives: (1) narrow forefoot width and repair the cleft; (2) provide a stable and functional weight-bearing foot; and (3) create an acceptable cosmetic result. Most authors agree that a better result is achieved if surgical repair is performed early, between 8 and 18 months of age.[82,93-96] Early repair tends to lessen the forefoot splaying and hook digit deformity that occurs within the first few years of life in the child with untreated cleft foot. Reconstruction often requires more than one operation. Each cleft foot deformity is unique and requires an individual approach. The initial procedure should repair the cleft and narrow or stabilize forefoot splaying. This often requires osteotomy of metatarsals on adjacent sides of the cleft. Reduction of digital deformity or syndactylized digits should be performed as a second stage not less than 6 weeks later in order to prevent vascular embarrassment. Parents of children with cleft foot deformity should be fully aware that a cosmetically normal foot cannot be obtained.

Several procedures have described for repair of cleft foot deformity. Tachdjian recommends excision of the cleft, osteotomy of adjacent metatarsals, and syndactylization of digits adjacent to the cleft to prevent recurrent

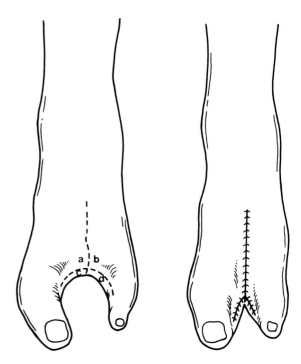

**Fig. 10-28.** Crossed-type incision with elevation of four skin flaps (a, b, c, and d) used for repair of cleft foot. (Adapted from Giorgini et al.,[93] with permission.)

splaying of the forefoot.[82] This is a simple one-stage procedure but results in a cosmetically unattractive cone-shaped foot. Barsky recommended a procedure for repair of cleft hand that is easily adapted to the foot.[83] Barsky's procedure does not require syndactylization of digits adjacent to the cleft, and the incision provides a skin flap for reconstruction of the web space (Fig. 10-27). Giorgini et al. in 1985 described a two-stage procedure for correction of mild atypical cleft foot.[93] The operation was performed on an 8-year-old child with a shallow cleft, and a good result was reported at 7-year follow-up. These authors used a crossed Kelikian-type incision with its intersection at the center of the cleft, creating four skin flaps, which could then be remodeled to narrow the cleft and reconstruct the web space (Fig. 10-28). They combined soft tissue repair with wedge osteotomy at the bases of the metatarsals adjacent to the cleft, using the excised bone wedges as a graft at the apex of the adjacent metatarsal bases to stabilize the forefoot and prevent further splaying. The second stage involved desyndactylization and any necessary structural digital repair.

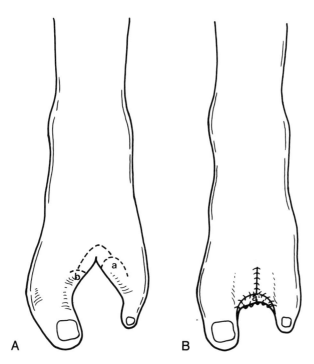

**Fig. 10-27.** **(A)** Barsky's operation for repair of cleft foot. A small distally based skin flap *a* is created to form the web space. **(B)** The cleft redundant skin is excised, and the cleft is repaired. A new web space is created by using the distally based skin flap. (Adapted from Barsky,[83] with permission.)

Weissman and Plaschkes described a repair technique, used in a 9-year-old child missing all three central rays, which might be valuable in dealing with an older patient with unrepaired cleft foot who already has marked digital deformity.[97] These authors believed that simple repair of the cleft when all three central rays were missing would create a "troublesome" skin pocket without osseous support. They used a transverse incision at the midpoint of the cleft, and after elevating full thickness soft tissue flaps, they turned one of the two claw-like digits from which all nail tissue had been excised, into the cleft. This technique eliminates the toes. The resulting foot resembles one that has undergone distal transmetatarsal am-

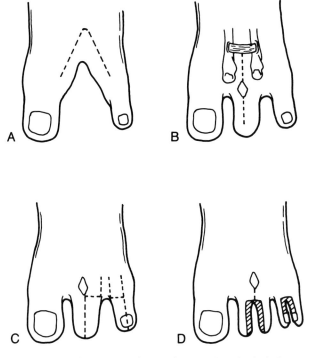

**Fig. 10-29.** Sumiya and Onizuka's staged method of plastic repair of cleft foot deformity. Simulated digits are created through elevation and division of a double pedicle skin flap. **(A)** Skin incision for creation of a double pedicle skin flap. The dorsal skin at the apex of this incision is turned plantarly to create one large middle "digit." **(B)** The foot is narrowed by metatarsal osteotomy and/or by tying the metatarsals together with a strip of fascia lata. The remaining dorsal defect is covered with a split thickness skin graft. **(C)** Skin incisions for division of the two lateral digits and creation of the web spaces. **(D)** Split thickness skin grafts are applied to open areas to create four digits.

putation. Continued growth of the immature phalanges could adversely affect the long-term result in this procedure, which therefore is not recommended for the younger child.

Sumiya and Onizuka reported a 7-year experience with the use of a new two-stage technique to reconstruct missing toes on 16 cleft feet in eight patients.[95,96] They believed that cosmesis was an extremely important consideration in their native Japanese population, whose feet were frequently exposed in traditional footwear. They used a double-pedicled flap created from an incision along the dorsal aspect of the cleft to create a middle digit (Fig. 10-29). The dorsal skin was then turned plantar and the cleft repaired. A split thickness skin graft was used to cover the small dorsal soft tissue defect. The second-stage procedure involved splitting the lateral and central digits to create four lesser toes, using a rectangular flap to reconstruct the web space. These authors reported good results in three children operated at ages 1, 3, and 4, with an average follow-up of 5½ years. Two of the children required repeat local transpositional skin flaps at the dorsum of the foot in the area of the old split thickness skin graft because of graft contracture that caused shortening of the newly created digits. Although this procedure has the potential to create a cosmetically more appealing result, it is also a staged procedure requiring creation of several flaps, with somewhat greater potential morbidity.

## CONSTRICTION BAND SYNDROME

Congenital constriction band syndrome is characterized by annular constricting bands about the extremities that are present at birth. These ligature-like bands may involve only the skin and subcutaneous tissue, or they may be substantially deeper, extending to fascia, deep compartments, or even bone. The most severe form of this syndrome is thought to result in autoamputation of a digit or limb in utero. Acrosyndactyly and clubfoot are commonly associated conditions. Constriction bands that involve deeper tissues may cause progressive strangulation of growing parts even after birth. Consequently, infants with this condition should be observed carefully, and surgical release of the bands may be necessary.

Von Helmont provided the first literature report of a child born with a healed amputation of the arm in 1652.

He believed that the condition occurred as the result of the mother having viewed a soldier with an amputated arm during her pregnancy.[98] Bartholini in 1673 was the first to report congenital clubfoot in association with congenital amputation,[99] and Montgomery in 1832 reported ligature-like "threads" about the extremities.[100] The first scientific theory of the etiology of congenital constriction bands was proposed in 1865 by Braun,[101] who believed that these ligature-like bands found encircling infant extremities at birth resulted from rupture of the amniotic membrane, possibly secondary to trauma during pregnancy. In 1930 Streeter made popular the endogenous etiologic theory that constriction bands occurred secondary to a germ plasm defect, which caused failure of mesodermal tissue to develop, resulting in necrosis and constrictive band formation.[102] In the past congenital constriction band syndrome has commonly been referred to as *Streeter's dysplasia.* Torpin's work in 1968 and most subsequent reports have substantiated Braun's original exogenous theory that congenital constriction bands are probably caused by changes in intrauterine environment related to amniotic membrane rupture.[103]

## Incidence and Associated Anomalies

Constriction band syndrome is a rare congenital condition, and its incidence is not well documented, but more than 500 cases have been reported in the world literature.[104] Tachdjian states that this condition occurs in one of 10,000 births.[105] Birch-Jensen reported a 1 in 48,500 incidence of constriction band syndrome of the upper extremity in the Danish population.[106] Most studies indicate that the upper extremity is affected up to twice as often as the lower extremity. Involvement tends to be unilateral and often may involve areas of an ipsilateral upper and lower extremity. In a study of 83 patients with congenital constriction band syndrome, Tada et al. found 224 affected limbs, with an average of 2.7 affected limbs per patient.[107] The distal extremity is much more frequently involved than the proximal extremity. Tada et al. found hand involvement in 89 percent of cases and foot involvement in 39 percent of cases, while the more proximal upper and lower extremities were affected 14 and 20 percent of the time, respectively.

A number of congenital anomalies have been associated with congenital constriction band syndrome, including syndactyly, acrosyndactyly, clubfoot, congenital dislocated hip, convex pes valgus, cleft palate, torticollis, pseudoarthrosis of the tibia, and umbilical hernia.[104,105,107] Clubfoot is the most frequently associated deformity next to acrosyndactyly, which is considered a direct result of the constriction band pathology. The incidence of clubfoot associated with congenital constriction band syndrome has been reported to be as high as 17 to 56 percent.[107-110] In Tada et al.'s series of 83 patients with constriction bands, 23 percent had clubfoot.[107] Approximately half of these had neurogenic clubfeet as a result of direct compression of the peroneal nerve just distal to the knee from a constriction band. The other half were thought to have idiopathic clubfoot. Most investigators have theorized that idiopathic clubfoot deformity develops in congenital constriction band syndrome secondary to oligohydramnios due to amnion rupture. This causes a decrease in uterine cavity size, which perpetuates the early fetal talipes equinovarus positional deformity. This theory is supported by the experimental work of DeMyer and Baird[111] and Poswillo,[112] who have produced clubbing deformity and constriction bands in the paws of laboratory rats following amniocentesis.

## Etiology and Pathology

The exact etiology of congenital constriction band syndrome is still unknown. No studies have shown familial tendencies, and the condition is not thought to be hereditary. The bulk of experimental and clinical evidence seems to implicate an intrauterine environmental event initiated by amniotic membrane rupture, which occurs after the fifth to sixth week of fetal development. One theory is that rupture of the amniotic membrane results in free-floating strands of amnion, which encircle and strangulate the moving extremities of the fetus. Rupture of the amniotic membrane also causes oligohydramnios and decrease in size of the uterine cavity. Kino also induced digital constriction band formation in laboratory rats by amniocentesis. Anatomic dissection of the rat fetuses showed that the malformations were caused by interdigital hemorrhage of marginal sinuses, which occurred within the first few hours after amniocentesis. These small interdigital hemorrhages then slowly progressed in size and eventually became necrotic, causing digital deformity (bands, acrosyndactyly, etc.)[113] The distal parts of the extremities are most exposed and are

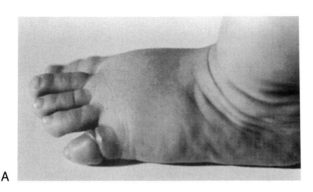
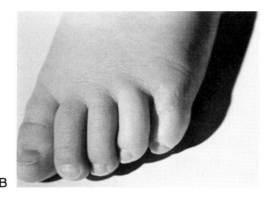

A

B

**Fig. 10-30.** (A) Congenital constriction band of the small toe. (B) Child in Fig. A after spontaneous resolution of constriction band.

therefore most frequently involved. The central digits are more frequently involved in the hand, and preaxial involvement is more common in the foot. Extremity or digital stumps have a typical "amputation" appearance rather than a congenital aplasia-type appearance. Stumps are transverse, with a distal scar and adequate soft tissue coverage. Metatarsals and metatarcarpals are rarely involved. Bands commonly encircle the digits distally, causing partial syndactyly with open spaces proximally (acrosyndactyly, fenestrated syndactyly), and multiple digits are frequently involved.

Constriction band syndrome is much more common in first pregnancies, and the prenatal complication rate is high, varying from 35 to 42 percent.[104,113,114] Premature rupture of membranes and premature delivery are also more common than would be expected.

## Clinical Appearance and Treatment

Constriction bands appear clinically as tight, thin constricting rings, which completely encircle the digits or extremity (Fig. 10-30). The depth of the thin groove varies. The ring may be superficial, involving only the skin and subcutaneous tissues, and may become less con-

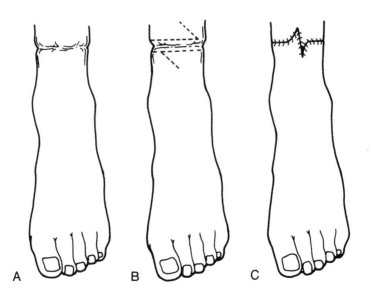

A                    B                    C

**Fig. 10-31.** Z-plasty release of congenital constriction band about ankle. (A) Constriction band. (B) Surgical excision of band. (C) After repair with transposition of Z-plasty skin flaps. (Adapted from Tachdjian,[115] with permission.)

strictive with time and require no treatment other than observation. Infants should be observed closely and frequently for progressive restriction of circulation during growth. When the constriction is deeper, lymphatic and venous drainage may be affected, causing a progressively worsening edema of the distal part of the extremity. When the neurovascular status is compromised, a staged excision of the band, with Z-plasty lengthening of the skin margins, should be performed. The band is excised via two transverse parallel incisions through normal skin on either side of the groove (Fig. 10-31). Not more than half of the band should be excised at one time to avoid circulatory compromise. The underlying fascia should be sectioned if any questions of constriction exists. Skin edges may then be lengthened by converting the transverse incision to multiple in-line Z-plasties along the course of the incisions. Desyndactylization is rarely necessary in the foot, but if indicated can be performed by standard techniques as a separate procedure.

# REFERENCES

## Polydactyly

1. Gould GM, Pyle WL: Anomalies and curiosities of medicine. Julian Press, New York, 1956
2. Masada K, Tsuyuguchi Y, Kawabata H, Ono K: Treatment of preaxial polydactyly of the foot. Plast Reconstr Surg 79:251, 1987
3. Frazier TM: A note on race-specific congenital malformation rates. Am J Obstet Gynecol 80:184, 1960
4. Wolf CM, Myrianthopolous NC: Polydactyly in American negroes and whites. Am J Hum Genet 25:397, 1973
5. Kromberg JGR, Jenkins T: Common birth defects in South African blacks. S Afr Med J 62:599, 1982
6. Neel JV: A study of major congenital defects in Japanese infants. Am J Hum Genet 10:398, 1958
7. Tetamy SA, McKusick VA: Synopsis of hand malformations with particular emphasis on genetic factors. Birth Defects 5(3):125, 1969
8. Phelps DA, Grogan DP: Polydactyly of the foot. J Pediatr Orthop 5:446, 1985
9. Meltzer RM: Poplydactyly. Clin Podiatr Med Surg 4:57, 1987
10. Venn-Watson EA: Problems in polydactyly of the foot. Orthop Clin North Am 7:909, 1976
11. Nogami H: Polydactyly and polysyndactyly of the fifth toe. Clin Orthop 204:261, 1986
12. Jahss MH, Nelson J: Duplication of the hallux. Foot Ankle 5:26, 1984

13. Cantu JM, Del Castillo V, Cortes R, Urrusti J: Autosoma' recessive post axial polydactyly: report of a family. p. 19. In Bergsma, D (ed): Limb Malformations. Grune & Stratton, Orlando, FL, 1974
14. Sverdrup A: Postaxial polydactylism in six generations of a Norwegian family. J Genet 12:217, 1922
15. Warkamy J: Notes and Comments. p. 978. In Congenital Malformation. Yearbook, Medical Publishers, Chicago, 1975
16. Scott WJ, Ritter EJ, Witson JG: Ectodermal and mesodermal cell death patterns in 6-mercaptopurine riboside-induced digital deformities. Teratology 21:271, 1980

## Syndactyly

17. Davis JS, German WJ: Syndactylism (coherence of the fingers or toes). Arch Surg 21:32, 1930
18. Bayne L: Congenital hand deformities. p. 1469. In Chapman MW (ed): Operative Orthopaedics. JB Lippincott, London, 1988
19. Dobbyns JH: Syndactyly. p. 281. In Green DP (ed): Operative Hand Surgery. Churchill Livingstone, New York, 1982
20. Bunnell S: Surgery of the Hand. 2nd Ed. JB Lippincott, Philadelphia, 1948
21. MacCollum DW: Clinical surgery—webbed fingers. Surg Gynecol Obstet 71:782, 1940
22. Barsky AJ: Congenital anomalies of the hand. J Bone Joint Surg [AM] 33:35, 1951
23. Milford L: Congenital anomalies. p. 423. In Crenshaw AH (ed): Campbell's Operative Orthopaedics. 2nd Ed. CV Mosby, St. Louis, 1987
24. Skoog T: Syndactyly. Acta Chir Scand 130:537, 1965
25. Warkany J: Congenital anomalies. J Pediatr 7:607, 1951
26. Coleman WB, Kissel CG, Sterling HD: Syndactylism and its surgical repair. J Am Podiatr Med Assoc 71:545, 1981
27. Tetamy SA, McKusick VA: Synopsis of hand malformations with particular emphasis on genetic factors. Birth Defects 5(3):125, 1969
28. Nogami H: Polydactyly and polysyndactyly of the fifth toe. Clin Orthop 204:261, 1986
29. Blackfield HM, Hause DPL: Syndactylism. Plast Reconstr Surg 16:37, 1955
30. Bouchard JL: Congenital deformities of the forefoot. p. 580. In McGlamry ED (ed): Comprehensive Textbook of Foot Surgery. Williams & Wilkins, Baltimore, 1987
31. Cangialosi BS, Polito MA: Surgical correction of congenital bilateral simple syndactylism. A case report. J Am Podiatr Med Assoc 65:465, 1975
32. Weinstock RE, Bass SJ, Farmer MA: Desyndactylization. A new modification. J Am Podiatr Med Assoc 74:458, 1984

33. Bauer TB, Tondra JM, Trusler HM: Technical modification in repair of syndactylism. Plastic Reconstr Surg 17:385, 1956

34. Losch GM, Hans-Rainer D: Anatomy and surgical treatment of syndactylism. Plastic Reconstr Surg 50:167, 1972

## Macrodactyly

35. Barsky AJ: Macrodactyly. J Bone Joint Surg 49:1255, 1967

36. DeValentine S, Scurran BL, Tuerk D, Karlin J: Macrodactyly of the lower extremity. A review with two case reports. J Am Podiatr Med Assoc 71(4):175, 1981

37. Swanson AB: Congenital limb defects: classification and treatment. Clin Symp 33(3), 1981

38. Inglis K: Local gigantism (a manifestation of neurofibromatosis): its relation to general gigantism and to acromegaly illustrating the influence of intrinsic factors in disease when development of the body is abnormal. Am J Pathol 26:1059, 1950

39. Edgerton MT, Tuerk DB: Macrodactyly, its nature and treatment. p. 103. In Littler JW (ed): Symposium on Reconstructive Hand Surgery. CV Mosby, St Louis, 1974

40. Kumar K, Kumar D, Gadegone WM, Kapahtia NK: Macrodactyly of the hand and foot. Int Orthop 9:259, 1985

41. Tsuge K: Treatment of macrodactyly. Plast Reconstr Surg 39:590, 1967

42. Tuli SM, Khanna MV, Sintra GP: Congenital macrodactyly. Br J Plast Surg 22:237, 1969

43. Minkowitz S, Minkowitz F: A morphological study of macrodactylism. J Pathol 90:323, 1965

44. Ben-Bassat M, Casper J, Kaplan I, Laran Z: Congenital macrodactyly. A case report with a three-year follow-up. J Bone Joint Surg [Br] 48:359, 1968

45. Turra S, Frizziero P, Cagnoni MD, Jacopetti T: Macrodactyly of the foot associated with plexiform neurofibroma of the medial plantar nerve. J Pediatr Orthop 6:489, 1986

46. Moore BH: Some orthopedic relationships of neurofibromatosis. Surg Gynecol Obstet 38:587, 1924

47. Alpenzeller O, Kornfield M: Macrodactyly and localized hypertrophic neuropathy. Neurology 24:767, 1974

48. McCarroll HR: Clinical manifestations of congenital neurofibromatosis. J Bone Joint Surg [Am] 32:601, 1950

49. Khanna N, Gupta S, Khanna S, Tripathi F: Macrodactyly. Hand 7:215, 1975

50. Elkeles A: Local gigantism of the right thumb and fourth fingers associated with multiple hemangiomiata of right chest wall. Proc R Soc Med 44:917, 1951

51. Jones KG: Megalodactylism. J Bone Joint Surg [Am] 45:1704, 1963

52. El Shami IN: Congenital partial gigantism. Surgery 65:683, 1969

53. Blais MM, Green WT, Anderson M: Lengths of the growing foot. J Bone Joint Surg [Am] 41:988, 1959

54. Clifford RH: Treatment of macrodactylism. Plast Reconstr Surg 23:245, 1959

55. Tsuge K: Treatment of macrodactyly. J Hand Surg [Am] 10A:968, 1985

55a. Diamond LS, Gould VE: Macrodactyly of the foot: surgical syndactyly after wedge resection. South Med J 67(6):645, 1974

## Hallux Varus

56. McElvenny RT: Hallux varus. Q Bull Northwestern Med School 15:277, 1941

57. Tachdjian MO: The Child's Foot. WB Saunders, Philadelphia, 1985

58. Sloane D: Congenital hallux varus, operative correction. J Bone Joint Surg 17:209, 1935

59. Haas SL: An operation for the correction of hallux varus. J Bone Joint Surg 20:705, 1938

60. Farmer AW: Congenital hallux varus. Am J Surg 95:274, 1958

61. Kleiner BC, Holmes LB: Brief clinical report: hallux varus and preaxial polysyndactyly in brothers. Am J Med Genet 6:113, 1980

62. Greig DM: Hallux varus. Edinburgh Med J 30:588, 1923

## Hallux Abductus Interphalangeus

63. Daw SW: An unusual type of hallux valgus (two cases). Br Med J 2:580, 1935

64. Gillett HG: Ungual phalanx valgus. J Am Podiatr Med Assoc 68:83, 1978

65. Barnett C: Valgus deviation of the distal phalanx of the great toe. J Anat 96:171, 1962

66. Sorto LA, Marshall GB, Weil LS, Smith SD: Hallux abductus interphalangeus, etiology, x-ray evaluation and treatment. J Am Podiatr Med Assoc 66:384, 1976

67. Bouchard JL: congenital deformities of the forefoot. In McGlamry ED (ed): Comprehensive Textbook of Foot Surgery. Vol 1. Williams & Wilkins, Baltimore, 1987

68. Hardy RH, Clapham JCR: Observations of hallux valgus. J Bone Joint Surg [Br] 33:376, 1951

69. Tachdjian MO: Pediatric Orthopedics. Vol 1. WB Saunders, Philadelphia, 1972

70. Tachdjian MO: The Child's Foot. WB Saunders, Philadelphia, 1985

## Brachymetatarsia

71. Tachdjian MO: The Child's Foot. WB Saunders, Philadelphia, 1985
72. Greenfield GB: Radiology of Bone Diseases. 2nd Ed. JB Lippincott, Philadelphia, 1975
73. Urano Y, Kobayashi A: Bone lengthening for shortness of the fourth toe. J Bone Joint Surg [Am] 60:91, 1978
74. Marcinko DE, Rappaport MJ, Gordon S: Post-traumatic brachymetatarsia. J Foot Surg 23:451, 1984
75. Harris RI, Beath T: The short first metatarsal. J Bone Joint Surg [Am] 31:553, 1949
76. Mah KS, Buegle TR, Falknor DW: A correction for short fourth metatarsal. J Am Podiatr Med Assoc 73:196, 1983
77. Biggs EW, Brahm TB, Efron BL: Surgical correction of congenital hypoplastic metatarsals. J Am Podiatr Med Assoc 69:241, 1979
78. Hosokawa K, Susuki T: Treatment of multiple brachymetatarsia; a case report. Br J Plastic Surg 40:423, 1987
79. McGlamry ED, Cooper CT: Brachymetatarsia; a surgical treatment. J Am Podiatr Med Assoc 59:259, 1969
80. Jimenez AL: Brachymetatarsia; a study in surgical planning. J Am Podiatr Med Assoc 69:245, 1979
81. McGlamry ED, Fenton CF: Brachymetatarsia: a case report. J Am Podiatr Med Assoc 73:75, 1983

## Cleft Foot

82. Tachdjian MO: The Child's Foot. WB Saunders, Philadelphia, 1985
83. Barsky AJ: Cleft hand: classification, incidence, and treatment. Review of the literature and report of nineteen cases. J Bone Joint Surg [Am] 46:1707, 1964
84. Hartsinck JJ: Beschryving van Guiana, of de wilde Kust in Zuid-America. Gerrit Tielenburg, Amsterdam, 1770
85. Martens FH: Ueber eine sehr complicirte Hasenscharte oder einen sogenannten Wolfsrachen, mit einer an demselben Subjekte befindlichen merkwürdigen Misstaltung der Hände und Füsse. EF Steinacker, Leipzig, 1804
86. Béchet JF: Essai sur les monstruosités humaines, ou vices congénitaux de conformation. Didot le Jeune, Paris, 1829
87. Geoffroy Saint-Hilaire I: Histoire générale et particulière des anomalies de l'organisation chez l'homme et les animaux. JB Baillière, Paris, 1832
88. Parker RW, Robinson HB: A case of inherited congenital malformation of the hands and feet: plastic operation of the feet: with a family tree. Clin Soc Lond 20:181, 1887
89. Birch-Jensen A: Congenital deformities of the upper extremities. Ejnar Munksgaard, Copenhagen, 1949
90. Walker JC, Clodius L: The syndromes of cleft lip, cleft palate and lobster claw deformities of hands and feet. Plast Reconstr Surg 32:627, 1963
91. Phillips RS: Congenital split foot (lobster claw) and triphalangeal thumb. J Bone Joint Surg [Br] 53:247, 1971
92. Majewski F, Kuster W, ter Haar B, Goeche T: Aplasia of the tibia with split-hand/split-foot deformity. Report of six families with 35 cases and consideration about variability and penetrance. Hum Genet 70:136, 1985
93. Giorgini RS, Capa CJ, Potter GK: Two-stage surgical correction of cleft foot. A seven year follow-up of one case. J Am Podiatr Med Assoc 75:481, 1985
94. Coleman WB, Aronovitz DC: Surgical management of cleft foot deformity. J Foot Surg 27:497, 1988
95. Onizuka T: Surgical correction of lobster-claw feet. Plast Reconstr Surg 57:98, 1976
96. Sumiya N, Onizuka T: Seven years' survey of our new cleft foot repair. Plast Reconstr Surg 65:447, 1980
97. Weissman SL, Plaschkes Y: Surgical correction of lobster-claw feet. Plast Reconstr Surg 49:89, 1972

## Congenital Constriction Band Syndrome

98. Van Helmont JB: Of material things injected or cast into the body. p. 597. In Ortus Medicinae Amsterodami, Oriatrike or Physick Refined, 1652
99. Bartholini T: De observationibus raris medicorum. Acta Med Phil Hafn 2:1, 1673
100. Montgomery FW: Observations on the spontaneous amputation of the limbs of the foetus in utero, with an attempt to explain the occasional cause of its production. Am J Med Sci 21:218, 1832
101. Braun G: Die strangformige Aufwickelung des Amnion um den Nabelstrang des feifen Kindes — eine seltene Ursache des intrauterinen Foetaltoedes. Oesterr Z Prakt Heilk 11:181, 1865
102. Streeter GL: Focal deficiencies in fetal tissues and their relation to intra-uterine amputation. Contrib Embryol Carnegie Inst 22:1, 1930
103. Torpin R: Fetal Malformations Caused by Amnion Rupture during Gestation. Charles C Thomas, Springfield, IL, 1968
104. Rossillon D, Rombouts JJ, Verellen-Dumoulin C, et al: Congenital ring-constriction syndrome of the limbs; a report of 19 cases. Br J Plast Surg 41:270, 1988
105. Tachdjian MO: The Child's Foot. WB Saunders, Philadelphia, 1985
106. Birch-Jensen A: Congenital Deformities of the Upper Extremities. Ejnar Munksgaard, Copenhagen, 1949
107. Tada K, Yonenobu K, Swanson AB: Congenital constriction band syndrome. J Pediatr Orthop 4:726, 1984

108. Cowell HR, Hensinger RN: The relationship of clubfoot to congenital annular bands. p. 41. In Bateman JE (ed): Foot Science. WB Saunders, Philadelphia, 1976
109. Patterson TJS: Congenital ring-constrictions. BR J Plast Surg 14:1, 1961
110. Moses JM, Flatt AE, Cooper RR: Annular constriction bands. J Bone Joint Surg [Am] 61:562, 1979
111. DeMyer W, Baird I: Mortality and skeletal malformations from amniocentesis and oligohydramnios in rats: cleft palate, clubfoot, microstomia, and adactyly. Teratology 2:33, 1969
112. Poswillo D: Observations of fetal posture and causal mechanisms of congenital deformity of palate, mandible, and limbs. J Dent Res 45:584, 1966
113. Kino Y: Clinical and experimental studies of the congenital constriction band syndrome, with an emphasis on its etiology. J Bone Joint Surg [Am] 57:636, 1975
114. Miura T: Congenital constriction band syndrome. J Hand Surg [Am] 9A:82, 1984
115. Tachdjian MO: Pediatric Orthopedics. Vol. 1. WB Saunders, Philadelphia, 1972, p. 237

## SUGGESTED READINGS

### Polydactyly

Bouchard JL: Congenital deformities of the forefoot. In McGlamry ED (ed): Comprehensive Textbook of Foot Surgery. Vol. 1. Williams & Wilkins, Baltimore, 1987

Giorgini RJ, Aquino JM: Surgical approach to polydactyly. J Foot Surg 23:221, 1984

Kapetanos GA: Mixed polydactyly. An unusual case of a patient with seven toed feet. Clin Orthop 186:220, 1984

Knecht JG: Polydactyly of the foot. J Foot Surg 22:23, 1983

Tozzi MA, Penny HL: Postaxial polydactyly with polymetatarsia. A case report. J Am Podiatr Med Assoc 71:374, 1981

### Macrodactyly

Boberg JS, Yu GV, Xenos D: Macrodactyly a case report. J Am Podiatr Med Assoc 75:41, 1985

Cavaliere RG, McElgun TM: Macrodactyly and hemihypertrophy: a new surgical procedure. J Foot Surg 27:226, 1988

DeGreef A, Petorius LKR: Macrodactyly: a review with a case report. S Afr Med J 63:939, 1983

Dennyson WG, Bear JN, Bhoola KD: Macrodactyly in the foot. J Bone Joint Surg [Br] 59:355, 1977

Figura MA: Practical approach to a rare deformity: macrodactyly. J Foot Surg 19:52, 1980

Herring JA: Macrodactyly. J Pediatr Orthop 4:503, 1984

Kalen V, Burwell DS, Omer GE: Macrodactyly of the hands and feet. J Pediatr Orthop 8:311, 1988

Keret D, Ger E, Marks HP: Macrodactyly involving both hands and both feet. J Hand Surg [Am] 12:610, 1987

O'Flanagan SJ, Moran V, Colville J: Brief report, congenital macrodactyly. Indian J Med Sci 156(5):151, 1987

Ofodile FA, Oluwasianmi J: Pedal macrodactyly—a report of seven cases. East Afr Med J 56:283, 1979

Pearn J, Block CE, Nelson MM: Macrodactyly simplex congenita. S Aft Med J 70:41, 1985

Perdiue RL, Mason WH, Bernard TN: Macrodactyly: a rare malformation. J Am Podiatr Med Assoc 69:657, 1979

Pho RWH, Patterson M, Lee YS: Reconstruction and pathology in macrodactyly. J Hand Surg [Am] 13(1):78, 1988

Rosenberg L, Yanai A, Mahler D: A nail island flap for treatment of macrodactyly. Hand 15:167, 1983

Sanchez AJ, Kamal B: Macrodactyly in the foot. Ann Acad Med 10:442, 1981

Winestine F: Relation of von Recklinghausen's disease (multiple neurofibromatosis) to giant growth and blastomatosis. J Cancer Res 8:409, 1924

# 11

# Related Congenital and Developmental Conditions of the Lower Extremity

## JAMES L. SHIVELY

## CONGENITAL DISLOCATED HIP

Congenital dislocation of the hip (CDH) is a loss of the normal articulating relationship between the head of the femur and the acetabulum of the ilium. Strictly speaking, a true CDH occurs in the neonatal or prenatal period and does not include spastic dislocations as frequently seen in children with cerebral palsy. Dislocations due to muscle imbalance in children with spina bifida and other diseases in which the muscle pull on the hip is abnormal are also not included in true CDH.

Typical CDH is common, ranging in incidence from 1.5 to 10 per 1,000 live births, depending on the criteria used to define the condition. Girls are affected about eight times more often than boys. The left hip is much more commonly involved than the right side. Overall, 60 percent of the dislocations are on the left side, 20 percent bilateral, and 20 percent right-sided, and 80 percent of patients with this problem are female.[1]

CDH is a relatively common problem in northern Italy, in Japan, and among certain American Indian tribes, particularly those that swaddle the hips in extension and adduction, a motion that is assumed to initiate dislocation. This same disease is relatively rare among blacks and Chinese. Particularly important is the increased incidence of CDH in children with metatarsus adductus, reported to be as high as 2 percent. Also, there may be as much as a 20 percent incidence of hip abnormalities in children with torticollis.

## Classification

A variety of terms have been used to describe CDH, and there is no consistent agreement as to the exact meaning of many of them. In newborns with a *dislocated* hip the femoral head is completely out of the acetabulum, and a reduction motion on the part of the examiner is required to place the hip back in the socket. A *dislocatable* hip exists when the femoral head is in the acetabulum but is easily dislocated by a provocative maneuver. The terms subluxed and subluxable usually refer to partial dislocation.

## Etiology

Three factors — genetic, hormonal, and mechanical — predispose to dislocation. It is known that as many as 50 dislocations per 1,000 live births will occur in children who have an older sibling with a dislocated hip. This risk is at least 10 times the expected average.

Hormonal factors have frequently been blamed as etiologic agents for CDH. While not all authors agree on the effect that estrogen breakdown products may have on the hip, this effect is assumed to be a predisposing factor in hip dislocations in some cases and may partially explain the sevenfold higher frequency in female infants. Female fetal tissue may be more responsive than male fetal tissue to hormonal influences.

Experience has shown that relative joint laxity in newborns lasts for several days. Many children with lax joints

261

have easily dislocatable hips, which if left untreated will develop stability in just a few days.

Mechanical factors markedly influence the occurrence of hip dislocation. Paterson[2] is credited with reporting a 30 percent incidence of hip instability in female breech infants at birth. Newborn girls also have a high incidence of hip problems when they are delivered by cesarean section. In the breech position in utero, the knees are held in hyperextension, which is assumed to add to hip instability. Studies in which the hips of rabbits were held in extension showed this same factor to contribute to a higher incidence of hip dislocation.

There is no uniform agreement as to why left hip involvement is much more frequent than right side or bilateral occurrence. It has been postulated that positioning in utero may cause the left hip to be held in adduction, thus contributing to the higher dislocation rate on the left side.

## Clinical Features

The diagnosis of CDH is not usually obvious; in examining newborns, specific attention must be given to looking for this problem. The importance of early detection and treatment must be emphasized. An initial normal examination at birth does not totally exclude CDH; repetitive examinations by experienced personnel are required throughout the first year of life.

The diagnosis of CDH in newborns is based on the clinical examination. With the quiet infant lying on its back on a firm surface, the examiner flexes the thigh to 90 degrees with one hand while stabilizing the pelvis with the other. The knee is then flexed to 90 degrees and the thumb of the examining hand placed over the lesser trochanter in the groin, while the index or long finger of the examining hand reaches down to the greater trochanter on the lateral side of the proximal femur. Gentle downward pressure is applied at the knee and, lateral pressure is applied on the inner thigh with the thumb (Fig. 11-1). The dislocatable hip then becomes displaced laterally with a "clunk." This is known as the Barlow test, a provocative test for an unstable hip.[3]

An additional valuable test in diagnosing hip dislocation in infants is Nélaton's line. This is an imaginary line connecting the anterior iliac spine and the tuberosity of the ischium. In a normal child the tip of the greater trochanter is palpable distal to Nélaton's line; hip dislocation should be suspected if the tip of the greater tro-

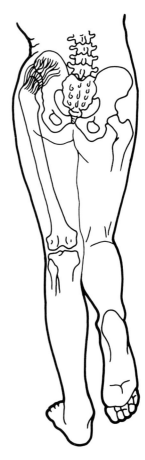

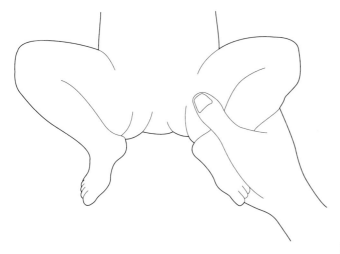

Fig. 11-1. Demonstration of the provocative maneuver of a Barlow Test to check for a dislocatable hip.

Fig. 11-2. This pelvis is lower on the right side during single leg stance owing to relative weak hip abductors on the left side due to a CDH.

chanter is proximal to Nélaton's line. The test for Nélaton's line may be particularly useful in children with bilateral hip dislocation; however, Nélaton's line may be difficult to localize in obese children.

In older children the classic signs of dislocation include limited abduction, asymmetric thigh folds, relative femoral shortening, and later, a limp. Children with the shortened leg usually walk on their toes on the involved side to make up for the proximally displaced and thus "shortened" femur. Asymmetric thigh folds may be present, but normal thigh folds in no way rule out dislocation; the presence of normal folds is a unreliable criterion for detecting hip dislocation.

Children with bilateral dislocation may have hyperlordosis of the lumbar spine when walking. In all children who are able to stand or walk, Trendelenburg's sign will be positive in the presence of dislocated hips or other hip pathology. This test allows the contralateral pelvis to drop when the child stands alone on the affected limb (Fig. 11-2).

## Radiologic Evaluation

Initial radiographic evaluation of newborn infants for CDH is unreliable. Efforts to shield the gonads usually result in repetitive radiographs and thus repetitive irradiation of reproductive tissue. In newborns the proximal end of the femur and parts of the acetabulum are cartilaginous and do not appear on routine radiographs. Generally, the diagnosis of hip dislocation can be made on a clinical examination; hip arthrograms, computed tomographic (CT) scans, and magnetic resonance imaging (MRI) are not indicated as routine diagnostic aids.

As infants mature, routine radiographs can be of use, and a variety of reference lines have been devised to facilitate the diagnosis.[4,5] These lines are drawn on the radiographs and used to help determine the location of the cartilaginous femoral head and acetabulum (Fig. 11-3). In skilled hands ultrasound can outline the underlying infant femoral head. Advantages of this study are a lack of radiation and usually no need for sedation of the patient. Other tests mentioned above, such as MRI and CT, also have their place in the management of CDH,[6] but when available, ultrasound is fast becoming the imaging technique of choice.[7,8]

## Treatment

A variety of devices exist for the treatment of hip dislocation in children. Treatment is usually age-dependent and begins as soon after the diagnosis as possible. In general, in infants and young children the success rate of treatment of hip dislocation is very high, and good results

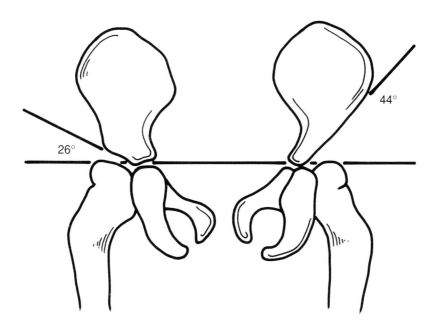

**Fig. 11-3.** Drawing of a radiograph, showing an increased acetabular angle on the involved left side.

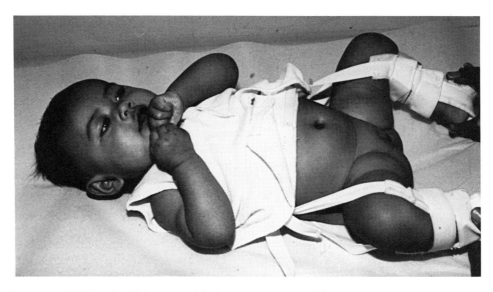

**Fig. 11-4.** Child in a Pavlik harness, with the correct amount of flexion and abduction of the femurs.

can be obtained. Once the child has begun to walk, good results are much more difficult to obtain, and residual deformity is frequent. In children in whom the hip can be reduced or in whom the hip is unstable, the Pavlik harness is frequently used to hold the hips in flexion and abduction (Fig. 11-4). With the femur in a flexed, abducted position, the femoral head usually is reduced into the acetabulum and with time becomes stable. In several reports a Pavlik harness has been used to *obtain* as well as maintain reduction of a dislocated hip.[9,10] Other splints and pillow devices can be useful in CDH treatment because they use a frogleg position of the patient to hold the unstable hip in a reduced position. As with almost all externally applied bracing devices, an anteroposterior radiograph of the pelvis in the Pavlik harness should be obtained to determine the position of the femoral head relative to the acetabulum (Fig. 11-5).

I believe that the use of a Pavlik harness is indicated full-time in children up to 6 months of age and that other devices are necessary when the child is past this age. The Pavlik harness requires moderate experience in its application, and parents need to be monitored in the application and adjustment of such a device. A Pavlik harness should be able to either obtain or maintain a hip reduction within 4 weeks; if reduction is not obtained, other methods are indicated. In newborns, stability of the hip should be obtained in 2 weeks or even less.

While use of multiple diapers as an abduction device

can be successful, this approach is generally criticized because diapers do not keep the hips in flexion. Careful, skilled follow-up is required if this method is used.

When a Pavlik harness or other device has been unsuccessful in obtaining or maintaining hip reduction and/or the child is more than 6 months of age, skin traction is indicated to obtain reduction. While the exact methods of application of traction vary, most authors agree that traction to obtain a reduction is indicated for 3 to 6 weeks.[4] If there is no improvement in the position of the femoral head or if the child persists in "kicking out" of the skin traction, skeletal pin traction is occasionally needed in selected children. With the knee in extension, a transverse skeletal traction pin is placed 1 cm above the proximal pole of the patella. Radiographic confirmation of the position of the pin is necessary. When traction alone is not successful in obtaining reduction, open reduction of the hip is indicated.[11]

Once reduction is obtained with any of the above methods, spica cast application is usually required to hold the reduced hip joint in children over 6 months of age (Fig. 11-6). While general anesthesia is not mandatory, its use does facilitate the application of the cast and allows the treating physician to place the hip joint in the most stable position possible without resistance from the patient. An adductor longus tenotomy may be carried out when the closed reduction is done and the child is placed in a cast.

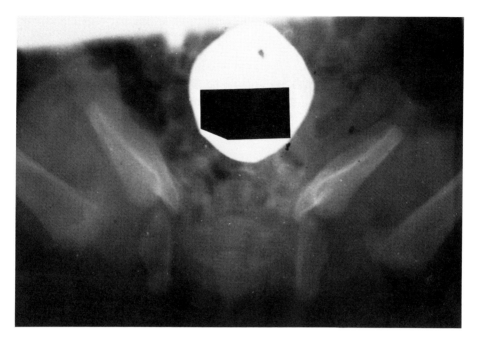

**Fig. 11-5.** Radiograph of child in a Pavlik harness, which is holding the hip joint reduced.

Prior to the age of walking, very few children will require open reduction to reduce the hip. Most hips, in children of this age category can be reduced by traction followed by closed reduction and spica cast. As the child becomes older, some authors would continue with skeletal traction while others believe that open reduction and/or femoral shortening as a primary procedure is indicated.[12]

Because of the poor results of treatment of CDH in older children compared with the results in infants, the

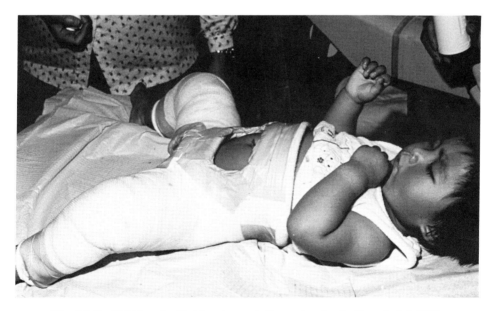

**Fig. 11-6.** Child in a double hip spica cast after a closed reduction of a left CDH.

importance of early diagnosis of this difficult problem cannot be overemphasized.

## LEGG-CALVÉ-PERTHES DISEASE

Following the discovery of radiography in 1895, the stage was set for improvement in diagnosis and treatment in many fields of medicine. In 1909 Waldenström described a form of benign juvenile tuberculosis of the hip. The next year Legg, Calvé, and Perthes all published their classic papers individually, describing a deformity in the hips of growing children. The disease is now generally known as *Legg-Calvé-Perthes disease,* although it sometimes is called *coxa plana,* a term given to the disease by Waldenström. While there is no uniform

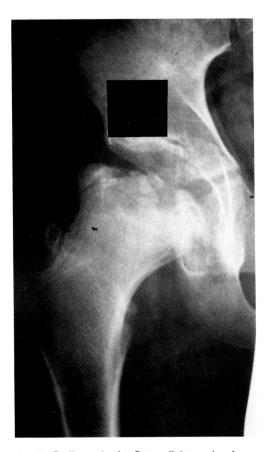

**Fig. 11-7.** Radiograph of a Catterall 3-type involvement of the right femoral head with Legg-Calvé-Perthes disease.

agreement on the name or etiology of this condition, many treatment regimens have been published in the world literature. This section will present the classification and some concepts concerning the etiology of this condition. In addition, the general clinical features and treatment plans will be discussed.

### Classification

The generally accepted classification of Legg-Calvé-Perthes disease was initially described by Anthony Catterall.[13] In this classification there are four groups based on the extent of involvement of the femoral head avascular necrosis. In group 1 there is no collapse of the femoral head, and no sequestrum or dead bone is seen. There is a sclerotic-appearing epiphysis on the anteroposterior radiograph. Although the epiphysis is sclerotic, its height is maintained. In the lateral (frog) radiograph there is a tongue of normal epiphysis reaching the anterior margin of the growth plate. Generally, this involvement of the femoral head runs a benign course, and there is a uniform good result.

Groups 2, 3, and 4 show further involvement of the epiphysis, the physis, and the adjacent metaphysis, with collapse of the femoral head and resultant deformity and early arthritic changes (Fig. 11-7). Whether treated or untreated, 92 percent of the poor results occur in Catterall groups 3 and 4.

### Etiology

It is generally accepted that the child with Legg-Calvé-Perthes disease develops changes in the hip joint as a consequence of vascular ischemia of the femoral head.[13] Attempts to repair the ischemia produce a growth disturbance in the head, which if uncontrolled leads to a deformity of the hip joint and sometimes to a painful arthritis.

Despite an increase in the volume of literature, the cause of this condition remains unknown. As far back as 1921 Phemister reported necrotic bone in the substance of the epiphysis in a case of Perthes disease.[14] Many theories have been advanced to explain the reasons for this necrosis and the subsequent changes that have evolved. It is generally thought that there may be a relationship between the higher incidence in boys and trauma to the hip. Many authors have commented on the personality of the involved youngsters and the fact that they seem to never sit still during an examination. Mothers have reported their children jumping off the back of the couch for 3 hours at a time. In addition to trauma, other factors such as inflammatory conditions, bacterial infections, and endocrine and nutritional causes have been implicated in the etiology of Legg-Calvé-Perthes disease.[15]

While each or all of these processes may explain the nature of individual cases of Perthes disease, the underlying nature of the disease remains unknown. It is of interest to note that its incidence is higher in cities than in rural communities. In many cases a strong family history of the disease, particularly of its bilateral occurrence, is more suggestive of some form of skeletal dysplasia, such as multiple epiphyseal dysplasia, than of a true case of Perthes. A number of authors have noted that children with Legg-Calvé-Perthes disease have abnormalities in height, weight, and skeletal maturation, as well as an unexpectedly high incidence of hernia, undescended testicle, and genitourinary disease.[16] Last, also for an unexplained reason, a greater than average proportion of children with Legg-Calvé-Perthes are born during the winter months.

## Clinical Features

It is generally accepted that Legg-Calvé-Perthes disease is more common among boys, although they have a better long-term prognosis than do girls. The average age at the time of presentation is between 4 and 9 years of age. The male to female ratio is 7 : 1. About 10 percent of the cases are bilateral.

The classic patient presenting with Perthes disease is a 6-year-old white boy of northern European ancestry with blond hair and blue eyes and often a painless limp. On clinical examination this youngster usually has a mild hip flexion contracture with further normal flexion of the hip. Internal and external rotation of the hip are markedly limited. The child typically cannot sit still on examination (i.e., he is fidgety), may be short for his age, and often is a first-born son. His bone age may be as much as 2 years behind his chronologic age. A higher than normal incidence of enuresis has been reported with this condition.

## Treatment

While various opinions about Legg-Calvé-Perthes disease have been presented thus far, a greater controversy exists regarding treatment than any other aspect of this disease. The treatment controversy exists because of the long duration of the disease and the concern for degenerative changes of the hip in early adult life.

While prolonged bed rest was initially considered the treatment of choice, treatment now has evolved to use the Scottish Rite abduction brace as the generally accepted early treatment in the Catterall groups 2 and 3 (Fig. 11–8). Catterall group 1 usually requires no treatment, while treatment of the unfortunate children with Catterall group 4 remains controversial.[17]

When an abduction brace is unsuccessful, surgery may be indicated to maintain coverage of the femoral head. Both upper femoral osteotomies and acetabular procedures have been used to increase the coverage of the femoral head. More recently, attention has been paid to

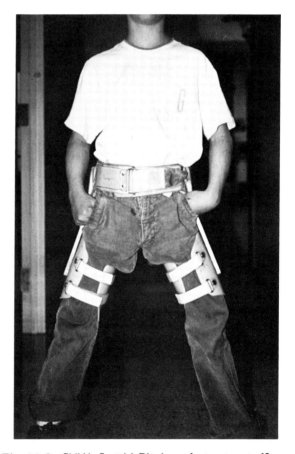

**Fig. 11-8.** Child in Scottish Rite brace for treatment of Legg-Calvé-Perthes disease.

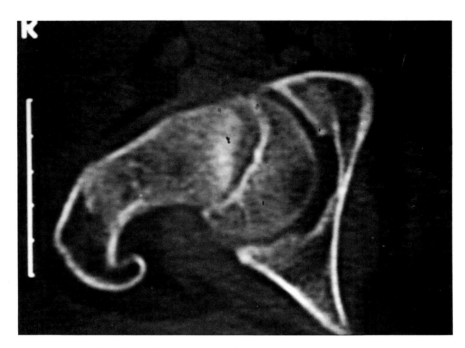

**Fig. 11-9.** CT lateral view of the femoral head and neck of a patient with slipped capital femoral epiphysis, showing a one-third posterior slip of the head in relation to the femoral neck.

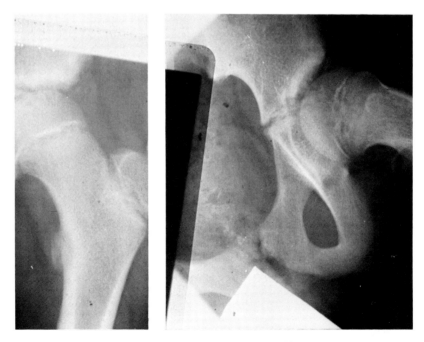

**Fig. 11-10.** Apparently normal anteroposterior radiograph of the hip. However, the lateral view shows a grade 1 slipped capital femoral epiphysis.

interruption of the growth of the proximal femoral physis with the resultant "pseudo-overgrowth" of the greater trochanter, which results in a progressive hip limp due to mechanical inefficiency of the hip abductors. This can best be treated before the child's eighth birthday by arrest of the growth of the greater trochanter. If the trochanteric transfer is not done before 8 years of age, a distal transfer of the greater trochanter must be carried out.[18]

A long-term residual effect of the hip severely involved with Legg-Calvé-Perthes disease is degenerative arthritis with painful hip motion. Salvage procedures, including total hip replacement, must sometimes be carried out to obtain optimal results.

## SLIPPED CAPITAL FEMORAL EPIPHYSIS

In slipped capital femoral epiphysis, also known as slipped upper femoral epiphysis or adolescent coxa vara, the epiphysis of the proximal femur displaces from the metaphysis in either an acute or a chronic condition. While the radiograph seems to show that the epiphysis moves inferiorly and posteriorly, actually the motion is in the metaphysis, which moves proximally and anteriorly. In about 30 percent of patients, slippage of the upper femoral epiphysis occurs in both hips. *Slips,* as they are generally known, are a problem that occurs in late childhood or adolescence, generally between the ages of 9 and 15 years. Boys are affected twice as commonly as girls. The disease is dramatically more common in blacks than in whites or Orientals.

### Classification

As implied above, slips are generally classified as either acute or chronic depending on the duration of the problem. Slips are also subdivided according to the degree of slippage, being termed first, second, or third degree on the basis of how much of the metaphysis and the femoral head are in contact when first seen by radiography (Fig. 11–9).

### Etiology

The etiology of slips is uncertain, though several factors relating to slipped epiphyses are well known. The proximal femur is considered to be mechanically weak in shear stress because of both local and systemic factors. Mechanical factors combine to dislodge the epiphysis from its normal position. In adolescence the periosteum of the femoral neck may be thinner than at an earlier age and thus weaker. The weakening may be affected by both mechanical and hormonal factors that allow the physis to move. Biomechanical studies have suggested that the weight-bearing of walking alone may be sufficient to cause a slipped upper femoral epiphysis.

Certainly in some patients a significant role is played by hormonal factors. In some of them excess levels of growth hormone are thought to cause widening and hence local weakness of some of the cartilaginous layers of the upper femoral physis. Other patients have shown a decrease in thyroid hormone (hypothyroidism), and this has been associated with slipped epiphysis.[19] Low levels of estrogen or of testosterone have been implicated in some patients who have developed slipped epiphyses.

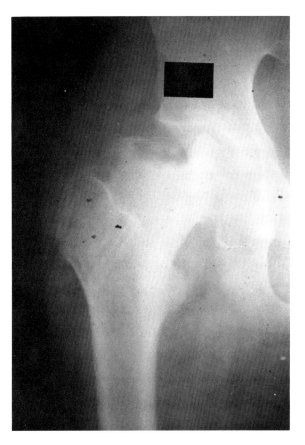

**Fig. 11-11.** Anteroposterior radiograph showing severe avascular necrosis as a result of a slipped epiphysis.

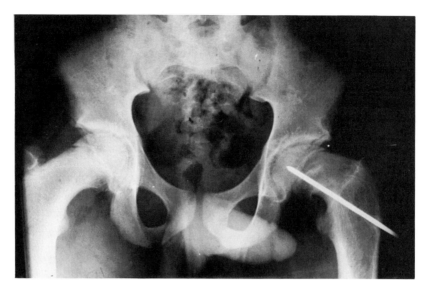

**Fig. 11-12.** Anteroposterior radiograph of pelvis showing a slipped capital femoral epiphysis stabilized with a single pin.

Some patients who are treated for slipped upper femoral epiphysis actually have an acute Salter 1 fracture of the proximal femur. These patients have all the usual complications of avascular necrosis, malunion, and nonunion that generally occur in femoral neck fractures in children. The classic slipped epiphysis actually is an "acute on chronic" slip, which brings the patient to treatment. This problem has generally been present for between 1 and 6 weeks, and pain somewhere in the lower extremity is the usual presenting complaint.

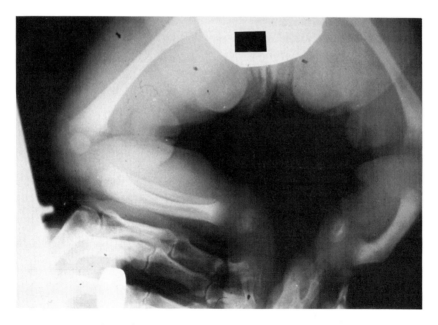

**Fig. 11-13.** Lateral radiograph of the left lower extremity in an infant, demonstrating anterolateral bowing of the tibia with total absence of the fibula.

Patients with an acute on chronic slip give a history of a gradual pain somewhere in the extremity, often at the knee and sometimes at the foot. The pain is generally vague in nature and not often associated with the hip itself. Although patients usually limp, they are often not aware of the limp. They usually walk with a mild Trendelenburg gait, with the entire affected leg held in external rotation.

## Clinical Features

The classic clinical presentation is that of an obese black male with a 3-week history of leg pain and a limp. On physical examination the affected leg usually is slightly shortened and held in external rotation. With the patient supine, passive hip flexion always produces acute external rotation of the hip; internal rotation, either active or passive, is not possible because the femoral head has in effect slipped inferiorly and posteriorly, although it is actually the femoral neck that has moved, as previously described. In addition to the loss of internal rotation, abduction of the hip is markedly diminished compared with the opposite side.

Radiographs of the hip must be taken in both the anteroposterior and lateral views; it is best to order an anteroposterior and a lateral (frog) view of the entire pelvis so that the correct view of the hips will be obtained. Often on initial anteroposterior radiographs of the hip, the femoral head will appear to be in normal relationship to the femoral neck. However, in the lateral view an imaginary line drawn along the lateral cortex of the neck of the femur should intersect the bony epiphysis; if this line does not intersect the epiphysis, the epiphysis may have slipped inferiorly. A slipped epiphysis is usually more noticeable in the lateral view, where the posterior displacement of the epiphysis can be appreciated (Fig. 11-10).

## Treatment

Untreated, the slippage of the femoral head progresses until there is marked displacement of the femoral head in relation to the neck. Premature degenerative arthritis then occurs in early adulthood, and in some circumstances avascular necrosis or cartilage necrosis of the femoral head may complicate this disease and/or its treatment (Fig. 11-11).

In mild to moderate slips (types 1 and 2), treatment is generally directed toward stopping the slip by placing a threaded pin or screw up the femoral neck, across the physis, and into the epiphysis. This fixation device is then left in place until the physis closes (Fig. 11-12). In strictly acute slips or slips that are acute on chronic, closed manipulation to reduce the slip may be carried out in selected patients. Some authors have popularized the idea of open reduction of the slipped epiphysis, although in many hands there is a higher incidence of avascular necrosis with this technique.

In severe slips osteotomy of the proximal femur is sometimes necessary to re-establish the relationship of the femoral head to the acetabulum.[20] Whatever the treatment of slipped epiphysis, initial management must be instituted upon recognition of the problem. Most authors recommend immediate cessation of weight-bearing, with either bed rest or crutches, upon diagnosis of

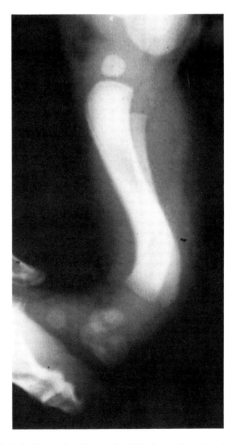

**Fig. 11-14.** Lateral radiograph of the lower leg showing posterior bowing of both bones with the foot in calcaneus.

this problem. Persistent weight-bearing may result in progression of the slip and further complications.

## ACUTE TOXIC SYNOVITIS OF THE HIP

Acute toxic synovitis of the hip, sometimes known as transient synovitis of the hip, is a nonspecific, self-limited, inflammatory process of the hip joint, which affects boys three times as often as girls. This relatively common cause of hip pain in children is most common between the ages of 3 and 6 years.

While the etiology is not known, patients frequently have a history of a recent upper respiratory infection, although the exact correlation is uncertain. Trauma is not usually considered to be an etiologic factor. As already described in the case of slipped epiphysis, the initial complaint is one of hip pain of a vague nature. The pain may be in the anterior thigh or even at the knee.

While motion of the hip is possible, motion is generally mildly limited on clinical examination. Laboratory tests are of no significant benefit, and even sedimentation rate and white counts are usually normal. In suspected synovitis, radiographs of the hip should be obtained to help differentiate this disease from other hip problems that

children develop. If septic hip arthritis or osteomyelitis cannot be ruled out, hip aspiration under fluoroscopic control is usually necessary. Bone scanning or MRI may be used to differentiate hip synovitis from infectious hip diseases or Legg-Calvé-Perthes disease.

Acute synovitis of the hip is a self-limited disease, which will eventually resolve if left alone. In most circumstances patients are treated with bed rest or some form of non-weight-bearing until the symptoms resolve. Improvement of the symptoms usually correlates with a normal hip examination and a resolution of the pain and limp. Follow up evaluation for possible infection or Legg-Calvé-Perthes disease is generally indicated in 1 to 2 months.

## TIBIAL AND FIBULAR DYSPLASIA

Although rare, both posterior and anterior bowing of the tibia and fibula can occur at birth and present uniquely different problems. Anterior and anterolateral bowing of the tibia and fibula are associated with congenital pseudarthrosis of the tibia, which has a high correlation with neurofibromatosis. In anterior bowing, both the tibia and the fibula are apex anterior or anterolateral. The apex of

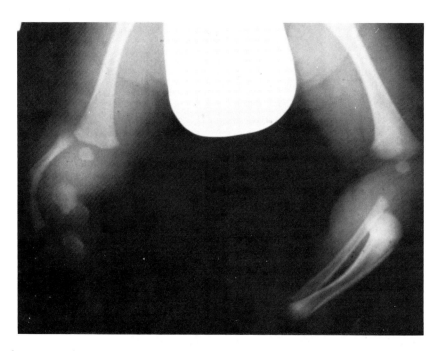

**Fig. 11-15.** Anteroposterior radiograph of the lower extremities demonstrating near total absence of the right tibia.

the bow is usually at the junction of the middle and distal thirds of the leg (Fig. 11-13). If there is anterior bowing of the tibia without fracture, use of an orthosis is indicated to help prevent fracture. Radiographs of the entire tibia and fibula are necessary to differentiate congenital bowing from other problems that are most likely acquired. In anterior bowing, the natural history without bracing is for progressive deformity and eventual fracture with resultant pseudarthrosis. Treatment of the pseudarthrosis is prolonged and difficult and frequently results in amputation.

Posterior bowing with the apex of the bones pointed posterior or posteromedial may also be present at birth. In this condition the foot is in calcaneus, and passive plantar flexion of the foot is limited (Fig. 11-14). Radiographs will again differentiate the congenital from other acquired conditions. The natural history of posterior bowing of the tibia is slow spontaneous improvement of the deformity. The primary residual problem for these patients is one of leg length inequality, which may require growth arrest of the longer side near the end of skeletal growth. In rare cases leg lengthening may be necessary in this condition.

Partial or complete absence of the fibula, generally termed *fibular hemimelia,* is not a common affliction in pediatric orthopedics. This entity is usually associated with a partial absence of the foot, although in rare cases the fibula alone may be absent. In addition to the specific problems with the fibula, this entity is usually associated with a short tibia on the same side.[21] Congenital dysplasia of the femur has a high association with fibular hemimelia.

The absence of the fibula produces gross ankle instability. While in some of these children the initial foot deformity may be one of equinovarus, calcaneovalgus usually ensues with weight-bearing because of the absent lateral structures. The combination of severe shortening below the knee with lateral instability of the foot makes this problem extremely difficult to treat. Many of these children eventually do best with Syme's amputation.[22]

Partial or complete absence of the tibia is much less common than congenital absence of the fibula (Fig. 11-15). Treatment of this condition may be by amputation, although in some centers a transfer of the fibula under the remaining tibia has produced acceptable results.

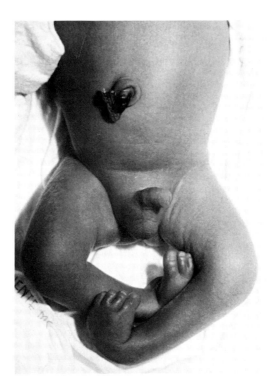

**Fig. 11-16.** Child with arthrogryposis with contractures of both knees and feet. The classic patient has smooth, shiny skin, dimples over the contracted extremity joints, and a small mouth and jaw.

# ARTHROGRYPOSIS

Arthrogryposis, which has been termed a "wastebasket diagnosis," is a collection of congenital contractures and deformities of the extremity. The arthrogryposis syndrome probably results from a variety of causes, including inherited disorders and anterior horn cell diseases. Multiple joint contractures in both the upper and lower extremities may be found in arthrogrypotic patients.

## Classification and Etiology

No single classification of this complex disorder is uniformly accepted owing to the variety of clinical manifestations that exist.

In generalized arthrogryposis, all four limbs and sometimes the spine are involved. Less severe forms such as Möbius syndrome and distal arthrogryposis, usually involve only the hands and feet. Pterygium syndrome with webbing of the popliteal space is also included as a form of arthrogryposis.

Any pathologic process that causes immobility of the extremities in utero can be considered an etiologic agent in arthrogryposis. Infectious agents, including polio virus, drugs, and uterine size and environment are among the etiologic factors. The most consistent finding is a decrease in anterior horn cells in the spinal cord.

Most patients demonstrate markedly thickened joint capsules and intra-articular fibrosis with decreased muscle mass.

## Clinical Features

The classical patient with arthrogryposis multiplex congenita has multiple stiff joints with dislocated hips and resistant clubfeet. Because of similarities, this disease can be thought of as an intrauterine polio with weak muscles, limited joint motion, and intact sensation. This classic patient has smooth, shiny skin, dimples over the joints, and a small mouth and jaw (Fig. 11-16).

Except in distal arthrogryposis, which is sex-linked, the family history is of no benefit in the diagnosis or workup. Affected families do not produce a second child with the classic form of arthrogryposis.

## Treatment

The management of the multiple musculoskeletal deformities of the arthrogrypotic syndromes requires years of perseverance and vigilance. The contractures and dislocations in this "diagnosis" are difficult to treat, and recurrence of the deformity even after optimal treatment is a common outcome.

As described in Chapter 6, aggressive management of

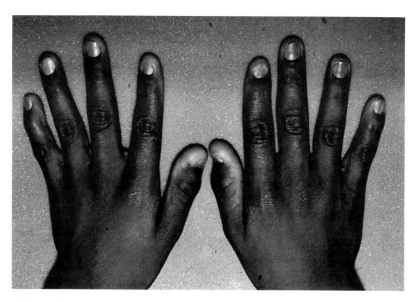

**Fig. 11-17.** Hands of a patient with nail-patella syndrome, showing the progressive radial dysplastic nails.

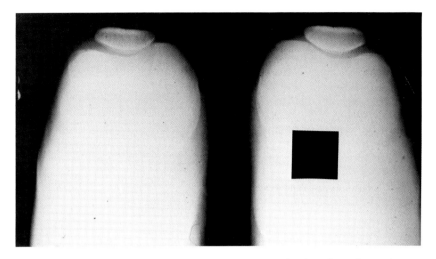

**Fig. 11-18.** Knee radiograph showing the small patellae in nail-patella syndrome.

the clubfoot deformity includes posterior medial release with excision of tendons and soft tissues. Talectomy is usually reserved for deformities that recur after an aggressive posterior and medial release.

The hip dislocations that are frequently found in arthrogryposis are likewise difficult to manage. The dislocations are referred to as teratologic, meaning that the dislocation did not occur in the perinatal period;[23] the hip joint may never have developed in a located position, making reduction impossible.[24] Some arthrogrypotic hips are best left in a dislocated position.

## NAIL-PATELLA SYNDROME

Although the nail-patella syndrome is not rare, affected children do not frequently seek medical management of their problems owing to the general benign nature of the syndrome. The syndrome includes small or even absent patellae, with dysplastic nails on the hands and feet (Figs. 11-17 and 11-18). There is a strong family inheritance in nail-patella syndrome. Various foot deformities, including clubfoot and resistant forefoot abduction, have been encountered. Knee symptoms with patellar dislocation secondary to instability are common.

Management of the deformities of nail-patella syndrome is similar to the care of these problems when they occur in an isolated situation.

## REFERENCES

### Congenital Dislocated Hip

1. Weinstein SL: Natural history of congenital hip dislocation (CDH) and hip dysplasia. Clin Orthop 225:62, 1987
2. Paterson DC: The early diagnosis and treatment of congenital dislocation of the hip. Clin Orthop 119:28, 1976
3. Barlow TG: Early diagnosis and treatment of congenital dislocation of the hip. J Bone Joint Surg [Br] 44:292, 1962
4. MacEwen GD: Treatment of congenital dislocation of the hip in older children. Clin Orthop 225:86, 1987
5. Tönnis D: Normal values of the hip joint for the evaluation of x-rays in children and adults. Clin Orthop 119:39, 1976
6. Bos FA: Treatment of dislocation of the hip, detected in early childhood, based on magnetic resonance imaging. J Bone Joint Surg [Am] 71A:1523, 1989
7. Exner GU: Ultrasound screening for hip dysplasia in neonates. J Pediatr Orthop 8:656, 1988
8. Castelein RM: Ultrasound screening for congenital dysplasia of the hip in newborns: its value. J Pediatr Orthop 8:666, 1988
9. Iwasaki K: Treatment of congenital dislocation of the hip by the Pavlik harness. J Bone Joint Surg [Am] 65:760, 1983
10. Filipe G: Use of the Pavlik harness in treating congenital dislocation of the hip. J Pediatr Orthop 2:357, 1982
11. Schoenecker MD: Congenital dislocation of the hip in children. J Bone Joint Surg [Am] 66:21, 1984
12. Galpin RD: One-stage treatment of congenital dislocation of the hip in older children, including femoral shortening. J Bone Joint Surg [Am] 71:734, 1989

## Legg-Calvé-Perthes Disease

13. Catterall A: The natural history of Perthes' disease. J Bone Joint Surg [Br] 53:37, 1971
14. Phemister PB: Perthes' disease. Surg Gynecol Obstet 33:87, 1921
15. Wamoscher Z: Hereditary Legg-Calvé-Perthes disease. Am J Dis Child 106:131, 1963
16. Abrams J: Legg-Calvé-Perthes disease. Contemp Orthop 10:27
17. Salter RB: Legg-Calvé-Perthes disease. J Bone Joint Surg [Am] 66:479, 1984
18. Stevens PM: Coxa breva: its pathogenesis and a rationale for its management. J Pediatr Orthop 5:515, 1985

## Slipped Capital Femoral Epiphysis

19. Hegerman W: Slipped epiphysis associated with hypothyroidism. J Pediatr Orthop 4:569, 1984
20. Herring JA: Slipped capital femoral epiphysis. J Pediatr Orthop 4:764, 1984

## Tibial and Fibular Dysplasia

21. Anderson L: Syme amputation in children: indications, results, and long-term follow-up. J Pediatr Orthop 4:550, 1984
22. Kruger LM: Amputation and prosthesis as definitive treatment in congenital absence of the fibula. J Bone Joint Surg [Am] 43:625, 1961

## Arthrogryposis

23. Gruel CR: Teratologic dislocation of the hip. J Pediatr Orthop 6:693, 1986
24. Staheli LT: Management of hip dislocations in children with arthrogryposis. J Pediatr Orthop 7:681, 1987

# 12

# Torsional and Frontal Plane Conditions of the Leg and Idiopathic Toe Walking

*RONALD L. VALMASSY*
*STEVEN J. DeVALENTINE*

Structural and positional developmental changes in the lower extremity occur in a continuous and dynamic fashion in the growing child. A thorough knowledge of those that may occur during normal physiologic development is required in order to successfully diagnose and manage any pediatric gait problem. The early years of growth represent the golden years of treatment, wherein the clinician may favorably influence lower extremity development and gait patterns that will be achieved by adolescence.

The clinician's most important function in the management of torsional and frontal plane leg conditions in the growing child is to identify those conditions that will probably not resolve spontaneously with growth. The vast majority of biomechanical lower extremity complaints in children involve flatfoot associated with either an in-toed or out-toed gait pattern. The true etiology of the problem may often lie outside the foot. This chapter attempts to discuss the various transverse and frontal plane developmental changes that occur in the growing child's leg, with particular emphasis upon the manner in which these conditions often influence the development of the child's foot and the resultant gait pattern.

## TRANSVERSE PLANE CONDITIONS

### Torsional and Positional Conditions of the Hip Joint and Femur

The four words most likely to precipitate some degree of anxiety or debate among practitioners dealing with pediatric patients are *antetorsion, anteversion, retrotorsion,* and *retroversion.* Although most clinicians are comfortable with the concept that these words represent, they are often confused when reviewing the literature, in which these four terms are often used interchangeably. For the purposes of this chapter the various rotational problems will be divided into two groups, torsional and positional developmental changes.

This concept can be easily understood if the infant femur is visualized as an isolated entity that is placed on a flat surface with the posterior aspect of the condyles flat against the surface. Closer inspection of the femur will indicate that there is an inherent 30-degree internal angulation of the condyles with respect to the head and neck of the femur. During normal growth, the femur undergoes a gradual external torsional growth of about 20 degrees by age 5 or 6, resulting in an average angle of antetorsion of 8 to 12 degrees.[1-3] If this change does not occur or occurs slowly, an in-toed type of gait will be present.

In some cases this torsional growth may occur very slowly, and the angle may not completely reduce until the age of 13 or 14 years. Gradual reduction may occur at a rate of 1 to 3 degrees per year until adolescence. This slow change explains why some youngsters who appear pigeon-toed for a long time will ultimately appear "normal" when they become teenagers. Approximately 90 percent of those youngsters possessing an internal femoral torsion will outgrow the pathology by adolescence unless, of course, there is a significant familial tendency toward this deformity. In these cases there is little likelihood of the torsional component improving spontaneously over time.

Additionally, it has been reported clinically that youngsters being treated for torsional problems of the femur often demonstrate readily observable angle of gait changes, which seem to correspond to overall growth spurts and increases in height.[1] It is postulated that growth spurts not only affect the length of the long bones but also may contribute in part to transverse plane alterations. In other instances there may be excessive external torsional growth (retrotorsion) of the femoral segment, which may result in external femoral torsion. As this represents an overgrowth, there is generally no treatment that can easily be provided to reverse this problem.[2,4] One must be cautious in informing parents which problems are most likely to resolve with time, as an external femoral torsion or position may appear potentially worse at age 13 to 14, depending on subsequent rotational tendencies.

The positional femoral component is associated with the soft tissue changes that occur during the first few years of development. The infant's femur undergoes a gradual internal rotation relative to the acetabulum from birth. Gradual internal rotation of the entire femoral segment occurs coincidentally with an external torsional growth of the femoral shaft, the overall net effect of which is to place the patella facing directly anterior and parallel to the frontal plane by the age of 5 or 6 years.[3-5] The external femoral position at birth is generally attributed to the externally rotated and abducted position of the fetal lower extremities in utero.[4,6] At birth the neonate will exhibit approximately three times as much ex-

ternal as internal rotation, with about 100 degrees total range of motion (ROM).[5-7]

A gradual reduction of external femoral position must be accompanied by changes in soft tissue structures about the hip, including capsule, ligaments, and muscle. Contracture of the ischiofemoral ligament will produce external femoral position, while contracture of the iliofemoral and pubofemoral ligaments will cause internal femoral position.[2,3] Contracture of the following muscles may be responsible for persistent external femoral position: gluteus maximus, obturator externus, obturator internus, gemelli, quadratus femoris, piriformis, sartorius, adductor magnus, adductor longus, and adductor brevis. Persistent internal femoral position may result from contracture of the iliopsoas, tensor fasciae latae, gluteus medius, and gluteus minimi.

Acetabular position may also influence rotational leg position. Skeletal variations in acetabular position have been reported.[2,6,8] The most common variation, and certainly a normal variant, is one in which the acetabulum is more externally rotated, which complements the overall externally rotated femoral position present in the infant. If, however, the acetabulum is significantly internally placed, it will contribute to an internally positioned limb, a factor that some authors consider to be significant, though commonly overlooked, in the overall development of the angle of gait.[2,4,8]

### Clinical Evaluation

Observation of a child's posturing and gait prior to examination can be very helpful in narrowing the focus of the musculoskeletal examination. The child should be allowed to walk independently while the examiner observes the position of the head, shoulders, and pelvis for signs of limb length discrepancy, scoliosis, muscle weakness, or gross musculoskeletal deformity. The examiner should note patellar position relative to the frontal plane, which normally should range from parallel to this plane (neutral) to slightly external until the age of 5 to 6 years. A neutral patellar position associated with an adducted foot position may indicate the presence of "pseudolack" of malleolar torsion, internal tibial torsion, metatarsus adductus, rigid forefoot valgus, or rigid plantar-flexed first ray deformity. Internal or external patellar position indicates that at least a portion of the transverse plane deformity is within the femoral segment. It is clinically difficult to determine the extent of the involvement at the various levels (femoral, tibial, and foot) solely by visualizing patellar position. Although it is difficult to determine whether an in-toed gait associated with internally facing patellae (often reported as the "squinting patellae" sign) is due to a positional or torsional problem, observation of the angle of gait can be helpful[8,9] (Fig. 12-1). If femoral antetorsion is present, the adducted gait pattern is typically consistent, with little angular deviation of the foot noted from one step to another. When internal femoral position due to tight internal rotator muscles is present, a dynamic adduction of the foot is noted during the late swing and contact phase of gait. A dynamic adduction movement of the foot is most typically associated with tight medial hamstring muscles. However, this movement is quite distinct from the marked adduction noted in children with spastic adductors or hamstrings associated with various types of neurologic deficits. The angle and base of gait, patellar posi-

tion, and extent of calcaneal eversion should all be recorded at the conclusion of this portion of the examination.

Once the gait evaluation is completed, the examiner should evaluate joints with the child unclothed from the waist down and supine either on the examining table or on the parent's lap. The examination should begin with the hip joints and progress distally. The importance of repeated hip examination to rule out dislocated or dislocatable hip in the infant and prewalking child cannot be too strongly emphasized.[9,10] Clinical signs indicative of a possible dislocated hip include redundant skin folds of the thigh, associated with an apparently shortened limb, and asymmetric gluteal folds. A Trendelenburg gait with associated mild shoulder and hip drop, along with a unilateral external leg position, is often noted in the ambulatory child with frank hip dislocation. The evaluation, physical diagnosis, and treatment of congenital dislocated or dislocatable hip is discussed in greater detail in Chapter 11.

Without question, there are numerous methods of determining the range of motion of the hips in the transverse plane. The child may be prone or supine, with knees either extended or flexed. The most accurate assessment of the functional range of hip rotation is obtained with the hip joint in extension. With the hip in flexion, the anterior hip joint capsule and ligament become loose and allow an increased external rotation. A general impression as to the actual available ROM may be achieved by envisioning the face of a clock proximal to the patella,[4,5,9] with an "hour hand" arising in a perpendicular fashion from the center of the patella. When the patella is parallel to the supporting surface, the imaginary hour hand typically reflects a position of 12 o'clock, or zero degrees. Thus, when the leg is internally or externally rotated, each hour designation on the clock represents a 30-degree angular change. For example, a child whose patella achieves a maximum externally rotated position of 2 o'clock would have a 60-degree external rotation of that hip. More accurate measurements of internal and external hip motion can be obtained by measuring the amount of motion available with a goniometer, first in the hip-flexed and then in the hip-extended position (Fig. 12-2). Elevation of the child's contralateral buttock from the examination table during external rotation or of the ipsilateral buttock during internal rotation indicates the end point of the ROM and can easily result in an inaccurate measurement. One should also note

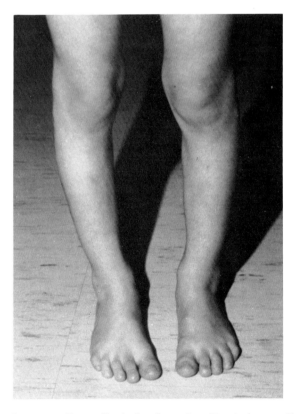

**Fig. 12-1.** Internally deviated patellae ("squinting patella sign"), indicating the presence of an internal rotation in the femoral segment (e.g., internal femoral position or torsion).

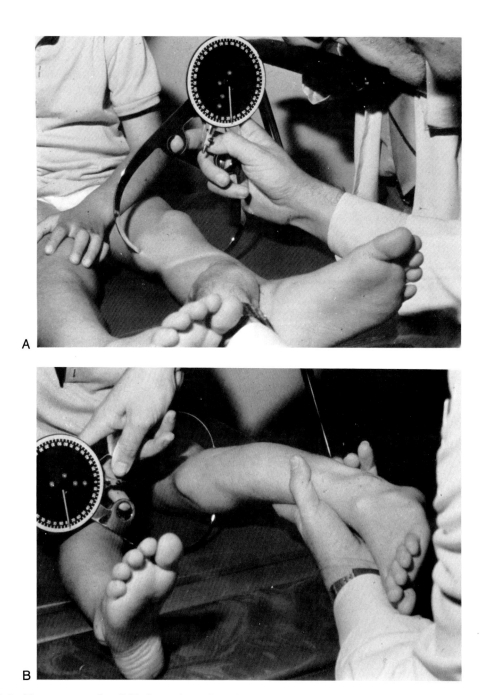

**Fig. 12-2.** Measurement of available femoral rotation using a goniometer. This child has (**A**) 25 degrees of external rotation and (**B**) near 80 degrees of internal rotation available in the hip-flexed position, which is consistent with internal femoral position or torsion.

whether the end of the ROM is soft and spongy or abrupt and bony in nature. Normally, children should demonstrate greater external than internal rotation of the femoral segment up to the age of 6 or 7, anywhere from two to three times as much external as internal rotation being present at that age. The total transverse plane ROM may be anywhere from 100 to 120 degrees at birth.[1,3] There is a gradual progression toward equalization of internal and external hip rotation from infancy to skeletal maturity, with reduction in total ROM to approximately 80 degrees. Any significant variation of these values may be accompanied by lower extremity gait disturbance.[3-5]

Evaluation of the quality of the end point ROM, as well as any quantitative variation in ROM between the hip-flexed and the hip-extended position, will help to differentiate between torsional (osseous) and positional problems. A ROM that remains essentially unchanged regardless of the hip position and is accompanied by a bony or abrupt feeling at its end typically indicates a femoral torsion problem (internal or external). Conversely, a ROM that varies with the hip in the flexed versus the extended position and is accompanied by a spongy feel at its end typically indicates a femoral position problem (internal or external).[3-5] For example, if one measured 80 degrees of internal hip rotation and 30 degrees of external hip rotation in both the hip-extended and the hip-flexed position and the end of the ROM were abrupt or "bony" in nature, that patient's clinical presentation would be consistent with an internal femoral torsion (antetorsion). Conversely, 90 degrees of external rotation with 10 degrees of internal rotation in both the hip-extended and the hip-flexed position, with that same bony feel at the end of the ROM, would be consistent with an external femoral torsion (retrotorsion).[3,4]

On the other hand, if examination revealed 60 degrees of internal rotation and 30 degrees of external rotation with the hip extended and a similar amount of internal rotation and 60 degrees of external rotation with the hip flexed, one should suspect soft tissue contracture. In this example, contracture of the pubofemoral, iliofemoral, or ligamentum teres should be suspected, since these structures, if contracted, will limit external rotation with the hip extended but are relaxed in the hip-flexed position and therefore will no longer limit external rotation. When external rotation is comparatively limited in the hip-flexed position, one should suspect a hamstring contracture. In this instance, specific evaluation of the ham-

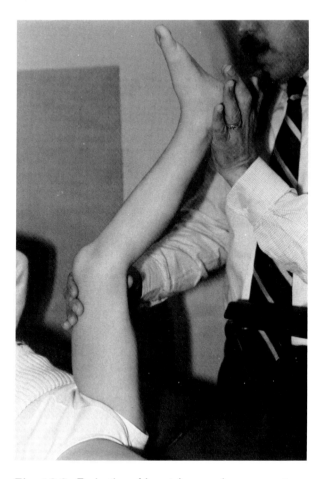

**Fig. 12-3.** Evaluation of hamstring muscle group contracture. The hip is flexed 90 degrees, and maximum knee extension is measured.

strings would be necessary to complete the examination[5] (Fig. 12-3). External femoral position may also result in a discrepancy in hip-flexed versus hip-extended ROM. If available internal rotation increases, with the hip moving from an extended to a flexed position or vice versa, or if a limited amount of internal rotation is noted only with the hip flexed and knee extended, a contracture of the lateral hamstring should be suspected. If limitation of internal rotation is present only with the hip in an extended position, one must suspect a contracture of the iliopsoas.[2,3]

Torsional and positional problems may also coexist in the same patient. Individuals whose initial problems are primarily positional are probably less likely to develop torsional abnormalities while children whose initial problems are torsional are more likely to develop secondary coexisting soft tissue contracture.

## Tibial Torsion

Most researchers agree that there is very little if any external rotation of the tibia relative to the fibula at birth. Postnatally, however, a gradual external torsional growth of the tibia relative to the fibula of approximately 18 to 23 degrees occurs.[1,3,11-13] True tibial torsion can be measured radiographically or by computed tomography (CT). As we are unable to clinically measure true tibial torsion, malleolar position, which is measured as the angle formed by a line bisecting the malleoli and a line parallel to the frontal plane, is used as an indicator of tibial torsion. Malleolar position (or *tibiofibular rotation,* as it has been termed by various authors) changes in a slow, gradual fashion from year to year, with approximately 13 to 18 degrees of external malleolar position being noted by the age of 7 to 8 years. Whereas external femoral rotation may occur up to 13 to 14 years of age, external rotation of the tibial component is generally completed by the age of 7 to 8 years.[12-14]

Additionally, one should distinguish between a low tibial or malleolar torsion and an internal tibial or malleolar torsion. Internal or negative tibial torsion (measuring less than zero) is certainly less likely to be outgrown, as the tibia has not even attained the position that should be present at birth. On the other hand, 5 degrees of external malleolar torsion in a 4-year-old who should possess approximately 8 degrees of tibial torsion is certainly a much less significant problem. Valmassy and Stanton, in a study of 281 schoolchildren between 1½ and 6 years of age, found a gradual and consistent increase in external malleolar position from 5.5 degrees at 1½ years to 11.2 degrees at 6 years of age.[15] Their data were consistent with the values reported by previous authors, indicating that a normal adult position of 13 degrees to 18 degrees of the transmalleolar position is usually achieved by the age of 7 to 8 years.

### Clinical Evaluation

Measurement of tibial or malleolar torsion is accomplished with the child lying supine or seated, with the knee in extension. If the measurement is performed with the knee flexed to 90 degrees and there is an element of internal tibial position present, then the measurement of true tibial or malleolar torsion may be altered. The femoral condyles are placed equidistant from the supporting surface, with the patella in the frontal plane. If the examiner's thumb and index fingers are placed anterior and posterior to each malleolus, visual interpretation of this finger position will allow initial determination of whether an internal or external tibial torsion is present (Fig. 12-4A). The foot should be positioned at a 90-degree angle to the leg with the subtalar joint in neutral position to facilitate visual determination of the transmalleolar axis and to avoid an artificial internal or external leg position such as may be produced by a retrograde closed kinetic chain pronation or supination of the foot.[15] A tractograph or goniometer may be utilized to document the actual amount of either internal or external tibial torsion that is present (Fig. 12-4B).

## Positional Conditions of the Knee Joint

As with most major joints of the upper and lower extremity, transverse plane motion at the knee joint is quite large at birth and throughout infancy but decreases rapidly over the first few years of life. The total range of transverse plane motion in infants and young children may be anywhere from zero to 15 to 20 degrees with the knee extended and may exceed 35 to 45 degrees with the knee in full flexion.[2,3] If the development of the knee as well as its surrounding ligamentous and muscular attachments proceeds in a normal fashion, there will be no interruption in the development of a normal angle of gait. However, if contracture of the medial ligamentous or muscular structures occurs through failure of reduction of the in utero position or through muscular imbalance, an asymmetry of the internal versus external ROM at the knee will occur. In these cases the tibia will develop and then function in an internally rotated position. Just as we can diagnose an internal femoral position versus an internal femoral torsion, we should be able to diagnose the presence of an internal tibial position versus an internal tibial torsion.

Internal tibial position has been referred to in the past as *pseudolack of malleolar torsion.*[3,9,10] This term, or the equivalent term *pseudomalleolar torsion,* is somewhat confusing at first, but it is an accurate description of the clinical presentation: the child's foot is adducted and the knee functions on the frontal plane, which gives the impression of a low or internal tibial torsion. In those

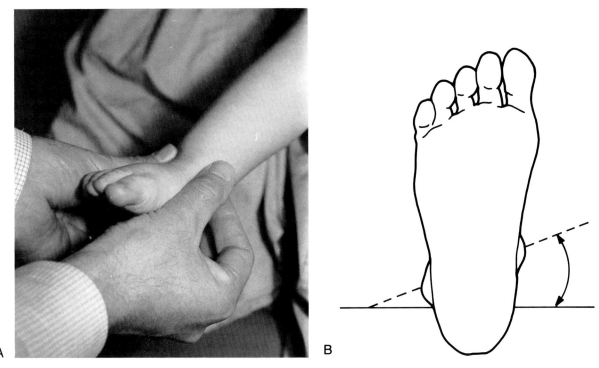

**Fig. 12-4.** (**A**) Evaluation of tibial torsion using malleolar position. The examiner's thumb and index fingers are placed anterior and posterior to each malleolus. (**B**) The angle between an imaginary line bisecting the malleoli and the frontal plane (with patella parallel to frontal plane) estimates the degree of tibial torsion. A tractograph or goniometer may be used to measure this angle.

cases in which normal tibial torsion is present, the resultant deformity has been attributed to a hypermobile or loose knee.

In a child with an in-toed gait, whose patella is parallel to the frontal plane, the cause of the in-toed gait must be distal to the femoral segment. If tibial torsion is normal and no abnormality of the foot is present, the in-toed gait must result from an internal position at the knee joint itself.

In a normally developing infant and child up to the age of 3 to 4 years, typically little rotation would be noted in the child's knee with full extension, as the knee would be locked in this position.

## Clinical Evaluation

With different steps the affected foot of a child with internal tibial position will often strike the ground in a slightly different position in the transverse plane. This is the effect of soft tissue contracture about the knee joint. Additionally, there may be a greater tendency toward tripping and instability in gait.[10] In the non-weight-bearing examination of the post-toddler child, minimal transverse motion should be detected at the knee joint with the knee extended. With minimal flexion, however, overall transverse plane motion usually increases markedly. The amount of internal and external rotation available at the child's flexed knee joint from the resting position should be approximately equal. If, however, more internal than external rotation is available, internal tibial position is present. If the relative amounts of internal and external rotation of the tibia at the knee joint change with hip extension and flexion, the contracture of muscles that cross the knee is the primary deforming force. However, if the tibial rotation remains essentially unchanged with hip extension and flexion, one would suspect knee ligament contracture as the primary etiology.

Internal tibial position is generally found only in the early walking child and is often considered to be self-limiting. The early walking child's gait pattern is one of knee flexion with whole foot contact at heel strike. Knee extension occurs much later than at heel contact and only for brief periods. Thus, if the knee remains flexed for a prolonged time, especially at heel contact and especially if the medial soft tissue structures are tight, one can easily envision the end result to be an in-toed gait.[2,4,5] As the child approaches 3 to 4 years of age, a more normal gait with full knee extension at heel contact will occur, thus usually eliminating the adducted gait associated with internal tibial position unless a soft tissue contracture has developed.

## FRONTAL PLANE CONDITIONS
### Coxa Vara and Coxa Valga

Coxa vara and coxa valga are relatively rare but are the clinically most significant frontal plane conditions affecting femoral segment alignment. Coxa vara and valga describe a varus or valgus alignment of the femoral head and neck relative to the femoral shaft and can be quantified by measuring the angle of femoral inclination, which is formed in the frontal plane between the long axis of the head and neck of the femur and the long axis of the femoral shaft. This angle is 140 to 150 degrees in neonates and normally reduces to 120 to 132 degrees (average 128 degrees) in the first 6 years of development.[3,16]

*Coxa valga* is defined as a lack of reduction of the angle of femoral inclination to a normal value (128 degrees). It may result from a lack of normal development of the head and neck of the femur relative to the femoral shaft (i.e., dysplasia, usually bilateral) or from some type of trauma (typically unilateral). Hip subluxation or dislocation is frequently present along with an awkward gait in this rare, usually congenital condition. Genu varum may occur secondary to coxa valga deformity.

*Coxa vara* is defined as an over-reduction of the angle of femoral inclination to a value significantly less than 128 degrees. It may be congenital or developmental and may be associated with slipped capital femoral epiphysis or may be secondary to overgrowth or trauma. Coxa vara is difficult to evaluate in radiographs of very young infants and is usually noticed when the child begins to walk. The leg is shorter on the affected side, and its abduction is restricted, as well as its internal rotation. Coxa vara may cause genu valgum.

## Genu Varum and Genu Valgum

Physiologic (normal) genu varum in infants and young children results from a combination of the small amount of normal lateral bowing of the femur and tibia combined with the physiologic coxa valga. It is commonly seen in the infant and early walker and may be present from birth until 4 years of age[4,17] (see Fig. 1-7). Physiologic genu varum may be exaggerated by either an internal rotation of the femoral segment or an internal tibial torsion, both of which will externally rotate the lateral aspect of the posterior calf musculature, thus tending to exaggerate the overall clinical appearance of a normal frontal plane bowing of the knee.[5] Diseases or dysplasias of the physes about the knee joint (e.g., rickets, Blount's disease, and asymmetric epiphyseal development) may also contribute to or mimic genu varum and must be considered within the differential diagnosis both when excessive bowing is present and when genu varum deformity fails to reduce significantly by the age of 4 years.[2,4,7]

Physiologic (normal) genu valgum occurs to some extent in most children. Usually, it is first noticed between 3 and 5 years of age, following the normal period of physiologic genu varum, and persists for several years before it is eventually outgrown by about 8 years of age[4] (see Fig. 1-7). Genu valgum that persists into adolescence is less likely to be outgrown when significant deformity is present, distal femoral epiphyseodesis or osteotomy may be necessary. Physiologic genu valgum probably develops owing to a varying rate of growth of the medial and lateral femoral condyles. Overgrowth of the medial femoral condyle in infants and toddlers as part of normal development and secondary to the differential compression effect of early weight-bearing on the physis probably contibutes to genu valgum in the post-toddler stage. Depending upon varying hereditary, physiologic, and local factors (e.g., weight, trauma, infection), varying degrees of genu valgum may develop.[4] With further growth and increasing pressure on the lateral physes of the knee joint, gradual spontaneous reduction of genu valgum usually occurs.

The clinician's primary task in the evaluation of children with genu varum and valgum is (1) to determine whether the condition is physiologic or secondary to some other disease process or mechanical abnormality; and (2) if it is physiologic, to determine if the degree of deformity is within acceptable developmental parameters to allow spontaneous correction. The clinician will also need to assess the extent to which the foot pronates in the child with genu valgum. The temporary use of orthotics and appropriate shoewear may be necessary to prevent the development of progressive or rigid pes valgus deformity.

### Clinical Evaluation

Angular measurement of genu varum or valgum can be accomplished either clinically or radiographically with the child supine or standing. Angular measurements greater than 15 to 30 degrees should be evaluated and followed closely. Measurements can be made by measuring the distance between the knee in genu varum or between the malleoli in genu valgum. When this indirect method is used, the knees or malleoli (depending upon whether genu valgum or varum is present) are brought together with the child supine, and the distance between the knees or malleoli is recorded and followed. Morley reported the following grading system for indirect measurement of genu valgum based upon a random examination of 1,000 children: grade I, intermalleolar distance less than 2.5 cm; grade II, 2.5 to 5.0 cm; grade III, 5.0 to 7.5 cm; and grade IV greater than 7.5 cm.[18] Additionally, Morley stated that approximately 74 percent of children between 3 and 3½ years of age had a greater than 2.5 cm distance between their malleoli, while 22 percent had 5.0 cm or more.

## Tibia Vara and Tibia Valga

Tibia vara often occurs in association with genu varum, contributing to the overall physiologic bowing of the legs that is common from birth to the age of 2 to 4 years. As much as 5 to 10 degrees of normal frontal plane bowing may be present at birth. This gradually reduces to 2 to 3 degrees (normal adult value) at approximately 2 to 4 years of age.[3,13] More than 5 degrees of tibial bowing will require some degree of compensation at the subtalar joint in order to allow the calcaneus to assume a vertical position with respect to the ground. In cases in which the degree of tibia vara exceeds the subtalar joint's range of pronation, the heel will remain in a varus attitude throughout the gait cycle. This may lead to chronic lateral instability or to the development of a retrocalcaneal exostosis, or "pump bump."

The differential diagnosis for severe bowing of the tibial segment must also include rickets and Blount's disease. Although rickets is not commonly seen, one must be aware of this possibility when evaluating the infant with marked genicular or tibial bowing. Rickets may be caused by chronic renal insufficiency and hypophosphatasia.[4,9] The resulting disturbance in calcium and phosphorus metabolism causes inadequate calcification of the soft tissue matrix, which is radiographically most evident at the ends of long bones, the most active sites of osteogenesis in the growing child. Generalized muscular weakness, lethargy, various skeletal abnormalities, and bowing of the lower extremity long bones are common clinical findings. Radiographic findings include thickening and haziness of the physis, widened epiphyses with "frayed" metaphyseal borders, coarse trabeculae, and decreased cortical density. Abnormalities of serum calcium and phosphorus may also be present.

Blount's disease is due to a growth disturbance of the medial aspect of the proximal tibial epiphysis, which results in progressive medial angulation of the tibia at the proximal medial epiphyses and metaphyses of the tibia. Blount's disease may occur in infancy and early childhood or in adolescence. The infant form is seen in the 1- to 3-year-old and is most classically associated with a chubby, active child who was an early walker (who typically began to walk prior to 9 months of age). Increased mechanical pressure at the proximal medial physis of the tibia is probably a significant factor in the development and/or progression of the tibia vara deformity. The adolescent type usually presents between 8 and 13 years of age and is probably due to partial physeal arrest. A history of trauma may be present. Radiographic characteristics of infantile Blount's include an acute medial angulation of the tibia just below the knee and widening and beaking of the medial metaphysis and physis.

Tibia valga is extremely rare. When it does occur, it generally results from a physeal injury or malunion of a tibial fracture. In evaluating the various possible etiologies of flexible flatfoot deformity, an anteroposterior view of the ankle is necessary to rule out any abnormal force generated by a valgus ankle joint, with or without tibia valga.

## TREATMENT OF TRANSVERSE AND FRONTAL PLANE CONDITIONS

The treatment of transverse and frontal plane variations of the lower extremity in children is a highly controversial subject. Recommendations by various authors and clinical researchers have run the gamut from aggressive splinting to benign neglect. The decision to prescribe some form of mechanical treatment should be based upon a sound knowledge of normal lower extremity development. One should ask the following questions before considering treatment: (1) Is the transverse or frontal plane variation physiologic and considered within the normal expected range for the child's age? (2) If the condition is physiologic and is expected to resolve spontaneously, will it do so without resulting in any significant permanent compensatory joint or foot deformity (e.g., pronated foot)? (3) Is reasonable evidence available that the proposed mechanical treatment is effective at the level of deformity and can be used with acceptable compliance?

## The Decision to Treat

If the physical examination of a child with an in-toed gait is consistent with a physiologic type of torsional or positional transverse or frontal plane leg condition that is appropriate for the child's age and development and if there is no gait instability or detrimental pronatory compensation, the child should not be treated but only followed. Parents should be provided reassurance that in-toeing will gradually improve (provided that it is not

familial and present in *adult* members of the family). Severe familial antetorsion may be treated with night splints (e.g., Denis-Browne bar or Ganley or Langer counter-rotation splints), but the effectiveness of these devices in treating the more severe hereditary types of in-toeing may be limited and has not been well documented. Children with severe hereditary types of antetorsion may eventually require derotational osteotomy.

Moderate to severe pronatory compensation of the foot associated with in-toeing due to transverse plane abnormalities (e.g., internal position or torsion) should probably be treated with a combination of night splints and custom foot orthoses so that the normal structural development of the child's foot may possibly be preserved.

## Splints

Traditional treatment of transverse plane variation has included the use of various types of night splints. Opinions concerning the effectiveness of such splints vary considerably. Most children with a transverse plane deformity assume sitting and sleeping attitudes that tend to be positions of comfort or reinforcement of their rotational problems (Fig. 12-5). Although parents may admonish children to stop sitting with legs tucked under-

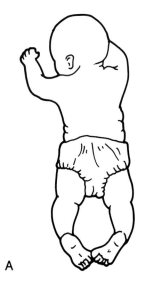 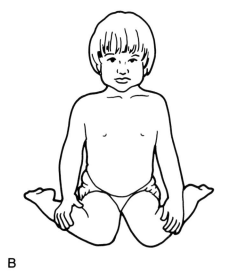

**Fig. 12-5.** Children with transverse plane rotational conditions of the legs tend to assume sleeping and sitting positions of comfort, which may perpetuate in-toeing or delay improvement. (**A**) Typical infant sleeping position that would contribute to internal femoral or tibial torsion or position. (**B**) Typical sitting position of the toddler or older child with internal femoral torsion (antetorsion).

neath their buttocks and encourage cross-legged or straight-legged position while playing, it is not easy to alter an abnormal sleeping position. I (R. L. V.) believe that night splints can often exert a positive influence in preventing children from assuming sleeping and resting positions that promote transverse plane abnormalities and thereby decrease the likelihood of normal spontaneous resolution.

Many authors agree that although a splint may be effective in cases of internal tibial position or internal tibial torsion, there is apparently no indication for the use of splints for femoral rotation problems. Although opinions vary as to whether or not the correction actually occurs within the long axis of the tibia or within the soft tissues surrounding the knee, the fact remains that one may generally attain a measurable clinical difference following the completion of therapy.[2,4]

### General Guidelines

Regardless of which of the available splints one chooses to utilize, a few general guidelines apply to all the devices. In treating internal rotation problems, one must be careful not to sublux any lower extremity joints, including those of the developing child's foot, which is one of the common abnormal sequelae of long-term night splint use. One must remember that when the child's foot is markedly abducted via a night splint, the first areas to be affected are the midtarsal and subtalar joints of the foot. Excessive, prolonged abduction can lead to a severe flatfoot deformity unless certain precautions are maintained. When more rigid splints are used, placing a varus wedge in the child's shoes or introducing a 10- to 15-degree varus bend into the bar may help prevent pronatory subluxation of the foot. Additionally, one should not vigorously exceed the normally available amount of external rotation present. Setting a splint at an extremely deviated position that greatly exceeds the total amount of external rotation present not only will make the bar uncomfortable for the child but also may lead to avascular necrosis of the head of the femur. The total range of external rotation available at the hip, knee, and tibia should be carefully assessed, and the foot position should be set accordingly.[9] Bar types of night splints should be used cautiously in infants with apparent external position or torsion, since these conditions are generally physiologic until at least 1 year of age and splinting of the hip in internal rotation can promote subluxation or dislocation, which may be very difficult to recognize.

If it is decided to utilize a splint, parents should be aware of the protracted nature of the treatment plan and be prepared to use the splint for at least 1 year in some cases. If marked, measurable change is not evident after 1 year of use, a change in the type of splint used or abandonment of splinting as a method of treatment should be considered. In any event, night splint therapy can be a useful modality in the overall management of the child with transverse plane pathology. The initial decision as to whether or not to splint should be based on the child's age, extent and level of deformity, and overall degree of compensation in gait.

## Developmental Changes

Significant variation in transverse and/or frontal plane alignment of the lower extremities generally results in the transmission of an abnormal pronatory force to the developing child's foot. A child's foot undergoes structural changes over the first 7 to 8 years of life. When a child first stands and ambulates, the feet are "fat, flat, and floppy," with no discernible arch and an apropulsive gait. This appearance and function reflect an everted calcaneus and an enlarged medial fat pad, along with a tendency to place the entire foot flat on the supporting surface with each step in order to attain greater stability. A child's foot may be everted by as much as 5 to 10 degrees (approximately 7 to 8 on the average) at the onset of weight-bearing (Fig. 12-6A). The everted calcaneus of the toddler normally reduces to neutral (perpendicular) by the age of 7 or 8. The enlarged arch fat pad gradually disappears, and the foot takes on the overall anatomic characteristics of the adult foot. At approximately 3 to 4 years of age, the child's improved proprioceptive capabilities allow a heel-to-toe type of gait, as opposed to the full foot contact type of gait associated with the early walker.[5,13]

There is a helpful clinical formula that may be used in screening a child's foot development to determine whether or not the amount of calcaneal eversion is appropriate for that particular child's age. The everted position of the toddler's heel generally reduces by about 1 degree per year until it reaches the perpendicular (to the ground) position at age 7 or 8. This information may be expressed by the following rule: 7 less the child's age equals the normal degree of calcaneal eversion in stance that should be present between the ages of 1 and 8 years. For example, if one were examining a 4-year-old child, the rule would indicate a 3-degree everted calcaneal po-

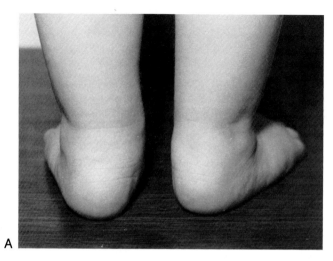

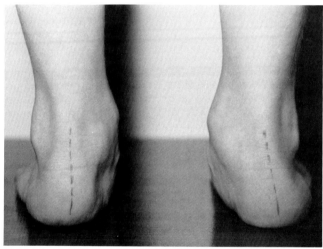

**Fig. 12-6.** (A) Normal calcaneal stance position and appearance of the early walking child. (B) Abnormal degree of calcaneal eversion in an older child.

sition (7 minus 4 years). This formula can be most helpful in evaluating the effect of abnormal transverse and frontal plane forces due to lower extremity torsional or positional problems in the child's foot (Fig. 12-6B).

An internal femoral or tibial torsion or position will also cause adduction of the talus. The internal position of the leg and talus precipitates a closed kinetic chain type of pronatory effect on the developing child's foot, which will maintain or aggravate the already pronated and everted attitude of the foot (Fig. 12-7). When a child reaches an age of self-awareness (4 to 5 years), the pronated foot position may also increase owing to a voluntary attempt to compensate for an in-toed gait.[1,2]

An external femoral or tibial torsion or position may also precipitate or aggravate a significant pes planus (Fig. 12-8). A markedly abducted gait secondary to an external rotational problem will certainly displace the subtalar joint axis farther away from the body, thus increasing the eversion force at the subtalar joint. A significant genu valgum will likewise impose an abnormal pronatory force on the developing child's foot.[15]

## Orthoses

If the lower extremity evaluation reveals that a pathologic pronatory compensation is occurring within a child's foot secondary to a transverse or frontal plane leg abnormality or if there is a history of unsteadiness or

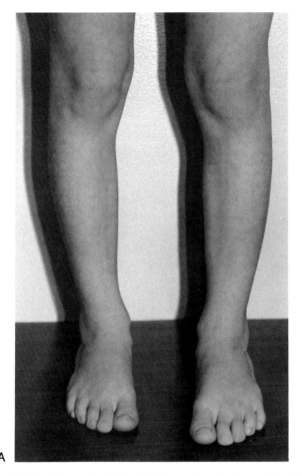 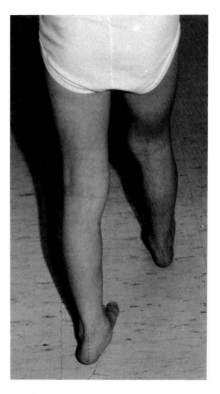

A        B

**Fig. 12-7.** Abnormal subtalar joint pronation in stance (**A**) and in gait (**B**), produced as a compensatory effect of internal femoral and tibial torsion.

fatigue with normal activities, some form of functional foot orthosis should probably be employed (see chapter 13). Although one might use a Root type of functional foot orthosis in these cases, the eversion force at the subtalar joint may be so excessive that a more aggressive type of control may be necessary. A University of California Biomechanic Laboratory (UCBL) orthosis has proved effective at controlling the abnormal pronation secondary to pedal compensation of transverse plane abnormalities of the leg. Two types of heel stabilizers have also been used to manage this type of problem. A type B stabilizer is useful if the foot is mildly or moderately pronated. A type C heel stabilizer, which has a larger medial and lateral flange, is appropriate if the foot demonstrates a greater degree of pes planus, with or without a torsional component.[2,4]

The Blake type of inverted foot orthosis, which relies on a cast modification that markedly inverts the calcaneus relative to the forefoot, is probably one of the most effective devices in managing the pediatric pronated foot secondary to compensation of transverse plane leg conditions.[19] This orthosis, typically structured with a deep heel cup of 20 to 25 mm and a rearfoot post, combines some of the best characteristics of the Root type of orthosis and a heel stabilizer both in improving function and in disallowing abnormal pronatory compensation.

In cases in which a child functions with an internal femoral position and an adducted gait, one may utilize either a gait plate or a type D heel stabilizer. Both of these will promote a more abducted gait. However, this may be accomplished at the expense of a mild increase in rearfoot pronation and for that reason should be utilized

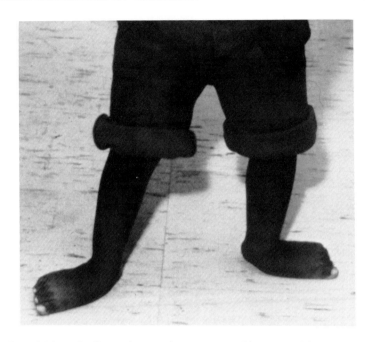

**Fig. 12-8.** Marked bilateral talipes calcaneovalgus aggravated by external femoral and tibial torsion.

selectively. Gait plates are fabricated with a rigid extension plantar to the fourth and fifth metatarsophalangeal joints, which alters propulsion so that the child is forced to pronate and abduct the foot in gait.[5] A gait plate orthosis is designed to improve the cosmetic appearance of the foot and to dynamically assist in stretching tight medial leg muscles that may be contributing to an internal femoral or tibial position. These devices may also be appropriate for the older child with a torsional component, who may function more efficiently in a more abducted position. Because these devices are ineffective once the lateral part of the orthosis is proximal to the fourth and fifth metatarsophalangeal joints, they require more frequent replacement than other types of orthoses.

If one chooses to utilize one of the functional foot orthoses to restrict abnormal pronation due to compensation of a transverse plane leg condition, the parents should be made aware that orthoses are likely to worsen the overall cosmetic appearance of the child. For example, the child with an adducted gait who demonstrates 7 degrees of calcaneal eversion during gait will exhibit an approximately 5- to 7-degree increase in adducted foot position if the heel is controlled in a vertical position. It is important to explain to parents that although in-toeing is worsened, overall foot function in gait is improved and

reduction of in-toeing can be expected with growth. Parents should also be made aware that orthoses will only be effective for approximately 1 to 2 years. Once the child's foot has grown enough that the distal aspect of the orthosis contacts the midshaft portion of the metatarsals, the orthosis becomes ineffective and uncomfortable and must be replaced.

## IDIOPATHIC TOE WALKING

Early walking patterns found in normal children are significantly different and vary considerably more among individuals than do typical adult gait patterns. The toddler usually walks with the hips and knees slightly flexed and the ankle neutral to slightly extended, with a more limited and primitive lower extremity movement pattern.[20] The entire sole of the foot contacts the support surface at the beginning of the stance phase of gait in the majority of children (as opposed to the normal adult type of heel contact) owing to the abnormal flexed hip and knee posture of the lower extremity.

The position in which the foot contacts the support surface (plantar-flexed, neutral, or dorsiflexed) varies considerably among children and even in the same child until a normal adult type of walking pattern has developed by the age of 3 to 4 years. Tiptoe walking is quite commonly seen at the onset of walking in normal children, but almost always yields to a normal heel-toe type of gait within 3 to 6 months.[21] Intermittent toe walking may be present in normal children until 7 years of age, but a well developed heel contact type of gait pattern is the rule by 1½ years of age.[22]

Toe walking may also be a presenting finding in children with various neuromuscular diseases, which have to be considered in the differential diagnosis and eliminated before a diagnosis of idiopathic toe walking (ITW) can be made. The differential diagnosis for ITW should include the following conditions: cerebral palsy, Duchenne muscular dystrophy, peroneal muscular atrophy, dystonia musculorum deformans, tethered cord syndrome, spinal cord tumor, acute myopathies, congenital gastrosoleus muscle contracture, and apparent (i.e., congenital dislocation of the hip [CDH]) or real limb length discrepancy.[22,23] A thorough perinatal and family history, as well as a complete neurologic examination, is essential. A serum creatinine phosphokinase screen should be considered to rule out muscular disease, and a magnetic resonance imaging (MRI) scan may be considered to rule out occult spinal dysraphism or tethered cord syndrome.

## Etiology and Results of Clinical Research

Persistent toe walking in children was first reported in 1967 by Hall et al.,[24] who described 20 toe walking children with an average age of 7½ years, all of whom had normal neurologic examinations. Seven of these children, who were initially suspected of having some neuromuscular pathology, had normal appearing electromyelograms (EMGs), and two had normal histologic findings upon muscle biopsy. Hall et al. termed this condition *congenital short tendo calcaneus* and believed that it represented a true Achilles tendon contracture. All of their patients underwent Achilles tendon lengthening, with good results reported in all cases.

Griffin et al. compared dynamic gait EMG studies of six children with ITW with those of six normal children who were asked to walk with a tiptoe gait.[25] They did not find abnormal swing phase gastrosoleus activity in either group during a normal heel-toe type of gait (children with ITW were able to walk heel-toe with concentration). Gastrosoleus activity was present, however, in both groups during 20 to 30 percent of swing phase during toe-toe gait, with no significant difference between normal children and those with ITW. The anterior tibial muscle demonstrated increased amplitude and prolonged duration of action as well as overlap of gastrosoleus activity in both groups during toe-toe gait. In summary, Griffin found no significant EMG differences in gait between normal children and those with ITW. All of the latter children also reverted to normal heel-toe gait EMG patterns after cast stretching with re-establishment of normal ankle ROM. They concluded that ITW was habitual or mechanical in etiology.

Kalen et al. studied 18 children with ITW and compared them with 14 normal controls (who were instructed to walk tiptoe) and 13 children with mild spastic diplegia.[22] They compared dynamic gait EMG data of all three groups with data on normal heel-toe gait and found the onset of gastrosoleus activity to be premature compared with normal gait in all three groups. The onset and cessation of gastrosoleus activity in the mildly spastic children and those with ITW were virtually identical, matching each other much more closely than the control group. Kalen et al. concluded that the behavior of patients with ITW as determined by EMG is similar to that of children with mild cerebral palsy and children with mechanical equinus (normal control group walking tiptoe). They suggested that ITW could be due to an as yet unknown central nervous system defect, but they could not rule out an entirely mechanical (equinus contracture) etiology.

A positive family history of toe walking and learning disabilities is not unusual. Kalen et al. found 10 (71 percent) of 14 children with ITW in their study to have a positive family history.[22] Of these 14 children, 6 (43 percent) had a history of learning disability. Accardo and Whitman found toe walking to frequently be present in children with developmental disabilities.[26] They reported the following frequency of toe walking in various subgroups of 799 developmentally disabled children: autism, 62.9 percent; communication disorders, 40.2 percent; mental retardation, 35.8 percent; and learning disabilities, 20 percent.

In summary, the etiology of ITW is unknown. It is possible that a clinically undetectable central nervous system abnormality may be responsible; however, it is equally possible that the condition may result from mild mechanical contracture in utero or from habitual early toe walking followed by mechanical contracture.

## Clinical Features

Most studies have shown idiopathic toe walking to be two to three times more common in boys than in girls.[22,27] The perinatal and developmental history and the physical and neurologic examination of children with ITW are generally unremarkable. These children begin walking at a normal age (about 12 months) but only walk tiptoe and generally do not exhibit improvement over time (Fig. 12-9). They are able to walk heel-toe upon command and occasionally will do so intermittently, but the toe-toe gait is more comfortable for them and requires less effort. The only finding on physical examination is a limitation of ankle dorsiflexion (usually zero degrees or less) in the knee-extended position. On the other hand, children with cerebral palsy and other upper motor neuron lesions usually display signs of spasticity, including hypertonic and pathologic reflexes and increased muscle tone. Children with muscular dystrophy may present as toe walkers and be difficult to distinguish from those with ITW. EMG and muscle biopsy may be helpful.

Hicks et al. published kinematic data obtained by three-dimensional motion studies comparing children with ITW and children with mild spastic diplegia.[27] They

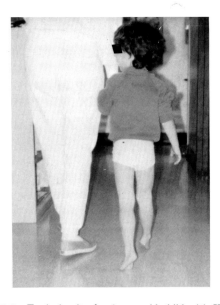

**Fig. 12-9.** Typical gait of a 6-year-old child with ITW. Although the child is able to make heel contact upon request, he has walked only on tiptoes since onset of walking at 12 months of age.

found that ankle motion during gait was considerably less but more varied in the ITW group. The children with ITW walked with the foot maintained in a plantar-flexed position, with the knee in extension or hyperextension, while the children with cerebral palsy walked with the foot in a less plantar-flexed or even neutral to dorsiflexed position, with the knee flexed. Neither group exhibited heel contact, but for different reasons; in the ITW group the cause was limited ankle dorsiflexion, and in the cerebral palsy group it was hamstring contracture. The primary modes of compensation in ITW were abducted gait (averaging 6 degrees greater than normal); and knee hyperextension (averaging 7 degrees greater than normal). Hicks et al. suggested that children with ITW may compensate for ankle equinus over time by developing external tibial torsion.

## Treatment

ITW is, by definition, a diagnosis of exclusion. The clinician should make every effort to rule out neurologic or other etiologies of toe walking before assigning a diagnosis of ITW. The clinical hallmarks of ITW (normal neurologic examination, constant and persistent toe walking since the onset of walking, and lack of normal ankle dorsiflexion) will help to distinguish occasional "normal" toe walking from ITW.

Some authors and clinicians have stated that ITW spontaneously resolves as children grow and increased body weight forces heel contact during gait. Although spontaneous resolution does occur in some cases, the clinician should not become complacent about this condition. Some children with ITW develop a progressively more rigid equinus contracture, which results in secondary compensation through knee hyperextension (genu recurvatum), external tibial torsion, and pronation of the foot. Very young children with ITW should be followed closely.

Manual stretching of the gastrosoleus muscles in the very young child can be carried out by parents. If spontaneous improvement does not occur or if secondary compensation or contracture is present, a trial of serial cast stretching is recommended. Short-leg walking casts are applied with the knee flexed to 90 degrees and with the foot in maximal dorsiflexion (Fig. 12-10). Because the gastrosoleus muscle group is biarticular, dynamic stretching of the muscles occurs during gait as the knee is extended. Casts are changed at 2-week intervals for 4

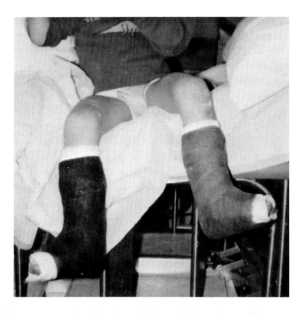

**Fig. 12-10.** Application of bilateral short leg walking cast with the knee flexed at 90 degrees and the foot in maximal dorsiflexion.

to 6 weeks, and cast treatment may need to be repeated periodically. This empirical serial cast treatment is almost always successful in the younger child. If a marked contracture is present or if serial casting is not successful in the older child (6 to 8 years), percutaneous sliding lengthening of the Achilles tendon should be considered.

# REFERENCES

## Torsional and Frontal Plane Conditions of the Leg

1. LaPorta G: Torsional abnormalities. Arch Podiatr Med Foot Surg 1:47, 1973
2. McCrea JD: Pediatric Orthopedics of the Lower Extremity. Futura Publishing Co, Mount Kisco, NY, 1985
3. Sgarlato TE: A Compendium of Podiatric Biomechanics. California College of Podiatric Medicine, San Francisco, 1971
4. Tax H: Podopediatrics. Williams & Wilkins, Baltimore, 1980
5. Valmassy RL: Biomechanical Evaluation of the Child, Clin Podiatr Med Surg 1:563, 1984
6. Shands AR, Steele MK: Torsion of the femur. Bone Joint Surg [Am] 40: ,1958
7. Staheli LT, Engel GM: Tibial torsion, a new method of assessment and a survey of normal children. Clin Orthop 86:183, 1977
8. Weseley MS, Berenfeld PA, Einstein AL: Thoughts on in-toeing and out-toeing. Twenty years experience with over 5,000 cases and review of the literature. Foot Ankle 2:(1):49, 1981
9. Tachdjian MO: Pediatric Orthopedics. WB Saunders, Philadelphia, 1972
10. Valmassy RL, Day S: Congenital dislocation of the hip. Podiatr Med Assoc 75(9):466, 1985
11. Hutter CG Jr, Scott W: Tibial torsion. J Bone Joint Surg [Am] 31:511, 1949
12. Rosen H, Sandwick H: The measurement of tibiofibular torsion. J Bone Joint Surg [Am] 37:847, 1955
13. Root ML: A discussion of biomechanical considerations for treatment of the infant foot. Arch Podiatr Med Foot Surg 1:41, 1973
14. Swanson AB, Greene PW, Allis HD: Rotational deformities of the lower extremity in children and their significance. Clin Orthop 27:157, 1963
15. Valmassy RL, Stanton B: Tibial torsion, normal values in children. J Am Podiatr Med Assoc 79(9):432, 1989
16. Schuster RD: In-toe and out-toe and its implications. Arch Podiatr Med Foot Surg 3(4):28, 1976
17. Kite J: Torsion of the legs in young children. Clin Orthop 16:152, 1960
18. Morley AJM: Knock knee in children. Br Med J 2:976, 1957
19. Blake RL: Inverted orthotic technique. J Am Podiatr Med Assoc 76(5):275, 1986

## Idiopathic Toe Walking

20. Statham L, Murray MP: Early walking patterns of normal children. Clin Orthop 79:8, 1971
21. Tachdjian MO: Pediatric Orthopedics. Vol. 2. WB Saunders, Philadelphia, 1972
22. Kalen V, Adler N, Bleck EE: Electromyography of idiopathic toe walking. J Pediatr Orthop 6:31, 1986
23. Shield LK: Toe walking and neuromuscular disease [letter]. Arch Dis Child 59:1003, 1984
24. Hall JE, Salter RB, Bhalla SK: Congenital short tendo calcaneus. J Bone Joint Surg [Br] 49:695, 1967
25. Griffin PP, Wheelhouse WW, Shiavi R, Bass BE: Habitual toe-walkers. J Bone Joint Surg [Am] 59:97, 1977
26. Accardo P, Whitman B: Toe walking: a marker for language disorders in the developmentally disabled. Clin Pediatr (Phila) 28:347, 1989
27. Hicks R, Durinick N, Gage JR: Differentiation of idiopathic toe-walking and cerebral palsy. J Pediatr Orthop 8:160, 1988

## SUGGESTED READINGS

### Torsional and Frontal Plane Conditions of the Leg

Barlow TG: Early diagnosis and treatment of congenital dislocation of the hip. J Bone Joint Surg [Br] 44:292, 1967

Crane L: Femoral torsion and its relation to toeing-in and toeing-out. J Bone Joint Surg [Am] 41A:421, 1959

Elffman H: Torsion of the lower extremity. Am J Phys Anthropol 3:255, 1945

Ganley JV: Lower extremity examination of the infant. J Am Podiatr Med Assoc 71(2):92, 1981

Root ML, Orien WD, Weed JH: Normal and Abnormal Function of the Foot. Clinical Biomechanics Corp. Los Angeles, 1977

Schoenhaus HD, Poss KD: The clinical and practical aspects in treating torsional problems in children. J Am Podiatr Med Assoc 67(9):620, 1977

Von Rosen S: Treatment of congenital dislocation of the hip in the newborn. Proc R Soc Med 56:801, 1963

# 13

# Evaluation and Nonoperative Management of Pes Valgus

KEVIN A. KIRBY
DONALD R. GREEN

The evaluation and conservative treatment of pediatric flexible flatfoot deformity, which will be referred to as *pediatric pes valgus deformity* throughout this chapter, has been an area of continued debate within the medical community for over a century. There are and probably will be, well into the future, a multitude of opinions as to when the pes valgus deformity in a child should be simply observed, treated conservatively with orthotic devices, or treated surgically.

This chapter includes sections on the history, biomechanics, evaluation, and conservative treatment of the pediatric pes valgus deformity in the hope that the reader will come to a better understanding of the complexity and seriousness of this common foot disorder. In this way physicians will be better equipped to deal with the many decisions that confront them when the flatfooted child seeks medical attention.

## HISTORY OF NONOPERATIVE TREATMENT

One of the earliest descriptions of the conservative treatment of pes valgus deformity was given by Durlacher, an English chiropodist.[1] In 1845 Durlacher described the use of a built-up leather inlay, which was used in the treatment of mechanical foot problems.

In 1874 Hugh Owen Thomas, an English surgeon, described the use of leather shoe sole additions in the treatment of foot disorders.[1] The Thomas heel, which is an elongation of the medial side of the heel of the shoe, is still used today either by itself or in combination with arch supports for the treatment of pediatric pes valgus deformity.

In 1888 Royal Whitman, an orthopedic surgeon, was one of the first to describe in detail the clinical pathomechanics of the pes valgus deformity.[2] One of his greatest contributions was in persuading the orthopedic community of his era to realize that severe foot deformities such as clubfoot or the polio foot were not the only foot deformities deserving of medical attention. He believed that "weakfoot" in itself should be considered a significant medical entity since he had long recognized that painful problems often developed as a result of "overwork" imposed upon the muscles and ligaments in flatfoot deformity.

Whitman's conservative treatment of weakfoot consisted of a metal foot brace, which had a medial and lateral flange and was designed to produce an inversion motion once the patient stepped down on it[3] (Fig. 13-1A). The inversion motion of the plate would cause the medial flange to press rather vigorously into the area of the navicular, thus causing a decrease in foot pronation either by force or by pain. According to Schuster,[1] P. W. Roberts, a physician, developed a metal brace in 1912 that was similar in function to the Whitman brace but smaller in size and that actually had a deep inverted heel and medial and lateral heel clips. Unfortunately, it seemed that the design of the Roberts brace was fairly extreme; it applied too much force through too little surface area and was difficult to adjust.

It was an orthopedic bracemaker turned podiatrist,

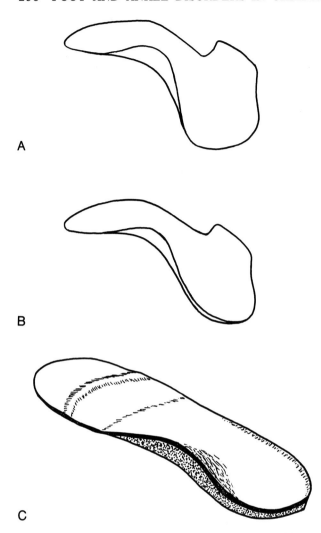

A

B

C

**Fig. 13-1.** (**A**) The Whitman brace, (**B**) the Roberts-Whitman brace, and (**C**) the Levy mold are all early forms of foot orthoses used in the treatment of pediatric pes valgus deformities.

Otto F. Schuster, who in the 1920s combined some of the better ideas of the Whitman brace and the Roberts brace into the Roberts-Whitman brace.[1] The Roberts-Whitman brace consisted of a metal brace, with a deep inverted heel cup, as in the Roberts brace, but which was made broader, like the Whitman brace (Fig. 13-1B). In effect, the deep inverted heel cup placed enough supination torque on the heel that the navicular would no longer

press as hard into the medial flange of the device, thereby improving medial arch comfort and improving pronation control of the foot.

In 1950 Ben Levy, a podiatrist, described a technique for producing an arch support (Fig. 13-1C) that incorporated a toe crest.[1] The resultant *Levy mold* consisted of a thick leather cover supported plantarly by a hardened latex mixture and filler, known as "rubber butter." The mold was easily adjustable and actually would shape itself to the foot over time.

In 1958 and 1959 Merton L. Root, a podiatrist, began work on an improvement of the Levy mold, which at the time was the most popular of the podiatric treatments for pes valgus deformity.[4] Root had found that the Levy mold could control excessive pronation, but it was not durable and soon became hygienically distasteful. His experimentation with thermoplastics led him to the thermoplastic material Rohadur, which could be heated and pressed over a plaster model of the foot to form an exceedingly durable and lightweight orthotic device (Fig. 13-2A). This new plastic orthosis, which was made from a non-weight-bearing cast of the foot held in the subtalar joint neutral position, is now known as the Root Functional Orthosis.[5] Today, there are many modifications of the Root Functional Orthosis, and these modified versions are the most common types of foot orthoses used within the podiatric medical community in the treatment of pes valgus deformity.

In 1967 W. H. Henderson and J. W. Campbell, while working at the University of California Biomechanics Laboratory (U.C.B.L.), developed a characteristically shaped thin polypropylene foot orthosis, the U.C.B.L., which has an extremely high heel cup and medial and lateral flanges.[6] Even though the "wrap-around" design of the U.C.B.L. has been widely accepted by the orthopedic community as one of the most effective conservative means of treating pediatric pes valgus deformity, the U.C.B.L. has not been nearly as popular as an orthotic device within the podiatric community (Fig. 13-2B).

## BIOMECHANICS OF PEDIATRIC PES VALGUS DEFORMITY

The clinical characteristics of the pediatric pes valgus deformity have been recognized by clinicians for over a century. In 1888 Dr. Royal Whitman wrote of his obser-

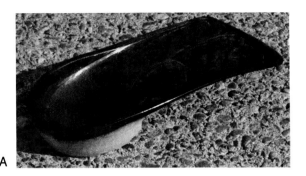 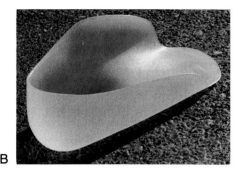

**Fig. 13-2.** (A) The Root Functional Orthosis and (B) the U.C.B.L. orthosis, the most common types of foot orthoses used today in the treatment of pediatric pes valgus deformities.

vations of 45 cases of flatfoot and described these feet as follows[2]:

> . . . the arch of the foot is lowered; or completely broken down, so that the entire sole rests upon the floor; on the inside of the foot the slight normal outward curve from the heel to the head of the first metatarsal is replaced by a bulging inwards, most prominent below and in front of the internal malleolus . . . the internal malleolus is abnormally prominent; when the patient stands the entire foot seems displaced outwards on the leg, . . . in walking the feet are turned out more than usual, and a short awkward step is sometimes observed . . .

Over 100 years later we still recognize that the pediatric pes valgus deformity involves, during standing, a complete to near complete collapse of the medial longitudinal arch and a talus that is so internally rotated and medially positioned on the calcaneus that the talar head bulges medially in the medial midfoot. Because the talus is so abnormally internally rotated and medially positioned on the calcaneus, the calcaneus and the rest of the foot appear externally rotated, laterally positioned, and everted in relation to the talus and tibia. The abnormal position of the talar head in relation to the calcaneus not only affects the clinical appearance of the pes valgus deformity but also causes significant abnormal biomechanical function of the foot during weight-bearing activities. Since much of the body's weight is transferred through the head of the talus during gait, the abnormal medial position of the head of the talus with respect to the weight-bearing surface of the foot results in a strong pronation force, which causes maximal pronation of the

subtalar joint and excessive calcaneal eversion. Indeed, if there is one structural abnormality that could be labeled the major contributor to the biomechanical pathology evident in the pes valgus deformity, it would have to be the internally rotated and medially located position of the talus on the calcaneus.

## Concept of Medial Deviation of the Subtalar Joint Axis

The idea that the abnormal position of the talus is a major contributing factor to the overall pathomechanics of pes valgus deformity has been appreciated by physicians for many decades. As Whitman noted over a century ago, the abnormal position of the talus in relation to the rest of the foot causes both an abnormal clinical appearance and abnormal function in the flatfoot, " . . . while its axis (the talus) should be in a line with the second toe, (the axis) may point inside the great toe." [2] Even though Dr. Whitman described a more generalized "talar head axis" rather than the subtalar joint axis (STJA) itself, his idea was clear: the abnormal plantar and medial position of the talar head relative to the calcaneus and the rest of the foot is of prime importance in the development of the pathologic pronation forces seen in the pes valgus foot.

The morphology of the talus and calcaneus are such that gliding movements between the two bones occur at the STJA, which on the average, is at a 16-degree angle from the sagittal plane and a 42-degree angle from the transverse plane of the foot.[7,8] Manter[7] and Root et al.[8] observed that the STJA passes through the head of the talus from posterolateral-inferior to anteromedial-supe-

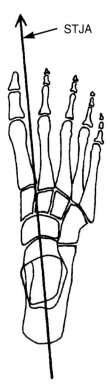
STJA

**Fig. 13-3.** Normal orientation of the subtalar joint axis within the transverse plane. Note that the subtalar joint axis passes through the talar head. (From Kirby,[9] with permission.)

rior (Fig. 13-3). Indeed, in clinical observation of hundreds of patients' feet and in many cadaver specimens, we have noted that the STJA does seem to pass through the talar head. Talar head position is very important to foot biomechanics because the relative position of the talar head to the calcaneus also determines the relative position of the STJA to the rest of the foot. If the talar head becomes positioned medially relative to the calcaneus, the STJA will also be medially positioned relative to the calcaneus.

The senior author (K.A.K.) developed a clinical examination technique that can be used to estimate the STJA position relative to the plantar aspect of the foot.[9] This examination technique can be used to clinically correlate foot function during gait with the STJA position (see Figs. 13-14 to 13-16). Kirby has also found that the STJA in feet that function normally in gait is positioned so that it passes through a point at the posterolateral aspect of the heel and through a point in the first intermetatarsal space.[9-11] Normal STJA position aids in producing nor-

mal biomechanical foot function (see Fig. 13-4A). However, abnormal medial or lateral deviation of the STJA results in abnormal pronation and supination forces. Based upon the examination of well over 1,000 feet, Kirby has found that those patients who have gross medial deviation of the STJA will stand and function during gait with the subtalar joint resting in the maximally pronated position (Fig. 13-4B) and those patients who have lateral deviation of the STJA will tend to stand and function during gait with the subtalar joint in a position that is either neutral or supinated from neutral[11] (Fig. 13-4C). Other researchers have also reported that the STJA is more medially deviated than normal in pronated feet and more laterally deviated in supinated feet.[12] The more medially deviated the STJA, the greater will be the pronation force on the foot with weight-bearing.

Since pronation movement is defined as occurring about an axis of rotation and is therefore an angular rather than a linear measurement, then a pronation *force* is more correctly described as a pronation *torque* or pronation *moment*.[9-11] The medially deviated STJA is located closer to the medial calcaneal tubercle and exits the posterior surface of the calcaneus more medially than normal (Fig. 13-4B). This abnormal STJA position decreases the moment arm that the ground reactive force (GRF) acts upon to cause a supination moment (through pressure against the medial calcaneal tubercle) and also decreases the moment arm acted upon by the Achilles tendon. The Achilles tendon normally causes a supination moment by its action on the posterior calcaneus.[9-11] As a result, during standing or walking the GRF on the medial calcaneal tubercle and the tension in the Achilles tendon produce a smaller than normal supination moment across a medially deviated STJA. A reduction in the supination moment acting upon the subtalar joint will cause the foot to be more susceptible to any additional pronation moments acting across the STJA, and the foot will tend to be more pronated during standing and during gait. In addition, medial deviation of the STJA causes the GRF against the lateral metatarsal heads to produce a much greater than normal pronation moment acting upon the STJA[9-11] (Fig. 13-4B).

The more medially deviated the STJA, the more difficult it is to supinate these feet away from the maximally pronated position of the subtalar joint either by internally generated forces (i.e., posterior tibial muscle contraction) or by externally generated forces (i.e., foot orthoses). Clinically this means that the more the talar head

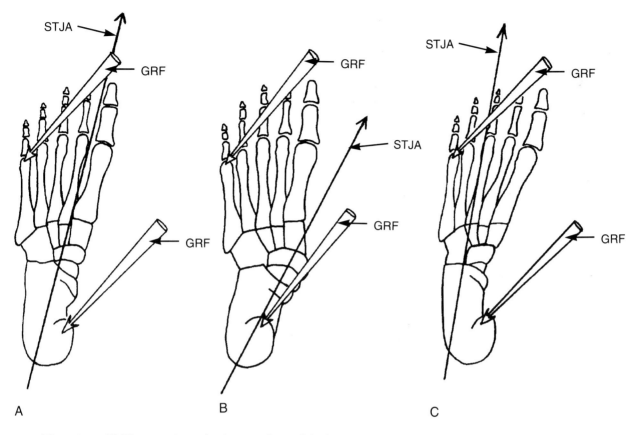

**Fig. 13-4.** **(A)** The ground reaction force on the medial calcaneal tubercle in a foot with a normally positioned STJA causes a supination moment across the STJA. The GRF on the lateral metatarsal heads and fifth metatarsal shaft causes a pronation moment across the STJA. This arrangement of the STJA results in a balance of the supination and pronation moments acting across the STJA so that neither excessive pronation nor excessive supination occurs during gait. **(B)** A medially deviated STJA alters the rotational effects of the GRF, which causes a net increase in the pronation moments acting across the STJA. This results in a foot that tends to pronate maximally at the subtalar joint during gait and that has pronation instability. **(C)** A laterally deviated STJA alters the rotational effects of the GRF, which causes a net increase in the supination moments acting across the STJA. This results in a foot that tends to have supination instability during gait. (From Kirby,[9] with permission.)

has rotated into a medial position in relation to the calcaneus, the greater will be the pronation instability of the foot and the greater will be the supination moment needed to supinate the foot out of the maximally pronated position.[11] A similar and useful method of portraying the effects of a medially deviated and internally rotated talar head position is to analyze the effects of the line of force through the talar head. If this line of force is grossly medial to the weight-bearing surface of the calcaneus because of a medial talar head position, a strong pronation moment is created during gait (Fig. 13-6). The more medial the location of the line of force through the talar head in relation to the calcaneus, the more difficult will be the supination force needed to push the talar head into a more lateral and externally rotated (i.e., more supinated) position.

## Biomechanical Effects of Ligamentous Laxity

The observation that the joints of the child's lower extremity have a greater range of motion (ROM) than the joints of an adult's lower extremity is clinically obvious to anyone actively involved in the treatment of structural or mechanical problems of the lower extremities. Specifically, the characterization of a child's foot as "fat, flat, and floppy" is certainly an excellent description of the overall clinical picture of "overflexibility," which all children's feet demonstrate off and on weight-bearing.[13] This greater degree of flexibility in the joints of the lower extremities of children is well documented in the literature. Engel and Staheli reported that total hip ROM decreased by 25 percent from birth to the age of 10 years.[14] Sgarlato reported that transverse plane rotational motion within the extended knee joint decreases from 15 degrees at birth to zero by 6 years of age.[15] Many authors feel that this excessive flexibility, or ligamentous laxity, may be one of the primary reasons that flatfoot is very common in children and less common in adults.[14,16-18] Of course, there are varying degrees of ligamentous laxity, and many of its most severe forms may actually be caused by hereditary disorders. Marfan syndrome, Ehlers-Danlos syndrome, and osteogenesis imperfecta are three of the more common connective tissue disorders characterized by ligamentous laxity that

frequently result in severe flatfoot deformities. In addition, many of the less severe cases of isolated joint hypermobility have been grouped into a set of disorders called *generalized familial ligamentous laxity.*[19]

Ligamentous laxity allows a greater than normal degree of subtalar joint motion (including pronation), which can result in the calcaneus assuming a more everted position relative to the tibia. As a result, any force that acts to pronate the subtalar joint will be able to evert the calcaneus to a greater degree than normal.

It is the medial longitudinal arch that is most affected by ligamentous laxity. This arch acts somewhat as a bridge functioning to support the body's weight as it passes through the talar head. The same mechanical concepts that affect the structural integrity and durability of a bridge's structure can be applied to the effects of ligamentous laxity upon the child's foot. For example, assuming that no muscular contraction occurs, a vertical force exerted in a plantarward direction upon the medial longitudinal arch causes one of two things to happen — either the bones and ligaments of the arch resist collapse

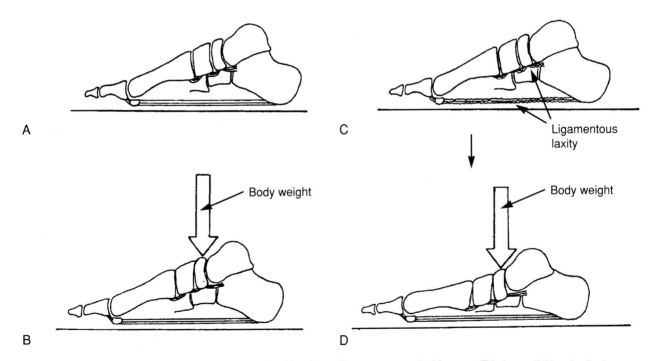

**Fig. 13-5.** In a foot that has **(A)** good integrity of its plantar ligaments, a vertical force on **(B)** the medial longitudinal arch will be resisted by the plantar ligaments and plantar fascia, with very little medial longitudinal arch collapse occurring. However, in a foot that has **(C)** excessive laxity of its plantar ligaments, a vertical force on the medial longitudinal arch will not be resisted effectively by the plantar ligaments or plantar fascia, and **(D)** significant medial longitudinal arch flattening will occur.

owing to the tensile strength of the supporting plantar ligaments and the plantar fascia, or the arch collapses (Fig. 13-5A–D). The greater the load applied to the arch, the greater is the tension force in the plantar ligaments and plantar fascia and the greater is the compression force within the bones of the arch.[20] Arch collapse (or gradual lowering of the arch) occurs, then, as a result of inherently loose ligaments (laxity), decreased ligament tensile resistance (e.g., due to connective tissue disorders), increasing loads (e.g., due to obesity), or a combination of those factors[21] (Fig. 13-5C and D).

Therefore increased ligamentous laxity, such as that seen normally in young children or abnormally in certain familial connective tissue disorders, causes the medial longitudinal arch of the foot to be much more susceptible to plantarly directed vertical forces acting upon it. The result is increased medial longitudinal arch collapse (Fig. 13-5D).

## Pathologic Biomechanical Forces

For nearly all weight-bearing activities, the principal force that acts externally on the foot is the GRF. Of course, the GRF is primarily caused by the action-reaction force of the ground responding to the gravitational attraction of the mass of the human body to the earth. The forces caused by the GRF that act on the foot and lower extremity during gait can be readily measured by use of a technically complex force transducer such as a force platform or of a technically simple apparatus such as a Harris footprint mat.[22-24] As would be evident with use of either a force platform or a Harris footprint mat, the major abnormality in the distribution of the GRF acting on the pes valgus deformity is the apparent shift of the GRF away from the lateral half of the plantar foot (i.e., the lateral metatarsal heads) to the medial half of the plantar foot (i.e., the medial metatarsal heads). This shift of the GRF toward the medial aspect of the plantar foot is caused by the medial deviation of the talar head, which causes the vertically directed line of force through the tibia and the talus during weight-bearing activities to be shifted medially in relation to the weight-bearing plantar structures of the foot[25] (Fig. 13-6).

Musculoskeletal injury is not always caused directly by the forces that act on the foot externally. Injury is often caused by conversion of these external forces into pathologic internal forces acting within the structures of the feet and lower extremities. Therefore, measurement of

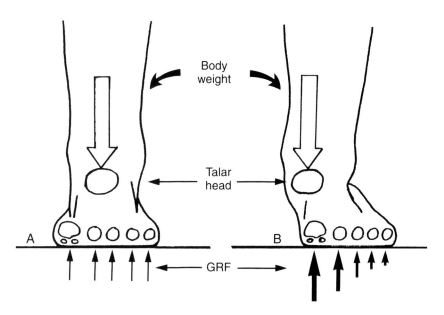

**Fig. 13-6.** (A) In a normal foot the more central location of the talar head causes the line of body weight through the talar head to allow an even distribution of the GRF through all the metatarsal heads. (B) However, in a pes valgus foot the talar head is positioned in a medial location, and thus the medial location of the line of body weight through the talar head results in a shift of the GRF toward the medial metatarsal heads and away from the lateral metatarsal heads.

external forces acting on the foot does not always predict what musculoskeletal injury will occur in a given subject. A better appreciation of these "hidden" abnormal internal forces, such as the pulling, pushing, or twisting forces that act on the bones, tendons, muscles, and ligaments of the lower extremity, is very important in determining the etiology of biomechanical symptoms in the child with pes valgus deformity.

In the pes valgus deformity pathologic internal forces resulting mostly from the excessive pronation moments acting on the subtalar joint, in turn cause excessive calcaneal eversion and excessive medial longitudinal arch collapse. The increase in the medial longitudinal arch flattening force causes an increase in the compressive forces within the talar head, navicular, cuneiforms, and three medial metatarsals and also causes increased tension within the plantar ligaments of the medial longitudinal arch and on the more medial bands of the plantar fascia (Fig. 13-7). Since the dorsal parts of the bones of the medial arch are under greater compressive loads than the plantar parts of the bones, early remodeling of the shapes of the bones is very likely to occur, especially while the young bones are more plastic and not yet completely ossified. Any remodeling of the bones of the me-

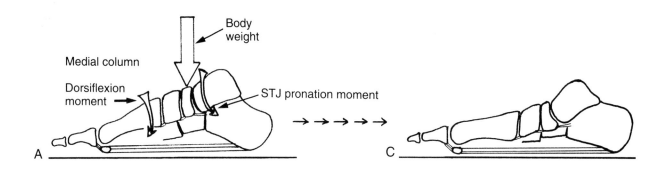

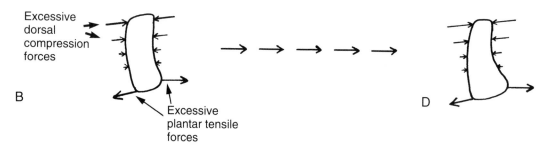

**Fig. 13-7.** At the age of 1 year the bones of the medial longitudinal arch are still largely cartilaginous. **(A)** When pronation forces act on the early walker's foot, they result in an increase in compression forces along the dorsal joint surfaces of the bones of the medial longitudinal arch and an increase in tension forces on the plantar aspects of the bones due to an increase in tension in the plantar ligaments. **(B)** Under the effects of these abnormal loads, the bones of the medial longitudinal arch, including the navicular, are compressed dorsally and pulled apart plantarly. **(C)** If these abnormal compression and tension forces on the navicular continue until the bones mature at approximately age 7, permanent changes in bone shape may occur, with dorsal narrowing and plantar widening of the bone. **(D)** The cumulative effect of abnormal pronation forces left untreated in an early walker's foot may lead to permanent structural changes in the bones of the medial longitudinal arch and to an adult flatfoot deformity.

dial longitudinal arch during the first decade of life that causes the dorsal half of the bones to decrease in size and/or the plantar half of the bone to increase in size will effectively decrease the height of the medial longitudinal arch (Fig. 13-7).

In addition, chronically increased tensile loads on the medial bands of the plantar fascia and within the plantar ligaments of the medial longitudinal arch may actually cause permanent elongation of these ligaments. The actual amount of elongation is dependent both on the magnitude and the duration of that pathologic stretch and on the elasticity of the ligaments.[21,26,27] Strong medial longitudinal arch flattening forces, such as those seen in pes valgus deformity, may then result in greater permanent flattening of the medial longitudinal arch as compared with the lateral longitudinal arch, depending on the intrinsic plasticity of the bones and ligaments of the medial arch. Because of this differential flattening of the medial as compared with the lateral longitudinal arch, either a forefoot varus deformity or a forefoot supinatus deformity may be created during childhood in feet with large

pronation moments acting across the STJA (see Fig. 13-17).

Many of the muscles of the lower extremity are also affected by the abnormal internal forces placed on the pathologically pronated foot. The posterior tibial muscle and the plantar intrinsic muscles are especially susceptible to strain when excessive pronation forces act on the foot. Symptoms such as shin pain, medial ankle pain, navicular tuberosity pain, and medial longitudinal arch pain may be caused by "overworking" of the posterior tibial or plantar intrinsic muscles.[28]

The sustentaculum tali has been mentioned frequently in the literature as a very important part of the overall supporting structure of the medial longitudinal arch of the foot.[29-33] The sustentaculum tali is subjected to quite severe interosseous compression forces from the head of the talus when an excessive pronation moment acts on the STJA. These severe interosseous compression forces created at an early age by the talar head slamming vigorously onto the sustentaculum tali with each step may very well induce deformation and/or hypoplasia of

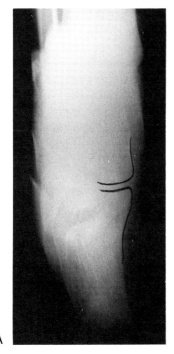
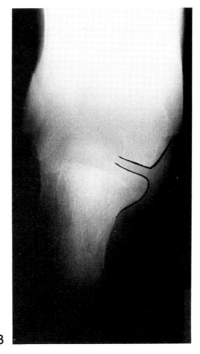

A B

Fig. 13-8. (A) In a child with a normal foot, a calcaneal axial projection of the foot shows a sustentaculum tali with a horizontal shelf to support the talar head. (B) However, in a child with pes valgus deformity, a calcaneal axial projection will often show an abnormally everted position of the sustentaculum tali, which offers poor support to the talar head.

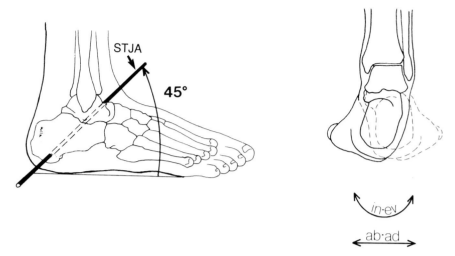

**Fig. 13-9.** If the foot has an STJA located halfway between the frontal and transverse planes, equal amounts of frontal plane motion and transverse plane motion will occur during subtalar joint motion (From Green and Carol,[34] with permission.)

the sustentaculum tali. In support of this theory, Kleiger and Mankin noted that both in normally arched feet and in flatfeet the sustentaculum tali remained cartilaginous until after the age of 12 months but that the ossification process of the sustentaculum tali developed more slowly in flatfeet than in normally arched feet. They also noticed that the superior articular surface of the sustentaculum tali remained abnormally sloped in an everted attitude throughout its development in the flatfoot[31] (Fig. 13-8).

The observations of Kleiger and Mankin seem logical, since any excessive pronation moment acting on the STJA during gait would tend to forcefully plantarflex the head of the talus onto the middle and anterior talar facets of the superior calcaneus. Any plastic deformation of the sustentaculum tali or of the middle or anterior talar facets of the calcaneus during early life could lead to permanent abnormally everted sloping of the osseous supporting structures of the talar head. It has not yet been demonstrated how much of the abnormal everted sloping of the sustentaculum tali or of the middle and anterior talar facets of the calcaneus is genetically predetermined and how much of it develops in the first

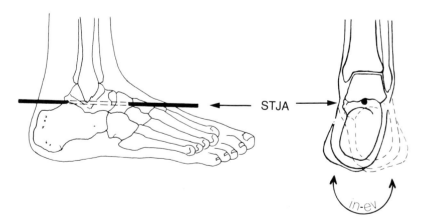

**Fig. 13-10.** If the foot has an STJA located within the sagittal and transverse planes, motion only within the frontal plane will occur during subtalar joint motion. (From Green and Carol,[34] with permission.)

decade of life as the result of abnormal, internally generated forces within the talocalcaneal joint of the pediatric flatfoot.

## Planal Dominance

In 1984 Green and Carol introduced the concept of *planal dominance,* which stresses the important fact that not all feet have similar angular relationships of the subtalar and midtarsal joint axes. As a result, every foot will display its own characteristic method of compensating for certain biomechanical faults within the lower extremities.[34] For example, a foot with its STJA at a 45-degree angle with respect to both the transverse plane and the frontal plane, and in line with the sagittal plane will allow equal amounts of transverse plane and frontal plane movement of the calcaneus on the talus with subtalar joint motion (Fig. 13-9). However, if a foot has an STJA located within an intersection of the transverse and sagittal planes, subtalar joint motion will allow only frontal plane movement of the calcaneus on the talus (Fig. 13-10). In this case the planal dominance around the STJA would be said to be in the frontal plane.[34] If the STJA is positioned vertically so that it lies within an intersection of the frontal and sagittal planes, then subtalar joint motion will allow only transverse plane movement of the calcaneus on the talus. In this example, the planal dominance around the STJA would be in the transverse plane.[34] These principles can be similarly applied to the joint axes of the midtarsal joint.

Individual patients may express a multitude of planal deformities at multiple joint axes. In the growing child the development of the planal dominant type of foot is dependent upon both the inherited foot type and the strength and plane of the deforming force. For example, an internal femoral torsion deformity will often cause transverse planal dominance of the subtalar and midtarsal joints with pronation compensation (Fig. 13-11). A severe sagittal plane deforming force such as gastrocnemius equinus may result in development of progressive dorsiflexion of the forefoot on the hindfoot, leading to a pronation compensation with sagittal plane dominance (Fig. 13-12). Extreme amounts of subtalar joint eversion ROM may allow development of a progressive inversion deformity of the forefoot on the rearfoot, leading to a frontal plane dominant pronation compensation (Fig. 13-13).

Identification of the plane of deforming force and the plane of compensation is important for determining an appropriate treatment plan. For example, in the gastrocnemius equinus deformity, appropriate conservative care would include gastrocnemius stretching exercises, heel lifts, and foot orthoses. Those cases unresponsive to conservative care may respond best to Achilles tendon lengthening. Whether conservative or surgical in nature, the treatment should always be directed toward decreasing the pathologic mechanical forces that are responsible for the primary plane of pronation compensation.

Planal dominance, though not an exacting measure of axis position within the foot, is an extremely useful con-

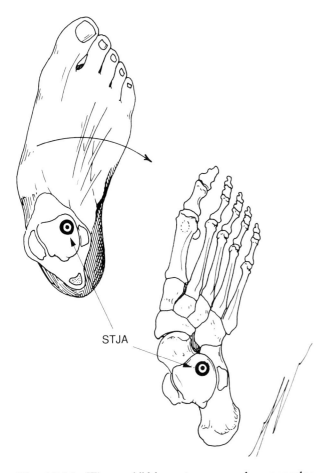

**Fig. 13-11.** When a child has a transverse plane musculoskeletal abnormality, such as internal tibial torsion, pronation compensation will primarily occur within the transverse plane, with abduction of the forefoot on the rearfoot. (From Green and Carol,[34] with permission.)

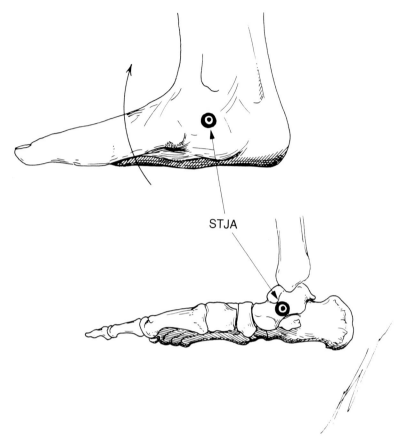

**Fig. 13-12.** When a child has a sagittal plane musculoskeletal abnormality, such as a gastrocnemius equinus deformity, pronation compensation will primarily occur within the sagittal plane, with dorsiflexion of the forefoot on the rearfoot. (From Green and Carol,[34] with permission.)

cept in the clinical setting. Determining the primary plane of pronation compensation within the pediatric pes valgus deformity, whether it be the transverse, sagittal, or frontal plane, is an important first step in recognizing the best conservative and/or surgical method of treatment.

## CLINICAL EVALUATION OF PEDIATRIC PES VALGUS

A thorough evaluation of the pediatric flatfoot deformity is of utmost importance in the formation of an accurate diagnosis and an appropriate treatment plan. In order to thoroughly evaluate the pediatric patient with pes valgus

deformity, a clinical history, physical examination, gait examination, and radiographic examination are all necessary.

### Clinical History

A complete clinical history of the pediatric pes valgus deformity is crucial in establishing both a differential diagnosis and the degree of patient's symptomatology. The history is best taken before the physical examination of the child starts, while the child, parent, and doctor are all in the examination room. After the history is taken, the physician should perform the physical examination as swiftly as possible to ensure the child's cooperation. The physician should obtain information from the parent and

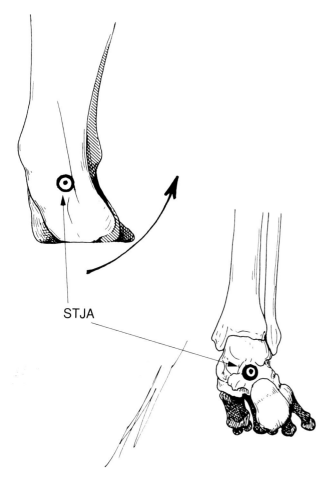

STJA

**Fig. 13-13.** When a child has a frontal plane musculoskeletal abnormality, such as an extreme eversion of the rearfoot, pronation compensation will primarily occur within the frontal plane, with inversion of the forefoot on the rearfoot. (From Green and Carol,[34] with permission.)

child concerning the history of the chief complaint, pre- and postnatal history, and developmental and family history.

The pre- and postnatal history should include any pre- or perinatal complication, the infant's gestational age at birth, and the type of delivery. Determination of the age at which certain developmental milestones occur, such as crawling and walking, help to rule out any neuromuscular pathology and also may indicate the overall coordination and lower extremity stability of the child.[35] Familial history of flatfoot is also of great importance and may

help predict the potential severity or disability of severe pes valgus with age. Indeed, the familial history of flatfoot often is the only information to which the parents can relate as far as future potential symptoms are concerned.

Any prior musculoskeletal trauma and/or treatment should be noted. The physician should specifically ask if the child has complained of foot, ankle, leg, knee, thigh, hip, or lower back pain or of fatigue with prolonged standing, prolonged walking, or running activities. Children over 3 years of age should be questioned directly concerning the location and duration of pain and any precipitating factors. Often the child may not be able to communicate adequately, and the parent may not be aware of subtle signs of foot or lower extremity pain or fatigue, such as limping, reluctance to bear weight or to walk, and constantly preferring to be carried by the parent. In addition, children who dislike weight-bearing activities that are universally enjoyed by children of similar ages (such as extended walking in an amusement park) should also be suspected of having lower extremity pain. Children should not normally experience long-lasting lower extremity fatigue with mild to moderate activity.[35]

There may be some validity to the argument that musculoskeletal pain in the pediatric patient is often the result of differential growth spurts of the long bones of the lower extremity relative to the surrounding muscular structures. Pain associated with such growth spurts is commonly referred to as "growing pains." However, since active growth in the bones of the lower extremities is normal from birth to adolescence and since many children have minimal symptoms within their lower extremities even during growth spurts, the presence of frequent lower extremity pain should be thoroughly investigated.

In 1934 J.C. Hawksley studied 115 children with growing pains and found that the pain was of muscular origin in 85 percent.[36] The children who complained of joint pain were usually found to have pain near the joint rather than in the joint. In addition, Hawksley found that many of these children had coexisting lower extremity deformities such as "flatfoot, knock-knee, scoliosis, or bad stance." Treatment of the lower extremity deformity nearly always relieved the growing pains, which has likewise been our finding; in 90 percent of the children in our studies who had lower extremity symptoms and some degree of overpronation of the feet, treatment with foot orthoses relieved the majority of "growing pains." Mechanical instability of the foot during weight-bearing activities may, therefore, be a substantial cause of growing pains in some children.

## Biomechanical Examination

The biomechanical examination is begun with the child sitting or lying supine on the examination table. Internal and external hip rotation should be evaluated with the hips both flexed and extended to determine if there are any osseous, ligamentous, or muscular abnormalities causing abnormal hip or knee joint position during gait,[15] after which malleolar torsion is the next parameter measured. The angle of the malleoli to the knee joint axis is normally zero at birth. The malleoli should normally twist externally in relation to the knee at a rate of 1 to 2 degrees per year up to the age of 7 or 8, with the adult normal external angle of 13 to 18 degrees being reached by the age of 8 years.[35] An internally positioned knee caused by an abnormality in the hip or femur (e.g., femoral anteversion) or a lack of normal malleolar torsion will tend to cause an adducted or pigeon-toed gait in the child. Even though an internally positioned knee or a lack of malleolar torsion is usually partially or completely outgrown by the time the child reaches adolescence, internal torsional abnormalities of the leg may contribute to the severity of the flatfoot condition before that time.

Foot orthosis control of the excessive foot pronation in these children will not improve their excessive intoeing and may actually cause more intoeing. However, nearly all these children report less pain and fatigue in the lower extremities, less clumsiness and tripping with walking and running activities, and improved shoe wear pattern with foot orthoses. In addition, the use of foot orthoses will help to counteract the severe pronation forces on the foot, which could further worsen the pes valgus deformity.

Ankle joint dorsiflexion should next be assessed while the patient is in the supine position with the knee both extended and flexed. It is important to make certain that the subtalar joint is in the neutral position while measuring ankle joint dorsiflexion in the pes valgus foot, since this type of foot is easily pronated when the foot is dorsiflexed, causing artificially high values of ankle joint dorsiflexion.[37] Restrictions in ankle joint dorsiflexion caused by osseous ankle equinus or gastrocnemius and/or soleus equinus can cause severe pronation moments across the subtalar and oblique midtarsal joints during gait, poten-

tially causing an excessively pronated foot. A genu recurvatum deformity in the child may also result from an excessively tight gastrocnemius muscle.[15] Any child who has less than 10 degrees of ankle joint dorsiflexion with the knee extended and the subtalar joint in the neutral position should be considered to have a potentially deforming equinus condition.

At this point in the biomechanical examination the position of the STJA relative to the plantar surface of the foot should be estimated. This can be done by finding the points on the plantar surface of the foot at which no subtalar joint rotation occurs when manual pressure is applied[8] (Figs. 13-14 to 13-16). In performing this technique, it is important that the foot be rotated about the STJA until the plane of the forefoot is parallel to the patient's transverse plane (Fig. 13-16). Even though the determination of STJA location is probably the most difficult biomechanical examination technique to master, it is perhaps the most fruitful in predicting the severity of the pronation moments acting on the foot during standing and during gait.[9]

The subtalar joint ROM, the forefoot to rearfoot relationship, and the planal dominance of the available subtalar joint and midtarsal joint ROM's are examined next, with the patient in a prone position.[34,37] Extreme care must be taken to ensure that the calcaneal bisections are drawn accurately on the posterior surface of the calcaneus, since if they are not, the measured subtalar joint neutral position, subtalar joint ROM, forefoot to rearfoot relationship, neutral calcaneal stance position (NCSP), and relaxed calcaneal stance position (RCSP) will all be inaccurate. Children with pes valgus deformity frequently display excessive subtalar joint pronation ROM, which can lead to excessive calcaneal eversion during stance.

When the forefoot is put through its ROM relative to the leg (which includes mostly subtalar joint but also midtarsal joint motion) the primary plane of motion should be identified. Usually the forefoot moves with equal amounts of transverse and frontal plane motion relative to the tibia. If transverse plane motion (abduction-adduction) predominates, then there is a more vertical STJA or midtarsal joint axis. If frontal plane motion (eversion-inversion) predominates, then there is a more horizontal STJA or midtarsal joint axis. It is quite uncommon for sagittal plane motion (dorsiflexion–plantar flexion) to predominate, since sagittal plane motion is readily available in the ankle joint.

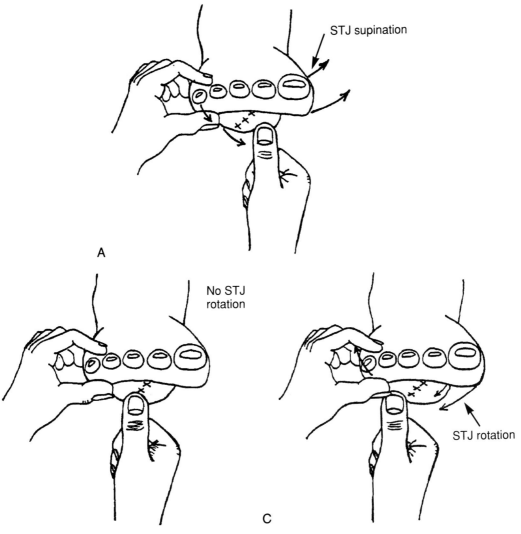

**Fig. 13-14.** STJA palpation technique. The position of the STJA in relation to the plantar surface of the foot may be determined by simply finding the point on the plantar foot at which no STJA rotation occurs with manual pressure. For the right foot, the examiner uses the left hand to sense subtalar joint motion and uses the right hand to produce subtalar joint motion by pressing on the plantar foot. **(A)** If thumb pressure is medial to the STJA, subtalar joint supination will occur. **(B)** If thumb pressure is directly on the STJA, no subtalar joint motion will occur. **(C)** If thumb pressure is lateral to the STJA, subtalar joint pronation will occur. The points of no rotation are marked on the foot to indicate the STJA location on the plantar foot. (From Kirby,[9] with permission.)

It is also quite common in the measurement of the forefoot to rearfoot relationship in children with pes valgus deformity to find an inverted forefoot to rearfoot alignment (Fig. 13-17). Since "structural" forefoot varus deformity causes excessive subtalar joint pronation and since excessive subtalar joint pronation causes

"positional" forefoot supinatus deformity, there is bound to be considerable overlap of these two conditions in the same foot. There is no accurate examination method that makes it possible to distinguish whether a foot with an inverted forefoot to rearfoot relationship has a forefoot varus or a forefoot supinatus deformity. However, it is

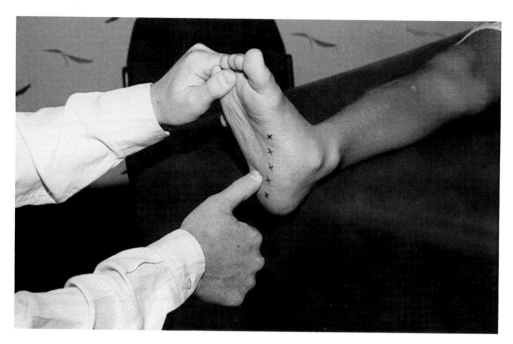

**Fig. 13-15.** Determining STJA location on the plantar foot by the palpation technique. It is important that very firm pressure be applied by the right thumb onto the plantar foot in order to produce noticeable subtalar joint rotation motion.

likely that all feet that do have an inverted forefoot to rearfoot relationship have a component of structural forefoot varus deformity, possibly genetically determined, and a component of positional forefoot supinatus deformity, caused by abnormal adaptation of the soft tissue structures to the flattened medial longitudinal arch position. If this is kept in mind, it is relatively unimportant whether the inverted forefoot position is termed a forefoot varus or a forefoot supinatus deformity, since treatment of both conditions is basically the same (i.e., by foot orthoses).

While the patient is still prone, the overall flexibility of the first, second, and third metatarsal rays (i.e., the medial column) within the sagittal plane should be assessed. Grumbine has described a technique for the measurement of medial column flexibility in which the second metatarsal head is gently dorsiflexed and loaded to resistance while the patient is in the prone position (Fig. 13-18). The combined varus components of this modified forefoot to hindfoot measurement technique added to the degree of rearfoot varus deformity is called *terra vara.*[38] Feet that allow more dorsiflexion of the medial column relative to the rearfoot and that allow greater

increases in the inversion of the forefoot to the rearfoot relationship during this maneuver will also allow greater medial longitudinal arch flattening during standing. This examination technique has special importance when surgical procedures are being considered in the pes valgus deformity and will be covered in Chapter 14 on the surgical treatment of pes valgus deformity. The ROM and relative position of the first ray relative to the second through fifth rays is next determined. If excessive first ray dorsiflexion motion is noted during the examination (which is quite common in pediatric pes valgus), the first ray will be relatively poor at supporting the medial longitudinal arch of the foot and at resisting pronation of the subtalar joint during weight-bearing activities. In general, excessive first ray dorsiflexion flexibility will result in increased subtalar joint pronation during gait.

The examination of the patient in the standing position often yields very useful information regarding the external and internal forces acting on and within the foot during weight-bearing activities. First of all, the child should be asked to stand either on the floor or on a raised stand with a flat top surface. With the feet positioned in the angle and base of gait (i.e., with the feet angled and

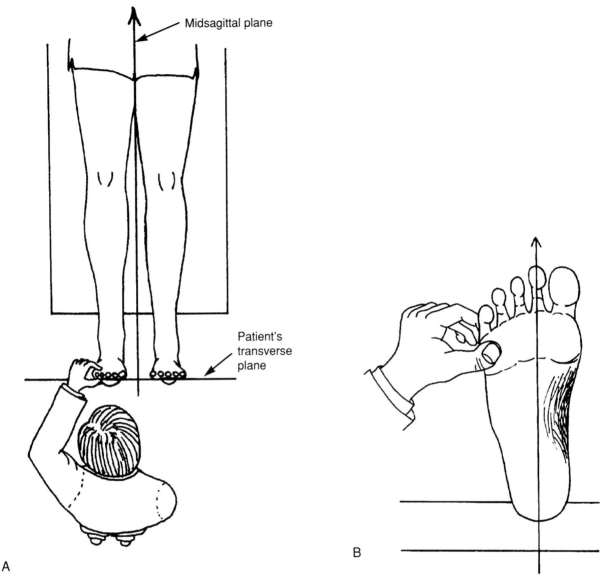

**Fig. 13-16.** (A) In the STJA palpation technique care must be taken that the patient is totally relaxed in a supine position, that the plane of the forefoot is placed parallel to the patient's transverse plane, and that the feet are spread apart on the table to their base of gait. (B) Finally, the patient's hip must then be rotated within the transverse plane until a bisector through the posterior heel and second digit is straight up and down. (From Kirby,[9] with permission.)

spread apart the same distance as occurs in walking), the child should be told to stand in a relaxed position. The heel bisection should then be measured relative to the ground to determine the RCSP. Children with pes valgus deformity will generally have an RCSP of 0 to 15 degrees everted, the more everted positions usually indicating more severe deformities. While still standing in the angle and base of gait the child is asked to supinate the feet until the subtalar joint is in the neutral position, which during standing is best determined by lo-

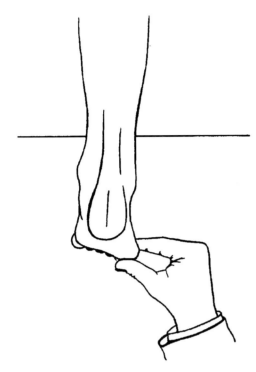

**Fig. 13-17.** Examination of the frontal plane forefoot to rearfoot relationship in a child with a forefoot varus deformity. Note that the subtalar joint is neutral and that both midtarsal joint axes are maximally pronated.

cating the congruent talonavicular joint position through palpation.

The NCSP is defined as the position of the calcaneal bisection relative to the ground with the subtalar joint in the neutral position. By definition, a calcaneus that is in an inverted position in the NCSP has a rearfoot varus deformity, and a calcaneus that is in an everted position while in NCSP has a rearfoot valgus deformity.[37] The NCSP is very helpful at demonstrating the neutral position at which the foot would function optimally. Even though feet with significant pes valgus deformities always function in a maximally pronated subtalar joint position during the midstance phase of gait, placing the foot in the NCSP gives both the examiner and the parent a better idea of the ideal morphology of that foot in the standing position (Fig. 13-19). This is a very convincing and graphic method of educating the parents about the sometimes extreme differences between the appearance of the neutral and maximally pronated positions in their child's feet. Comparison of radiographs in the RCSP and the NCSP further documents these differences.

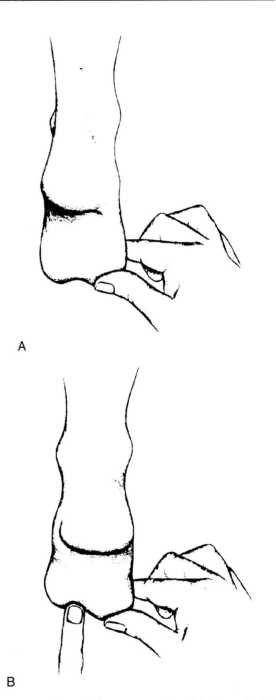

A

B

**Fig. 13-18.** Method of assessment of medial column flexibility. **(A)** Initially the foot is positioned so that the subtalar joint is neutral and both midtarsal joint axes are maximally pronated. **(B)** The second ray is then gently dorsiflexed to resistance to determine the degree of dorsiflexion available at the medial column. Care must be taken to avoid movement of the subtalar joint or calcaneocuboid joint when dorsiflexing the second ray. (From Grumbine,[38] with permission.)

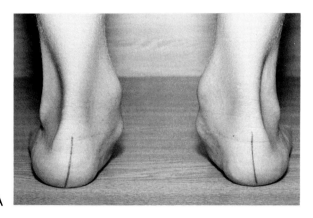 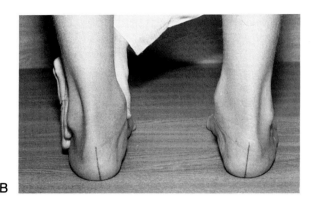

A                                                          B

**Fig. 13-19. (A)** Child with significant pes valgus deformity in the RCSP shows excessive calcaneal eversion and medial bulging of the talar head in the midfoot. **(B)** With the same child positioned in the NCSP, the parent can be shown the ideal clinical appearance, which one would hope to achieve with either conservative or surgical therapy.

Two of the most important tests in the physical examination of the pes valgus deformity are next performed, with the child again in RCSP. The first of these tests, the *maximum pronation test,* is a maneuver designed to determine whether the foot is standing in the maximally pronated subtalar joint position. The child is first asked to stand in a totally relaxed position without using any muscles to help support the medial longitudinal arch. Observation of the posterior tibial and anterior tibial tendons for any abnormal tension or bowstringing is

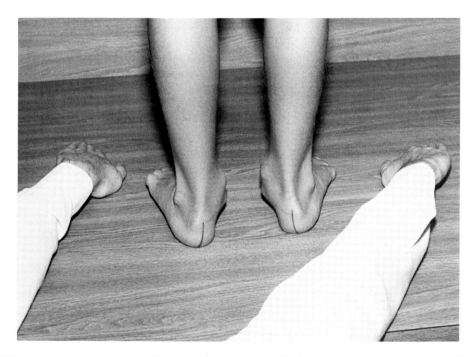

**Fig. 13-20.** Maximum pronation test. The patient is instructed to lift the lateral forefeet as much as possible without flexing the knees, which causes maximal subtalar joint pronation. It is often helpful to demonstrate this maneuver with the examiner's hands or feet. If the eversion motion of the calcaneus from the relaxed calcaneal stance position to the maximally pronated position during the test is less than 2 degrees, then the subtalar joint can be considered to be resting in its maximally pronated position when in the relaxed stance.

helpful. The child, while in the relaxed stance position, should be asked to try to lift up the lateral sides of the forefoot without flexing the knees (Fig. 13-20). If the maximum pronation test is done correctly, the child will use the peroneus brevis muscle in attempting to pronate the subtalar joint. If this joint is not already maximally pronated, the calcaneus will evert further. The physician should observe for heel motion from the back. Any calcaneal eversion of less than 2 degrees occurring during the test signifies that the child is standing in the maximally pronated position while in RCSP. It is important to determine whether or not a foot in RCSP is maximally pronated at the subtalar joint because the risk of significant future biomechanical pathology is much less if the child's foot is not maximally pronated.

An estimate of the magnitude of the excessive pronation moments acting at the subtalar joint during standing can be obtained by the *supination resistance test,* which is performed with the patient in the angle and base of gait in relaxed stance. The supination resistance test is a subjective measurement of the amount of lifting force required to cause supination motion at the subtalar joint (Fig. 13-21). The child must be instructed not to assist the examiner with even the slightest extrinsic muscular contraction or any lower extremity movement. The test is invalid if any patient assistance occurs.

The greater the force required to produce supination about the STJA, the greater is the pronation moment acting across that axis and the more difficult that foot will be to control with foot orthoses. In a normal foot during standing, the STJA is in a relatively lateral location relative to the medial navicular bone. Supination of the subtalar joint then becomes relatively easy when the examiner exerts a lifting force under the navicular, since the lever arm is relatively long. If, however, the STJA is medially deviated, as in a pes valgus deformity, then the much shorter lever arm will necessitate a much greater lifting force under the medial navicular to produce even small increases in supination moment across the STJA. In many of the more severe pes valgus deformities, the supination resistance test will produce no subtalar joint supination since the talar head is so medially deviated that the lifting force on the navicular from the examiner's fingertips acts directly inferior to the STJA. In this situation the lifting force has no lever arm and will produce no subtalar joint supination. Like any clinical test, the supination resistance test requires practice and observation on numerous patients. It is the one clinical test that most

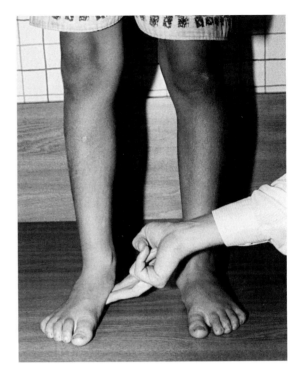

**Fig. 13-21.** Supination resistance test. The patient is instructed to stand relaxed without any attempt to move the foot or lift the arch. The examiner's fingertips are then placed plantar to the medial half of the navicular, and the examiner exerts a significant lifting force on the navicular. A normal foot will demonstrate subtalar joint supination with minimal lifting force. A pes valgus deformity will need extreme amounts of lifting force in order to produce little, if any, subtalar joint supination motion.

reliably unmasks many of the "unseen" pathologic internal forces acting within the feet of children with pes valgus deformity.

## Gait Examination

A detailed gait examination usually provides the most dramatic evidence of pathologic biomechanical function in pediatric pes valgus deformity. It is important to have the child as relaxed as possible and to instruct the parent not to assist by touching the child in any way. A gait examination in which the child gives the examiner "a performance" is not helpful to the child or the examiner. The following description will provide a brief review of

the most common abnormal gait examination in the child with a pes valgus deformity.

The child with pes valgus deformity generally exhibits minimal subtalar joint pronation motion during the contact phase of walking, because at heel contact the subtalar joint is already very close to the maximally pronated position. The abnormally pronated position of the foot at the initiation of the contact phase is the result of the foot being carried in a pronated position during the latter half of the swing phase of gait. Normally, the foot should be supinating at the subtalar joint during the latter half of the swing phase. During midstance the child with pes valgus deformity will invariably exhibit a maximally pronated subtalar joint, which either does not resupinate or may undergo further pronation during late midstance. Late midstance pronation probably contributes most to structural failure of the medial longitudinal arch, since it occurs at a time when nearly all the body's weight is on the forefoot. This in turn causes an extreme dorsiflexion force on the medial metatarsal rays, which may lead eventually to further medial longitudinal arch flattening.

Heel lift in the stance phase should normally occur at about the same time as heel contact of the contralateral foot. Early heel lift indicates either an osseous equinus deformity, a tight Achilles tendon, or idiopathic toe walking. Only in the most severe pes valgus deformities does heel lift occur without at least some supination of the subtalar joint. In any case heel lift should produce a rapid raising of the whole lateral border of the foot as one unit. If there is evidence of a "banana peeling" effect, in which the heel first lifts off the ground to be followed a moment later by the styloid process of the fifth metatarsal, then the child has sagittal plane subluxation of the oblique midtarsal joint (Fig. 13-22). Excessive dorsiflexion subluxation of the forefoot on the rearfoot is most commonly seen in pes valgus deformities coexisting with a severe gastrocnemius equinus deformity.

In children with more severe pes valgus deformities, the propulsive phase of gait will constitute a smaller percentage of the stance phase of gait than normal. Flattening of the medial longitudinal arch in severe pes valgus will result in decreased forefoot stability, making the forefoot an inefficient propulsive lever. In addition, the more severe the pronation of the foot, the more medial will be the propulsion force that occurs at the hallux and first metatarsal head and the more normal propulsion pattern of force transmission through the central hallux and second, and third digits will be lost.

The transverse plane positions of the knees and feet should always be noted to rule out any torsional abnormalities. During walking the angle of gait should be between 0 and 10 degrees, abducted to the line of progression, and the patellae should face straight ahead. Another common coexisting problem in children with pes valgus deformity is *genu valgum*,[34] which causes the medial knees to rub against each other in walking as the swing phase limb passes the stance phase limb. Genu valgum during gait is also often magnified in pes valgus deformity owing to the excessively internally rotated position of the knee joint, which results from closed kinetic chain subtalar joint pronation. Use of foot orthoses to decrease the subtalar joint pronation during gait can decrease the apparent genu valgum by decreasing the internally rotated knee position. One of the most pleasing events in prescribing effective foot orthoses for these patients is watching the knock-kneed appearance virtually disappear when the child first walks in the orthoses.

## Radiographic Evaluation

Radiographs can be very helpful in the evaluation of pediatric pes valgus deformity. They provide quantitative information concerning the severity of deformity and the degree of osseous adaptation, and they also provide information about the primary plane in which pronation compensation has occurred. Green and Carol's concept of planal dominance of pronation compensation can be most easily illustrated by radiographs.[34] Standard radiographic projections for the evaluation of pes valgus include dorsoplantar, lateral, and medial oblique views. Weight-bearing dorsoplantar and lateral views are used to determine pronation compensation and joint subluxation within, the transverse and sagittal planes, respectively. The medial oblique view is helpful in ruling out the possibility of calcaneonavicular coalition.

The extent of transverse plane compensation is determined by the degree of increase in the talocalcaneal, cuboid abduction, and forefoot abduction angles and by the decreased percentage of talonavicular congruence in the dorsoplantar projection.[40] In addition, a marked anterior break in the cyma line caused by anterior displacement of the talar head in relation to the calcaneocuboid joint is also a sign of transverse plane pronation compensation. The degree of dominance of sagittal plane pronation compensation is best identified by increased lateral talocalcaneal and talar declination angles and by a navi-

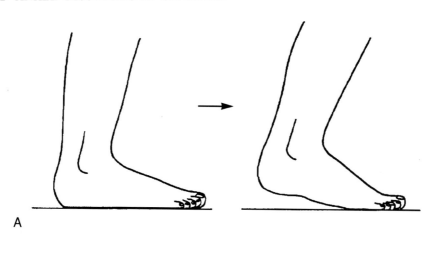

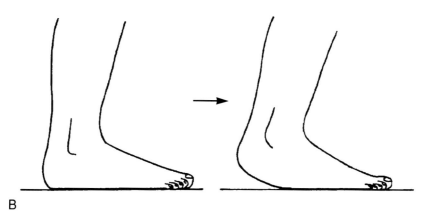

**Fig. 13-22.** **(A)** During the propulsive phase of a gait in a normal foot, raising of the heel off the ground occurs simultaneously with raising of the forefoot off the ground. **(B)** In a foot that has dorsiflexion subluxation of the midtarsal joint, however, raising of the heel will occur before lifting of the lateral forefoot off the ground, producing something of a "banana peeling" effect. This commonly occurs in pes valgus deformity with coexisting gastrocnemius equinus.

culocuneiform breach on the lateral projection.[40] Also, a decrease in the first metatarsal declination angle will be evident as pronation compensation increases within the sagittal plane. Frontal plane compensation is not directly demonstrated by standard radiographic projections of the foot but can be identified indirectly on dorsoplantar and lateral projections. An increase in the osseous super-imposition of the lesser tarsus and metatarsal bases, a decrease in height of the sustentaculum tali of the cal-caneus, and a decrease in height of the navicular relative to the cuboid on the lateral view indicates frontal plane pronation compensation. On the dorsoplantar projection, a decrease in the osseous superimposition of the lesser tarsus and the metatarsal bases indicates frontal plane dominance of pronation compensation.[40]

A new radiographic projection, the anterior axial view, which delineates the frontal plane relationship of the talar dome relative to the weight-bearing surface of the calcaneus, shows considerable promise in its ability to directly demonstrate abnormal frontal plane relation-ships in the rearfoot in the pes valgus deformity.[10] Fu-ture research will be needed in order to determine how well measurement parameters in this view will correlate with the severity of pes valgus deformity. Even so, this projection already has been shown to be quite helpful in determining the true frontal plane relationship of the talus to the calcaneus.

## NONOPERATIVE TREATMENT OF PEDIATRIC PES VALGUS

As mentioned earlier, the treatment of flatfoot deformities with shoe inserts has been evolving for at least the past 150 years. Foot orthoses have been consistently useful in the treatment of pain and/or fatigue in the feet, ankles, legs, knees, thighs, hips, and even lower backs of children. Improvement of the abnormal gait function of the lower extremities is the prime reason that foot orthoses are so helpful in relieving the abnormal externally and internally generated forces on the lower extremities that cause much of the musculoskeletal pain associated with pes valgus deformity.

However, much of the medical literature seems to support the idea that foot orthoses are useless in the treatment of the pes valgus deformity since many studies have shown no more change in the arch height of the child than what would be expected from normal growth. We hope that the following critical analysis of these studies will help the physician to realize why treatment of pes valgus deformity with foot orthoses is truly a valuable service for the child.

### Analysis of Research

A number of studies on the effects of foot orthoses and shoe corrections have been published. There is, however, one insurmountable problem with all the research. Every study that we have reviewed that sought to determine whether foot orthoses or shoe corrections produced any short- or long-term improvement of pes valgus in children looked only at the structure of the foot in a static state. The actual function of the foot during weight-bearing activities was never quantitatively assessed.[17,41-44] Typical methods of measurement have included lateral and dorsoplantar radiography of the foot, photography of the foot, and measurement of the plantar footprint in standing.[17,41-44] Static measurements of the standing foot provide little evidence of how the foot will function in gait or of the extent to which abnormal pro-

nation forces within that foot have been neutralized by a foot orthosis. Cinematographic and force plate analysis of the lower extremity during gait, with and without foot orthoses inside the child's shoes, would be a much more appropriate method of determining whether the orthoses were helping to decrease the pathologic forces on the child's foot and lower extremity during weight-bearing activities.

A number of experimental studies by sports medicine researchers found that foot orthoses not only reduce the symptoms associated with an overpronating foot but also the magnitude, velocity, and acceleration of rearfoot pronation that occurs within the foot during the support phase of running gait. Analysis of rearfoot movement within the frontal plane by digitization of high-speed cinematography has shown significant decreases in rearfoot movement with orthoses inside the shoes in most individuals. Therefore many researchers have concluded that foot orthoses do indeed have a positive impact on the reduction of overpronation in the foot.[23,45-48]

Because it is clinically obvious that children with pes valgus deformity do show marked improvement in gait function with foot orthoses, we feel that orthoses are warranted in those children who have significant pes valgus deformity or symptoms related to overpronation. Until clinically pertinent research that objectively measures gait function in children with pes valgus deformity with and without foot orthoses is carried out, the long-term effects of foot orthoses on the pediatric pes valgus foot will remain undetermined, and their potentially beneficial effects will remain unappreciated by the majority of the medical community.

### Foot Orthoses

The Whitman plate, the Roberts-Whitman brace, the Levy mold, the U.C.B.L., and the many modifications of the Root Functional Orthosis are all effective in controlling the excessive pronation of the subtalar joint that is common to children with pes valgus deformity. With different materials, different shapes, and different shoe fit characteristics, all these foot orthoses work in varying degrees to help prevent the pronation forces acting on the foot that cause biomechanically related symptoms. Since we believe that it would be unfair to comment on the effectiveness of the devices with which our experience is limited, this discussion will be limited to those devices with which we have the most experience. The

Root Functional Orthosis will be discussed in detail, and the usefulness of a modified version of it, the Blake Inverted Orthosis, will also be explored.

## Root Functional Orthosis/Functional Foot Orthosis

The Root Functional Orthosis was developed by a podiatrist, Merton Root, in the late 1950s. This orthosis (Fig. 13-2A), along with its many design variations, has since become the most popular type of foot orthosis used by podiatrists for the treatment of pes valgus deformity in both adults and children. Even though modified designs have been shown to work well at controlling pronation in the foot, the design criteria of the Root Functional Orthosis are so strict that many other useful thermoplastic foot orthoses can not be labeled true Root orthoses. Therefore the many other design variations of the Root Functional Orthosis that are also effective in the treatment of pes valgus deformity in children will be grouped in this chapter under the more general descriptive term *functional foot orthoses* (FFO).

All foot orthoses that are effective in controlling the excessive foot pronation seen in pes valgus deformity share a common characteristic, namely, they all increase the supination moment acting across the STJA. Those orthoses that are better at increasing the supination moment across the STJA are better at controlling excessive pronation of the foot. A FFO acts to control the excessive subtalar joint pronation of a pes valgus deformity by converting the GRF exerted on the heel, the fifth metatarsal shaft, and the metatarsal heads of the plantar foot into an orthotic reactive force (ORF) distributed over the whole plantar foot from the posterior heel to the metatarsal necks. The ORF is defined simply as that force which exists at the interface between the orthotic device and the foot (Fig. 13-23). In order for an FFO to exert a supination moment at the subtalar joint, it must change the distribution of forces acting on the plantar foot from lateral to medial. In other words, an FFO must alter the GRF acting on the plantar foot so that the resulting ORF is distributed more medially on the plantar foot (Fig. 13-23). If a foot orthosis is to effectively generate a supination moment across the subtalar joint, it must cause the ORF to be positioned medial to the STJA. Since greater forces and increasing lever arms both cause increased moments of rotational force across a joint axis, the greater the ORF that acts medial to the STJA on the plantar foot, the greater will be the supination moment

generated across the STJA (Fig. 13-24). Any ORF exerted by the orthosis on the plantar foot that is located lateral to the STJA will generate an unwanted pronation moment across the STJA.

Ideally, if the FFO has been designed to cause increased control of pronation in the flatfoot, the GRF will be transferred from a relatively lateral position on the plantar foot into an ORF that is distributed as close to a medial position on the plantar foot as possible. Common alterations in the FFO, such as deep medial heel cups, medial flanges, higher medial longitudinal arches, and an inverted balancing position of the positive cast, all tend to increase the ORF on the more medial portions of the heel and medial arch. In effect, these orthosis modifications cause more ORF to be exerted medial to the STJA and less ORF to be exerted lateral to the STJA. An increased supination moment at the STJA and increased pronation control from the orthosis are the direct results.

It becomes apparent, however, that if the pes valgus deformity is relatively severe and the talar head has become largely medially positioned relative to the plantar aspect of the foot, then the STJA will likewise be excessively medially deviated. Medial deviation of the subtalar joint causes the orthosis to lose effectiveness at producing an antipronation effect since the ORF has only a very short lever arm by which to produce a supination moment across the STJA. Feet that have normal STJA position have relatively long lever arms available for an ORF to produce a supination moment (Fig. 13-25A).

Any ORF directly plantar to the talar head produces more of a compression effect and less of a rotational supination effect across the STJA. This will cause the soft tissues under the talar head to be compressed excessively in a pes valgus deformity and may lead to pain or callus formation on the medial edge of the arch of the orthosis. The net effect on a pes valgus deformity is that the decreased supination moment at the STJA caused by medial deviation of the STJA will cause the orthosis to have little effect in improving the pronated position of the flatfoot (Fig. 13-25B).

It is important when trying to control excessive pronation in the pes valgus deformity with an FFO that care be taken not to allow too much dorsiflexion force to be exerted by the orthosis on the medial metatarsal rays. Excessive dorsiflexion force on the medial column can easily occur if large amounts of either extrinsic or intrinsic forefoot varus posting is added either to the orthosis shell or to a forefoot extension. Ganley believes that if forefoot posting is continued throughout childhood, the

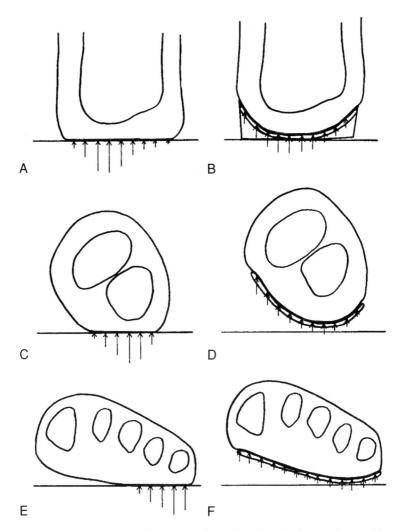

**Fig. 13-23.** (**A,C,&E**) The force the ground exerts against a bare foot in the standing position or during weight-bearing activities is the GRF; (**B,D,&F**) the force that a foot orthosis exerts against a foot is the ORF. (**A**) At the level of the medial tubercle of the calcaneus, the GRF is distributed primarily under the medial tubercle. (**B**) When an orthosis acts on the heel, the ORF is distributed more evenly from the medial to the lateral heel. (**C**) At the level of the distal talus and distal calcaneus (i.e., the midtarsal joint), the GRF is distributed primarily under the calcaneocuboid joint. (**D**) When an orthosis acts on the midtarsal joint, the ORF is lessened under the calcaneocuboid joint and widely increased under the talar head and navicular. (**E**) At the level of the midshafts of the metatarsals, GRF is distributed primarily under the fourth and fifth metatarsal bases. (**F**) When an orthosis acts at the midshafts of the metatarsals, the ORF is decreased under the fourth and fifth metatarsals and increased under the first, second, and third metatarsals. It is this conversion of a laterally positioned GRF to a more medially positioned ORF that allows a foot orthosis to exert supination moment across the STJA and resist subtalar joint pronation.

time when the orthosis can be permanently removed from patient's shoes will never occur.[32] There should be concern that continued severe dorsiflexion forces on the medial column of the forefoot from excessive forefoot varus posting will cause a permanent decrease in arch height and a permanent inverted forefoot to rearfoot deformity in the adult.

In order to eliminate this risk of excessively dorsiflex-ing the medial column, or supinating the longitudinal midtarsal joint axis with the orthosis, the child with pes

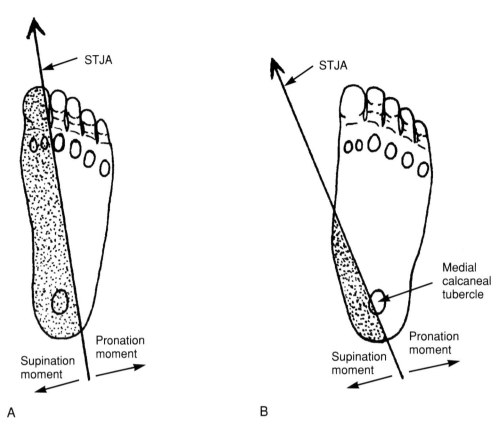

A                                                      B

**Fig. 13-24.** **(A)** The STJA in a normal foot passes from the posterolateral heel to the first intermetatarsal space. **(B)** In a pes valgus deformity, the STJA is medially deviated in relation to the plantar foot owing to the medial position of the talar head. Any GRF or ORF acting medial to the STJA will exert a supination moment across the STJA and any GRF or ORF acting lateral to the STJA will exert a pronation moment across the STJA. A normal foot has much more area available on the plantar foot for a foot orthosis to exert ORF medial to the STJA than does a pes valgus foot with a medially deviated STJA. This is one of the main reasons why foot orthoses are more effective at producing subtalar joint supination in a normal foot than they are in a pes valgus deformity.

valgus deformity should be casted for orthoses by the standard non-weight-bearing suspension casting method for the neutral subtalar joint position,[5] but with the medial column plantar-flexed to increase the medial longitudinal arch height in the cast (Fig. 13-26). This is accomplished by applying light digital pressure dorsal to the bases of the first and second metatarsals during the neutral suspension casting procedure until the plane of the metatarsal heads everts by approximately 4 to 8 degrees. This medial column plantar flexion technique decreases the inverted forefoot to rearfoot relationship (i.e., decreases the amount of forefoot varus or increases the amount of forefoot valgus) within the negative and

positive cast of the foot and increases the medial longitudinal arch height of the casts. The resulting cast is then balanced with the heel at a 5- to 10-degree inverted position so that the resulting orthosis will not only cause less medial column dorsiflexion but also will cause greater independent rearfoot control of pronation.

Other standard orthosis modifications for children's pes valgus deformities include use of rigid thermoplastic shells, 20-mm deep heel cups, and full-length rigid rearfoot posts. Medial arch flanges may also be used effectively as long as navicular tuberosity irritation does not occur. Again, all these modifications are used to mechan-

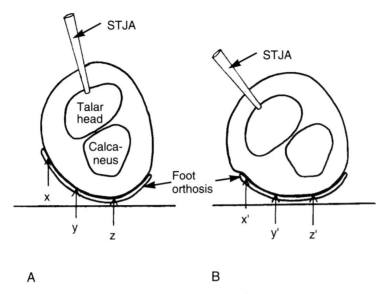

A                                              B

**Fig. 13-25.** A foot with a normally positioned STJA reacts differently to foot orthosis forces than does a foot with a pes valgus deformity with a medially deviated STJA. Three points on two sets of foot orthoses at the midtarsal joint level have been chosen for comparison: points $x$ and $x'$ are at the medial edge of the orthosis, points $z$ and $z'$ are at a point directly under the cuboid, and points $y$ and $y'$ are halfway between, respectively, points $x$ and $z$ and points $x'$ and $z'$. **(A)** In the foot with a normally positioned STJA, the ORF acting at $x$ has a long lever arm and the ORF acting at $y$ has a short lever arm to produce supination moments across the STJA. ORF acting at $z$ has a medium length lever arm, which produces a pronation moment across the STJA. **(B)** In the pes valgus foot with a medially deviated STJA, the ORF acting at $x'$ has only a very short lever arm to produce a supination moment across the STJA. The ORF at $x'$ in this foot will produce little STJA rotational effect and will produce mostly a compression effect on the soft tissues between the orthosis and the osseous structures. Since the ORF at $y'$ has a medium length lever arm and that at $z'$ has a very long lever arm to produce the pronation moment across the STJA, then the ORFs acting at $x'$ and $z'$ will both produce large pronation moments across the STJA. Therefore, the ORFs that produce a slight net supination effect when acting at three given points on the normal foot will produce a large net pronation effect when acting at these same points on a pes valgus deformity.

ically generate a greater supination moment across the STJA without causing unwanted excessive dorsiflexion of the medial column of the forefoot.

## Blake Inverted Orthosis

In the early 1980s Richard Blake, a podiatrist, began working on a modified version of the FFO, which involved actually pouring and balancing the positive cast of the foot in extremely inverted positions in order to gain more control of foot pronation in runners. The resulting orthosis, the Blake Inverted Orthosis (BIO), is actually very similar in shape to an FFO. However, the modified positive cast construction techniques used give the BIO a heel cup area that may be inverted by 15, 25, 35, or even

45 degrees. The BIO acts as an orthosis with an extreme varus heel wedge. Somewhat surprisingly, this extreme heel varus correction does not cause lateral ankle instability since the arch height of the BIO is at about the same height as would be evident in a more standard FFO. Other standard modifications of the BIO include a flat rearfoot post, a 20-mm heel cup height, and a standard accommodation for the medial band of the plantar fascia (Richard Blake, personal communication). The reason that the BIO is often more efficient than a standard FFO in controlling excessive pronation in feet is that its inverted heel cup redirects more of the ORF from the more lateral aspects to the more medial aspects of the plantar heel (Fig. 13-27). The result is that the BIO can generate larger subtalar joint supination moments than

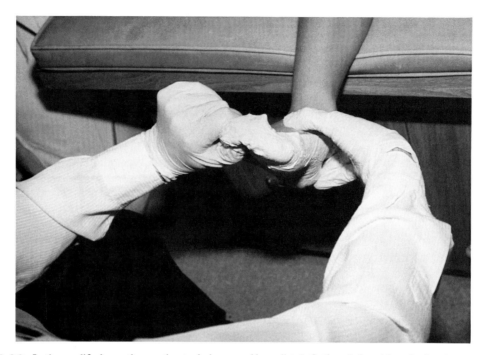

**Fig. 13-26.** In the modified negative casting technique used in pediatric flatfoot deformities, the foot is grasped at the fourth and fifth digits to position the subtalar joint in the neutral position and the midtarsal joint axes in their maximally pronated position. In addition, the other hand is positioned so that light pressure may be applied to the dorsal aspects of the first and second metatarsal bases to plantar-flex the medial column during the casting procedure. The resulting negative cast has a higher medial longitudinal arch than usual.

the FFO since the BIO has longer moment arms available to produce the supination moment.

The BIO is very useful in the more severe cases of pes valgus deformity in which the STJA is so adducted or medially deviated that there is little area available on the plantar foot for an orthosis to produce a supination moment across the STJA (Figs. 13-24, 13-25, and 13-27). In addition, children with greater amounts of ligamentary laxity seem to show the best response with the BIO since orthosis control of such feet is especially difficult. We prefer the 35-degree inverted BIO for children with the more severe cases of hyperflexible flatfeet.

Even though the BIO was originally designed for runners, it has also been used successfully by us for over 5 years in the treatment of pes valgus deformity in children. The design features of the BIO help to provide the clinician with that extra measure of pronation control that is sometimes necessary to show clinical improvement in the floppy jointed pediatric flatfoot.

## Shoe Recommendations and Shoe Modifications

Modification of existing shoes or use of prescription shoegear for the treatment of pes valgus deformity has been practiced since the 1870s when the Thomas heel was introduced.[1] However, in today's world of high-technology athletic shoes and children's increased desire to wear only shoes that are "in style," "orthopedic shoes" may soon become practical only in the infant. Rather than prescribe an orthopedic shoe, we choose to treat pes valgus deformity in children with commonly available shoegear that is cosmetically acceptable to both the parent and child and is functionally useful. Compliance of both the parent and child is also greatly improved.

In general, shoes alone (without custom arch supports of some design) are relatively poor at controlling excessive foot pronation. Most shoes have minimal support to prevent the medial longitudinal arch collapse that occurs in pes valgus deformities. However, even the best foot orthosis will not maintain its efficiency at controlling excessive foot pronation if the shoe does not have a relatively firm sole and counter. Placing the rigid, well designed orthosis made for the severely pronating foot into a soft-soled shoe can be likened to trying to build a skyscraper on a foundation of sand. Any excessive pronation force on the foot is transferred to an eversion force on the orthosis, which then simply compresses the medial sole of the shoe and allows the foot to continue pronating (Fig. 13-28). Even a rigid heel counter is quite ineffective in a soft-soled shoe since eversion compression of the sole will also cause eversion of the heel counter of the shoe. Therefore the prime consideration in shoes for children with pes valgus deformity who are being treated with foot orthoses is to make sure that the shoe has a firm sole. Next, it is helpful for the shoe to have a relatively firm heel counter and to be reinforced with leather or hard rubber where the upper attaches to the sole. Finally, added control of the medial ankle displacement seen with foot pronation can come from a high-top shoe that is appropriately laced or strapped. Many of the high-top leather basketball-style shoes or "fitness" shoes currently available in children's sizes make excellent complements to foot orthoses (Fig. 13-29). Children's running-style shoes are to be generally avoided since their midsoles are usually too soft to offer good orthosis support.

If foot orthoses are not warranted because of minimal pes valgus deformity or minimal symptoms of the deformity, then a high-top athletic-style shoe with a firm sole is often recommended. Once the shoes have been purchased, an adhesive felt or cork varus heel wedge and medial longitudinal arch support is added to the shoe to help control the heel eversion and medial arch collapse. Clinically this is often enough to greatly relieve the patient's mechanical symptoms.

## Treatment Goals and Protocol

Determining the age at which foot orthoses are recommended for the patient with pes valgus deformity requires biomechanical, technical, and financial consideration. We believe that ideally there is much more likelihood of producing permanent positive structural change in the flatfooted child if orthosis treatment is

initiated as soon the child starts walking at the age of about 1 year. Unfortunately, at this young age the frequent replacement of orthoses that would be necessary to accommodate foot growth would be financially prohibitive for most parents. Treatment with varus heel wedges and medial longitudinal arch supports, triplane heel wedges, or some form of heel stabilizer inside the child's supportive shoes from the age of 1 to 2 becomes a more practical solution to prevent excessive pronation in this young age group. It must be emphasized that effective treatment with varus heel support and medial arch support from the age of the child's first few steps gives the practitioner a golden opportunity to alter abnormal function and structure while the osseous foot skeleton is still relatively plastic.

Rigid thermoplastic foot orthoses should be instituted from the age of 2 years. Even though this may be before the child has achieved normal heel to toe gait pattern, to wait to initiate orthosis treatment until the child with significant pes valgus deformity is 3 or 4 years old could mean a poorer prognosis. Foot orthoses should be changed every one-and-a-half to two shoe sizes or when the foot has grown enough in length and width to cause the child increased discomfort when wearing the foot orthoses. Parents should be instructed to continue orthosis use either until the foot has gained more acceptable heel and arch alignment or until the child's foot growth has ended. Since adult foot length is reached generally in the midteens, we prefer to allow teenage patients to decide whether to continue their treatment with foot orthoses into adulthood. Most nonsedentary teenagers who have significant pes valgus deformity will elect to continue wearing foot orthoses well into their adult years.

As mentioned earlier, the main goal of conservative treatment of pes valgus deformity is reduction or elimination of the lower extremity symptoms that frequently accompany this common deformity of the feet. Allowing the flatfooted patient to be athletically active in school and play without continual pain is both physically and psychologically healthy for the growing child. It is obvious why it is so common for children with untreated symptomatic pes valgus deformities to grow up preferring indoor activities to outdoor play and athletic activity. Parents are told at the beginning of foot orthosis therapy that the main goal in treating their child is symptom reduction by relief of the pathologic internal stresses

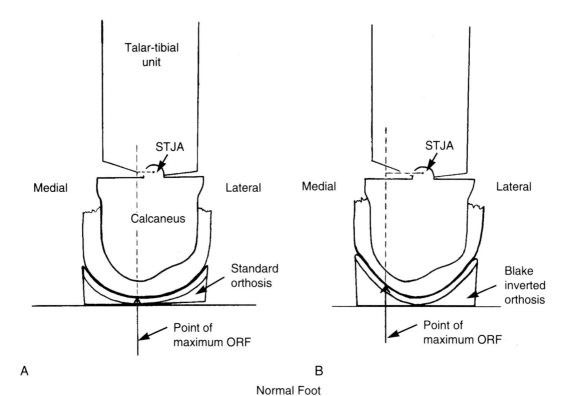

Talar-tibial
unit

STJA

Medial                    Lateral

Calcaneus

Standard
orthosis

Point of
maximum ORF

A

STJA

Medial                    Lateral

Blake
inverted
orthosis

Point of
maximum ORF

B

Normal Foot

STJA

Medial                    Lateral

Standard
orthosis

Point of
maximum ORF

C

STJA

Medial                    Lateral

Blake
inverted
orthosis

Point of
maximum ORF

D

Medially Deviated
STJ Axis Foot

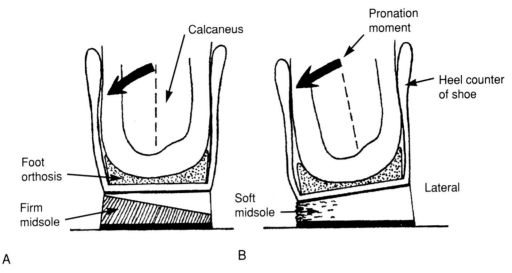

**Fig. 13-28.** **(A)** Pronation forces acting on a foot and orthosis inside a shoe with a relatively firm, incompressible sole produce little compression of the medial midsole material. **(B)** However, these same pronation forces acting on a foot and orthosis inside a shoe with a spongy, compressible sole produce excessive compression of the medial midsole material and cause the foot, orthosis, and heel counter of the shoe to evert excessively to the ground.

on the lower extremities. They are further told that the orthoses will probably not increase arch height by themselves but will allow more normal development of the child's arch by preventing the abnormal pronation compensation that tends to cause persistence of the flat-footed structure into adulthood. These explanations are fair assessments, which are based on our clinical observations and the prevailing medical literature and are well accepted by nearly all concerned parents.

The decision to perform foot surgery is a very difficult one, especially in pediatric patients. In the vast majority of cases foot surgery should be considered only after various foot orthoses and shoes have been tried and have

proved ineffective. In a smaller number of patients with the more severe deformities, the practitioner and the parents may decide that foot surgery is in the best interest of the child even without extensive attempts at conservative control of the excessive foot pronation. The practitioner must always keep in mind that a bad pair of shoes or orthoses can always be discarded, usually with minimal destructive effect, whereas a bad surgical result may remain with the child, parents, and practitioner for the rest of their lives. On the other hand, failure to consider a surgical alternative may condemn a child with severe deformity to an adulthood of pain and suffering and a more sedentary existence. Utilization of the

**Fig. 13-27.** Models of the posterior aspect of the right foot with an STJA connecting the talotibial unit to the calcaneus. **(A)** A foot with a normally positioned STJA is shown resting on a standard functional foot orthosis. The point of maximum ORF is plantar to the medial calcaneal tubercle; this orientation produces a slight supination moment across the STJA. **(B)** In the same foot with a Blake inverted orthosis, the point of maximum ORF is on the more medial aspect of the medial calcaneal tubercle, which produces a significantly larger supination moment than with a functional foot orthosis. **(C)** In a foot with pes valgus deformity with a medially deviated STJA, the point of maximum ORF is again plantar to the medial calcaneal tubercle in a functional foot orthosis. However, since the STJA position is now more medial, the ORF produces a slight pronation moment across the STJA. **(D)** In the same foot with pes valgus deformity with a medially deviated STJA resting on a Blake inverted orthosis, the point of maximum ORF is now on the medial side of the STJA and produces a supination moment across the STJA. Therefore, the Blake inverted orthosis can exert a greater supination effect on feet than would be possible with a standard functional foot orthosis by shifting its point of maximum ORF on the calcaneus and thus effectively increasing the length of its supination lever arm.

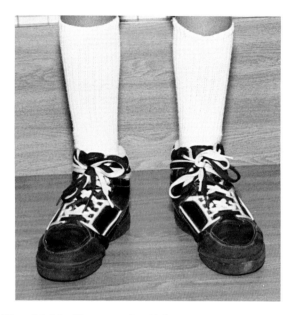

**Fig. 13-29.** Many popular high-top athletic shoes with uppers extending above the ankle joint are quite effective at improving the control of the excessive pronation by foot orthoses and improving shoe fit of the orthoses in pes valgus deformities.

growth potential for more normal musculoskeletal development can produce remarkable results. However, failure to neutralize the deforming forces in the growing child can lead to disaster. In general, when surgery is likely to be required, the earlier it is performed, the less surgery will be required, and, as with orthosis therapy, the more effective the surgery will be in neutralizing the deformity. To paraphrase Lenoir: Every day of delay in treating the pediatric deformity is a golden opportunity lost forever.

## REFERENCES

1. Schuster RO: A history of orthopedics in podiatry. J Am Podiatr Med Assoc 64:332, 1974
2. Whitman R: Observations of forty-five cases of flat-foot with particular reference to etiology and treatment. Boston Med Surg J 118:598, 1888
3. Whitman R: The importance of positive support in the curative treatment of weak feet and a comparison of the means employed to assure it. Am J Orthop Surg 11:215, 1913
4. Root ML: How was the Root functional orthotic developed? Podiatr Arts Lab Newslett, 1981
5. Root ML, Weed JH, Orien WP: Neutral Position Casting Techniques. Clinical Biomechanics Corp., Los Angeles, 1978
6. Henderson WH, Campbell JW: U.C.B.L. Shoe Insert Casting and Fabrication. Technical Report 53. Biomechanics Laboratory, University of California at San Francisco and Berkeley, 1967
7. Manter JT: Movements of the subtalar and transverse tarsal joints. Anat Rec 80:397, 1941
8. Root, ML, Weed JH, Sgarlato TE, Bluth DR: Axis of motion of the subtalar joint. J Am Podiatr Med Assoc 56:149, 1966
9. Kirby KA: Methods for determination of positional variations in the subtalar joint axis. J Am Podiatr Med Assoc 77:228, 1987
10. Kirby KA, Loendorf AJ, Gregorio R: Anterior axial projection of the foot. J Am Podiatr Med Assoc 78:159, 1988
11. Kirby KA: Rotational equilibrium across the subtalar joint axis. J Am Podiatr Med Assoc 79:1, 1989
12. Close JR, Inman VT, Poor PM, Todd FN: The function of the subtalar joint. Clin Orthop 50:149, 1967
13. Valmassy RL: Biomechanical evaluation of the child. Clin Podiatr 1:563, 1984
14. Engel GM, Staheli LT: The natural history of torsion and other factors influencing gait in childhood. Clin Orthop 99:12, 1974
15. Sgarlato TE (ed): A Compendium of Podiatric Biomechanics. California College of Podiatric Medicine, San Francisco, 1971
16. Gould N, Moreland M, Alvarez R et al: Development of the child's arch. Foot Ankle 9:241, 1989
17. Wenger DR, Mauldin D, Speck G et al: Corrective shoes and inserts as treatment for flexible flatfoot in infants and children. J Bone Joint Surg [Am] 71:800, 1989
18. Staheli LT, Chew DE, Corbett M: The longitudinal arch. J Bone Joint Surg [Am] 69A:426, 1987
19. Kirk JA, Ansell BM, Bywaters EGL: The hypermobility syndrome: musculoskeletal complaints associated with generalized joint hypermobility. Ann Rheum Dis 26:419, 1967
20. Hicks JH: The three weight-bearing mechanisms of the foot. p. 161. In Evans FG (ed): Biomechanical Studies of the Musculoskeletal System. Charles C Thomas, Springfield, IL, 1961
21. Wright DG, Rennels DC: A study of the elastic properties of the plantar fascia. J Bone Joint Surg [Am] 46A:482, 1964
22. Cavanagh PR, Lafortune MA: Ground reaction forces in distance running. J. Biomechan 13:397, 1980

23. Nigg BM (ed): Biomechanics of Running Shoes. Human Kinetics Publishers, Champaign, IL 1986
24. Brand PW: The insensitive foot (including leprosy). p. 1266. In Jahss MH (ed): Disorders of the Foot. SB Saunders, Philadelphia, 1982
25. Morton DJ: Mechanism of the normal foot and flat foot. J Bone Joint Surg [AM] 6:368, 1924
26. Smith JW: Elastic properties of the anterior cruciate ligament of the rabbit. J Anat 88:369, 1954
27. Sears FW, Zemansky MW, Young HD (eds): University Physics. 5th edition. Addison-Wesley, Menlo Park, 1976
28. Root ML, Orien WP, Weed JH: Normal and Abnormal Function of the Foot. Clinical Biomechanics Corp., Los Angeles, 1987
29. Selakovich WG: Medial arch support by operation: sustentaculum tali procedure. Ortho Clin North Am 4:117, 1973
30. Harris RI, Beath T: Hypermobile flat-foot with short tendo Achillis. J Bone Joint Surg [Am] 30A:116, 1948
31. Kleiger B, Mankin HJ: A roentgenographic study of the development of the calcaneus by means of the posterior tangential view. J Bone Joint Surg [Am] 43A:961, 1961
32. Ganley JV: Calcaneovalgus deformity in infants. J Am Podiatr Med Assoc 65:407, 1975
33. Morton DJ: Physiological considerations in the treatment of foot deformities. J Bone Joint Surg [AM] 19:1052, 1937
34. Green DR, Carol A: Planal dominance. J Am Podiatr Med Assoc 74:98, 1984
35. Valmassy RL: Pediatric biomechanics. Podiatry Today. May 1989, p. 86
36. Hawksley JC: The nature of growing pains and their relation to rheumatism in children and adolescents. Br Med J: 155, 1939
37. Root ML, Orien WP, Weed RH, Hughes RJ: Biomechanical Examination of the Foot. Clinical Biomechanics Corp., Los Angeles, 1971
38. Grumbine NA: The varus components of the forefoot in flatfoot deformities. J Am Podiatr Med Assoc 77:14, January 1987
39. Hoppenfelds: Physical Examination of the Spine and Extremities. Appleton-Century-Crofts, East Norwalk, CT, 1976, p. 172
40. McGlamry ED (ed): Comprehensive Textbook of Foot Surgery, Vol. 1. Williams & Wilkins, Baltimore, 1987, p. 403
41. Gould N, Moreland M, Alvarez R et al: Development of the child's arch. Foot Ankle 9:241, 1989
42. Pennau K, Lutter LD, Winter RD: Pes planus: radiographic changes with foot orthoses and shoes. Foot Ankle 2:299, 1982
43. Mereday C, Dolan CME, Lusskin R: Evaluation of the University of California Biomechanics Laboratory shoe insert in "flexible" pes planus. Clin Orthop 82:45, 1972
44. Bordelon RL: Correction of hypermobile flatfoot in children by molded insert. Foot Ankle 1:143, 1980
45. Smith LS, Clarke TE, Hamill CL, Santopietro F: The effects of soft and semi-rigid orthoses upon rearfoot movement in running. J Am Podiatr Med Assoc 76:227, 1986
46. Bates BT, Osternig LR, Mason B, James LS: Foot orthotic devices to modify selected aspects of lower extremity mechanics. Am J Sports Med 7:338, 1979
47. Cavanagh PR, Clarke TE, Williams KR, Kalenak A: An evaluation of the effects of orthotics on pressure distribution and rearfoot movement during running. American Orthopaedic Society for Sports Medicine Meeting, Lake Placid, N.Y., June 1978
48. Frederick EC (ed): *Sports Shoes and Playing Surfaces.* Human Kinetics Publishers. Champaign, IL 1984

# 14

# Operative Treatment of Non-neurogenic Pes Valgus Feet

*ALAN S. BANKS*
*THOMAS F. SMITH*

The majority of children with nonparalytic pes valgus deformity may be treated successfully by conservative means; however, not all those who need treatment will be afforded an opportunity for appropriate care. Despite a large volume of information that details the serious nature of pes valgus deformity, a great many physicians still adhere to the incorrect assumption that this condition is benign. In addition to local symptoms, many patients may suffer for years from a variety of leg or postural complaints and yet never appreciate the relationship of these maladies to their pes valgus deformity. For the vast majority of individuals, adult symptoms do not represent an acute event but rather the additive effects of conditions that have been present since childhood. Therefore the misconceptions regarding pes valgus deformity may result in a delay in treating some patients until an age at which conservative means have limited efficacy. Other patients will fail to respond to conservative means despite concerted attempts.

McGlamry et al. suggest that the failure of many physicians to recognize that nonparalytic pes valgus deformity is pathologic may be related to confusing nomenclature. Many knowledgeable people still refer to a collapsed, pathologically pronated foot as pes planus or flatfoot. These terms denote a benign condition in which the foot has a depressed arch but congruous rearfoot joints. Pes valgus deformity possesses most of the following characteristics: an everted heel; an abducted forefoot relative to the rearfoot; a collapsed medial column; and a flexible deformity, which may be reduced.[1] Pes valgus deformity is directly related to other pediatric foot problems as well. Kalen and Brecher have noted that patients with juvenile hallux valgus have an incidence of pes valgus that is 8 to 24 times as great as normal.[2] Other authors have also noted the correlation between these two conditions.[3,4]

Pathologic pronation may be a source of knee pain in many individuals. The excessive medial rotation of the tibia that accompanies pes valgus deformity alters the vector of contraction for the quadriceps tendon and may lead to chondromalacia patellae, or chronic subluxating patella. One of the ways that humans adapt to the stress of bipedal locomotion is through mild physiologic pronation at heel strike. However, in the patient who pronates to excess, the ability to withstand this shock is greatly reduced and may contribute to symptoms in the foot, knee, hip, or lower back.

Children may not complain of specific foot symptoms despite the presence of a significant pes valgus deformity. Herein lies another reason that many individuals may not receive early evaluation and treatment. However, the lack of localized symptoms may be secondary to acquired habits in which activity known to create discomfort is avoided. Pediatric patients with significant pes valgus deformity are less likely to be active and may tend to prefer indoor play as opposed to activities requiring walking or running. The fact that some of these children are overweight may reflect this sedentary lifestyle. Younger children will request to be carried when required to walk for extended periods or else they will constantly complain of being tired. They may also tend to remove their shoes. A history of more general symptoms such as fatigue or leg cramps may be elicited if the patient is thoroughly interviewed. Otherwise it is not until

329

adolescence or later, when the patient's activity is forcibly altered, that true foot symptoms may become evident. Giannestras firmly believed that all children with pronated feet should be treated regardless of symptoms. He noted that once the patient was exposed to "the uses and abuses of modern living," this foot type would "inevitably become symptomatic."[5]

There should be no doubt that pes valgus deformity is pathologic at any age. A cursory review of the multitude of surgical procedures that have been developed to address this condition will attest to the fact that knowledgeable sources consider this to be a substantial problem.

## CRITERIA FOR SURGICAL INTERVENTION

Previous authors have supplied criteria for determining which patients with pes valgus deformity should be considered surgical candidates. Sgarlato used a point system based upon clinical findings and symptoms. The three elements deemed most important were a maximally pronated foot in stance and gait, a positive familial history for similar deformity, and unsatisfactory improvement with functional orthoses. Interestingly, patient symptoms were assigned a relatively lower score, which confirms the issues discussed previously.[3] McGlamry et al. stated that at least one of four criteria should be met: (1) continued pain or fatigue despite adequate mechanical control; (2) severe conditions, in which the degree of deformity could be expected to progress regardless of mechanical support; (3) conditions in which abnormal stress is transferred to adjacent anatomic areas; or (4) sufficiently severe deformity to make it possible or impractical to attempt conservative control.[1]

Giannestras recommended conservative approaches in most girls until age 10 to 12 and in most boys until age 12 to 14 years. At the time the "totally pronated foot" that had not responded to conservative measures was deemed to warrant surgery even if asymptomatic.[5,6] However, we do not feel that strict age guidelines should be employed for determining the appropriate time for surgical intervention. Many factors must be considered, but in the younger child it would be ill-advised to allow deformity and symptoms to progress while awaiting a chronologic milestone. It is at this time, prior to complete osseous adaptation, that reconstructive operative techniques may be most advantageous. A surgical approach may be more conservative when compared with the measures that are required for correction in adulthood or late adolescence. Specific correction may be attained, symptoms improved or prevented, and subordinate deformities arrested or averted.

Concurrent evidence of juvenile hallux valgus or progressive hammertoe contractures indicates a more advanced condition and may imply a need for more aggressive care. A structural deformity such as a persistent compensated metatarsus adductus will be very difficult to accommodate conservatively if moderate to severe in nature. Certainly the issues discussed here provide the reader with the necessary elements for forming a basic impression as to whether or not surgery should be entertained.

## EXAMINATION OF THE PES VALGUS PATIENT
### General Examination

An initial part of the general examination will be to evaluate whether other disease states or more proximal origins of pathology are associated with the pes valgus condition. An accurate history, with specific attention paid to the perinatal period and developmental progress, will help in developing a basic impression. The influence of these conditions in the development, progression, and resistance of deformity will need to be considered. A thorough biomechanical examination is necessary for a full understanding of all factors that may be related to the pes valgus deformity. Proximally, one should rule out torsional influences in the hip, thigh, and leg. Rotational imbalance, be it medial or lateral, will be very difficult to neutralize if it is moderate to severe. Surgical intervention within the foot may need to be postponed until these factors can be properly addressed. Should extreme flexibility be noted, one should examine other joints to determine if generalized ligamentary laxity is present. At times the procedural selection may have to be altered from what would be selected under other circumstances. For the purposes of discussion, the emphasis of the chapter will be restricted to forms of pes valgus deformity that are independent of other systemic or developmental conditions, except as noted.

## Clinical Examination of the Foot and Ankle

### Ankle

One of the more common findings associated with pes valgus deformity is ankle equinus. *Equinus* is defined as the failure to achieve adequate dorsiflexion of the foot with the knee fully extended and the subtalar joint in a neutral or slightly supinated position. It is generally accepted that approximately 10 degrees of dorsiflexion is required in the average patient just prior to heel lift.[7] Should limitation of ankle motion be present, the patient will simply compensate in other areas. Equinus may be due to several factors, but it is classified into three basic types; namely, muscular, osseous, or a combination of these types.[8,9] In children osseous equinus is extremely rare; therefore, the majority of patients will have soft tissues that restrict motion. Isolated spasticity (spastic diplegia) of the gastrosoleal complex may be a subtle finding and at times is unsuspected until the patient is examined by a physician.

As there are two major muscles that constitute the tendo Achilles (and the lesser plantaris), one needs to determine the exact role of each muscle-tendon unit in perpetuating equinus. The Silverskiold test is utilized to differentiate the specific components of muscular equinus.[10] The foot is first dorsiflexed with the subtalar joint in a neutral to a slightly supinated position and the knee extended. If the patient fails to achieve adequate dorsiflexion, the knee is then flexed and the foot dorsiflexed again. The gastrocnemius muscle takes its origin proximal to the knee joint on the femoral condyles; accordingly, when the knee is flexed, the gastrocnemius aponeurosis is relaxed and its influence obviated, so that the examiner is determining if the soleus muscle is also preventing motion. If motion is limited only when the knee is extended, then only the gastrocnemius muscle is involved, and the patient is described as having a *gastrocnemius equinus* (Fig. 14-1). If sufficient dorsiflexion is not achieved with the knee extended or flexed, then both the gastrocnemius and soleus are restricting motion, and the patient has a *gastrosoleal* and/or an *osseous equinus* (Fig. 14-2).

A special consideration to keep in mind when examining for equinus is genu recurvatum. The knee must be maintained in its fully extended and functioning position, not straight relative to the thigh and leg. Genu recurva-

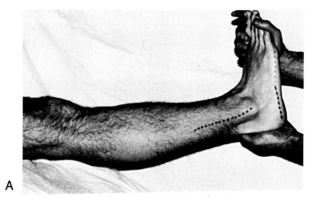

A

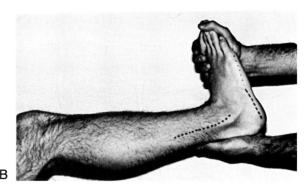

B

**Fig. 14-1.** Clinical demonstration of gastrocnemius equinus. **(A)** With the knee fully extended the foot can only be dorsiflexed to a position perpendicular to the leg. **(B)** With the knee flexed and the gastrocnemius relaxed, adequate dorsiflexion is achieved. (From Downey,[8] with permission.)

tum is a compensatory mechanism for equinus, and in gait the knee is typically maximally extended, not necessarily neutral. Failure to fully extend the knee to this end range of motion (ROM) will elicit more ankle dorsiflexion than is truly available from a functional standpoint and therefore may result in failure to diagnose this additional deformity.[9]

The foot itself should also be inspected during this maneuver. Many times in a flexible pes valgus deformity, the end range of dorsiflexion at the ankle will be achieved, and further dorsiflexion will be obtained at the midtarsal joint. Once again, the measurement of ankle motion will not be accurate. Therefore the midtarsal joint needs to be firmly stabilized and the lateral border of

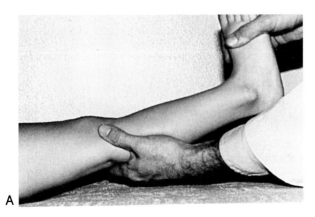

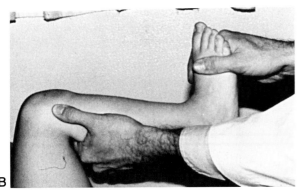

**Fig. 14-2.** Failure to achieve adequate dorsiflexion is noted both (**A**) with the knee extended (**B**) with the knee flexed, indicating gastrosoleal and/or osseous equinus. (From Downey,[8] with permission.)

the foot proximal to this level used as the reference for ascertaining ROM.

Failure to achieve adequate motion at the ankle will result in compensatory changes proximally and/or distally.[8,9] Proximal changes, which are less common, may consist of genu recurvatum, hip flexion, or lumbar lordosis. Distal compensation occurs as the foot deforms in an attempt to provide enhanced sagittal plane mobility. When the subtalar joint pronates, the midtarsal joint unlocks and is subjected to its end ROM about the oblique axis. Since one of the components of pronation is dorsiflexion, additional sagittal plane motion may be obtained from within the foot itself. Understandably, pes valgus deformity may result from the hypermobility of these joints.

The first ray becomes hypermobile when the midtarsal joint pronates; therefore medial column instability is another characteristic of compensated equinus. In the child this may lead to the development of juvenile hallux abductovalgus, callus formation plantar to the lesser metatarsals, and lesser digital contractures.[11] Arch strain or plantar fasciitis is also noted, due to the pathologic elongation of the medial column. Equinus is also a common irritating factor when calcaneal apophysitis is encountered.

## Subtalar Joint

Two specific factors to evaluate with regard to the subtalar joint are its quality and its ROM. Most importantly, it is necessary to rule out limitation of motion due to other pathologic conditions such as tarsal coalition or congenital vertical talus. Second, the joint should be evaluated for any abrupt changes in the vector of motion. This may indicate displacement of the talar head plantarly off the sustentaculum tali. Previous authors have questioned whether or not atrophy of the sustentaculum may encourage development of pes valgus deformity.[12] However, we believe that chronic pressure from a medially displaced talar head is a more plausible etiology for a dystrophic sustentaculum, especially in a patient with an untreated calcaneovalgus. In either case it may be difficult to achieve adequate correction and avoid arthrodesis if the sustentaculum is not capable of supporting the talus in the reduced position (Fig. 14-3). Additionally, adaptive change, which may be impossible to overcome, may have occurred in the posterior subtalar joint.

The subtalar joint should also be examined for any gross discrepancies in planal dominance.[1,13] In other words, does motion occur primarily in one plane? If present, pronounced uniplanar dominance may help to dictate which surgical procedure(s) to use. For example, a calcaneal osteotomy, which primarily produces a more varus alignment of the heel, may not be adequate to correct a foot in which the subtalar joint axis is high and motion occurs primarily in the transverse plane.

## Midtarsal Joint

The midtarsal joint should be evaluated for any limitation of motion that might indicate evidence of a tarsal coalition. It should be noted whether adequate freedom is available or whether the motion is "trackbound," indicating adaptation to the deformed position. The transverse plane alignment of the midtarsal joint may be indic-

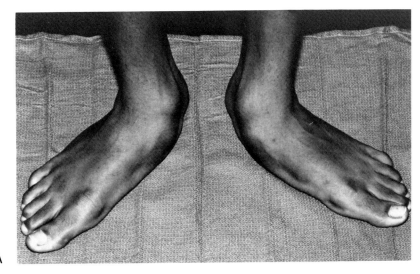

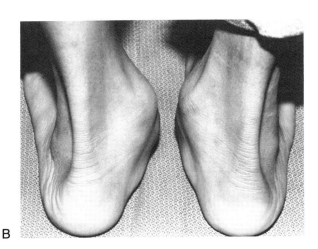

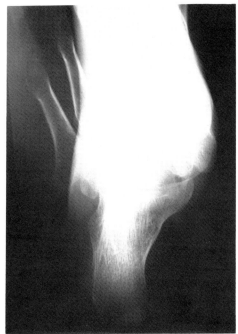

**Fig. 14-3. (A&B)** Severe collapsing pes planus valgus deformity in a 13-year-old boy. **(C&D)** Calcaneal axial radiographs demonstrate a severely adducted talar head. Chronic pressure upon the sustentaculum may induce deformity or atrophy at this level.

ative of planal dominance. A moderate to severe degree of abduction will be noted with a significant transverse plane component. An everted heel with a straight lateral border is more representative of frontal plane dominance.

**First Ray**

The term *first ray* refers to the medial column of the foot distal to the midtarsal joint. Hypermobility of the first ray would certainly serve as a cause of pes valgus deformity and is a concomitant finding in many individuals. However, we believe that first ray instability is more than likely to be secondary to equinus and/or rearfoot instability in most instances. In either case, a distinction needs to be made between the hypermobile ray, which is otherwise fairly anatomic, and a forefoot varus or supinatus. In the former condition suitable stabilization of the rearfoot may render the medial column manageable by conservative means. However, forefoot supinatus or high degrees of forefoot varus will typically require surgical intervention regardless of the concomitant procedures.

### Weight-Bearing Examination

The weight-bearing examination should be performed in static stance as well as in gait. In pes valgus deformity uncomplicated by neurologic, muscular, or significant superstructural defects, a more thorough evaluation may be made as to the planal components involved in the overall condition. One should determine whether specific aberrations that are noted represent primary deformities or secondary compensation.

Viewing the foot in static stance provides the examiner with an opportunity to compare non-weight-bearing findings with initial compensatory mechanisms. The ankle is a relatively uniplanar joint, and the primary plane of deformity will be manifested in the sagittal plane. Deformity that occurs at the ankle level may not be directly visible initially in the weight-bearing mode. The compensatory findings associated with equinus have already been discussed. The examiner should not neglect to evaluate the patient for genu recurvatum and lumbar lordosis. The heel may actually not sustain full contact with the ground in more severe cases of equinus. Ankle valgus malalignment will be difficult to discern clinically and is more often determined by radiographic examination. The position of the malleoli may indicate a proximal torsional aberration of the transverse plane. Compensation will primarily occur thorough abduction at the subtalar and midtarsal joints, creating a false impression of a normal angle of gait.

Unlike the ankle joint, the subtalar joint demonstrates substantial motion in all three planes. However, one plane of deformity can generally be identified as primary. Sagittal plane deformity at the subtalar joint is usually a response to equinus. A prominent talar head with only mild valgus or abduction of the rearfoot is characteristic.

Frontal plane deformity manifests as heel valgus, the presence of which generally indicates the existence of a forefoot varus. Transverse plane dominance will produce a prominent talar head medially with concomitant abduction. The medial prominence should not be confused with an enlarged navicular.

The midtarsal joint more commonly is associated with multiplanar deformity. Transverse plane abduction occurring at the calcaneocuboid level will be the most noticeable component clinically while in stance.

Several details noted in gait may also serve to indicate planar involvement. Medial alignment of the patellae may be due a torsional problem, which might otherwise be unappreciated because of compensation within the foot. The patient who strikes with the heel pronated, keeps the heel pronated throughout stance and, whose resupinatory effort is weak and abbreviated will usually fare poorly with conservative treatment alone. The angle of gait may be abducted in response to equinus, or the length of each stride may be shortened. An early heel-off may also be seen with equinus.

## Radiographic Examination of the Foot and Ankle

The standard radiographic views for evaluating pes valgus deformity are weight-bearing dorsoplantar and lateral views in the angle and base of gait. These views will generally provide all the information necessary to properly evaluate a patient when combined with a good clinical examination. Surgical procedures for pes valgus deformity are usually selected on the basis of clinical findings, radiographs being used to either confirm or refute these impressions. The specific radiographic changes associated with differences in planal dominance have previously been discussed. It is important to consider these factors prior to surgery to select the procedures(s) that will be most effective.

There are several other parameters to observe in addition to determining the planar components of the deformity. On the dorsoplantar view the degree of forefoot abduction should be noted and correlated with clinical motion. Another variable that many clinicians fail to assess is the degree of metatarsus adductus, which may not be clinically evident. Compensation for this deformity may lead to a significant pes valgus deformity. Surgical repair of the more obvious pes valgus condition may unmask the metatarsus adductus. Failure of the reconstructive procedures or other forms of compensation may result in moderate to severe cases. This "serpentine foot" is very difficult to manage with or without operation.

Sagittal plane influences are primarily reflected in the lateral radiograph, where they typically manifest as a depressed calcaneal inclination angle. Forefoot supinatus will also be evident in the lateral projection. The metatarsals will essentially parallel each other in the transverse plane.

Of interest is the dorsal naviculocuneiform breach, which will be evident in a large number of individuals. Several authors in the past have felt that this reflected a primary medial column fault, which allowed development of pes valgus deformity.[14,15] However, this radiographic finding represents compensatory change secondary to equinus and is therefore not a primary source of deformity in the vast majority of cases.[16,17] As the foot attempts to dorsiflex upon itself, buckling forces are directed dorsally as the plantar joint structures gap. Eventually this results in resorption of bone and adaptation at the dorsal joint interface.

Metatarsus primus elevatus is also a consequence of pes valgus deformity. Excessive pronation of the rearfoot results in subsequent hypermobility of the first ray and subsequent sagittal plane dorsiflexion. The weight-bearing function of the medial column is further impaired, which exacerbates more proximal pronatory influences.

Lateral radiographs may also be used to document flexibility and the neutral position of the foot prior to surgery. This may be helpful in the adolescent when attempting to decide exactly which means of surgical intervention is most appropriate. The foot may be placed in the neutral position or else the hallux may be dorsiflexed (Jack test) to determine the potential degree of reduction.

Calcaneal axial (Harris-Beath) radiographs will provide visualization of the posterior and middle subtalar facets as well as the sustentaculum tali. Normally these two joints should be parallel. Deviation from this orientation is indicative of a functional subtalar coalition.

In severe pes valgus deformities one may consider making anteroposterior ankle radiographs to rule out valgus deformity of the ankle. Extensive compression against the lateral aspect of the distal tibial physis or traumatic partial physeal arrest may create an uneven growth pattern with subsequent angular deformity at the distal tibia. In addition, exaggerated lateral pressure against the fibular malleolus may encourage a loss of congruity between the epiphysis and diaphysis of the fibula. Instability of the ankle mortise develops and allows the talar head to displace more medially, accentuating the abduction and valgus attitudes of the foot.[18] Ankle valgus is seen with some frequency in patients with neuromuscular disease and at times may be mistaken for a rearfoot valgus deformity.[19] Malalignment of this form may make conservative management of the foot much more difficult and if not recognized may result in the failure of a pes valgus repair.

## SURGICAL PROCEDURES

When selecting the surgical approach to pes valgus deformity the surgeon should consider only procedures that specifically address the primary plane(s) of deformity. Not all patients will possess uniplanar dominance, and several procedures may be required to provide adequate correction. In other instances surgical stabilization of one component of deformity may make the others manageable by conservative means. Although a multitude of procedures have been described for the repair of pes valgus deformity, this discussion will be limited to those that are commonly employed or have sufficient documentation to prove or disprove their efficacy.

### Gastrocnemius Recession/Tendo Achilles Lengthening

A large number of patients with pes valgus deformity will have some degree of ankle equinus. The association of ankle equinus with pes valgus deformity has been discussed by numerous authorities for years.[1,7,14,16,20-22] Pes valgus deformity may develop as compensation for triceps contracture. In fact, early surgical intervention for moderate to severe ankle equinus may prevent further destructive changes in the foot. Furthermore, if adequate growth remains, appropriate supportive measures may result in improvement in the structure of the foot.[9,23] Patients with more advanced pes valgus conditions may require additional reconstructive procedures. However, failure to release an ankle equinus may compromise the success of any other surgical procedure. Although numerous modifications and new techniques have evolved since about 1960 to 1970 for the repair of

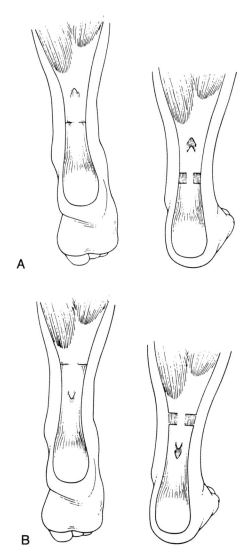

A

B

**Fig. 14-4. (A)** The traditional Baker procedure for surgical treatment of gastrocnemius equinus. **(B)** Inverted Baker technique. This approach is no longer employed, as the medial gastrocnemius head tended to undergo some degree of atrophy postoperatively. This was attributed to uneven loading due to the relatively narrow central aponeurotic band that remained following this operation. (From Downey and Banks,[9] with permission.)

pes valgus deformity, the only constant during this entire period has been the surgical treatment of equinus.[24]

Historically, numerous procedures have been described for lengthening the gastrocnemius aponeurosis for spastic conditions.[25-27] Fulp and McGlamry were the

first to describe selective gastrocnemius recession for treatment of nonspastic gastrocnemius equinus. Prior to this a complete tendo Achillis lengthening was performed regardless of whether or not the soleal fibers were involved in the contracture. Obviously, Fulp and McGlamry's modification provided a more logical approach to the deformity and a reduced recovery time. Lengthening was performed by a tongue-in-groove technique similar to that advocated by Baker.[28] Today this remains the preferred technique for surgical treatment of gastrocnemius equinus. Attempts to invert the Baker procedure may lead to mild atrophy of the medial gastrocnemius muscle mass due to uneven loading of the aponeurosis[9] (Fig. 14-4).

When both the gastrocnemius and soleal fibers are restricting dorsiflexion, a complete tendo Achillis lengthening is indicated. Sgarlato et al. noted excellent results in 78 percent of 158 patients who underwent tendo Achillis lengthening. Improved foot structure was demonstrated in children for whom orthotic support was instituted postoperatively provided 3 years of growth remained at the time of surgery. Symptomatic improvement was also demonstrated in a number of conditions.[23]

A variety of means are available for lengthening the tendo Achillis; however, we prefer open frontal plane Z-plasty. This has been found to provide more accurate

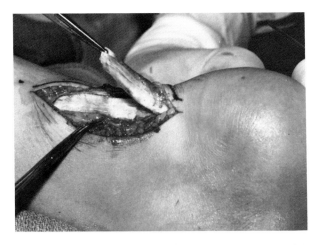

**Fig. 14-5.** Open frontal plane tendo Achilles lengthening following incision of the tendon. The foot is then dorsiflexed to an appropriate level and the tendon sutured. Direct visualization and complete exposure afford a more precise measure of correction for gastrosoleal equinus than do to other techniques.

correction with less opportunity for overlengthening. (Fig. 14-5).

## Postoperative Care

When a gastrocnemius recession or tendo Achilles lengthening is performed as an isolated procedure, patients are maintained in a below-knee walking cast for 4 weeks. Orthotic support should be instituted as soon as possible once the cast is removed. Compressive stockings such as Tubigrip will be comforting to the patient, as weakness of the triceps will be noticeable. The compression also helps to minimize scar formation. Activity such as running and jumping is avoided for another 1 to 2 months.

Normal strength will return in a matter of weeks for younger patients and in several months for adolescents. Initial exercises are isometric in nature; these are followed by toe raises, which are initially performed with the assistance of the arms and then gradually progress to unilateral, unassisted efforts. Enlargement of the tendon or aponeurosis will be palpable for several months at the surgical area. Compressive stockings will help this to resolve more rapidly.

Individual triceps lengthening procedures serve to alleviate a deforming force but do not create improved foot structure. Other problems such as forefoot varus will not be addressed. Supportive measures must be instituted to ensure that adaptive growth occurs in a favorable manner.

## Medial Column Procedures

### Young Procedure

In 1939 Young described the transposition of the tibialis anterior tendon into a slot in the navicular for the repair of pes valgus deformity. Young felt that the new position of the tibialis anterior helped to augment the tibialis posterior tendon in supporting the foot. As the tendon was not detached from its insertion, a strong plantar ligament was created for the medial arch. Following surgery the foot was said to resist abduction as well. Young recommended the procedure for patients over 10 years

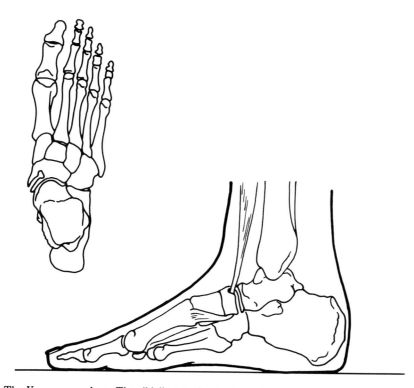

**Fig. 14-6.** The Young procedure. The tibialis anterior tendon is transposed into a slot created in the navicular.

of age, in whom suitable ossification of the navicular would be present. In younger children a suture would be necessary to secure the tendon in position. Originally the procedure was performed on adolescents, but the author later successfully performed the surgery on one adult[29] (Fig. 14-6).

Crego and Ford performed the Young procedure on six patients, who were re-examined at an average of 5½ years following surgery; four excellent and two good results were reported.[30] The benefits of the procedure were later confirmed by Beck and McGlamry. Satisfactory clinical and radiographic improvement was noted with the tendosuspension and surgical release of equinus. Enhanced stance and gait function was said to result from a more supinated position of the subtalar joint. Concomitant stabilization of the transverse axis of the midtarsal joint provided a more stable lateral column for the peroneus longus to plantar-flex the first ray while the rerouted tendon supported the medial arch. Slight adduction of the foot was recognized.[31]

Further experiences began to reveal the shortcomings of the Young tendosuspension. Patients with marked abduction were noted to have inadequate correction. Additional advancement of the tibialis posterior or transfer of a portion of the flexor digitorum longus into the tibialis posterior made little difference in reducing the transverse plane abduction at the midtarsal joint.[24]

The Young procedure is indicated for medial column stabilization of flexible sagittal plane deformity. However, the transposition serves to distinctly plantarflex the first ray and will have the added benefit of reducing frontal plane forefoot varus or supinatus. Not only is the first ray stabilized, but the tendency for dorsal joint space breach is eliminated if ankle equinus is addressed concomitantly. The procedure should not be expected to correct transverse plane deformity, and the efficacy of the procedure in patients beyond adolescence is not as reliable. At this point osseous adaptation to the deformed position may be difficult to overcome with tendosuspension. Despite additional lateral column stabilization, Jacobs and Oloff noted two satisfactory and two unsatisfactory results in patients in whom the Young procedure was utilized to reduce forefoot supinatus. The average age of these patients was 19.7 years.[32]

In younger patients in whom the navicular is not sufficiently ossified to allow a suitable drill hole for anchoring the tendon, the tibialis anterior may be sutured into the tibialis posterior plantarly. Greater reinforcement may be achieved by suturing the transposed tendon into the lateral branch of the tibialis posterior within the midarch. A groove is created in the medial aspect of the navicular prior to final placement in order to encourage tenodesis. Should the navicular fracture during surgery on an older patient, this same technique may be employed successfully.

## Kidner Procedure

The association of the symptomatic accessory navicular (os tibiale externum) with pes valgus deformity led Kidner to propose that the presence of this ossicle directly contributes to an anomalous insertion of the tibialis posterior, thereby preventing the tendon from performing the requisite function of supporting the arch. To counteract this fault Kidner recommended that the tibialis posterior tendon be rerouted beneath the navicular whenever syptomatic ossicles were excised. He proposed that a more effective support mechanism is thus created and the pes valgus deformity thereby improved[33,34] (Fig. 14-7).

Evaluation of the Kidner procedure entails assessment of two different parameters, namely, whether or not local symptoms are alleviated and whether or not the structure of the foot is altered. Veitch performed the Kidner procedure in a number of patients, 15 of whom had pes valgus deformity. Although symptoms resolved postoperatively, he noted that there was no radiographic or photographic evidence to suggest a change in arch appearance.[35] Sullivan and Miller examined radiographs of 179 patients without and 49 patients with an os tibiale externum. There was no significant difference in the radiographic measurement of arch height between the two groups. They concluded that there was no evidence that the os tibiale externum disrupted the integrity of the tibialis posterior.[36] Macnicol and Voutsinas reported that the course of the tibialis posterior tendon was not abnormal in patients with an accessory navicular. However, these authors did report improvement in foot structure in 14 of 22 patients following the Kidner procedure.[37] Lawson et al. noted a normal arch in the 10 patients undergoing excision of painful os tibiale externum.[38]

The basic premise underlying the use of the Kidner procedure to correct pes valgus deformity has not been substantiated. The insertion of the tibialis posterior is quite expansive and involves much more than an attach-

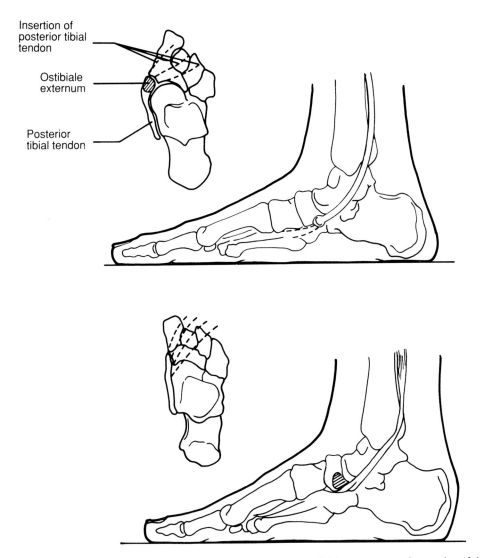

Insertion of
posterior tibial
tendon

Ostibiale
externum

Posterior
tibial tendon

**Fig. 14-7.** The original Kidner procedure consisted of excision of the os tibiale externum and rerouting of the tibialis posterior tendon.

ment to the navicular tuberosity. Basmajian and Stecko have further shown that the muscles and tendons are not required for arch support in the normal foot.[39] It is only in the pathologic setting, when hypermobility is present, that the tibialis posterior attempts to perform this function. Lemont et al. demonstrated a synovial joint between the navicular and the os tibiale externum, and this may account for inflammatory symptoms in the area.[40] Therefore, patients with pre-existing pes valgus deformity and this accessory ossicle in whom overuse of the

tibialis posterior is also present are more likely to develop symptoms. As clinicians are much more likely to examine patients with complaints than those without, the association of os tibiale externum with pes valgus deformity is more anecdotal than scientific. Most clinicians will vouch for the fact that the accessory navicular is most often an incidental radiographic finding in a variety of foot types.

Theoretically, advancing the tibialis posterior would adduct the midtarsal joint and assist in reducing transverse plane abduction. More strength could be provided if the spring ligament were to be advanced as well. However, experience has demonstrated that medial column tendon procedures generally are not alone able to sustain correction of the transverse plane component of pes valgus deformity. Therefore, the isolated use of the Kidner procedure in a primary reconstruction of pes valgus deformity is an exception. The Kidner procedure can be useful, however, as a method of plicating the posterior tibial tendon after excision of a symptomatic os tibiale externum.

## Medial Arch Tendosuspension

By combining and modifying the Young and Kidner procedures into a single technique, a more effective soft tissue correction may be provided than by using either alone. Young originally transposed the tibialis anterior

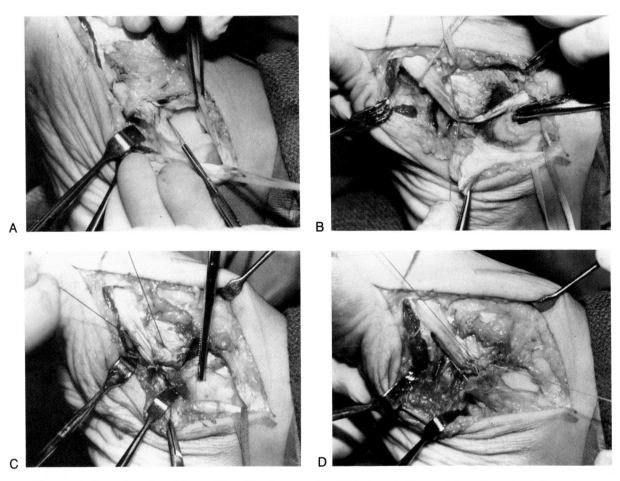

**Fig. 14-8.** Deep dissection of the medial arch tendosuspension. **(A)** An inverted L capsulotomy is created in the spring ligament once the medial expansion of the tibialis posterior is incised and retracted. The talonavicular joint is now visualized, as well as the very thick nature of the spring ligament. **(B)** The tibialis anterior is tagged with a 0 gauge suture into the lateral expansion of the tibialis posterior tendon and then transposed into the navicular slot. **(C)** Once the tibialis anterior is transposed the spring ligament (held by the hemostat) is advanced into the tibialis anterior and the lateral slip of the tibialis posterior. **(D)** The medial slip of the tibialis posterior is similarly advanced and sutured into position. *(Figure continues.)*

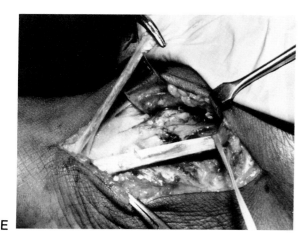
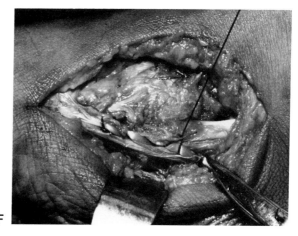

**Fig. 14-8** *(Continued).* **(E)** Alternatively, the tibialis anterior may be hemisected prior to transfer. **(F)** The free tendon piece is then used medially as a reinforcement for the previously transposed portion of the tibialis anterior and tibialis posterior.

and lengthened the tendo Achilles but did not address any of the other structures of the foot. Kidner advanced the tibialis posterior on itself but really did not involve other anatomic structures that could aid in maintaining correction. There are several key steps that help to distinguish the medial arch tendosuspension. First, the tibialis anterior may be split longitudinally, with one half subsequently being detached proximally. The medial insertional slip of the tibialis posterior tendon is severed at the level of the navicular and dissected free proximally. The spring ligament is thus exposed, and an inverted L capsulotomy is created in the talonavicular joint.

The intact half of the tibialis anterior tendon is then routed through the slot in the navicular. While the foot is maintained in an adducted position, the spring ligament is advanced and sutured into the lateral tendinous slip of the tibialis posterior and the transferred portion of the tibialis anterior. The medial section of the tibialis posterior is then advanced along its original course and sutured distally. The free slip of the tibialis anterior may then be laid on top of the new tendinous complex medially as a reinforcement (Fig. 14-8).

The medial arch tendosuspension has proved to be a highly effective means of stabilizing the medial column. Sagittal plane improvement is provided by the transfer of the tibialis anterior. Advancement of the tibialis posterior also tends to recreate good soft tissue support in the arch. Frontal plane improvement will be noted as the

tension on the transferred tibialis anterior tendon will plantar-flex the first ray. Advancement of the spring ligament and the medial slip of the tibialis posterior serves to enhance transverse plane stabilization to a far greater extent than the Kidner procedure alone. However, one should not rely on the medial arch procedure to provide the principal means of transverse plane stabilization.

Generally the medial arch reconstruction is combined with an appropriate lateral column procedure, but in patients between the ages of 3 and 6 it may be used alone or in conjunction with subtalar arthroereisis.

### Hoke Arthrodesis

Hoke was the first to describe arthrodesis of the navicular and first and second cuneiform joints for pes valgus deformity. This was performed in conjunction with tendo Achilles lengthening. Hoke felt that the integrity of the arch was maintained by the muscles and arthrodesis enhanced their ability to function[14] (Fig. 14-9).

Butte performed 138 procedures and reported only 50 percent as satisfactory at follow-up. He noted that the operation was most successful in patients with naviculo-cuneiform sag on the lateral radiograph. Relative contraindications included obesity, severe pronation, deformity within the tarsus, and arthrosis of the foot and ankle.[22] Unfavorable results were also noted by Crego

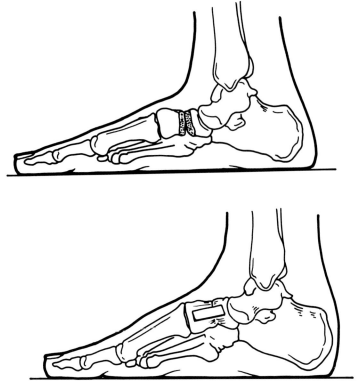

**Fig. 14-9.** The Hoke arthrodesis.

and Ford, who concluded that fusion of this single joint was not sufficient to support the arch, confirming the earlier thoughts of Butte.[30]

The use of the Hoke arthrodesis for naviculocuneiform sag was also espoused by Jack and later by Giannestras.[5,41] Jack modified the arthrodesis by utilizing a strut of autogenous tibial metaphyseal graft; 38 or 46 feet were judged to have a good or excellent result at initial follow-up 15 months to 5 years after surgery. All patients were between the ages of 11 and 14 at the time of surgery. A tendo Achilles lengthening was not performed in this series, and in fact a number of patients were reportedly casted in equinus.[41]

Seymour examined 17 of Jack's original patients 16 to 19 years following surgery, using the same grading scale as Jack. During the intervening period the patients had undergone distinct deterioration, about half of those feet examined demonstrating an unsatisfactory result. The radiographs of this group all demonstrated degenerative changes in the subtalar and midtarsal joints. Seymours's conclusion was similar to the conclusions of earlier au-

thors, namely, that fusion of one segment of the arch can not be expected to prevent collapse of the remaining medial joints. Furthermore, Seymour postulated that the Hoke procedure had actually hastened arthritic changes in adjacent joints.[42]

Giannestras, who held an opposing view, combined the Hoke procedure with transposition of the tibialis anterior and posterior. He also used an osteoperiosteal flap to reinforce the medial column.[5] Jacobs and Oloff reported either an excellent or a satisfactory result in all 16 patients undergoing Hoke arthrodesis. However, each was evaluated 5 years or less postoperatively. The average age at the time of surgery was 13.2 years. In each instance the Hoke arthrodesis was used as a medial column adjunct to lateral column stabilization, and equinus was addressed simultaneously.[32]

Success or failure with the Hoke procedure is predicated upon several key factors. The first is the view that naviculocuneiform sag is representative of compensation for other deforming forces and not a primary cause of medial column instability. Ankle equinus is the usual deformity that leads to this radiographic finding. Therefore, arthrodesis of this joint as a single procedure is not usually indicated, as compensation for the primary deformity will only occur elsewhere. Second, the resection of bone required for arthrodesis will result in adduction of the foot, which may encourage excessive stress in the lateral column. This may account for continued pain or later degenerative changes. Although the follow-up period was rather brief, those patients reported by Jacobs and Oloff stand the best chance to achieve overall satisfactory results as equinus and lateral column stabilization were both addressed simultaneously.[32] However, one should note the historical inadequacies of the procedure prior to implementation.

## Miller Procedure

The Miller procedure, first described in 1927, involves arthrodesis of the naviculo-first cuneiform and first cuneiform-first metatarsal joints. A medial osteoperiosteal flap was also used and advanced distally following ar-

throdesis[15] (Fig. 14-10). In 15 patients examined 9½ years following surgery, Crego and Ford noted three excellent and eight good results.[30] Today there are very limited indications for the Miller procedure in the child or adolescent, as other measures have proved to be equally effective without sacrificing joint motion. Specific considerations are neuromuscular disease, severe ligamentary laxity, and post-traumatic degeneration.

## Talonavicular Arthrodesis

Talonavicular arthrodesis, rarely performed today for pediatric or adolescent pes valgus deformity, has been used in the past primarily as an adjunctive procedure. Lowman combined this technique with tendo Achilles lengthening and rerouting of the tibialis anterior through the navicular.[43] Tachdjian recommends the procedure primarily for symptomatic post-traumatic arthrosis.[44]

It is preferable to avoid talonavicular arthrodesis in the child if suitable alternative procedures are available. Arthrodesis of this one joint effectively eliminates rear-

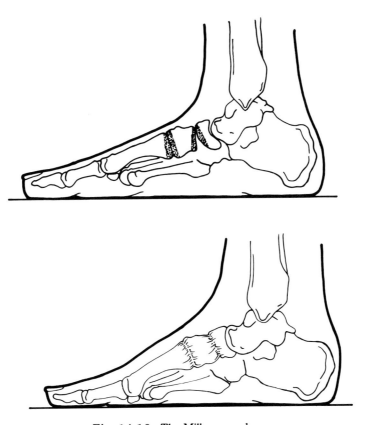

**Fig. 14-10.** The Miller procedure.

foot motion. There is a question as to whether the fusion of the talonavicular joint encourages later degenerative change at the subtalar or calcaneocuboid level. Fogel et al. examined 11 patients who had undergone talonavicular arthrodesis for isolated arthrosis 9.5 years previously on average. Their ages at the time of surgery ranged from 2.5 to 21 years. Asymptomatic arthrosis was noted radiographically in adjacent joints in 3 of the 11 patients.[45] Conversely, it is interesting to note that talonavicular coalitions are generally asymptomatic.[46] On this basis the failure of isolated talonavicular arthrodesis may be related to the degree of shortening, residual deformity following surgery, or inadequate appreciation of the primary deforming influences.

Arthrodesis at this level allows for derotation of the forefoot to correct unreduced forefoot varus or supinatus. However, as an isolated procedure this may induce stress on the lateral column, which may later prove symptomatic. Care should be taken to adduct the foot as little as possible, which may require the use of grafting techniques. Certainly alleviation of pain resulting from arthrosis is one indication for this procedure. However, arthrosis at the talonavicular joint in the patient with pes valgus deformity may also be representative of a tarsal coalition. One must be careful to evaluate patients for the presence of other pathology, as many coalitions do not become symptomatic until an injury occurs to the foot. Preoperative radiographs while performing the Jack test may also be helpful. If a talonavicular fault reduces with this maneuver, then the deformity is flexible and may be corrected just as well by other means. However, failure of the talonavicular joint to relocate following hallux dorsiflexion indicates that a talonavicular arthrodesis should be strongly considered.

## Surgical Approach

The surgical approach for the medial arch tendosuspension, Young, Kidner, Hoke, and Miller procedures as well as talonavicular arthrodesis may all be achieved through the universal dissection process described by Ruch (Film, The Podiatry Institute, Tucker, GA, 1986) and McGlamry et al.[1] For visualization of the entire medial column, an incision is extended from the inferior aspect of the medial malleolus to a point distal to the first metatarsal base. This incision is shortened as required for lesser degrees of exposure. Dissection is carried through the skin and subcutaneous tissues, where numerous branches of the great saphenous vein will be encountered. The superficial fascia is then bluntly separated from the underlying deep fascia with a moist sponge. Adequate clearance can be achieved for harvesting the tibialis anterior or for any of the fusion techniques. The deep fascia overlying the abductor hallucis muscle is identified at the base of the first metatarsal. This layer is punctured with a Metzenbaum scissors, which is then directed within this layer proximally until it reaches the tibialis posterior sheath. Complete visualization of the access to any structure of the medial arch are now available (Fig. 14-11).

The Hoke and Miller procedures, as well as talonavicular arthrodesis, are generally reserved for patients with either fixed or rigid deformities. In fixed deformities the medial column retains some degree of flexibility and yet can not be fully reduced, or the medial column elevatus is reducible but retains a fair degree of resistance. Sometimes these deformities may appear flexible while non-weight-bearing, but the arch will not appreciably change in stance with the Jack test. Obviously, rigid deformity will not respond well to soft tissue techniques. However, in pediatric and adolescent patients with flexible and reducible conditions, the medial arch tendosuspension is superior. Necessary correction is achieved and abnormal motion is controlled without sacrificing all mobility of the affected joints.

One should be careful when carrying out the medial column fusion techniques as isolated procedures. Excessive shortening may place stress on the lateral column, which may result in a variety of complaints. The degenerative changes noted following the Hoke procedure may be evidence of this. Either grafting of the medial column arthrodesis to preserve length or concomitant lateral column procedures appear to be indicated.

## Postoperative Care

Postoperative care for the soft tissue procedures should consist of a non-weight-bearing cast for 6 weeks. Orthotic support is essential once weight-bearing is resumed; otherwise some loss of correction may occur. Supportive measures may also enhance long-term correction by allowing the foot to adapt with growth to the new alignment.

Medial column arthrodesis procedures should also be managed in a non-weight-bearing cast for 6 to 12 weeks. The length of casting depends upon the age of the indi-

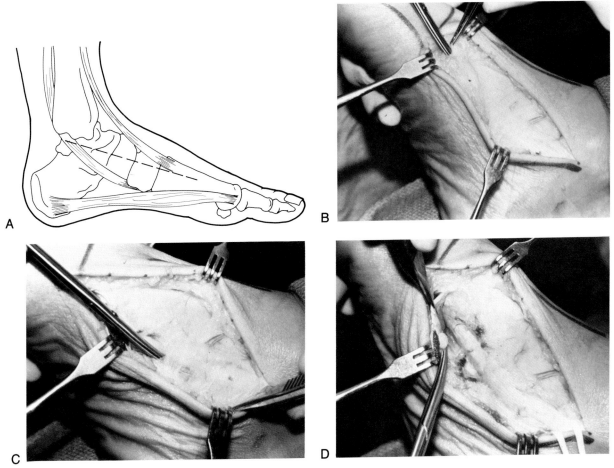

**Fig. 14-11.** Universal soft tissue dissection for the medial arch structures. **(A)** The incision commences proximally just inferior to the medial malleolus and extends distally beyond the first metatarsocuneiform articulation, generally besecting the osseous structures in between. The incision may be shortened appropriately depending upon the procedure to be performed. **(B)** The deep fascia is punctured at the level of the first metatarsal between the bone and the abductor hallucis muscle. **(C)** Dissection is followed within this plane proximally into the sheath of the tibialis posterior. **(D)** Further separation of the deep fascia overlying the navicular and cuneiform will reveal the full extent of the medial band of the tibialis posterior. Full access to any of the medial arch structures may now be obtained.

vidual and whether or not bone grafts were used. Compressive stockings will be helpful to counteract edema once the cast is removed.

## Lateral Column Procedure — Evans Calcaneal Osteotomy

Evans devised his calcaneal osteotomy procedure after noticing that excessive removal of bone from the lateral column of a foot with pes cavus deformity resulted in the opposite pes valgus condition. Therefore he proposed

that lengthening the lateral column of a patient with pes valgus deformity would improve the shape of the foot.[47] Evans believed that the lateral column of the foot was the foundation of the skeletal structure and that restoration of appropriate length could be used to treat either supinated or pronated feet. With regard to pes valgus deformity, he believed that shortening of the lateral structures of the foot occurs as an adaptation to aberrant pronating forces acting upon immature bone. Therefore patients were treated by osteotomy of the calcaneus with insertion of a bone graft to lengthen the lateral

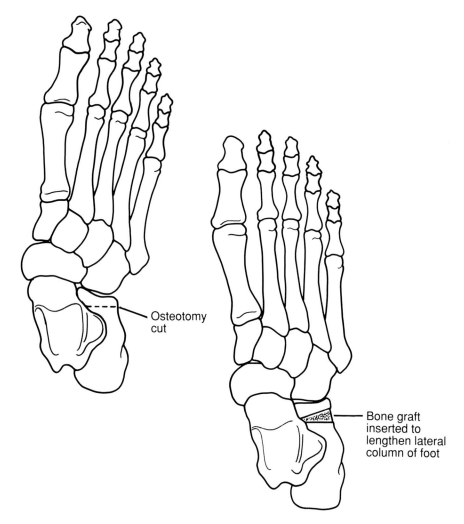

Osteotomy
cut

Bone graft
inserted to
lengthen lateral
column of foot

**Fig. 14-12.** The Evans osteotomy with bone graft.

column (Fig. 14-12). The specific indications proposed by Evans included overcorrection of talipes equinovarus, calcaneovalgus following poliomyelitis, rigid flatfoot, and idiopathic calcaneovalgus. He considered the procedure to be relatively contraindicated in patients with spasticity or spina bifida.[47]

## Results

Phillips published a report of patients who had undergone surgery by Evans 7 to 20 years prior to follow-up examination. Of the 23 feet in this series, 17 were judged to

have a very good or good result. Interestingly, Phillips noted that the procedure had been performed on a number of spastic patients, but none were included in the follow-up study.[48] Dollard et al. reported favorable results in 50 feet undergoing the Evans procedure, although each was examined less than 3 years postoperatively.[49] Anderson and Fowler examined nine feet 6 years following Evans osteotomy surgery and reported only one poor result. Posterior tibial tendon advancement was also performed in each instance. These authors recommended that the procedure be performed on patients between 6 to 10 years of age to allow time for remodeling of the tarsal joints to the new position prior to maturity. In some instances forefoot supinatus was addressed through additional medial column procedures.[50] Mahan and McGlamry reported on 21 patients representing a total of 35 feet. Most of these patients had undergone surgery to alleviate equinus as well as medial arch tendosuspension. Significant improvement was noted clinically, radiographically, and symptomatically, although the average time elapsed since surgery was only 11 months. The correction was noted to be superior to the results achieved by the Young procedure alone.[51]

The Evans procedure remains an effective means of providing permanent reliable correction for pes valgus deformity. It is primarily indicated in patients with a transverse plane abduction, as evidenced clinically and in the dorsoplantar radiograph. The benefits of the anterior calcaneal graft are many. The enhanced stability of the midtarsal complex resists deformity in the medial column and forefoot. The forefoot will adduct and create a more congrous talonavicular joint.[49] In the younger patient

this may prevent adaptive joint alignment, which tends to perpetuate the pes valgus condition. Following surgery the calcaneus is noted to assume a more vertical position.

### Technique

The surgical technique has been described by numerous authors. Originally the approach was through a linear incision paralleling the peroneal tendons. This was later changed to an oblique incision overlying the anterior calcaneus and parallel to the relaxed skin tension lines. This incision provides good exposure, and yet there is less risk of hypertrophic scar formation (Fig. 14-13).

Dissection is carried through the superficial fascia, with care to avoid damage to the intermediate dorsal cutaneous and sural nerves, which may be identified as the dorsal and plantar ends of the incision, respectively. The superficial fascia is thin over the center of the incision, overlying the extensor digitorum brevis. It is preferable to bluntly separate this tissue layer to avoid disturbing the deep fascia investing the muscle. The

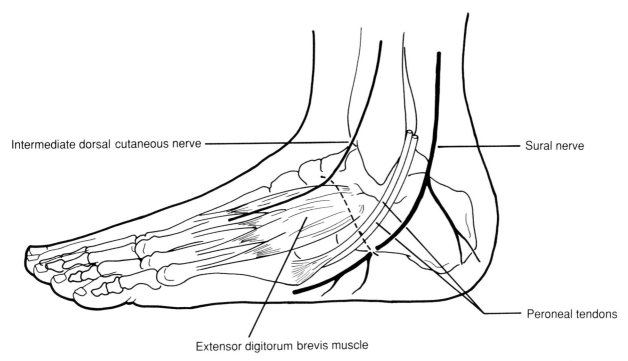

Intermediate dorsal cutaneous nerve

Sural nerve

Peroneal tendons

Extensor digitorum brevis muscle

**Fig. 14-13.** Surgical approach for the Evans procedure. Care should be exercised at the dorsal and plantar ends of the incision to avoid damage to neural structures. The peroneal tendons will need to be retracted prior to osteotomy.

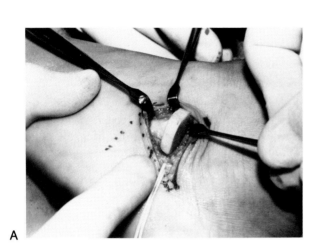 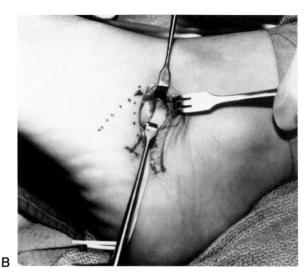

A                                                                    B

**Fig. 14-14.** Appearance of the allogeneic bone graft **(A)** before and **(B)** after seating. The lateral dorsal cutaneous nerve is retracted inferiorly with a vessel loop.

peroneal tendons should be identified inferiorly. An L-shaped incision is made in the deep fascia at the anterior edge of the lateral talar process. The extensor digitorum brevis is then dissected free from the calcaneus and reflected anteriorly. The periosteum is then undermined plantarly, the peroneal tendons being contained within the flap. Care should be exercised to preserve the ligaments of the calcaneocuboid joint while dissecting the soft tissues. Compromise of these ligaments may result in displacement of the distal calcaneal fragment following insertion of the graft.

The osteotomy is then performed in the anterior aspect of the calcaneus, approximately 1 to 1.5 cm proximal to the calcaneocuboid joint. Excessive dorsal excursion of the saw during this process may result in damage to the talar head. Once the bone has been cut, an osteo-

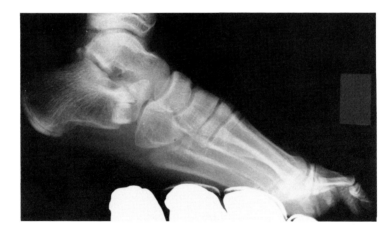

**Fig. 14-15.** Dorsal displacement of the distal aspect of the calcaneus may occur if the calcaneocuboid joint ligaments are compromised or if very wide sections of graft are used. The buildup of linear tension created by impaction of the graft wedges the less stable section of the calcaneus dorsally.

tome is introduced and twisted from side to side to break free any ligamentous tether caused by the long and short plantar ligaments. The osteotomy may then be pried open and an estimate made of the required width of the graft.

The bone graft may be taken from the patient's proximal tibia, from the iliac crest, or from freeze-dried allogeneic specimens. Experience over the past 10 years has proved that additional invasive procedures are not required, as the allogeneic bone bank material is quite suitable. No problems have been experienced with regard to healing or rejection. A piece of bone approximately 5 to 8 mm wide is usually appropriate. Although some authors have described cutting the graft into a T shape to enhance stability, in more recent years this has proved unnecessary, as the compression against the graft has been found to be secure. The surgeon may choose to make the graft wedge-shaped or trapezoidal. The wedge graft is primarily used for patients requiring lesser degrees of correction, as this is not quite as effective as lengthening of the entire lateral column (Fig. 14-14).

Fixation is not necessary unless visible instability is recognized. Options include the use of a lateral staple or a Kirschner wire. Prior to closure the foot should be assessed to ensure that there has been no overcorrection of the pes valgus deformity, which might be manifested either as excessive forefoot adduction or rearfoot varus.

## Postoperative Care

Postoperatively the patient is maintained in a non-weight-bearing cast for 12 weeks. By this time the graft will have been assimilated, although it may be several months before the cortical portions of the graft are fully resorbed radiographically. The cast may be bivalved after 5 to 6 weeks to allow for hydrotherapy and gentle ROM exercises of the ankle. The patient should be placed in an orthotic device after cast removal.

We are aware of only two cases of delayed union following allogeneic bone graft for the Evans osteotomy. Each of these patients eventually progressed to complete healing without complications. Occasionally one may notice that the distal fragment of the calcaneus will appear to be slightly dorsally displaced as compared with the preoperative radiograph. This has so far not proved to be a problem. Potential irritation of the peroneal tendons by contact with a prominent graft or be-

cause lateral column lengthening has not been confirmed (Fig. 14-15).

## Combination Procedures

Originally the Evans osteotomy was described as an isolated procedure. However, McGlamry and Downey[52] and Dockery[53] noted that forefoot varus or supinatus did not reduce adequately without supplemental procedures. Failure of this forefoot deformity to reduce will cause excessive stress on the lateral column and may result in symptoms similar to those of fixed forefoot varus. Therefore, the Evans osteotomy is most commonly combined with medial column procedures to enhance correction (Figs. 14-16 and 14-17).

## Posterior Calcaneal Osteotomies

### Silver Calcaneal Osteotomy

Silver et al. first described the lateral insertion of a wedge of bone graft into the body of the calcaneus for the treatment of valgus feet associated with cerebral palsy. They believed that the procedure was superior to the Grice procedure, as the patients retained subtalar motion. These authors performed 20 osteotomies for the correction of valgus deformity in conjunction with requisite soft tissue techniques.[54] Later the procedure was extended for use in 22 patients with severe idiopathic valgus, with good results. Patients with idiopathic deformity were between the ages of 6 and 17, the majority being 3 to 10 years old. Silver noted that the osteotomy was not the solution for all valgus feet and that some would require additional soft tissue procedures[55] (Fig. 14-18). Marcinko et al. described good results in 10 patients between the ages of 4 and 16 at the time of surgery,[56] which they claimed closely approximated those of Beck and McGlamry with the Young suspension.[31] Allogeneic bone bank graft material was employed in all cases without complications. These authors recommended that cortical allogeneic bone be utilized to prevent later collapse of the graft with potential loss of correction.

The Silver osteotomy plus graft is a useful technique for the treatment of the frontal plane component of structural rearfoot deformity. This may be shown by placing the foot in the neutral position and noting the heel position. Failure of the calcaneus to approximate a vertical position is an indication for the Silver procedure.

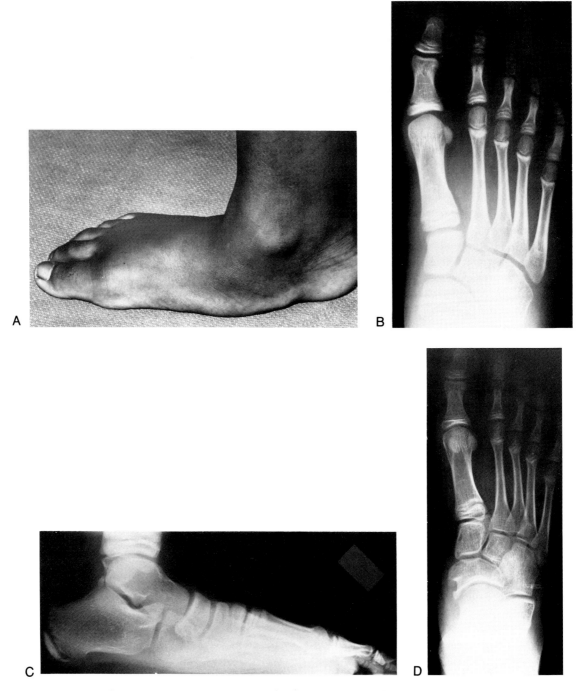

**Fig. 14-16.** **(A)** Preoperative clinical appearance of 11-year-old boy. **(B&C)** Preoperative radiographs. **(D&E)** Postoperative radiographs 2 years following Evans, medial arch tendosuspension, and gastrocnemius recession. *(Figure continues.)*

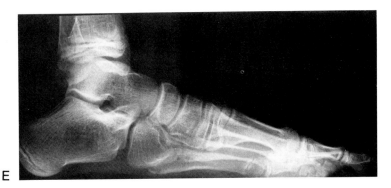

E

**Fig. 14-16** *(Continued)*.

The operation is technically easy to perform, and complications are not commonly encountered. It involves a curvilinear incision over the lateral aspect of the heel just posterior to the peroneal tendons. Dissection is uncomplicated once the surgeon has ensured that the sural nerve and lateral calcaneal artery are avoided. Adequate reflection of the soft tissues must be provided laterally, dorsally, and plantarly, as only the medial cortex of the calcaneus will be left intact. The calcaneal periosteum is incised and reflected slightly to provide clearance for the saw. The osteotomy should be made as far anteriorly as possible without compromising the subtalar joint. This will ensure the maximum degree of correction as it provides a longer lever. Wedging with an osteotome following completion of the bone cuts may help to enhance flexibility.

Allogeneic graft material is preferred for this procedure. Iliac crest wedges, similar to those for the Evans osteotomy, are used. The cortical margins of these wedges have been found to be adequately strong to resist collapse. Several pieces, 5 to 8 mm in width at the lateral margin, are required to fill the void. The compressive forces of the medial cortical hinge provide sufficient compression to prevent graft displacement. However, a staple may be employed in questionable cases (Fig. 14-19). Postoperative care consists of 9 to 12 weeks in a non-weight-bearing cast.

### Transpositional Calcaneal Osteotomies

Several authors have described transpositional osteotomies of the calcaneus for the treatment of pes valgus deformity. Lord reproduced the technique of Gleich.[57,58] Following osteotomy of the body of the calcaneus, the posterior fragment was shifted medially so that the center of gravity would strike in a more lateral position, thereby relieving stress to the arch. Koutsogiannis reported on 34 feet treated by his displacement osteotomy technique, with a follow-up period of 6 years to several months. He noted success in reducing the valgus position of the heel in 30 of the 34 feet. However, a lesser degree of improvement was noted in the longitudinal arch, especially in more advanced cases. Only two of Koutsogiannis's patients were over age 17 at the time of surgery[59] (Fig. 14-20).

Jacobs et al. considered posterior calcaneal osteotomies for patients in whom the facets of the subtalar joint were adapted to a deformed position. The rationale for selecting this approach was that once the posterior aspect of the calcaneus was translocated, the available ROM would be oriented in a more beneficial direction. Subtalar pronation was reported to be reduced by an average of 25 to 40 percent. In addition, the medial and/or plantar position of the heel reduced the pronating effects of the triceps, and a subsequent improvement in forefoot supinatus was noted. Patients with a great degree of transverse plane deformity were treated by Evans osteotomy rather than by this method. Jacobs et al. reported good results in 20 cases, although only 2 patients were less than 16 years old.[60] Tachdjian states that medial displacement osteotomies are highly recommended to correct severe rearfoot valgus deformities in the child.[44]

We have not had any experiences with translocation osteotomies. The rationale for using this approach in patients with fixed articular deviation of the subtalar joint appears to be sound, as it may provide a means of avoiding arthrodesis. McGlamry et al. note that even though

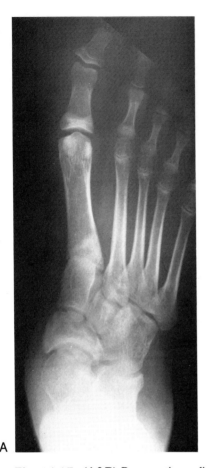
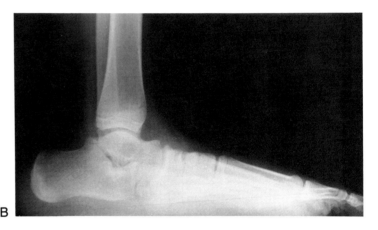

A                    B

**Fig. 14-17. (A&B)** Preoperative radiographs of a 15-year-old girl with symptomatic pes valgus deformity, gastrocnemius equinus, and metatarsus adductus. (*Figure continues.*)

the calcaneus may be shifted so as to favor supination, the subtalar joint may continue to function in maximal pronation. This would still leave the midtarsal joint unlocked and unstable. Additionally, the patient may continue to experience postural symptoms due to the incapacity to adequately absorb the shock of heel strike.[1] Therefore, other procedures are generally favored in this patient population.

## Additional Procedures

### Triple Arthrodesis

In the child every consideration should be given to avoiding arthrodesing procedures. However, there will arise certain situations in which it is obvious that reconstructive techniques will not be adequate to maintain correc-

tion. Triple arthrodesis provides the surgeon with an opportunity to permanently correct all three planes of deformity. Crego and Ford disagreed with their contemporaries, who felt that triple arthrodesis should not be performed for the correction of pes valgus deformity. They reported excellent or good results in 20 of 26 feet undergoing this procedure. In fact, these authors concluded that any arthrodesing procedure(s) performed for the correction of pes valgus deformity should involve the subtalar joint.[30]

Some authors have stated that degenerative joint changes are likely to occur in the ankle following triple arthrodesis. In fact, this has yet to be supported by objective study provided that the foot is placed in the proper position at the time of fusion. Duncan and Lovell, in reviewing 109 cases at 1 to 28 years following surgery, were not able to show any excessive incidence of

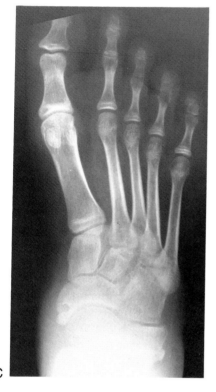
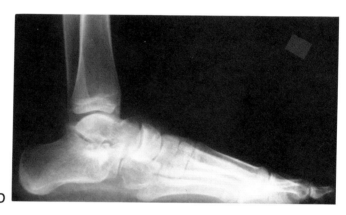

**Fig. 14-17** (*Continued*). **(C&D)** Postoperative radiographs 6 months following the Evans calcaneal osteotomy, medial arch tendosuspension, and gastronemius recession. The metatarsus adductus was not addressed surgically, and attempts will be made to accommodate this deformity in a conservative manner.

degenerative changes at the ankle. Those patients who did demonstrate marked degenerative arthrosis at this level all showed the same findings prior to surgery. The authors concluded that "perhaps the severe foot deformity, present preoperatively, places more stress on the ankle joint than was present after the triple arthrodesis."[61]

The rearfoot must be fused in a slightly valgus position and the forefoot must be similarly placed in a neutral to slightly valgus position relative to the heel. Support for this premise may be found in the long-term review by Angus and Cowell, who examined 80 feet an average of 13 years following triple arthrodesis. Degenerative joint changes were seen in 31 ankles, and 49 feet were noted to possess residual deformity. In fact, all 15 feet with preoperative planovalgus or calcaneovalgus deformity were considered to possess residual deformity postoperatively. There were no good results in this subset of patients, with only fair or poor conditions seen at follow-up[62,63] Southwell and Sherman found that increased load concentration under one or more metatarsal heads was common following triple arthrodesis. However, increased loading of the first and second metatarsals due to forefoot valgus was found to be asymptomatic. Painful hyperkeratoses were noted when forefoot varus was present postoperatively.[64]

Ankle arthrosis following triple arthrodesis may also result from uncorrected muscular equinus.[65] Many patients with pes valgus deformity compensate for the lack of adequate ankle motion by dorsiflexion at the midtarsal joint. Following fusion this mode of compensation is eliminated, and jamming can be expected later at the ankle joint level. Stress may also be transferred to the lesser tarsal and tarsometatarsal articulations.[65]

Our approach for triple arthrodesis is that previously demonstrated by McGlamry et al.[65] A medial and a lateral incision are employed. The lateral incision is used for exposure of the subtalar and calcaneocuboid joints. It

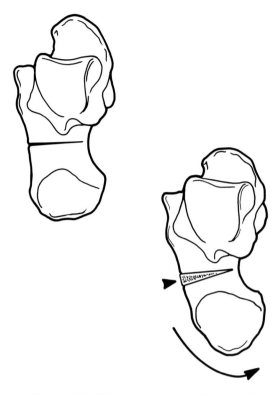

**Fig. 14-18.** Silver osteotomy with bone graft.

begins just inferior to the distal tip of the fibular malleolus and extends distally along the lateral margin of the floor of the sinus tarsi and across the calcaneocuboid joint to the junction of the fourth and fifth metatarsal bases. The medial incision begins at the junction of the anterior edge of the medial malleolus and the medial talar dome. It is carried distally across the lower margin of the navicular and ends at the lower edge of the naviculocuneiform joint. This additional incision provides direct access to the talonavicular joint for joint resection and fixation and improved visualization of the neck of the talus for fixation.

Internal fixation is preferred and is effected with a 6.5-mm AO/ASIF screw across the talocalcaneal joint space. Alternatively, the midtarsal joint may be fixed with 6.5-mm screws medially and laterally. However, staple fixation is more commonly employed at the midtarsal level because of ease and speed of insertion of staples.

Postoperatively the patient is maintained in a non-weight-bearing cast for 12 weeks. Once the cast is re-moved, a compressive wrap is used for several weeks to minimize edema. An orthotic is usually prescribed as well. At times a slight heel raise may be necessary in the shoe to prevent irritation of the malleoli from the shoe counter, which happens on occasion as a result of the shortening produced by the joint resection necessary for fusion.

As a general rule, triple arthrodesis will be more reliable than most other procedures in patients with neuromuscular disease. Individuals with ligamentous laxity or obesity may also require triple arthrodesis as opposed to reconstruction, or else correction may not be maintained. We agree with those who prefer to delay triple arthrodesis until adolescence. Arthrodesis at an earlier age during active growth has been reported to contribute to additional shortening of the foot. The Grice procedure (discussed below) may be a suitable alternative in the younger patient and may be combined with medial column procedures to address forefoot deformity.

We have found triple arthrodesis to be a gratifying procedure in the adolescent whose condition is not amenable to other techniques, provided the foot is arthrodesed in an adequate position. Improved dissection techniques have eliminated the excessive swelling and wound complications encountered in the past. Aseptic necrosis of the talus has been seen only once in the several hundred operations performed by many surgeons at our institution in the past 10 years. In contrast, a much higher incidence is reported in the literature. Nonunion or delayed union is a rare problem postoperatively; in current experience it almost always involves the calcaneocuboid joint. It is most frequently seen in patients who ambulate prematurely (Fig. 14-21).

## Grice Extra-Articular Arthrodesis

In 1952 Grice described his initial finding regarding extra-articular arthrodesis of the subtalar joint.[66] Although he stated that the procedure had been used for severely pronated feet, rocker bottom clubfoot, and congenital flatfoot, he discussed only those patients suffering from severe paralytic valgus foot deformity. Autogenous graft from the tibia was fashioned into two struts, which were placed laterally in the sinus tarsi and fitted into superficial grooves created in the talus and calcaneus. Arthrodesis and subsequent stabilization were achieved without interfering with growth. Patients aged 4 to 7 were considered well adapted, although successful

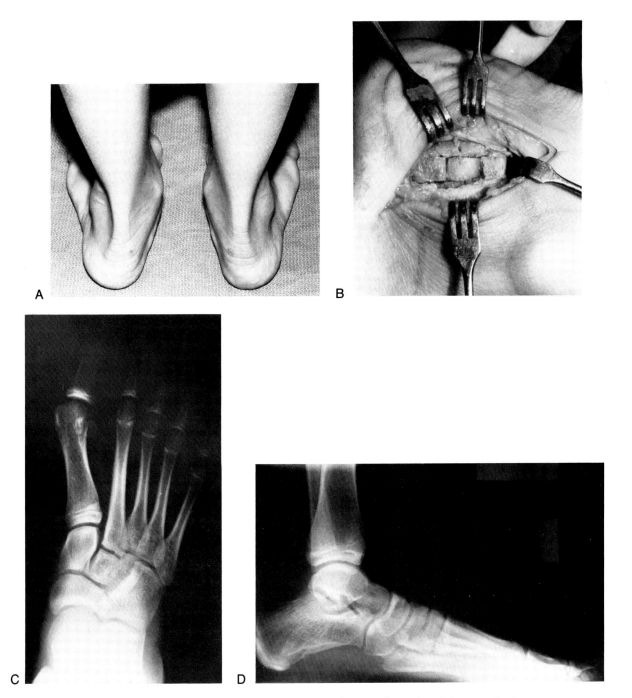

**Fig. 14-19.** (A) Clinical appearance of a 14-year-old girl with a fixed rearfoot valgus deformity. (B) Allogeneic graft material in position. (C&D) Preoperative radiographs. *(Figure continues.)*

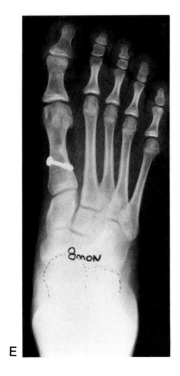

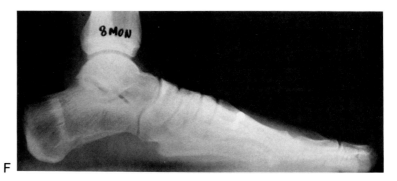

**Fig. 14-19** *(Continued).* **(E&F)**

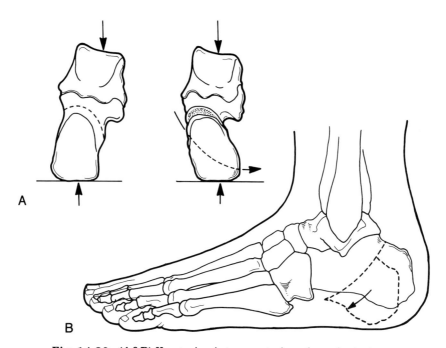

**Fig. 14-20. (A&B)** Koustogiannis-type posterior calcaneal osteotomy.

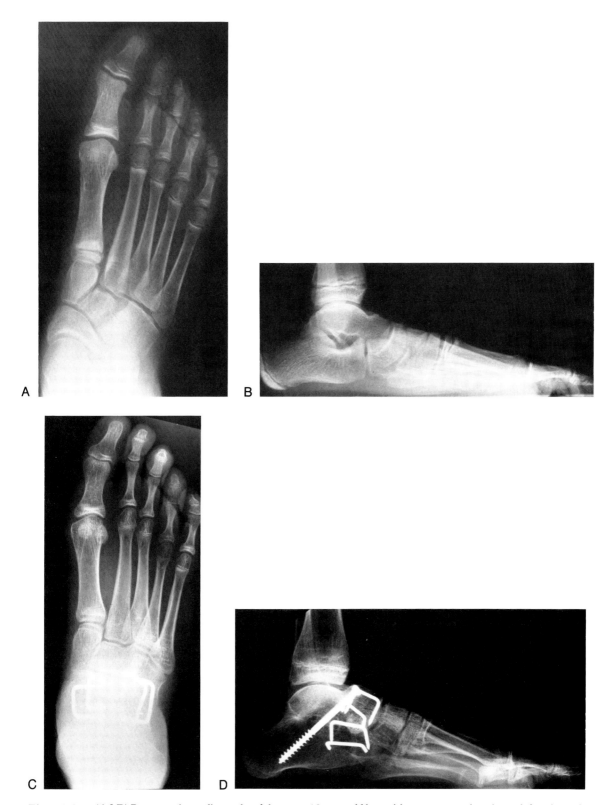

**Fig. 14-21.** (**A&B**) Preoperative radiographs of the same 13-year-old boy with severe pes valgo planus deformity and gastrocnemius equinus shown in Figure 14-3. (**C&D**) The patient 1 year following triple arthrodesis with solid fusion and a rectus foot.

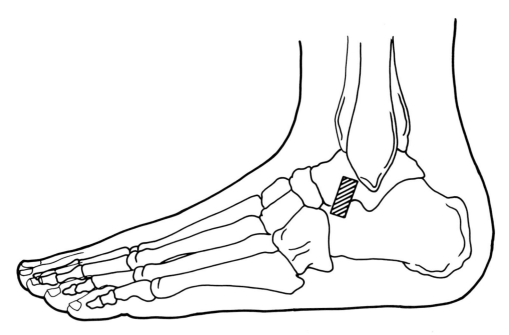

**Fig. 14-22.** Grice extra-articular arthrodesis. Note the anterior angulation of the graft within the sinus tarsi.

results had been attained in patients 10 to 11 years old[66] (Fig. 14-22). Three years later Grice noted good results in 41 of 52 patients undergoing the surgery.[67] Appropriate tendon transfers were also performed to re-establish muscle balance in the paralytic states.

Since that time numerous authors have reported results achieved with the procedure. Complications have been reported frequently and usually have consisted of recurrence of deformity, shift of the graft, and overcorrection. In most instances the recurrence of deformity appears to be due to the surgeon's failure to recognize the presence of an ankle valgus deformity preoperatively. Either the pronated alignment recurs or the heel is placed into varus to overcompensate.[68,69] In fact, Ross and Lyne found that inability to control ankle instability was the primary reason for failure in their patients.[70] Therefore there was no inherent problem with the procedure itself, only in the patient selection. Recurrence of the valgus heel is also associated with displacement of the graft. Grice noted that the struts needed to be oriented with the inferior margin slightly distal. This alignment is more effective in blocking subtalar motion, as it is more nearly perpendicular to the

joint axis and therefore limits the potential for graft displacement.[66,67] Scott et al. noted that 56 percent of the anteriorly oriented grafts resorbed.[69] The technique of using cylindrical iliac crest plugs to achieve arthrodesis seems to be fairly reliable and obviates the need for strict attention to graft orientation.[71]

Vogler has noted that many postoperative problems appear to be related to failure to address ankle equinus.[72] Following surgery, unresolved equinus places an excessive load upon the graft, encouraging graft resorption, displacement, and ultimately loss of correction.

The Grice procedure is primarily indicated for stabilization of severe rearfoot deformity in children who are so young that triple arthrodesis would distinctly affect future growth. The most common indication still appears to be neuromuscular imbalance. In patients with this problem arthrodesis combined with necessary tendon transfers and equinus release will provide a more reliable means of correction than will tendon procedures alone. However, the Grice procedure should be viewed as a part but not all of what is required to stabilize any foot type. This procedure does not address midfoot or medial column deformity. Therefore, other procedures may be re-

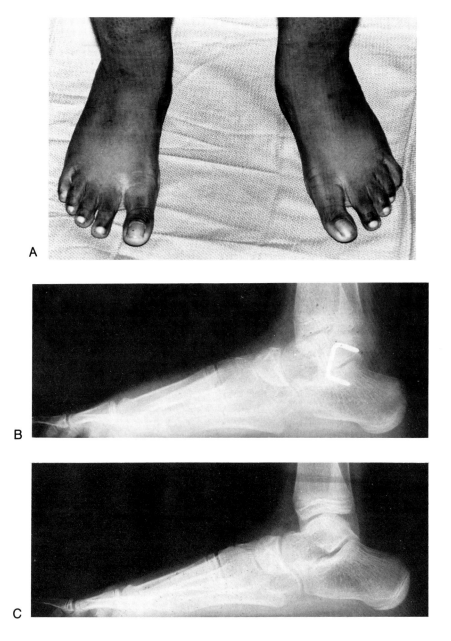

**Fig. 14-23.** (A) An 11-year-old girl with flaccid paralysis. Previous attempts at reconstruction have failed to alleviate the left pes valgus deformity and concomitant symptoms. (B) Preoperative lateral radiograph. (C) Postoperative lateral radiograph following Grice procedure with allogenic bone graft.

quired in conjunction with the Grice arthrodesis to ensure adequate correction and to minimize the risks of adverse sequalae.

## Techniques and Postoperative Care

The surgical approach is similar to that of the Evans procedure but with the incision placed slightly more proximal so as to facilitate exposure of the sinus tarsi. The contents of the sinus tarsi are evacuated so that clear visualization is attained. The cortical margins of the talus and calcaneus are grooved to improve seating of the graft and to encourage more rapid incorporation. The graft is then fashioned and placed in the sinus tarsi with the distal end angled slightly anteriorly. The calcaneus is everted until impaction is achieved. The graft is then modified until the calcaneus is slightly everted with maximal impaction. A lateral staple or a Kirschner wire may be used to maintain the position (Fig. 14-23).

Various graft materials have been used with success. Grice recommended autogenous tibial material,[66,67] which seems to have been the general trend reported in subsequent papers. Vogler recommended that bone be removed from the middle third of the fibula and replaced with allogeneic material.[72] Grice noted that Malvarez had achieved good results in 18 cases with bone bank material.[66] Successful incorporation of allogeneic bone has been noted by other authors as well.[69,73] Although autogenous bone may have a theoretical advantage, we feel that allogeneic material can be employed without complications or inordinate delays in healing.

Follow-up care consists of a non-weight-bearing cast until adequate consolidation of the arthrodesis site is demonstrated. At times this may necessitate above-knee immobilization to completely eliminate torque to the subtalar joint area. Orthotic support may be instituted upon resumption of weight-bearing.

## Arthroereisis

Arthroereisis procedures initially seem to offer a simple, minimally invasive, yet effective means of treating the juvenile patient with pes valgus deformity. The rationale of subtalar arthroereisis techniques is to allow normal joint motion while blocking the extreme pronation range associated with the pes valgus deformity. The joint blocking technique was first described by LeLievre in 1970 as an alternative to the Grice procedure.[74]

## Types of Arthroereisis Devices

Vogler lists three basic types of arthroereisis devices. The first is a self-locking wedge whereby the opposing surfaces of the talus and calcaneus are separated by a block of material. The subtalar joint axis is not changed, but pronational motion is restricted. Axis-altering devices serve to redirect the joint axis for a patient with a predominance of frontal plane motion. Direct impaction

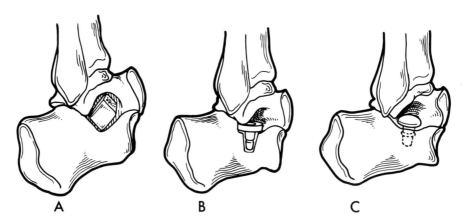

Fig. 14-24. The three types of arthroereisis devices. (A) Self-locking wedge. The talus and the calcaneus are separated by the sinus tarsi implant, which limits pronation. (B) STA-peg device, which is an example of an axis-altering design. The lateral process of the talus impinges upon the dorsal surface of the implant, redirecting a low subtalar joint axis. (C) Direct-impact device of Sgarlato. The lateral process of the talus impinges upon the device, thereby limiting anterior displacement of the talus and pronation. (From Vogler,[72] with permission.)

devices impinge on the anterior margin of talus once the desired end range of pronation is achieved (Fig. 14-24).

*Self-Locking Wedge Devices.* Within the podiatric profession several authors have inserted a Silastic device within the sinus tarsi as a self-locking wedge. The devices were carved by Subotnick[75] and Smith and Rappaport[76] from Silastic blocks, whereas Lanham used the stem from the Swanson great toe implant. In 1979 Lanham reported gratifying results in 51 cases representing 102 procedures. Patients aged 2 through 9 underwent arthroereisis along with appropriate release of equinus when required. Those aged 9 through 13 also underwent a Young procedure.[77] In 1981 Lanham published a brief update indicating continued success with this approach in another 22 cases.[78] When combined, the two groups exhibited a success rate of 89 percent. Smith and Rappaport reported the results of 68 surgeries surveyed via questionaire along with their clinical experience with 40 feet. Better than 50 percent improvement in symptoms was reported by 94 percent of the patients, and good clinical and radiographic improvement was also noted.[76]

The Valente arthroereisis is a threaded self-locking device made from ultrahigh molecular weight polyethylene. Langford et al. described the basic concepts of this technique based upon their experience with over 200 patients. The best candidates for the procedure were considered to be patients between the ages of 6 and 12. Individuals with little or no calcaneal eversion seemed to do better with other procedures. The most common postoperative problem appeared to be pain at the lateral aspect of the sinus tarsi. These symptoms were attributed to the use of an implant too large or to temporary adjustment of the subtalar joint to the restriction of excessive pronation.[79]

*STA-Peg Device.* In 1975 Smith and Miller described the STA-peg device, which was milled from ultra-high molecular weight polyethylene. This was the first uniform device available for implantation and represented an axis-altering mechanism. When 53 feet in which it was used were examined at 3 and 9 years following surgery, calcaneal eversion was reduced to 3.19 degrees from 10.31 degrees preoperatively, and forefoot varus was reduced from an average of 8.4 to 2.4 degrees.[80] Smith and Wagreich reported on 11 patients (18 feet) who had received STA-peg devices 11 to 42 months prior to fol-

low-up.[81] The average age of the children at the time of surgery was 6.54 years. Calcaneal eversion was reduced from 12.17 to 5.83 degrees postoperatively. Forefoot varus was reported to have improved to an extent similar to that noted in Smith and Miller's study.[80]

Lundeen reported 78 percent good results in 96 patients seen an average of 46 months following STA-peg implantation. Both the talonavicular and metatarsocuneiform breaches were effectively controlled and reduced following surgery. However, the naviculocuneiform breach proved to be somewhat resistant. Lundeen felt that this was indicative of equinus or ligamentous laxity. Equinus was treated by the appropriate tendon lengthening procedure. However, for those patients without evidence of equinus, a split tibialis anterior tendon transfer and Kidner procedure were recommended to stabilize the midtarsal joint. Metatarsus adductus was also observed to persist following use of the STA-peg device alone.[82]

*Complications*

Transient synovitis has been noted at the surgical site in a number of patients following arthroereisis. This reportedly resolves spontaneously most of the time. Complications specific to the blocking device have been reported but are few in number. Lanham noted extrusion of the device from the sinus tarsi laterally in a few cases and attributed this to incomplete severance of the interosseous talocalcaneal ligament. Transection of this structure is essential to allow full supination of the subtalar joint and to minimize compressive forces upon the device.[77] Smith and Rappaport noted extrusion of the hand-carved Silastic plug in the 20 percent of their patients until changes were made in the shape of the device and suture was used to secure the device to the deltoid ligament medially. With these modifications no further evidence of extrusion was noted.[76] Oloff et al. observed that 6 of 23 patients developed signs and symptoms referred to the surgical sites following the use of the STA-peg. Three of these individuals had normal findings upon computed tomography (CT) scan, but in three others improper position, implant failure, or detritic matter was noted.[83] Kuwada and Dockery described three complications in patients with STA-peg devices following traumatic incidents. Two of the three had damaged devices with cartilage disruption of the anterior edge of the talus.[84]

## Indications for and Selection of Arthroereisis Devices

Criteria for the selection and use of arthroereisis have been described by Vogler.[72] The self-locking devices are best applied in the adolescent, as the congruity of the subtalar and midtarsal joints is not as greatly disturbed. This may be important in a patient who is close to skeletal maturity with little ability to compensate for or adapt to gross changes in the alignment or axis of motion in either area. The joint axis alteration techniques seem best suited for younger patients, who have the potential to adapt. Direct-impact devices may be used in either age group. Vogler has noted that the pronated foot must be flexible and reducible and that the midtarsal joint must be free of fixed adaptive change.[72]

Dockery prefers the custom Silastic plugs in very young patients or in those who are teenage or older provided that they are not obese.[53] Advantages of the Silastic plug are the softer nature of the material and elimination of the need for osseous remodeling to implant the device. The STA-peg is selected in patients with moderate to severe deformity prior to the teenage years and in the child who is overweight. This is based upon Dockery's observations that more consistent correction and less chance of extrusion is likely with the STA-peg arthroereisis.[53]

## Long-Term Effects

Significant questions still remain regarding the long-term effects of arthroereisis devices. In particular, will there be any tendency for subtalar joint arthrosis at some later point in time? Theoretically, the materials utilized today are fairly inert and nonreactive, but the long-term effects of implanting these materials into the body have yet to be determined. Oloff et al. indicate that ultrahigh molecular weight polyethylene is not a static material but undergoes dynamic change in vivo, including increased crystallinity.[83] Fatigue resistance and durability are thereby changed, which presumably makes the material prone to cracking and fissuring. Clinically, the long-term durability of silicone polymer implants has often proved unsatisfactory when this material is exposed to substantial mechanical strain (as in radial head, carpometacarpal, metacarpophalangeal, and metatarsophalangeal joint implants), and the general trend at present is toward avoidance of these materials except in very limited situations. Furthermore, the methyl methacrylate cement that may be required for adequate stability in some cases of arthroereisis may lead to complications such as cement hepatitis or pulmonary leak.[85,86] Theoretically, the intermediate metabolites of polymethylmethacrylate are reported to be mutagens.[87] However, these complications have not been reported as a sequela of foot surgery of this type and in most instances methyl methacrylate is not required.

We would consider arthroereisis in very young children between the ages of 2 and 5, who lack sufficient osseous maturity to allow other procedures. After this time osseous reconstruction is preferred to address rearfoot deformities.

## Treatment of Skewfoot

*Skewfoot* and *serpentine foot* are equivalent terms used to describe the syndrome of an adducted forefoot, an abducted midfoot, and a pronated rearfoot. Radiographically a Z configuration is recognized. Simple stated, a skewfoot possesses the components of both metatarsus adductus and pes valgus deformity. The contradictory pathologic conditions make successful conservative management difficult and surgical treatment complex and challenging.

Several etiologies have been proposed for this condition. Peterson states that skewfoot was first noted following serial casts for either clubfoot or metatarsus adductus. Therefore, inappropriate casting techniques causing the heel to be positioned in valgus have been implicated.[88] Congenital metatarsus adductus with calcaneovalgus has also been cited.[89] Another proposed etiology is the development of subtalar joint pronation to compensate for a residual metatarsus adductus.[90] This is probably the most common source of skewfoot, as many still subscribe to the errant belief that all infants outgrow metatarsus adductus. Therefore, the tarsal malalignment persists into childhood, and the patient eventually compensates. Rearfoot pronation may also be present in response to other deformities in conjunction with metatarsus adductus.

Most sources in the literature agree that if surgery is performed, aggressive steps are required.[88,90,91] Generally, both metatarsal realignment and rearfoot stabilization procedures are performed. The age of the patient may dictate which procedures are preferable in some cases. Metatarsus adductus may be dealt with by a variety of techniques, which have been discussed in Chapter

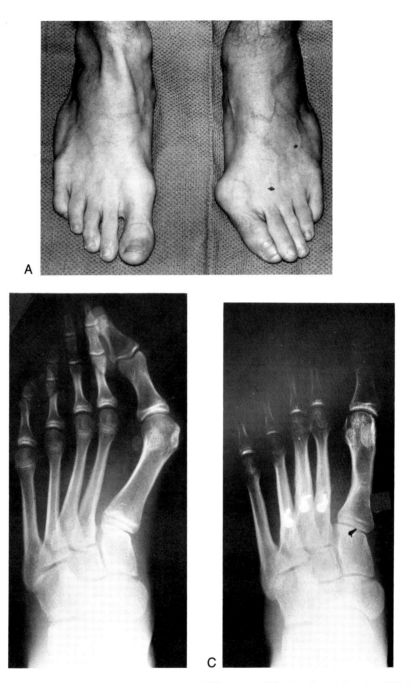

**Fig. 14-25.** **(A)** Preoperative appearance of a 14-year-old boy with left skewfoot deformity. **(B)** Preoperative radiograph. Note the degree of metatarsus adductus. **(C)** Radiographic appearance 20 months following abductory metatarsal osteotomies and Evans procedure.

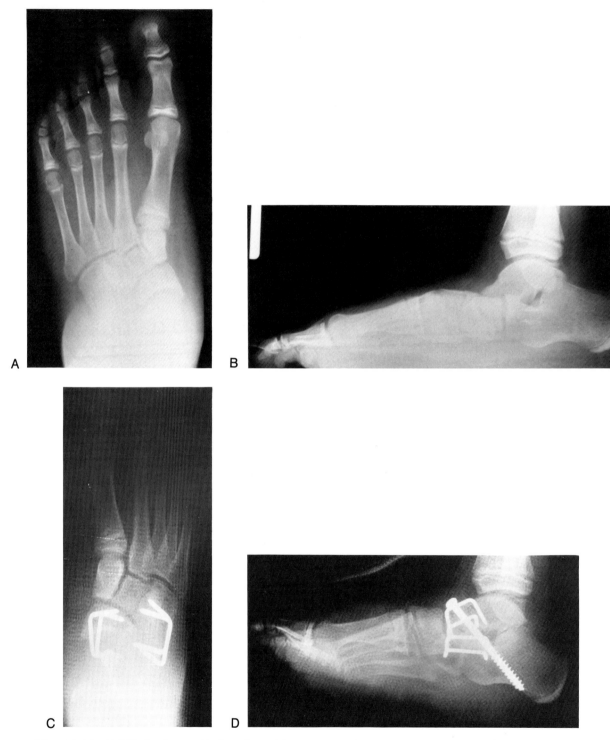

**Fig. 14-26. (A&B)** A 12-year-old obese boy with severe skewfoot and ligmentous laxity. **(C&D)** Radiographic appearance following triple arthrodesis and tendo Achilles lengthening. This should allow for triplane correction of deformity, including the accommodation of metatarsus adductus. *(Figure continues.)*

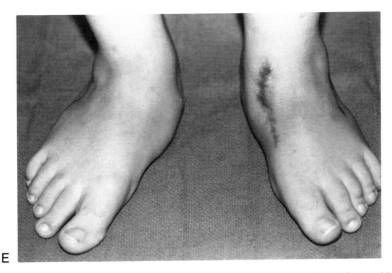

**Fig. 14-26** *(Continued).* **(E)** Clinical photograph 8 months following surgery on the left foot and before surgery on the right.

8. The next consideration is to select appropriate stabilization of the rearfoot. A high degree of transverse plane deformity is fairly characteristic at this level, and Evans osteotomy is certainly indicated in this instance. The talus usually demonstrates a high degree of adduction and may contribute to significant medial column laxity. Therefore medial arch tendosuspension may also be required (Fig. 14-25).

However, the question arises as to how much intervention is required and whether or not staging of procedures is advantageous. If staging is a consideration, then which aspects of the deformity are addressed first? Generally the metatarsus adductus repair and the Evans procedure are performed first. The patient is monitored closely, and should medial column instability be noted, this may be addressed later. In older children adaptation may be so ingrained as to require triple arthrodesis. One may create a more suitable rearfoot alignment and also wedge the midtarsal joint to better accommodate the adducted forefoot. Failure to achieve suitable abduction of the metatarsals will result in stress on the lateral ankle, as the means of compensation in the rearfoot has been eliminated by arthrodesis (Fig. 14-26).

Another consideration arises in the patient who demonstrates moderate metatarsus adductus with pes valgus deformity in association with other conditions. In such instances it may be difficult to determine how much the metatarsus adductus has influenced the development of pes valgus deformity. Therefore, rearfoot stabilization may be performed first and the patient then be monitored to determine if later repair of the metatarsus adductus in necessary.

## REFERENCES

1. McGlamry ED, Mahan KT, Green DR: Pes valgo planus deformity. p. 403. In McGlamry ED Textbook of Foot Surgery. (ed): Williams & Wilkins, Baltimore, 1987
2. Kalen V, Brecher A: Relationship between adolescent bunions and flatfeet. Foot Ankle 8:331, 1988
3. Sgarlato T: Pediatric foot surgery. Clin Podiatr Med Surg 1:709, 1984
4. Scranton PE, Zuckerman JD: Bunion surgery in adolescents: results of surgical treatment. J Pediatr Orthop 4:39, 1984
5. Giannestras NJ: Static foot problems in the pre-adolescent and adolescent stages. p. 134. In Giannestras NJ (ed): Foot Disorders. Medical and Surgical Management, 2nd Ed. Lea & Febiger, Philadelphia, 1973
6. Giannestras NJ: The pronated foot in infancy and childhood. p.108. In Giannestras NJ (ed): Foot Disorders. Medical and Surgical Management. 2nd Ed. Lea & Febiger, Philadelphia, 1973
7. Root ML, Orien WP, Weed JH: Normal and Abnormal Function of the Foot. Vol. 2. Clinical Biomechanics Corp., Los Angeles, 1977

8. Downey MS: Ankle equinus. p. 369. In McGlamry ED (ed): Textbook of Foot Surgery. Williams & Wilkins, Baltimore, 1987

9. Downey MS, Banks AS: Gastrocnemius recession in the treatment of nonspastic ankle equinus. J Am Podiatr Med Assoc 79:160, 1989

10. Silfverskiold N: Reduction of the uncrossed two-joints muscles of the leg to one-joint muscles in spastic conditions. Acta Chir Scand 56:315, 1924

11. Amarnek DL, Jacobs AM, Oloff LM: Adolescent hallux valgus: its etiology and surgical management. J Foot Surg 24:54, 1985

12. Selakovich WG: Medial arch support by operation. Sustentaculum tali procedure. Orthop Clin North Am 4:117, 1973

13. Green DR, Carol A: Planal dominance. J Am Podiatr Med Assoc 74:98, 1984

14. Hoke M: An operation for the correction of extremely relaxed flat feet. J Bone Joint Surg 13:773, 1931

15. Miller OL: A plastic flat foot operation. J Bone Joint Surg 9:84, 1927

16. McGlamry ED: Equinus related deformities. p. 12. In Doctors Hospital Podiatric Education and Research Institute 14th Annual Surgical Seminar Syllabus. Podiatry Institute Book Co., Tucker, GA, 1985

17. Gamble FO, Yale I: Acquired foot fault syndromes. p. 209. In Clinical Foot Roentenology. 2nd Ed. Krieger Publishing Co., Huntington, NY, 1975

18. Oberling RE: Ankle valgus. Its relationship to rearfoot instability. J Am Podiatr Med Assoc 73:405, 1983

19. Stevens PM: Effect of ankle valgus on radiographic appearance of the hindfoot. J Pediatr Orthop 8:184, 1988

20. Hibbs RA: Muscle bound feet. NY State J Med 17C:798, 1914

21. Harris RI, Beath T: Hypermobile flat-foot with short tendo Achillis. J Bone Joint Surg [Am] 30A:116, 1948

22. Butte FL: Navicular-cuneiform arthrodesis for flat-foot: an end-result study. J Bone Joint Surg 19:496, 1937

23. Sgarlato TE, Morgan J, Shane HS, Frenkenberg A: Tendo Achillis lengthening and its effect on foot disorders. J Am Podiatr Med Assoc 65:845, 1975

24. McGlamry ED: Evolution of flatfoot surgery. p. 124. In Schlefman BS (ed): Reconstructive Surgery of the Foot and Leg. Doctors Hospital Surgical Seminar Syllabus, Tucker, GA, 1982

25. Valpius O, Stoffel A: Orthopädische Operationslehre. Ferdinand Enke, Stuttgart, 1913

26. Strayer LM: Recession of the gastrocnemius: an operation to relieve spastic contracture of the calf muscles. J Bone Joint Surg [Am] 32:671, 1950

27. Baker LD: A rational approach to the surgical needs of the cerebral palsy patient. J Bone Joint Surg [Am] 38:313, 1956

28. Fulp MJ, McGlamry ED: Gastrocnemius tendon recession: tongue in groove procedure to lengthen gastorcnemius tendon. J Am Podiatr Med Assoc 64:163, 1974

29. Young CS: Operative treatment of pes planus. Surg Gynecol Obstet 68:1099, 1939

30. Crego CH, Ford LT: An end-result study of various operative procedures for corrective flatfoot in children. J Bone Joint Surg [Am] 34:183, 1952

31. Beck EL, McGlamry ED: Modified Young tendosuspension technique for flexible flatfoot. J Am Podiatr Med Assoc 63:582, 1973

32. Jacobs AM, Oloff LM: Surgical management of forefoot supinatus in flexible flatfoot deformity. J Foot Surg 23:410, 1984

33. Kidner FC: The prehallux (accessory scaphoid) in its relation to flatfoot. J Bone Joint Surg 11:831, 1929

34. Kidner FC: The prehallux in relation to flatfoot. JAMA 101:1539, 1933

35. Veitch JM: Evaluation of the Kidner procedure in treatment of symptomatic accessory tarsal scaphoid. Clin Orthop 131:210, 1978

36. Sullivan JA, Miller WA: The relationship of the accessory navicular to the development of the flat foot. Clin Orthop 144:233, 1979

37. Macnicol MF, Voutsinas S: Surgical treatment of the symptomatic accessory navicular. J Bone Joint Surg [Br] 66:218, 1984

38. Lawson JP, Ogden JA, Sella E, Barwick KW: The painful accessory navicular. Skeletal Radiol 12:250, 1984

39. Basmajian JV, Stecko G: The role of muscles in arch support of the foot. An electromyographic study. J Bone Joint Surg, 45:1184, 1963

40. Lemont H, Travisano VL, Lyman J: Accessory navicular. Appearance of a synovial joint. J Am Podiatr Med Assoc 71:423, 1981

41. Jack EA: Naviculo-cuneiform fusion in the treatment of flat foot. J Bone Joint Surg [Br] 35:75, 1953

42. Seymour N: The late results of naviculo-cuneiform fusion. J Bone Joint Surg [Br] 49:558, 1967

43. Lowman CL: An operative method for correction of certain forms of flatfoot. JAMA 81:1500, 1923

44. Tachdjian MO: Flexible pes planovalgus (flat foot). p. 556. In Tachdjian MO (ed): The Child's Foot. WB Saunders, Philadelphia, 1985

45. Fogel GR, Katoh Y, Rand JA, Chao EYS: Talonavicular arthrodesis for isolated arthrosis. 9.5 year results and gait analysis. Foot Ankle 3:105, 1982

46. Schlefman BS: Tarsal coalition. p. 483. In McGlamry ED (ed): Textbook of Foot Surgery, Williams & Wilkins, Baltimore, 1987

47. Evans D: Calcaneo-valgus deformity. J Bone Joint Surg [Br] 57:270, 1975

48. Phillips GE: A review of enlongation of the os calcis for flat feet. J Bone Joint Surg [Br] 65:15, 1983

49. Dollard MD, Marcinko DE, Lazerson A, Elleby DH: The Evans calcaneal osteotomy for correction of flexible flatfoot syndrome. J Foot Surg 23:291, 1984

50. Anderson AF, Fowler SB: Anterior calcaneal osteotomy for symptomatic juvenile pes planus. Foot Ankle 4:274, 1984

51. Mahan KT, McGlamry ED: Evans calcaneal osteotomy for flexible pes valgus deformity. Clin Podiatr 4:137, 1987

52. McGlamry ED, Downey MS: Evans calcaneal osteotomy. p. 53. In Doctors Hospital Podiatric Education and Research Institute 15th Surgical Seminar Syllabus. Doctors Hospital Podiatry Institute, Tucker, GA, 1986

53. Dockery GL: Surgical treatment of the symptomatic juvenile flexible flatfoot condition. Clin Podiatr 4:99, 1987

54. Silver CM, Simon SD, Spindell E et al: Calcaneal osteotomy for valgus and varus deformities of the foot in cerebral palsy. A preliminary report on 27 operations. J Bone Joint Surg [Am] 49:232, 1967

55. Silver CM, Simon SD, Litchman HM: Long term follow-up observations on calcaneal osteotomy. Clin Orthop 99:181, 1974

56. Marcinko DE, Lazerson A, Elleby DH: Silver calcaneal osteotomy for flexible flatfoot: a retrospective preliminary report. J Foot Surg 23:191, 1984

57. Lord JP: Correction of extreme flatfoot. Value of osteotomy of os calcis and inward displacement of posterior fragment (Gleich procedure). JAMA 81:1502, 1923

58. Gleich A: Beitrag zur operativen Plattfussbehandlung. Arch Klin Chir 46:358, 1893

59. Koutsogiannis E: Treatment of mobile flat foot by displacement osteotomy of the calcaneus. J Bone Joint Surg [Br] 53:96, 1971

60. Jacobs AM, Oloff L, Visser HJ: Calcaneal osteotomy in the management of flexible and nonflexible flatfoot deformity: a preliminary report. J Foot Surg 20:57, 1981

61. Duncan JW, Lovell WW: Hoke triple arthrodesis. J Bone Joint Surg [Am] 60:795, 1978

62. Angus PD, Cowell HR: Triple arthrodesis. A critical long-term review. J Bone Joint Surg [Br] 68:260, 1986

63. Seitz DC, Carpenter EB: Triple arthrodesis in children: a ten year review. South Med J 67:1420, 1981

64. Southwell RB, Sherman FC: Triple arthrodesis: a long term study with force plate analysis. Foot Ankle 2:15, 1981

65. McGlamry ED, Ruch JA, Mahan KT, DiNapoli DR: Triple arthrodesis. p. 126. In McGlamry ED (ed): Reconstructive Surgery of the Foot and Leg, Update '87. Podiatry Institute Publishing Co., Tucker, GA, 1987

66. Grice DS: An extra-articular arthrodesis of the subastrangular joint for correction of paralytic flat feet in children. J Bone Joint Surg [Am] 34:927, 1952

67. Grice DS: Further experience with extra-articular arthrodesis of the subtalar joint. J Bone Joint Surg [Am] 37:246, 1955

68. Moreland JR, Westin GW: Further experience with Grice subtalar arthrodesis. Clin Orthop 207:113, 1986

69. Scott SM, Janes PC, Stevens PM: Grice subtalar arthrodesis followed to skeletal maturity. J Pediatr Orthop 8:176, 1988

70. Ross PM, Lyne ED: The Grice procedure: indications and evaluation of long term results. Clin Orthop 153:194, 1980

71. Guttmann GG: Subtalar arthrodesis in children with cerebral palsy: results using iliac bone plug. Foot Ankle 10:206, 1990

72. Vogler HW: Subtalar joint blocking operations for pathological pronation syndromes. p. 447. In McGlamry ED (ed): Textbook of Foot Surgery, Williams & Wilkins, Baltimore, 1987

73. Aronson J, Nunley J, Frankovitch K: Lateral talocalcaneal angle in assessment of subtalar valgus: follow-up of seventy Grice-Green arthrodeses. Foot Ankle 4:56, 1983

74. LeLeivre J: The valgus foot: current concepts and correction Clin Orthop 70:43, 1970

75. Subotnick SI: The sub-talar joint lateral extra articular arthroereisis: a preliminary report. J Am Podiatr Med Assoc 64:701, 1974

76. Smith RD, Rappaport MJ: Subtalar arthroereisis, A 4-year follow-up study. J Am Podiatr Med Assoc 73:356, 1983

77. Lanham RH: Indications and complications of arthroereisis in hypermobile flatfoot. J Am Podiatr Med Assoc 69:178, 1979

78. Lanham RH: Arthroereisis update. J Am Podiatr Med Assoc 71:693, 1981

79. Langford JH, Bozof H, Horowitz BD: Subtalar arthroereisis. Valente procedure. Clin Podiatr Med Surg 4:153, 1987

80. Smith SD, Millar EA: Arthrorisis by means of a subtalar polyethylene peg implant for correction of hindfoot pronation in children. Clin Orthop 181:15, 1983

81. Smith SD, Wagreich CR: Review of postoperative results of the subtalar arthrorisis operation: a preliminary study. J Foot Surg 23:253, 1984

82. Lundeen RO: The Smith STA-peg operation for hypermobile pes planovalgus in children. J Am Podiatr Med Assoc 75:177, 1985

83. Oloff LM, Naylor BL, Jacobs AM: Complications of subtalar arthroereisis. J Foot Surg 26:136, 1987

84. Kuwada GT, Dockery GL: Complications following trau-

matic incidents with STA-peg procedures. J Foot Surg 27:236, 1988

85. Ritter M, Gioe T, Sieber J: Systemic effects of polymethylmethacrylate. Acta Orthop Scan 55:411, 1984

86. Safwat A, Dror A: Pulmonary capillary leak associated with methylmethacrylate during general anesthesia: a case report. Clin Orthop 168:59, 1982

87. Poss R, Thilly W, Kaden D: Methylmethacrylate is a mutagen for *Salmonella typhimurium.* J Bone Joint Surg [Am] 61:1203, 1979

88. Peterson H: Skewfoot (forefoot adduction with heel valgus). J Pediatr Orthop 6:24, 1986

89. Kite H: Congenital metatarsus varus. J Bone Joint Surg [Am] 49A:388, 1967

90. Phillips AJ, McGlamry ED: Skewfoot. p. 251. In McGlamry ED (ed): Reconstructive Surgery of the Foot and Leg, Update '89. Podiatry Institute Publishing Co., Tucker, GA, 1989

91. Berg E: A reappraisal of metatarsus adductus and skewfoot. J Bone Joint Surg [Am] 68:1185, 1986

# 15

# Juvenile and Adolescent Hallux Abducto Valgus Deformity

GERARD V. YU
PATRICK A. LANDERS
KAREN G. LO
JEFFREY E. SHOOK

Juvenile or adolescent hallux abducto valgus deformity is routinely recognized and diagnosed in the typical podiatric practice. The treatment of this deformity, however, is often a challenge to the same physician because of the lack of specific and well accepted guidelines for treatment, whether conservative or surgical. The deformity is not infrequently complicated by other, concomitant deformities, which may or may not influence the development and propagation of the bunion deformity regardless of the degree of symptomatology.

Controversy exists not only concerning the treatment of the hallux abducto valgus deformity but also concerning the treatment, if any, of other concomitant deformities (equinus, pes plano valgus, or metatarsus adductus). Any treatment program, conservative or surgical, should have as its end result the restoration of a pain-free, normally functioning first metatarsophalangeal joint. Selection of the most appropriate approach should be based on a number of factors, including the nature and severity of the deformity, the rate of development and progression of the deformity, the clinical and radiographic findings, patient and parent expectations, and finally, the surgeon's own ability, experience, and expertise. Limited surgical experience on the part of the practitioner should not be the reason for avoiding definitive treatment.

Every attempt should be made to identify underlying contributing factors that potentially have a significant influence on the hallux abducto valgus deformity itself, including neuromuscular diseases such as cerebral palsy,

systemic diseases such as rheumatoid arthritis, and congenital deformities involving malformation of bone such as Down syndrome. The purpose of this chapter is to provide a review of juvenile and adolescent hallux abducto valgus deformity, with emphasis on the selection of appropriate surgical procedures that will ensure permanent structural correction with restoration of normal function.

## DEFINITION AND DESCRIPTION

A precise definition of juvenile or adolescent hallux abducto valgus deformity is lacking. Goldner and Gaines have arbitrarily classified the deformity as occuring in an individual aged 20 years or less because of the relatively plastic nature of the components of the deformity.[1] Some authors have simply referred to the deformity as manifesting itself during the formative years of life.[2-5] The deformity may also be seen in early infancy alone or, more commonly, in conjunction with another condition, which itself may go unrecognized until the hallux abducto valgus deformity has been recognized and identified (Fig. 15-1). *Dorland's Illustrated Medical Dictionary* defines adolescence as "the period of life beginning with the appearance of secondary sex characters and terminating with the cessation of somatic growth, roughly from 11 to 19 years of age."[6] The term *juvenile*, on the other hand, refers more typically to the period of child-

369

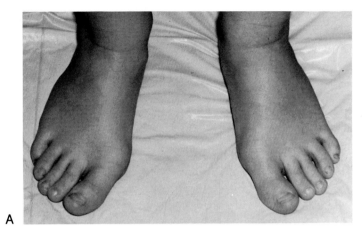

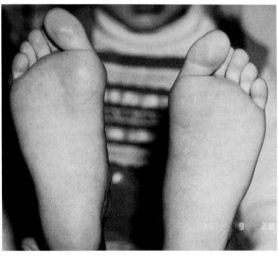

**Fig. 15-1.** **(A)** Dorsal and **(B)** plantar views of 3-year-old child with early juvenile hallux abducto valgus deformity secondary to an underlying uncorrected metatarsus adductus deformity. Notice significant underlapping of the hallux and second toe in non-weight-bearing attitude of both feet.

hood from infancy to puberty. With this in mind, it is preferable to refer to the adolescent hallux abducto valgus deformity as occurring in individuals under 20 years of age who are experiencing or have completed puberty; individuals who do not meet this criterion would then be referred to as patients with juvenile hallux abducto valgus deformity.

Of more importance is the understanding that an adolescent or juvenile with a hallux abducto valgus deformity is presenting with a condition that is not merely a precursor to the everyday adult condition but is rather a progressive deformity, which may ultimately result in

severe distortion of the first metatarsophalangeal joint and first ray segment. Furthermore, it is intimately related to other components of the human foot and as such may adversely affect the foot's entire structure and function, resulting in increased disability and pain.

The juvenile and adolescent hallux abducto valgus deformity is different from the adult form. While transverse plane abduction may be mild, moderate, or severe, rarely is frontal plane valgus rotation of the hallux a major finding in this age group. In addition, chronic tissue reactions such as degenerative joint disease, medial bursal formation or thickening, and related hammer toe deformities or lesser metatarsalgia are rarely present. When such findings are present, they most commonly indicate a rapidly progressing deformity, with other major deformities present more proximally, such as equinus at the ankle, pes plano valgus, or compensated metatarsus adductus.

Although seldom the reason for seeking professional care, metatarsus adductus, a severe pes plano valgus deformity, or an equinus deformity may be intimately related and deserves a thorough and comprehensive evaluation to determine its relationship to the bunion deformity. Many authors have noted an intimate relationship between these conditions, indicating that failure to treat them appropriately may adversely affect the outcome of any treatment of the bunion deformity.[1,3,7-11]

The juvenile and adolescent hallux abducto valgus deformity is typically of concern between the ages of 11 and 15 years. It is during this time that children, especially girls, are becoming increasingly aware of their own bodies and their perception by others. Any distinguishing deformity, including a bunion deformity, may be a serious concern in relation to self-image. The child may be unable to wear stylish shoes comfortably or fear wearing open shoes such as sandals. In such cases the pain is more psychological than physical. The cosmetic concern of such adolescent girls is realistic and must be handled with appropriate sensitivity and empathy by the treating physician.

Parents may seek professional care, desiring an opinion as to whether treatment should be undertaken promptly or deferred. There may be a family history of the condition and a concern or fear that the child's deformity will progress to or surpass the severity of the parents' or grandparents' condition. Frequently the hope of learning of a definitive solution to the problem leads to questions such as: Will the condition worsen? Can something be done to prevent if from worsening? Should certain shoes be worn? Will it recur if it is operated on now?

In spite of the fact that juvenile and adolescent hallux abducto valgus is not an uncommon problem, treatment continues to be controversial. Many factors must be taken into consideration in dealing with the deformity, including

1. The age of the patient and the status of the growth plate (open or closed)
2. The rigidity or flexibility of the deformity
3. The onset and progressive nature of the deformity
4. The presence of coexisting etiologic factors powerful enough to initiate and propagate the deformity
5. The presence of coexisting deformity that may contribute to recurrence of a juvenile or adolescent hallux abducto valgus deformity if left untreated
6. The family history of such deformity
7. The degree of symptomatology, both psychological and physical
8. Patient and parent expectations

For the convenience of the reader, the term *juvenile hallux valgus deformity* will be used to represent both the juvenile and the adolescent hallux abducto valgus deformities described above.

## INCIDENCE

The true frequency of juvenile hallux valgus deformity is unknown for obvious reasons. Various authors have reported a wide range in limited studies. The condition, however, is common and has received considerable attention over the years.

Cole reported an incidence of 36 percent in a study of schoolchildren between the ages of 8 and 18 years; 75 percent of the children with a juvenile hallux valgus deformity were girls, and the deformity ranging from mild to severe.[12] Piggott reported that 57 percent of adult patients with hallux valgus recalled the deformity being present in their teens or even earlier,[5] and Hardy and Clapham stated 46 percent of their adult patients recalled the deformity as being present before the age of 20 years.[10] Similar results have been reported by other authors. Helal found that 92 percent of all his juvenile hallux valgus patients, ranging in age from 9 to 19 years, were girls with 75 percent of all cases occurring bilaterally.[4]

## ETIOLOGY

Controversy surrounds the etiology of the juvenile hallux valgus deformity. Many theories have been published suggesting a myriad of factors as being responsible for its development and propagation. While some authors favor malposition of the metatarsophalangeal joint as the sole etiology,[2,5,13,14] others have blamed structural abnormalities of the metatarsal bone, the cuneiform bone, or the metatarsocuneiform joint.[1,3,15-19] Many authors have recognized the presence of a severe flatfoot deformity, equinus, or other structural or functional abnormality as commonplace.[1,7,8,11,20-23] In all probability, the etiology is multifactorial in nature, although in some cases one specific factor may have a dominant role. In many cases the etiology is unknown.

Hereditary factors are perhaps the most commonly cited cause. This viewpoint has been supported by several authors.[13,24-26] Meier and Kenzora have reported a positive family history in over 80 percent of their studied cases.[27] An incidence of familial history in 68 percent of cases was reported in 1980 by Glynn and associates.[28] The factor predisposing to the evolution of a hallux valgus deformity may, indeed, be transmitted by an autosomal dominant trait showing incomplete penetrance. Perhaps full penetrance results in a much earlier onset and a more severe deformity. Some congenital cases may represent a limb bud deficiency or actual developmental anomaly.[1]

Studies have demonstrated the presence of hallux valgus deformity in non-shoe-wearing populations.[29,30] A higher incidence in girls has also been reported, especially around the age of 14 years.[13,31,32] This however, may simply reflect greater awareness of and concern about the deformity in girls than in boys. Although footwear might presumably be a necessary prerequisite, the deformity clearly appears in the unshod as well as the shod populations. There must, therefore, be some intrinsic factor(s) predisposing those who wear moderately deforming shoes or are normally unshod to hallux valgus deformity.

Footwear is perhaps the most common extrinsic factor contributing to a hallux valgus deformity. The incidence of juvenile hallux valgus deformity has been shown to be higher in the generally shod population than among those who walk barefooted.[33,34] In addition, it has been shown that ill-fitting shoes may be a contributing factor in the progression of the juvenile hallux valgus deformity.[35] Perhaps, this deformity becomes more noticeable to the 12- to 14-year-old girl because of an increased self-awareness, a desire to wear stylish shoes, or the cultural emphasis placed on appearance by our society. A foot with either the proper predisposing factors or an already present deformity, even one mild in nature, would then conceivably develop symptoms.

Great controversy surrounds the question of whether the primary event is abduction or deviation of the great toe or whether it is the increased spread between the first and second metatarsals. Hardy and Clapham[13] as well as Bonney and MacNab[31] have observed a strong correlation between hallux valgus deformity and increased intermetatarsal angle and contend that hallux abductus is the primary deformity and that the increased separation between the first and second metatarsals is a secondary feature. In many cases abduction of the hallux is the more severe component, with the metatarsus primus adductus clearly developing secondarily and as a sequela (Fig. 15-2). The classic studies of Hardy and Clapham demonstrated the highest incidence of hallux valgus deformity to occur in patients under the age of 14 years, in contrast to the increased intermetatarsal angle, which showed its greatest incidence after the age of 15 years.[13] Furthermore, Piggott in 1960 found that subluxation of the first metatarsophalangeal joint occurred with intermetatarsal angles as low as 7 degrees.[5] In a

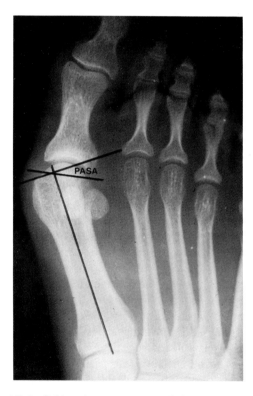

**Fig. 15-2.** Subluxation at metatarsophalangeal joint in adolescent with hallux abducto valgus deformity indicated radiographically by abnormal PASA (proximal articular set angle). Note the relatively low intermetatarsal angle. Also note the significant displacement of the sesamoid apparatus. Early adaptation of the first metatarsal head is seen.

more recent (1988) study, metatarsus primus varus was nearly absent in adolescents; only 27 percent had an increased intermetatarsal angle, while the hallux was almost always in a position of valgus alignment.[21]

The opposite view, that metatarsus primus varus is the primary deformity and results in secondary hallux valgus deformity, has also been proposed by many authors with some variation.[3,15-18] In 1925 Truslow advocated the term *metatarsus primus varus* to describe the abnormal obliquity of the first metatarsal bone in relation to the remaining lesser metatarsals, as determined through a retrospective radiographic review, in which a distinct angular divergence of the first metatarsal from the second metatarsal was identified. This divergence was thought to be an anatomic variation and to represent the primary deformity in the juvenile or adolescent patient with a hallux abducto valgus deformity. It was not thought to be an acquired deformity.[15]

In 1912 Ewald suggested that an abnormal obliquity of the first metatarsocuneiform joint leads to an excessive medial deviation of the first metatarsal. A higher intermetatarsal angle or atavistic cuneiform with medial angulation could conceivably affect the development of a hallux valgus deformity[19] (Fig. 15-3).

Lapidus described the atavistic cuneiform as a deformity in which a large intermetatarsal angle presents similarly to the prehensile great toe of higher primates. He also pointed out that girls around 13 to 14 years of age with this type of foot would tend to develop a bunion, especially if they began to wear narrower and less physiologically desirable shoes. He believed that there is an inherent instability in the medial column of the foot, predisposing the foot to the development and propagation of a bunion deformity.[18,36]

Other authors have hypothesized that the architectural configuration of the first metatarsal bone may be a contributing factor to the evolution of hallux valgus deformity. Both a short and a long first metatarsal bone have been suggested as contributing factors[13,37-39] (Fig. 15-4). A flat shape of the first metatarsal base is thought to be more resistant to the deforming forces at the level of the metatarsophalangeal joint than the relatively unstable rounded shape[40-42] (Fig. 15-5). The presence of an enlarged or an accessory bone at the lateral aspect of the base of the first metatarsal or cuneiform may also promote medial angulation of the metatarsal bone, although this phenomenon is presumed to be less common.[43,44] Definitive evidence that the aforementioned architectural variations definitively contribute to a juvenile hallux valgus deformity is still lacking. At the very least, cadaveric studies are necessary to define conclusively the true shape of the first metatarsal base and/or medial cuneiform bone.

The etiology of the juvenile hallux valgus deformity has also been classified as static or dynamic. In cases classified as static, there is early appearance of metatarsus primus adductus, which is considered to be the primary cause and therefore the focus of correction. The bunion deformity in this group manifests itself while the child is still growing. Splaying occurs because of asymmetric growth at the epiphysis of the first metatarsal base or because of excessive obliquity at the first metatarsocuneiform joint, a condition termed *atavistic cuneiform* by Lapidus.[18] Excessive adduction of all the me-

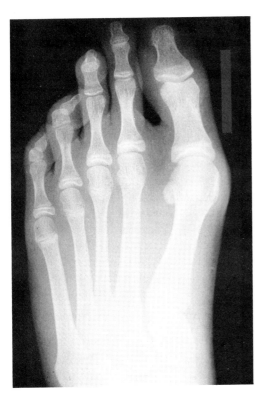

**Fig. 15-3.** Juvenile bunion deformity with excessive obliquity of the metatarsocuneiform joint on dorsoplantar radiograph.

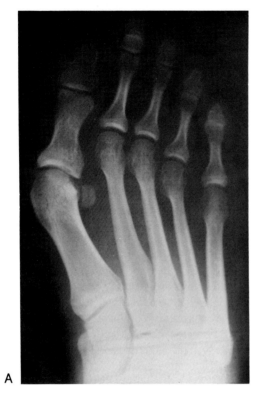
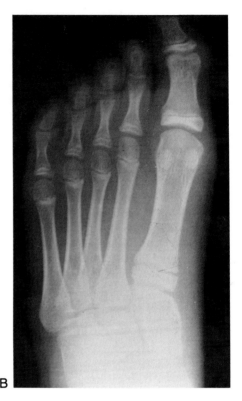

**Fig. 15-4.** **(A)** Juvenile hallux abducto valgus deformity with extremely short first metatarsal bone. Also, note atypical appearance of the medial cuneiform and increased obliquity of the metatarsocuneiform joint. Residual metatarsus adductus is also present. **(B)** Long first metatarsal in juvenile patient. Also present is an abductus deformity at the level of the interphalangeal joint of the great toe. This has been postulated as a contributing cause of the juvenile or adolescent bunion deformity.

tatarsal bones also falls within this category. Such conditions require realignment of the first metatarsal as the focus of correction. Realignment of the metatarsophalangeal joint is secondary. Correction in this situation may occur at the base of the first metatarsal, within the metatarsocuneiform joint, or within the medial cuneiform itself.

In dynamic juvenile hallux valgus, the deformity occurs at the end of growth of the first metatarsal but may occur sooner. In these cases there is normal development of the bones; the deformity occurs as a result of abnormal motion through the first ray, with resultant tendon and ligament malposition and failure. This is most often seen in the severely pronated or hypermobile flatfoot with associated equinus at the ankle joint. It is also seen in patients with a long first ray segment and ligamentous laxity. In each case the flexor hallucis longus

tendon becomes a major deforming force as the hallux is forced against the first metatarsal, with resulting splaying between the first and second metatarsals (Fig. 15-6). Metatarsus primus adductus is then secondary to deviation of the hallux. Corrections in these situations are aimed at realignment of the hallux and control or correction of excessive hypermobility and pronation.

## Concomitant Flatfoot Deformity

Both the orthopedic and the podiatric literature strongly suggest a correlation between more proximal pathology and the severity of the juvenile hallux valgus deformity.[7,11,45-48] In 1954 Hohman stated, "Hallux valgus is always combined with pes planus, and pes planus is always the predisposing factor in hallux valgus."[22] While this statement is certainly an oversim-

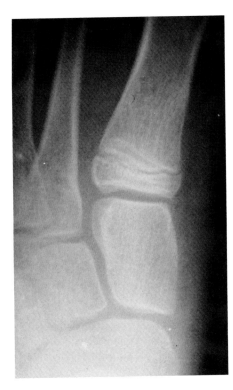

**Fig. 15-5.** Flat first metatarsocuneiform joint, thought to be more resistant than a rounded joint to deforming forces and splaying between the first and second metatarsal bones.

plified summation, it clearly identifies the coexistence of pes plano valgus and hallux valgus deformity. This correlation has been observed by many authors. A pronated foot type or hypermobile flatfoot has been cited frequently as the cause or predisposing factor in juvenile hallux valgus deformities.[1,3,8-10,20,21,49,50] Sgarlato[51] and Root et al.[52] have provided detailed descriptions of the influence of excessive and abnormal pronation of the rearfoot on the evolution of a hallus valgus deformity.

The coexistence of hallux valgus with flatfoot deformity is believed to be 8 to 24 times its occurrence in members of the same population who do not have pes planus deformity.[21] In 1984 Scranton and Zuckerman, in a major study, demonstrated a 51 percent incidence of hypermobile flatfoot syndrome based on a study of 50 feet of juvenile or adolescent patients with hallux valgus deformity. A long first metatarsal was identified in 32 percent of the patients.[8] In 1931 Hiss reported on 1,812 patients, of whom 60.3 percent had "everted" feet and 82.1 percent "malpositioned arches."[46] Hardy and

Clapham found the severity of hallux valgus to be significantly correlated with arch height, subcutaneous prominence of the talus, eversion of the calcaneus, and pronation of the foot.[10] It appeared that any pronatory abnormalities that result in hypermobility of the first ray may cause a hallux valgus deformity. These include both forefoot and rearfoot varus deformities, tibia vara, tight posterior muscle groups, and abnormal rotation or torsion of the leg segment. Flexible forefoot valgus and compensated equinus deformities may be the earliest manifestations of hallux valgus deformity (Fig. 15-7).

## Concomitant Metatarsus Adductus

Metatarsus adductus is also frequently associated with the juvenile or adolescent hallux valgus deformity.[23,41,53,54] The recognition of an underlying metatarsus adductus deformity has received little attention in the orthopedic or podiatric literature until recently. We have recognized the intimate relationship between these deformities since about 1980 and recently published several brief articles introducing and proposing mathematical relationships to improve understanding of the two deformities[7,55-57] (Figs. 15-8 and 15-9). It is our contention that a long first metatarsal segment, often referred to as an underlying cause of juvenile hallux valgus deformity, may be merely a manifestation of an underlying metatarsus adductus. When a long first metatarsal segment is identified, careful evaluation, both clinical and radiographic, is in order to determine if metatarsus adductus is in fact, coexistent. Such deformity may be masked by excessive abduction at the midtarsal joint level and/or subtalar joint pronation, which are not uncommonly seen as compensation for metatarsus adductus.

Failure to recognize the influence of metatarsus adductus in the juvenile or adolescent with a hallux valgus deformity can result in complications following surgical correction of the bunion, especially recurrence of the hallux valgus deformity. We have seen patients in whom apparently adequate surgical procedures failed to provide long-term structural correction (Fig. 15-10). The primary reason for this failure is the deceptive intermetatarsal angle measured on standard dorsoplantar radiographs, which is typically very low in the patient with metatarsus adductus. The radiographically low intermetatarsal angle usually results in the selection of a distal metaphyseal osteotomy, which would appear to be an

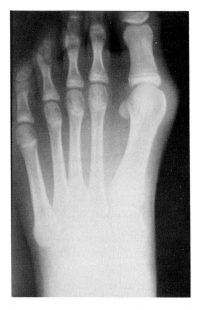
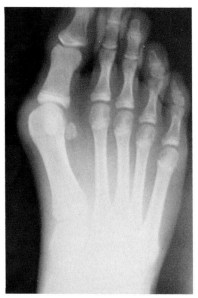

**Fig. 15-6.** Significant metatarsus primus adductus with concomitant hallux abductus. Significant displacement of the sesamoid apparatus implies displacement of the long flexor tendon. Note that significant adaptation has not taken place in the cartilage of the first metatarsal head or base of the phalanx. Increased obliquity at the metatarsocuneiform joint may be a contributing factor.

appropriate procedure. Later the deformity recurs, causing frustration to both the patient and the surgeon.

The true or effective intermetatarsal angle can be defined mathematically by the formula

$$IMA + (MAA - 15°) = IMA_t$$

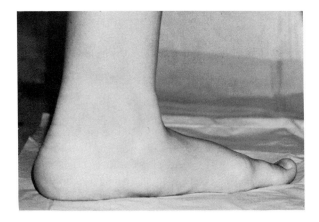

**Fig. 15-7.** Severe collapsing pes valgo planus deformity in an adolescent patient with significant hallux abducto valgus deformity. Notice complete and total collapse of the medial longitudinal arch with bulging of the talar head.

where IMA is the intermetatarsal angle and MAA is the metatarsus adductus angle, both as measured on the dorsoplantar radiograph.[57] When this formula is employed, a proximal first metatarsal base wedge osteotomy will more frequently be selected as the procedure of choice and will result in a more definitive structural and clinical correction. A paper dealing solely with the complex but intimate interrelationship of metatarsus adductus and hallux abducto valgus deformity is presently in progress (1991) and will be published in a separate text in the near future.

In summary, the precise etiology of the juvenile hallux valgus deformity appears to be multifactorial. While hereditary factors clearly play a role, the relationship between hallux abductus and metatarsus primus varus (adductus) still remains controversial. The coexistence of an underlying flatfoot syndrome, equinus deformity, or other osseous deformity such as metatarsus adductus has clearly been shown to be related to the juvenile hallux valgus deformity. In many cases, perhaps, the hallux valgus deformity should be regarded as a sign or symptom of another underlying major deformity rather than as an isolated deformity in and of itself. In any event, treatment should be based upon a comprehensive ap-

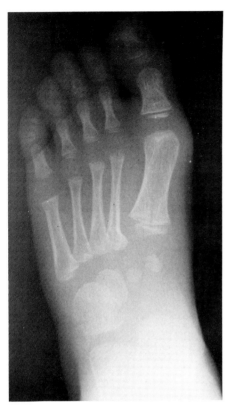

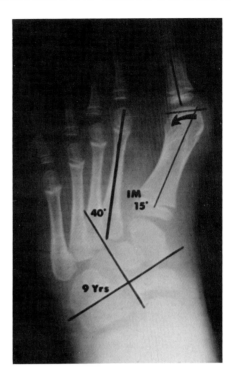

**Fig. 15-8.**  Dorsoplantar radiograph of the patient seen in Fig. 15-1. Note early juvenile hallux abducto valgus deformity and early adaptation of the first metatarsal head. Significant splaying between the first and second metatarsal bones is not seen; however, significant metatarsus adductus deformity is present.

**Fig. 15-9.**  In this 9-year-old patient, severe underlying metatarsus adductus is a contributing factor to the juvenile bunion deformity. Note excessive obliquity of the metatarsocuneiform joint as well as significant adaptation of the first metatarsal head as a result of the severe deformity.

proach, with every effort made to identify an underlying etiology. We believe that only rarely should treatment focus solely on the clinical manifestations of the bunion itself. In all cases in which surgery is undertaken, it is our recommendation and strong belief that a purely symptomatic approach should be avoided. Procedures should be selected to provide the best possible structural correction of the deformity and correction of any underlying etiologic factors.

## RADIOGRAPHIC EVALUATION

Radiographic assessment involves the evaluation of weight-bearing dorsoplantar and lateral views taken in angle and base of gait. A sesamoid axial view should also be obtained. A medial oblique radiograph is optional and may be helpful in assessing any significant metatarsus primus elevatus deformity, both prior to and following surgical correction.

The following radiographic parameters should be assessed:

Hallux abductus angle (HA)
Intermetatarsal angle (IM)
Metatarsus primus adductus (MPA) (varus) angle
Tibial sesamoid position
Metatarsus adductus angle (MA)
Proximal articular set angle (PASA)
Distal articular set angle (DASA)
Hallux abductus interphalangeus angle (HAI)

These radiographic parameters will be helpful in determining the most appropriate surgical procedure(s) (Figs. 15-11, 12). The normal values of the above angles,

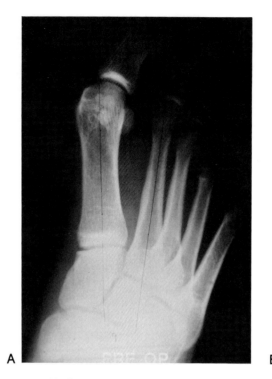
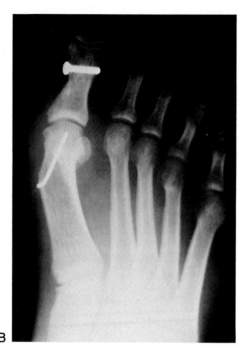

**Fig. 15-10. (A)** Preoperative and **(B)** postoperative radiographs of juvenile bunion deformity corrected by distal metaphyseal osteotomy and Akin osteotomy. Notice recurrence of the deformity 2 months following surgery.

as well as the methods for determining them, are not within the scope of this chapter.

We place primary emphasis on the intermetatarsal angle, metatarsus primus varus angle, tibial sesamoid position, and hallux abductus angle. Less emphasis is placed on the proximal and distal articular set angles and the hallux abductus interphalangeus angle, as these are considered secondary parameters. They become of key importance in those situations in which a rapidly progressive or severe deformity has resulted in adaptation of articular surfaces. One should also assess the overall shape of the first metatarsal and observe the presence or absence of any accessory bone(s) between the first and second metatarsal bases or their corresponding cuneiforms. An asymmetric appearance of the first metatarsal in which the lateral cortex is longer than the medial cortex and/or the metatarsal appears rhomboidal rather than rectangular in shape suggests the need for a proximally based osteotomy for correction of the intermetatarsal angle.

Significant displacement of the sesamoid bones implies a gain in the mechanical advantage of the adductor hallucis tendon, lateral head of the flexor hallucis brevis, and less commonly the flexor hallucis longus tendon itself. It is important to realize that this is, in reality, a medial migration of the first metatarsal head rather than an actual displacement of the sesamoid apparatus. The sesamoid bones lie within the substance of the intrinsic musculature, which is essentially fixed within its position relative to the other soft tissues of the foot. Clinically a displaced sesamoid apparatus manifests itself as frontal plane valgus rotation in addition to transverse plane abduction of the great toe as the deformity becomes more long-standing and rigid. Relocation and repositioning of the sesamoid bones beneath the metatarsal head constitute a primary focus and goal of surgical reconstruction. Persistent malposition of the sesamoid apparatus and thus the flexor hallucis tendon greatly increases the likelihood that the deformity will recur, as the normal retrograde forces across the joint have not been reestablished.

A significant increase in the proximal articular set angle indicates functional adaptation of the first metatarsal due to chronic malpositioning of and abnormal forces

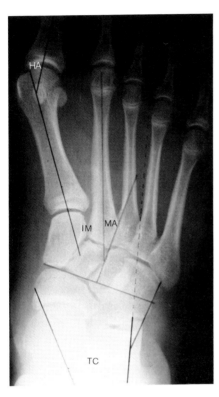

**Fig. 15-11.** Dorsoplantar radiograph demonstrating commonly measured angular relationships, in both the forefoot and rearfoot, in the assessment of the juvenile or adolescent with a bunion deformity. HA, hallux abductus angle; IM, intermetatarsal angle; MA, metatarsus adductus angle; TC, talocalcaneal.

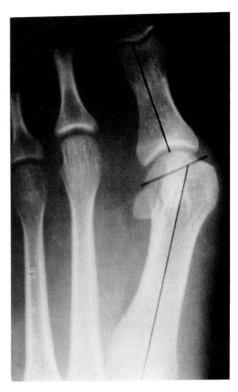

**Fig. 15-12.** Dorsoplantar radiograph of juvenile bunion deformity. Notice significant adaptation of the first metatarsal head as a result of hallux drifting and retrograde force on the first metatarsal bone. If confirmed intraoperatively, an osteotomy for correction of the proximal articular set angle would be required in addition to a procedure to reduce the intermetatarsal angle.

on the great toe (Fig. 15-12). In certain circumstances it may correlate clinically with an irreducible hallux valgus deformity, which is typically referred to as being "track-bound."[58] Final determination of the proximal articular set angle, however, should be made intraoperatively, as this angle can be quite deceiving on standard radiographs alone.

The overall relative length of the first metatarsal should be determined. An excessively long or short first metatarsal may influence the final selection of procedures (Fig. 15-4). A long first metatarsal segment may be the only evidence of an underlying metatarsus adductus deformity and thus, when observed, should suggest its presence. As previously mentioned, a significant underlying metatarsus adductus deformity will mask the true intermetatarsal angle and may falsely influence the

selection of procedure(s). A metatarsus adductus angle greater than 15 to 18 degrees with a long first metatarsal as determined on the dorsoplantar radiograph deserves very careful assessment. The previously discussed formula should be employed to more accurately determine the effective or true intermetatarsal angle. Correction of metatarsus adductus may be required in addition to aggressive correction of the intermetatarsal angle by osteotomy of the metatarsal base or cuneiform.

The extent of closure or ossification of the epiphyseal growth plate at the base of the first metatarsal should be evaluated. In patients under the age of 14 to 16 years, an open and viable plate should be readily observed on conventional radiographs, especially on the dorsoplantar view.[59] On occasion a secondary distal epiphyseal growth plate at the head of the first metatarsal has been reported.[60] The presence of a secondary growth plate may influence the selection of procedures and/or the timing of surgery at both the head and the base of the metatarsal.

In addition to determining the angular relationships of the first ray, the rearfoot should be assessed to determine any significant structural or positional abnormalities that might influence the juvenile hallux abductus deformity. This is especially true in patients in whom a significant collapsing pes valgo planus or equinus deformity has already been identified clinically. Such radiographic parameters (Fig. 15-13) would include:

Calcaneal inclination angle
Talar declination angle
Talocalcaneal angle
Medial column breaches
Talonavicular congruity
Cuboid abduction
Talar neck exostosis formation
Blunting of the lateral process of the talus

On the basis of radiographic findings, the juvenile hallux valgus deformity can be classified as either static or dynamic. As previously discussed, the dynamic form results from hypermobility of the forefoot due to biomechanical abnormalities. The primary deformity, then, exists at the level of the first metatarsophalangeal joint, as evidenced by abduction or lateral deviation of the great toe. The extent of this lateral deviation is impor-

tant for two reasons. First, the articular surface of the first metatarsal possesses adaptable and plastic qualities in the juvenile or adolescent foot; chronic eccentric loading of the first metatarsophalangeal joint by a laterally subluxed hallux will eventually produce a corresponding lateral articular cartilage deviation and adaptation, referred to as an increased *proximal articular set angle* (PASA). Radiographically these long-term adaptive changes are reflected by an abnormal measurement of the proximal articular set angle and a lateral displacement of the subchondral bone plate on the first metatarsal head. Second, the greater the abduction of the great toe on the first metatarsal, the greater the retrograde buckling force placed against the first metatarsal head. This results in increased splaying between the first and second metatarsals. The dynamic deformity eventually contains two components: abnormal abduction of the hallux and an increase in the intermetatarsal angle.

The static form presents primarily as a deformity of the metatarsal itself or the metatarsocuneiform joint. Both levels of the deformity present with an abnormally high intermetatarsal angle, with or without abduction of the great toe. A rhomboid shape of the metatarsal can result from an abnormally wide and hyperplastic lateral epiphyseal growth plate. The lateral side of the metatarsal will be longer than the medial side in such cases.[61] The obliquity of the metatarsocuneiform joint is defined by determination of the metatarsus primus varus angle, which in turn is determined by the angle formed by the

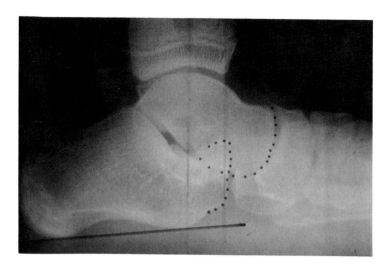

**Fig. 15-13.** Lateral radiograph demonstrating significant flatfoot deformity. Notice the decrease in calcaneal inclination angle and medial column breaching. Forward and downward migration of the talus is also present.

bisector of the medial cuneiform and the bisector of the first metatarsal. If this angular measurement is greater than 25 degrees, it is considered abnormal, and a metatarsus primus varus deformity is said to exist.[15]

The intermetatarsal angle may also be abnormally increased in the static or dynamic juvenile hallux valgus deformity. In 1957 Stamm stated that an abnormal intermetatarsal angle adds to "the breakdown of the mechanical integrity of the forefoot and often causes more pain and dysfunction than the valgus deformity of the great toe."[62] We agree that the severely increased intermetatarsal angle adds greatly to the overall instability of the foot, especially the medial column. Once this angle exceeds 15 degrees, it becomes a deforming force on the entire foot and will require aggressive surgical treatment (Fig. 15-11).

## THERAPY

### Conservative Treatment

A well defined protocol for the conservative management of the juvenile hallux valgus deformity is clearly lacking. Furthermore, the short- or long-term outcome of any such treatment is unclear and lacks documentation; to date (1990) there have been no published data to substantiate the effectiveness of such treatment. On the other hand, Hardy and Clapham have documented the outcome of the condition in a random study of 3,642 feet of children between the ages of 4 and 15. This study, performed in 1952, concluded that there is a progressive increase of the lateral displacement of the great toe with increasing age.[13] Can one then draw the seemingly logical conclusion that the painful degenerative hallux valgus deformity so frequently seen in the adult foot represents the long-term outcome of the mismanaged or untreated bunion of adolescents? Traditionally, the orthopedic community has emphasized nonoperative treatment modalities. Helal has stated that "the shape of the shoe can be adapted to that of the foot, or the shape of the foot can be altered,"[4] and Coughlin and Mann have suggested that "most adolescents with a bunion deformity do not require aggressive surgical treatment."[49] Trott believed that if an adequately wider shoe were worn, surgical intervention could be avoided.[26]

The changing of shoe type has been frequently recorded as a conservative treatment modality; however, this treatment does little or nothing to prevent further progression of the deformity or to control the deforming forces responsible for the development and propagation of the hallux valgus deformity itself.[63] Admittedly, pain resulting from shoe pressure will resolve with a wider shoe or no shoe at all. While the avoidance of narrow or pointed shoes will conceivably decrease the progression rate of deformity of the juvenile or adolescent foot already predisposed to such deformity, actual correction of the deformity does not occur. In short, alteration of foot gear is primarily symptomatic treatment.

Other conservative treatment modalities are palliative in nature and include hallux splints, toe wedges, bunion shields, and pads.[4,63,64] Their use should be selective and limited to those patients with only mild deformity and minimal symptomatology and in whom progression of the deformity has been slow.

Stretching and manipulation have also been reported but are not likely to result in any significant correction. In the best case scenario, they may help to stretch the lateral periarticular structures, which tighten and contract with time and thereby maintain or create some flexibility in the deformity. This, of course, is, again, purely hypothetical and has yet to be proved.

In some cases an aggressive stretching program may prove helpful in patients with a gastrocnemius or gastrocnemius-soleus equinus deformity. If this program proves unsuccessful, surgical correction of the equinus deformity may be necessary.

More aggressive conservative treatment focuses on biomechanical control of the foot by utilizing orthotic devices. Such devices should control or limit excessive pronation of the foot and thereby reduce hypermobility of the first ray. It should be emphasized that such devices have their limits. Orthotic devices cannot adequately control the foot indefinitely, especially in cases of a strong familial history of similar deformity, a concomitant major structural deformity such as severe pes planus or metatarsus adductus, or an overwhelming biomechanical force as in the equinus deformity. Functional orthotic devices are recommended and indicated under the following conditions:

1. Mild to moderate deformity, which is flexible in nature
2. Biomechanical etiology of the deformity (e.g., flexible forefoot valgus, moderate pes planus deformity, or mild equinus)
3. Minimal symptomatology
4. Slow progression of the deformity

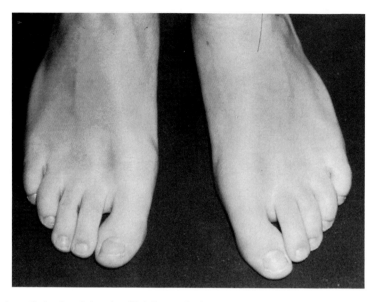

**Fig. 15-14.** Early juvenile bunion deformity. This is a typical presentation of a foot that should be monitored closely. Immediate surgical intervention is not warranted.

Any patient treated nonoperatively should be monitored periodically for progression of the deformity or adaptive changes. Baseline and then periodic radiographs should be obtained to document the course of the deformity, as clinical monitoring alone is not adequate to assess the progress of deformity or lack thereof[3,7,8,52] (Fig. 15-14).

In summary, with the exception of orthotic devices, all conservative treatment modalities essentially represent a symptomatic approach to the management of the juvenile hallux valgus foot. Orthotic devices affording biomechanical control may prevent or slow the progression of deformity. Further clinical and radiographic studies, however, are clearly needed to document the effectiveness of such treatment. In other than mild cases with minimal symptomatology, surgical intervention will more than likely be necessary. Orthotic devices postoperatively, however, will be critical to prevent recurrence of the deformity in those patients with contributory biomechanical pathology, especially in those with severe pes planus deformity.

## Surgical Management

### Indications and Considerations

The decision whether to treat the juvenile or adolescent hallux abducto valgus deformity conservatively or surgically has often been made on the basis of other than objective criteria. In many cases physicians completely ignore the problem and refuse to acknowledge the concern of the child or parents. Any surgical treatment is strongly discouraged owing to the lack of experience in treating this deformity, lack of knowledge of the known progression of the deformity, and fear of the open epiphyseal plate.

Two basic and divergent philosophies have been advocated concerning the surgical treatment of the juvenile bunion deformity. The traditional and conservative school of thought advocates delaying any surgery until skeletal maturity has been attained, as evidenced by radiographically demonstrated closure of the epiphyseal growth plate. Bonney and McNab[31] reported a complication rate involving recurrence in 10 of 14 children who underwent surgical correction prior to closure of the epiphyseal plate; they attributed the recurrence to execution of an osteotomy distal to this plate. Following surgery, growth of the first metatarsal continued in a varus direction, resulting in recurrence of the deformity.[31] A 20 percent recurrence rate was reported by Scranton and Zuckerman[8] when surgery was performed on five adolescents in the presence of an open epiphyseal plate. This, however, may be totally insignificant, as the recurrence involved one of five cases in which a soft tissue procedure alone was performed for correction of the deformity.[8]

A more logical approach to surgery advocates evaluation and assessment of a myriad of factors associated with the juvenile bunion deformity. It does not isolate any one component as the sole factor determining whether to treat the deformity surgically or conservatively. The following factors should be thoroughly assessed prior to deciding whether surgical intervention is appropriate and if it is, which procedure should be performed and when:

Symptoms
Extent or severity of deformity
Rate of progression of the deformity
Family history
Etiology and associated deformities
Age (skeletal maturity)

Many authors have reported the absence of pain in the juvenile patient with a hallux abducto valgus deformity.[7,9,11,65,66] Only 21 percent of Carr and Boyd's patients reported pain associated with the deformity.[2] The presence of pain, however, is likely to indicate and be associated with more severe deformity. When present, it is often aggravated by conventional footwear, especially the stylish shoes worn by the female patient. This may be one factor explaining the somewhat higher incidence of juvenile bunion deformities among girls as reported by several authors. Significant adaptation of the first metatarsophalangeal joint, especially the cartilage of the first metatarsal, may be suggested by conventional radiographs.

Not uncommonly, parents express concern over the disfiguring appearance of the child's foot even when symptomatology attributed to the deformity is minimal. On further questioning, a clear history of pain and disability in the remainder of the foot may be elicited. Constant or easy fatigue, a lack of enthusiasm for normal recreational activities, and other postural complaints about the knee, hip, or leg may be signs and symptoms related to a bunion deformity in the juvenile or adolescent. These complaints are often due to major bimechanical dysfunction or to structural deformities such as metatarsus adductus, severe collapsing pes plano valgus, or equinus. In these situations the juvenile or adolescent bunion deformity should be considered a sign of a significant deformity deserving complete evaluation and, most probably, aggressive treatment, whether conservative or surgical.[11] The presence of pain directly attributable to the bunion prominence itself should not be considered

an absolute or strict prerequisite to surgical management. To rely solely on such a symptom as a surgical indication may ultimately result in substantial deterioration of the first metatarsophalangeal joint and other components of the first ray complex. The presence of significant pain and an inability to tolerate conventional footgear comfortably indicates a need for surgical correction.

The severity of the bunion deformity as assessed clinically and radiographically will also influence the decision of whether or not to operate (Fig. 15-15). This is most commonly assessed by determining the degree of hallux abductus, the extent of frontal plane valgus rotation, and the degree of splaying between the first and second metatarsals. There is clearly a strong relationship between abduction of the hallux and medial deviation of the first metatarsal, as previously discussed.

With extensive lateral drifting of the hallux, there is

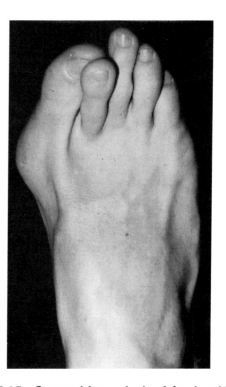

Fig. 15-15. Severe adolescent bunion deformity with secondary dorsal migration of the second digit. A comprehensive evaluation is necessary to rule out other underlying deformities in the rearfoot or leg that may be contributing factors to the rapidly progressive bunion deformity. This deformity most likely would require surgical intervention consisting of multiple procedures.

progressive subluxation of the metatarsophalangeal joint and a resultant increase in the retrograde force against the metatarsal head. Once the intermetatarsal angle exceeds 15 degrees, the deformity should be considered severe in nature. Medial column stability is lost, and collapse of the medial longitudinal arch, if not already present, is likely to ensue. In addition, the hallux abducto valgus deformity can be expected to progress. Scranton and Zuckerman[8] and others have clearly shown a relationship between excessive pronation and the likelihood of recurrence of deformity on the basis of several studies.

The presence of adaptive changes in the first metatarsal head is directly proportional to the extent and severity of the deformity. These changes are best identified on the weight-bearing dorsoplantar radiograph, on which a lateral shift in the subchondral bone plate is seen, corresponding to a lateral deviation of the articular surface of the first metatarsal head (i.e., an increase in the PASA). This remodeling or functional adaptation, if confirmed surgically, requires a technically more complicated and complex procedure in order to achieve correction of the deformity. In very young, skeletally immature patients, adaptive changes may occur without direct surgical correction of the articular cartilage if the joint congruity and the metatarsal splaying are satisfactorily corrected. Individuals with significant adaptation of the first metatarsal head tend to have what has been referred to as a "trackbound" deformity. These persons are more likely to experience pain upon manual reduction of the deformity with dorsiflexion and plantar flexion at the metatarsophalangeal joint.

The juvenile and adolescent hallux abducto valgus deformity rarely demonstrates degenerative arthritic changes, clinically or radiographically, at the first metatarsophalangeal joint itself. When present, however, such changes provide a strong argument for surgical correction. While osteophytic lipping may not be identified, erosions of the central cristae, subchondral sclerosis, medial cystic changes in the metatarsal head, and progressive elevation of the first ray segment are not infrequently encountered. An early hallux limitus deformity also supports the need for early surgical intervention. We have encountered degenerative changes of the first metatarsal head on numerous occasions during surgical correction of the juvenile or adolescent bunion deformity.

The rate of progression should be assessed when evaluating the juvenile or adolescent patient with a bunion deformity. A clear history can usually be obtained and documented by interviewing not only the patient but the parents as well. Identification of the deformity in early childhood with subsequent progressive increase in the deformity, especially a rapid increase, is another indication for surgical intervention. This is especially true when a strong influencing biomechanical force or deformity such as excessive pronation, metatarsus adductus or equinus is also present, as is not infrequently the case.

Piggott[5] emphasized the importance and significance of a congruous, deviated, or subluxed joint in relation to progression of the hallux abductus deformity in a juvenile (Fig. 15-2). In a small study of 216 patients, Piggott found 20 congruous, 18 deviated, and 114 subluxed first metatarsophalangeal joints. Because only 8 of the 18 deviated joints demonstrated signs of progression, he surmised that progression of the deformity in patients with a deviated joint was unlikely. He also theorized that subluxed metatarsophalangeal joints would progress and deteriorate in the future but that congruous joints would not.[5] The presence of an etiologic factor such as excessive pronation, hypermobility, or equinus can be expected to accelerate progression of the deformity. Conversely, a child with near normal biomechanical function and similar joint relationships is likely to demonstrate slow progression of the deformity. Perhaps such an individual will present later in life with a symptomatic bunion deformity.

It is clear that the juvenile bunion deformity is frequently associated with other structural or functional abnormalities. While the relationships are complex, they are logical and comprehensible. In addition, the juvenile hallux abducto valgus deformity, if severe enough, may itself result in secondary deformities including lesser metatarsalgia, single or multiple digital deformities such as digiti abducti, and further collapse and instability of the medial longitudinal arch.

Furthermore, the juvenile or adolescent hallux abducto valgus deformity may be only one component of a splayfoot deformity and as such a contributing factor to the well known ailments of such feet. The child with a significant splayfoot deformity is more likely to require surgical intervention at an earlier age (Fig. 15-16).

If surgical intervention is not undertaken, the child should be monitored on a periodic basis, both clinically and radiographically. Sudden changes in the radiographic parameters previously discussed should alert the practitioner to an increasing need for surgical intervention.

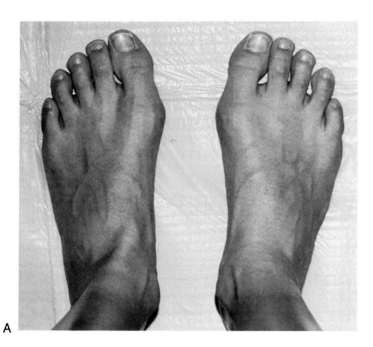
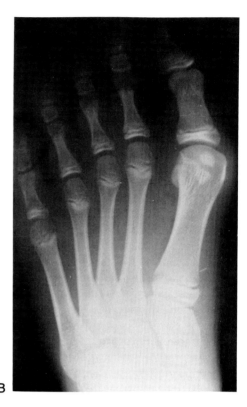

A

B

**Fig. 15-16.** (A) Clinical and (B) radiographic presentation of juvenile bunion deformity in an 11-year-old girl. This is typical of the early splayfoot deformity. Note widening of the forefoot. Underlying residual metatarsus adductus is also present.

Likewise, a sudden increase in the symptoms of a progressive deformity is also an indication for surgical intervention prior to osseous maturity.

More important than chronologic age in deciding when surgical intervention is best undertaken is the degree of skeletal maturity. Closure of the epiphyseal growth plate is well known to occur by the age of 16 years in both boys and girls, (somewhat earlier in girls).[59] Any surgical procedure performed at the base of the proximal phalanx or first metatarsal could conceivably result in damage to the growth plate and thereby in distorted growth; abnormal shape or abnormal position could ensue, causing an even more difficult problem. While proper selection of the procedures determines the expected correction, it is surgical expertise and the technical execution of the procedures that ensure a final successful outcome. Operating in close proximity to the epiphyseal growth plate requires the surgeon to have considerable experience, skill, and judgment to ensure

that damage to the growth plate does not occur. Inadvertent damage to the growth plate could conceivably create a "cure worse than the original disease." Knowledge of the growth rate of the first metatarsal may provide insight regarding the timing of surgical intervention. Nelson[59] has studied and charted the average skeletal maturity of the first metatarsal in boys and girls ranging from age 1 to 16. In children 6 years old and younger, 40 to 50 percent of the total growth of the first metatarsal has taken place, while in children between 6 and 9 or 10 years of age, 60 to 80 percent of the metatarsal length has been attained. In this age category the first metatarsal resembles that of the adult in its overall shape and therefore lends itself to surgical procedures more readily.[59]

Surgery in children under the age of 10 years is generally avoided unless the deformity is severe, rapidly progressive, and/or associated with other major structural or functional abnormalities unresponsive to conservative treatment modalities. It is also indicated in cases in which significant adaptation is identified radiographically. If surgery is pursued, special precautions to protect the epiphyseal plate from surgical insult are required.[4,7,65] Age between 10 and 15 years is considered by many to represent the ideal time. By the age of 12 years, 90 percent of the first metatarsal length has been achieved in boys and 95 percent in girls.[59] The bone structure is usually of significant maturity to allow execution of osseous procedures that readily permit fixation by a number of modalities. Our experience would recommend surgical intervention in this age group when a severe deformity is present with or without significant symptomatology, when the deformity demonstrates rapid progression or adaptation in either the metatarsophalangeal joint or metatarsocuneiform joint, or when significant structural or functional abnormalities are present and are believed to constitute a significant etiologic factor underlying the juvenile or adolescent bunion deformity.

By the age of 16 years most children have attained full skeletal maturity, with very little growth remaining in the first metatarsal. There is, in essence, minimal risk of damage to the epiphyseal area. Surgical procedures can be planned as in the adult, and surgery can be performed with confidence.

In summary, the presence of a juvenile or adolescent hallux abducto valgus deformity may represent an isolated clinical pathologic problem or, more commonly, may be part of a symptom complex indicating significant functional or structural pathology. If allowed to persist, it may result in to more serious deformity with both physical and psychological sequelae. Although the patient's and parents' concern may only be cosmetic in nature, the physician's concern must be the overall function of the patient's entire lower extremity. In some cases surgery involves only the first ray segment; in others it may entail surgical correction of an equinus, metatarsus adductus, or pathologic collapsing pes plano valgus deformity. Selection of the most appropriate procedure or combination of procedures, as well as the timing of the surgery, clearly depends on a myriad of factors, all of which require a detailed and comprehensive approach to a seemingly simple problem.

The optimal treatment, however, has not been generally agreed upon; it remains at the discretion of the surgeon and depends on the surgeon's training and experience. There are an estimated 100 surgical procedures for correction of the bunion deformity. In spite of this, however, there is general agreement regarding the need for adequate correction of both the osseous component of the deformity and the muscular imbalance about the joint. The overall goals of the surgery on the first ray are to re-establish a congruous joint, reposition the sesamoid apparatus beneath the metatarsal head, and reduce splaying and deviation between the first and second metatarsal bones. Failure to achieve these parameters is likely to result in recurrence of the deformity over time.

## Surgical Procedures

### Soft Tissue Procedures

With the development of the juvenile or adolescent hallux abducto valgus deformity, there is a lateral drift of the sesamoid apparatus with respect to the first metatarsal head, as the great toe deviates in both the transverse (abduction) and frontal (valgus) planes. In addition, there is a weakening and stretching of the medial periarticular structures and a secondary contracture of the lateral periarticular structures. As the sesamoid bones displace, the central crista separating the medial and lateral sesamoid bones is eroded and smoothed, which decreases the resistance to further displacement. As this further displacement occurs, the lateral intrinsic musculature (adductor hallucis and flexor hallucis brevis) clearly gains a mechanical advantage, causing further progression of the deformity (Fig. 15-17). This has been clearly demonstrated in electromyographic studies by Shimazaki and Takebea.[32] The greater the displacement of the sesamoid apparatus, the greater the imbalance that occurs between the intrinsic musculature medially and laterally. The study by Shimazaki and Takebe has also shown greater sesamoid displacement in the hyperpronated flatfoot.[32] In addition, there is a loss of pure sagittal plane pull by the long flexor and long extensor tendons with pronation of the great toe and sesamoid displacement. Snijders and Philippens showed, through electromyographic studies in 1986 that the long flexor tendon increases the valgus positioning of the hallux and varus positioning of the first metatarsal with progressive sesamoid displacement.[67]

The surgical repair of the adolescent or juvenile hallux

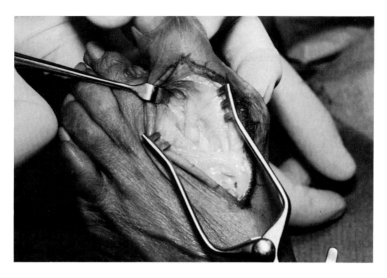

**Fig. 15-17.** Intraoperative photograph demonstrating the conjoined tendon of the adductor hallucis muscle. This muscle is believed to be the most important muscle contributing to the development and propagation of a bunion deformity in the adult or juvenile patient.

abducto valgus deformity by soft tissue procedures alone is likely to be met with poor success.[7,11] This has been clearly demonstrated in the orthopedic literature.[8,68,69] While such results support the need for osseous correction, soft tissue procedures are, nevertheless, an important component of any surgical procedure. A goal of the surgery should be to relocate the sesamoid apparatus to its normal anatomic position beneath the first metatarsal head, thereby centralizing the flexor hallucis longus tendon and directing its actions toward proper sagittal plane movements of the great toe (Fig. 15-18).

Current techniques of soft tissue procedures involve anatomic dissection about the first metatarsophalangeal joint, with a systematic approach to release the contracted structures and augmentation by tendon transfer when necessary. The proper surgical sequence includes

1. Release of the conjoined tendon and the adductor hallucis muscle from the base of the proximal phalanx and fibular sesamoid
2. Identification and sectioning or release of the contracted fibular sesamoidal ligament (Fig. 15-19A)
3. Sectioning or release of the lateral head of the flexor hallucis brevis tendon between the leading edge of the fibular sesamoid bone and the base of the proximal phalanx

4. Plication or shortening of the tibial sesamoidal ligament and medial collateral ligaments *or*
5. Transfer of the adductor hallucis tendon beneath the capsule, periosteum, and extensor hallucis longus tendon into the tibial sesamoidal ligament or medial capsular tissues (Fig. 15-19B)
6. Occasionally, release of the lateral metatarsophalangeal joint capsule
7. Rarely, excision of the fibular sesamoid itself

The specific surgical techniques outlined above have been well described.[7,70] The extent of dissection and manipulation of the soft tissues will depend upon the extent of derangement of the periarticular structures about the joint. In those cases in which the sesamoid apparatus has remained in relatively normal position, minimal soft tissue manipulations will be necessary. In such cases a simple lateral capsulotomy and medial capsulorrhaphy are all that may be necessary. In cases in which significant fibular sesamoidal deviation is identified, transfer of the adductor tendon is commonly performed. True fibular sesamoidectomy is seldom, if ever, indicated in the juvenile or adolescent patient. Sesamoidectomy should be performed only when adaptation of the central plantar crista on the lateral aspect of the first metatarsal head is so extensive that soft tissue releases

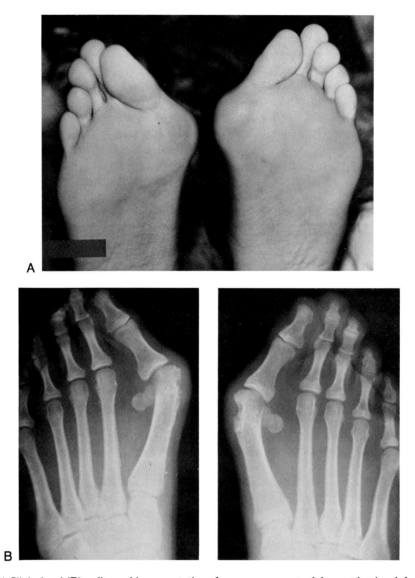

**Fig. 15-18.** (A) Clinical and (B) radiographic presentation of severe recurrent adolescent bunion deformity secondary to inadequate correction at the time of initial surgery. Specifically, there has been an overly aggressive resection of the medial eminence, with failure to relocate the sesamoid apparatus beneath the first metatarsal head. Inadequate medial capsulorrhaphy may also have been a contributing factor, as well as failure to completely correct the splaying between the first and second metatarsal bones.

and transfers prove insufficient in maintaining the sesamoid apparatus beneath the metatarsal head. When necessary, intraoperative radiographs should be obtained to confirm the realignment and positioning of the sesamoid apparatus. When performed with appropriate osseous procedures, the muscle-tendon rebalancing component

of the surgery removes the deforming forces, repositions the long flexor tendon centrally beneath the first metatarsal head, and thus assists in the restoration of normal structure and function to the joint (Fig. 15-20).

Finally, all soft tissue procedures (McBride, Silver, Hiss, etc.) involve resection of the medial bunion promi-

JUVENILE AND ADOLESCENT HALLUX ABDUCTO VALGUS DEFORMITY    389

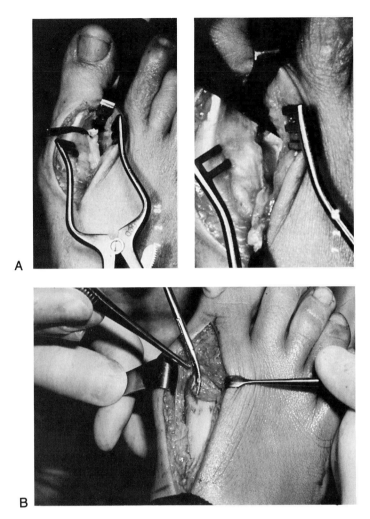

**Fig. 15-19. (A)** Intraoperative photograph demonstrating the completed release of the conjoined tendon of the adductor hallucis muscle. Also seen is the fibular dorsal surface of the fibular sesamoid following release of the fibular sesamoidal ligament and the tendon of the lateral head of the flexor hallucis brevis at the distal edge of the sesamoid bone. **(B)** Adductor tendon being transferred over the dorsal aspect of the first metatarsal head for attachment to the medial capsular structures to assist in the derotation and maintenance of proper sesamoid position.

nence. Emphasis is placed on preservation of the medial sagittal groove to allow normal articulation of the base of the proximal phalanx with the metatarsal head and provide a proper gliding surface for the tibial sesamoid bone (Fig. 15-21). In most cases the clinically apparent bunion prominence represents the normal first metatarsal head in an abnormal position, and rarely is there significant bone proliferation requiring removal. When exuberant bone formation is identified, it is carefully resected with either an osteotome and mallet or a rongeur and appro-

priately smoothened so as to provide a normal shape to the first metatarsal head.

### Distal Metaphyseal Osteotomies

Distal metaphyseal osteotomy has been widely used for correction of the juvenile or adolescent hallux abducto valgus deformity.[2,11,47,66,71-75] While specific indications are lacking, it is commonly performed for individuals with mild to moderate increase in the intermetatarsal

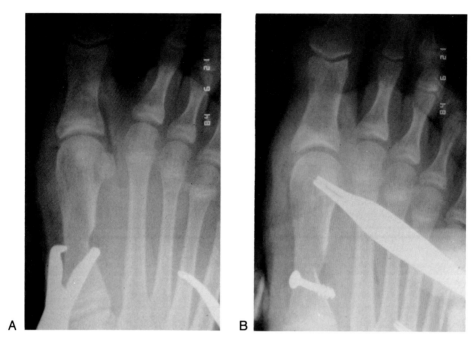

**Fig. 15-20.** **(A)** Intraoperative radiograph following reduction of the metatarsus primus adductus by use of an oblique base wedge osteotomy. Notice persistent malposition of the sesamoid apparatus. **(B)** Sesamoid apparatus has now been repositioned centrally beneath the metatarsal head by a simulated adductor tendon transfer, which will ensure relocation of the sesamoid apparatus and centralization of the long flexor tendon.

angle. Correction of the intermetatarsal angle by distal metaphyseal osteotomy has been reported to vary from 2 to 13 degrees.[76,77] Use of such procedures is generally reserved for individuals in whom the intermetatarsal angle does not exceed 12 degrees.

The most commonly reported distal metaphyseal osteotomies are the Mitchell, Wilson, and Austin procedures. Poor results have been reported with such osteotomies in the juvenile or adolescent patient; problems have included excessive shortening and elevatus deformity resulting in complaints of lesser metatarsalgia.[2,66,78] Allen et al. reported a significant incidence of callus formation and associated pain beneath the second and third metatarsal bones following use of the Wilson osteotomy for repair of the juvenile and adolescent bunion deformity.[75] While some of the procedures produce shortening inherently and by design, such symptoms may be the result of inadvertent dorsal displacement due to inadequate fixation of the osteotomy or inappropriate postoperative management.

The Austin procedure is a particularly valuable procedure for correction of the juvenile or adolescent bunion deformity, especially when shortening is to be avoided (Fig. 15-22). By utilizing current technical concepts of the apical axis guide, the surgeon can control lateral shift, plantar displacement, and subtle changes in length when performing this procedure.[58] The specific techniques have been well described. When the Austin procedure is performed, fixation of the capital fragment by use of one or two 0.062-inch Kirschner wires, although not mandatory, is strongly recommended. Other acceptable means of fixation for the Austin osteotomy include small staples, small cortical or cancellous screws, and, more recently, absorbable pins. We do not recommend the use of the Austin procedure to achieve significant shortening or lengthening or correction of the PASA, as other distal metaphyseal osteotomies achieve these goals more accurately.

The Mitchell osteotomy results in a reduction of the intermetatarsal angle similar to that of the Austin osteotomy. The Mitchell procedure, however, causes a predictable shortening of the first metatarsal bone, which may be desired when an excessively long first metatarsal has been previously identified. The procedure, however,

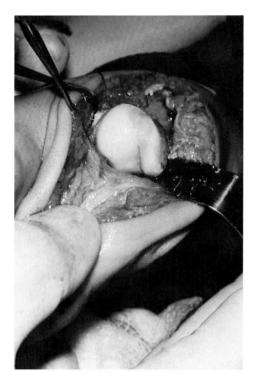

**Fig. 15-21.** Intraoperative photograph showing proper remodeling of the dorsomedial eminence. Note preservation of the medial sagittal groove for articulation of the base of the proximal phalanx and the tibial sesamoid plantarly.

should not be performed when the excessive length of the first metatarsal is due to a severe underlying metatarsus adductus deformity. Predictable shortening can be achieved by appropriate measurement of the first, second, and third metatarsals preoperatively. Because of the inherent design of the osteotomy itself, internal fixation is strongly recommended to avoid dorsal migration and resultant elevatus of the first metatarsal. We recommend the use of one or two 0.062-inch Kirschner wires directed from dorso proximal to plantar distal in a crossing fashion. When shortening of the first metatarsal is desired as well as a correction of an increased PASA, the cuts are modified so that a trapeziodal rather than the normal rectangular section of bone is removed. This procedure has been previously described and is referred to as a Roux osteotomy.[41]

The Reverdin osteotomy and its modifications are designed primarily for correction of significant lateral deviation of the cartilage that is identified intraoperatively.

This is often identified on preoperative radiographs as an increase in the PASA. While the Reverdin osteotomy is effective in restoring the normal alignment of the distal articular cartilage of the first metatarsal, it is not effective in reducing the intermetatarsal angle to any significant extent. This procedure is most commonly combined with a basal type of osteotomy for the reduction of the intermetatarsal angle (Fig. 15-23A-D). Our preference for fixation of this osteotomy is a small scaphoid staple at the medial aspect of the first metatarsal head. Significant lateral deviation of the articular cartilage of the first metatarsal head has been identified in older patients and indicates a rapidly progressing deformity in which severe splaying between the first and second metatarsal bones occurs with significant adaptation at the metatarsophalangeal joint level. In such cases significant displacement of the sesamoid apparatus is usually seen and requires aggressive soft tissue muscle-tendon balancing procedures.

Significant advances have been made in the technical execution of these osteotomies. When the osteotomy has been properly performed and fixed, complications of delayed union, nonunion, pseudoarthrosis, or malunion are uncommon. Aseptic necrosis of the distal metatarsal fragment has not been reported as a complication of juvenile and adolescent hallux valgus repair. It is the responsibility of the surgeon to follow sound mechanical principles of osteotomy design, rigid or stable internal fixation, and logical postoperative care to avoid disruptive forces that may alter the desired position as healing of the distal metaphyseal osteotomy occurs.

*Proximal Metaphyseal Osteotomies*

Several procedures in the proximal metaphyseal area of the first metatarsal have been described in both the orthopedic and podiatric literature for the correction of the juvenile or adolescent hallux abducto valgus deformity; these include the opening wedge, transverse closing wedge, oblique closing wedge, and crescentic osteotomies.[4,7,11,15,16,26,36,41,62] Osteotomy procedures in the proximal metaphysis produce the truest structural correction of a metatarsus primus varus or adductus deformity and are typically recommended in patients with an intermetatarsal angle of 15 degrees or greater. These procedures are also strongly recommended in patients with an underlying structural metatarsus adductus deformity, in whom the intermetatarsal angle may mea-

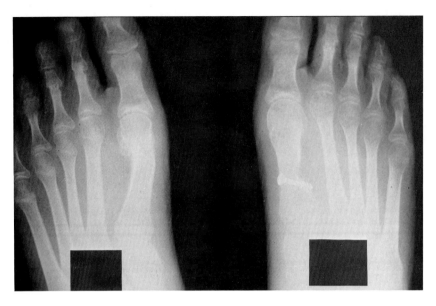

**Fig. 15-22.** Postoperative radiograph of left foot 4 months following correction of juvenile hallux valgus deformity by use of the Austin procedure on the left foot and basal osteotomy on the right foot. Although clinically both deformities are similarly corrected, the basal osteotomy provides a truer structural correction than does the Austin procedure.

sure only 8 to 13 degrees. The goal of each of these procedures is to create a parallel relationship between the first and second metatarsal bones without damage to the open epiphyseal plate.

Historically, opening wedge osteotomies have met with limited success. Common complications include early recurrence of deformity and limitation of motion at the first metatarsophalangeal joint.[4,8] However, some authors have reported success with this procedure.[26,65] Early closure of the epiphyseal plate has been reported as a possible sequela of the opening wedge osteotomy.[65] It is our belief that opening wedge osteotomy of the first metatarsal is rarely needed; however, it should be considered in situations in which an extremely short first metatarsal has been identified in conjunction with significant splaying between the first and second metatarsal bones. When this procedure is performed, it is important to understand the mechanics of the hinge axis concept in order to accurately predict movement of the distal portion of the metatarsal. In addition, because a bone graft must be inserted, appropriate fixation techniques must be employed. An autogenous corticocancellous graft is preferred and will require 8 to 12 weeks of non-weight-bearing cast immobilization. When an opening wedge osteotomy of the first metatarsal is necessary, the graft

should not be procured by an overaggressive resection of the medial eminence of the first metatarsal bone. In addition, an Akin procedure or similar type of wedge osteotomy should not be performed solely in order to obtain a graft for insertion at the base of the metatarsal bone. Instead, a graft may be obtained from the body of the calcaneus, iliac crest, or a tricortical allogeneic corticocancellous graft may be used.

Closing base wedge osteotomies have been advocated by many authors as the most successful techniques for correction of the juvenile or adolescent bunion deformity.[1,7,8,77,79,80] Whether the osteotomy is performed in a transverse or oblique manner will depend upon the preference, skills, and experience of the individual surgeon. In either case the osteotomy must be placed distal to the epiphyseal growth plate to avoid damage. Because the fixation devices should not penetrate or cross the epiphysis itself, the transverse osteotomy is usually located approximately 1 cm distal to the epiphyseal plate. The transverse osteotomy may be fixed by use of Kirschner wires, stainless steel wire, small staples, or the Osteoclasp. As with the opening wedge osteotomy, the principles of mechanical design and proper orientation of the medial cortical hinge are critical for avoiding elevatus deformity of the metatarsal head while simultaneously

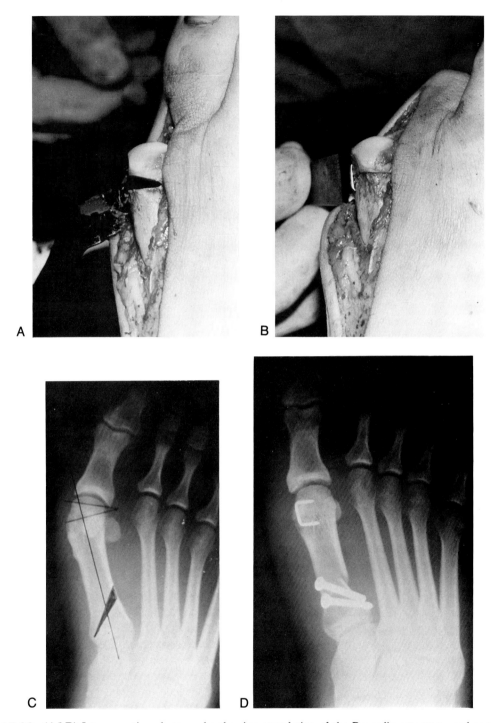

**Fig. 15-23.** **(A&B)** Intraoperative photographs showing completion of the Reverdin osteotomy and appropriate wedge resection of bone. A lateral cortical hinge has been preserved. The osteotomy is then reduced and fixed with a small scaphoid bone staple. Notice that the cartilage is now oriented at 90 degrees to the long axis of the first metatarsal bone. **(C&D)** Preoperative and postoperative radiographs of the same patient. Note that procedures have been selected so as to structurally reduce the intermetatarsal angle and the increase in the proximal articular set angle. A distal metaphyseal osteotomy cannot provide the same structural correction.

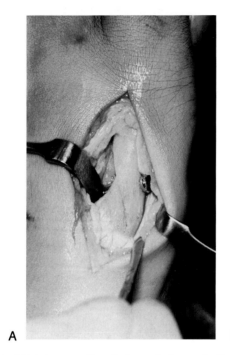
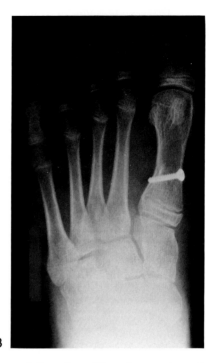

A                                                        B

**Fig. 15-24.** **(A)** Intraoperative photograph demonstrating completion of an oblique base wedge osteotomy with preservation of a medial cortical hinge approximately 2 mm distal to the epiphyseal plate. **(B)** Postoperative radiograph 2 years following surgery shows no violation or damage to the epiphyseal growth plate and continued normal growth pattern. An excellent reduction of the bunion deformity has been achieved.

reducing the intermetatarsal angle. Because the osteotomy will tend to be placed more in the diaphyseal portion of the metatarsal bone, the rate and quality of osteotomy healing may be less than optimal.

It is our experience that the oblique closing wedge osteotomy in the proximal metaphysis provides the most anatomic correction of intermetatarsal splaying. The medial cortical hinge may be placed in close proximity to the epiphyseal growth plate (Fig. 15-24). This osteotomy most effectively employs the radius arm concept and is most amenable to manipulations of the apical axis in the frontal plane to achieve plantar flexion with simultaneous reduction of the intermetatarsal angle. In addition, the oblique osteotomy allows rigid internal compression fixation with one or two small cortical or cancellous screws without violation of the epiphyseal plate (Figs. 15-25 and 15-26). This procedure is technically demanding and should not be performed by the novice surgeon. A working knowlege of rigid internal compression fixation is critical for a successful outcome.

Because of the design of the osteotomy, patients must be maintained in non-weight-bearing status for 5 to 6 weeks to avoid the disruptive forces of weight-bearing.

*Metatarsocuneiform Fusion*

In 1934 Lapidus described a procedure consisting of fusion of the metatarsocuneiform joint to address the metatarsus primus varus component of hallux abducto valgus deformity.[18] The procedure was designed to fuse the metatarsocuneiform joint and the adjacent bases of the first and second metatarsal bones in a corrected position. This procedure is rarely indicated in correction of the juvenile or adolescent bunion deformity and is reserved for those situations in which the intermetatarsal angle is exceedingly high (greater than 25 to 30 degrees) or an underlying major congenital deformity or neurologic condition is present (Fig. 15-27). The procedure should be performed with extreme caution in any patient in whom closure of the epiphyseal growth plate

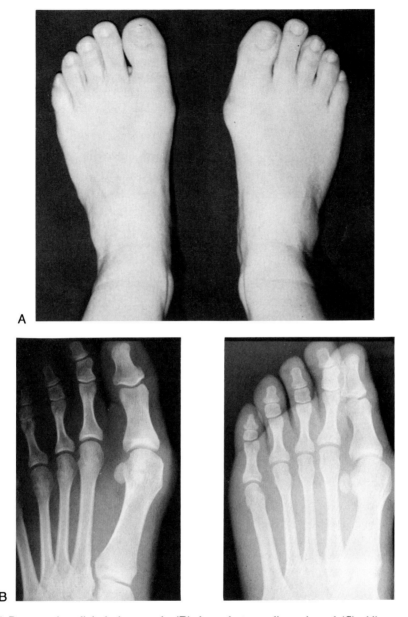

**Fig. 15-25.** (A) Preoperative clinical photograph, (B) dorsoplantar radiograph, and (C) oblique radiograph of a patient with a juvenile bunion deformity. *(Figure continues.)*

has not taken place. Excessive shortening of the metatarsal is not uncommon, and we recommend that consideration be given to the insertion of a corticocancellous graft to offset shortening when resecting the adjacent cartilaginous surfaces. The procedure should be avoided in the young patient without an underlying neurologic condition, major congenital deformity, or excessive first ray hypermobility. In such cases the oblique closing wedge osteotomy is selected and has proved quite successful over the years (Fig. 15-27).

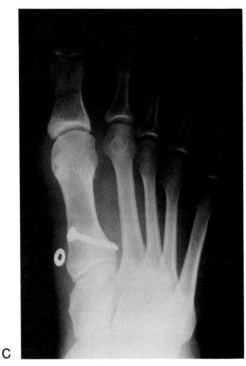

C

Fig. 15-25 *(Continued)*. (C) A 2-year follow-up radiograph demonstrates complete relignment of the first ray, with excellent reduction of the intermetatarsal angle, restoration of the congruous metatarsophalangeal joint, and normal alignment and positioning of the sesamoid apparatus.

## Medial Cuneiform Osteotomy

In 1909 Riedl recommended a closing wedge osteotomy of the medial cuneiform to address an "atavistic" deformity.[41] This procedure clearly would be technically demanding and is rarely, if ever, performed today.

In 1958 Joplin proposed an opening wedge osteotomy of the medial cuneiform for the same condition. This procedure involves insertion of a corticocancellous graft and is designed to correct for excessive obliquity of the metatarsocuneiform joint.[41] While we have not had the occasion to use this procedure for the correction of splaying between the first and second metatarsals in association with a juvenile or adolescent bunion deformity, the procedure seemingly would have merit in certain patients. Subluxation of the metatarsocuneiform joint has been seen postoperatively following base wedge osteotomy of the first metatarsal for correction of metatarsus adductus deformity in which excessive obliquity

at the metatarsocuneiform joint was present preoperatively. This would suggest that the opening wedge osteotomy of the medial cuneiform would be a more appropriate procedure for correction of both the intermetatarsal splaying and the abnormality of the joint. It may be done as an isolated procedure or, less commonly, in combination with a base wedge osteotomy (Fig. 15-28).

## Hallucal Osteotomy

Proximal phalangeal osteotomies such as the Akin procedure are rarely performed for correction of the juvenile or adolescent bunion deformity; these procedures are more commonly performed in the mature adult foot to correct structural or positional abnormalities. Abnormalities and distortion of the overall shape of the proximal phalanx are rarely significant components of the deformity in the juvenile or adolescent patient. Such procedures may be appropriate in some cases, in which there is a significant increase in the hallux abductus interphalangeal angle clinically and radiographically. In such cases a distal transverse or oblique osteotomy is appropriate. Significant deviation of the proximal articular surface of the proximal phalanx as determined by the DASA on a dorsoplantar view may also indicate the need for a proximal Akin osteotomy, but the procedure should only be performed after skeletal maturity has been achieved because of the presence of the open epiphyseal plate in younger patients.

We recommend performing proximal phalangeal osteotomies only after positional and structural corrections have been achieved more proximally and there is a residual abductus deformity distal to the joint. The use of the "cheater" Akin cannot be recommended in the juvenile or adolescent patient with hallux valgus (Fig. 15-29). When the procedure is necessary, the same basic principles and surgical techniques are recommended. Care should be taken to avoid any violation or injury to an open epiphyseal plate in the base of the proximal phalanx.

## Metatarsophalangeal Joint Arthrodesis

First metatarsophalangeal joint arthrodesis is rarely performed for the correction of the juvenile or adolescent bunion deformity. Arthrodesis of the joint is appropriate in patients who have an underlying neuromuscular disease such as cerebral palsy or polio myelitis, in whom the intrinsic and extrinsic musculature to the great toe

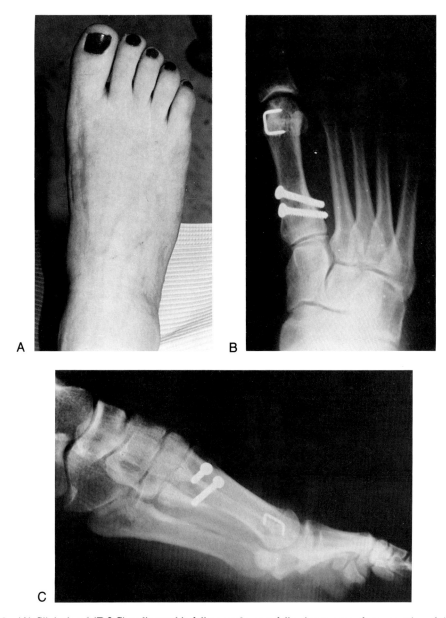

**Fig. 15-26.** (A) Clinical and (B&C) radiographic follow-up 2 years following surgery for correction of the recurrent hallux valgus deformity seen in Fig. 15-23C. although some shortening has resulted, the first metatarsal has been maintained in a weight-bearing attitude.

may have an unpredictable effect on the position of the toe. We believe that this procedure should also be considered in patients with chromosomal abnormalities such as Down syndrome, as fusion may provide the best structural and functional correction to the first ray. In such cases one can expect a simultaneous reduction of the intermetatarsal angle without the need for an osteotomy of the first metatarsal or medial cuneiform or, fusion of the metatarsocuneiform joint. The recommended position of fusion is one of slight dorsiflexion from the

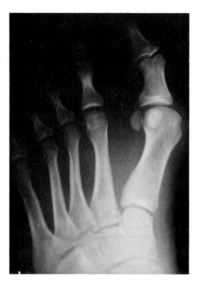
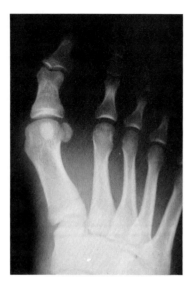

**Fig. 15-27.** Dorsoplantar radiograph of a juvenile patient with Down syndrome. Notice the atypical configuration of the bone and soft tissue about the first ray. A first metatarsocuneiform arthrodesis may be an appropriate procedure to reduce the excessively high intermetatarsal angle.

ground supporting surface (15 to 20 degrees), with the toe placed in a position parallel to the second digit. When performing arthrodesis of the first metatarsophalangeal joint, the method of fixation will depend upon the experience and preference of the surgeon.

*Ancillary Procedures*

An integral part of the surgical reconstruction of the juvenile or adolescent hallux abducto valgus deformity includes removal, correction, or control of deforming forces considered to constitute a major contributing factor to the deformity. Surgical procedures may be designed to correct an underlying equinus, severe collapsing pes plano valgus, or metatarsus adductus deformity. Conservative treatment modalities should be exhausted prior to recommending surgical correction of these deformities. However, when the condition is unresponsive to conservative treatment, surgical correction is strongly recommended. The intimate relationship between these deformities and the juvenile or adolescent bunion deformity have been clearly recognized and reported in the orthopedic literature.[1,7,8,11,20-23,47,81] Failure to address the deforming forces may result in early recurrence of deformity or a less than optimal surgical outcome.[7,8,47,81]

An underlying equinus deformity is addressed by either a gastrocnemius recession or a tendo Achillis lengthening (Fig. 15-30). The particular procedure selected will depend upon the individual preference and experiences of the surgeon. Our preference for a gastrocnemius recession is the Vulpius or Strayer technique or a modified Baker procedure. Tendo Achillis lengthenings are accomplished by either a percutaneous technique or open frontal plane slide lengthening.

Correction of an underlying flatfoot deformity depends heavily upon the clinical, biomechanical, and radiographic assessment. Emphasis is placed on identification of the primary plane of dominance of the deformity. Transverse plane flatfoot deformities, usually seen in conjunction with an underlying metatarsus adductus, are corrected by use of an Evans calcaneal osteotomy (Fig. 15-31). Frontal plane flatfoot deformity is most commonly addressed by a subtalar joint arthroereisis. Regardless of whether the flatfoot deformity is of a transverse or frontal plane nature, medial arch reconstruction by a modified Kidner procedure, alone or in combination with a modified Young's tenosuspension, is not uncommonly performed to help stabilize medial column breaching.

Metatarsus adductus deformity is not uncommon in a child with a juvenile or adolescent bunion deformity and

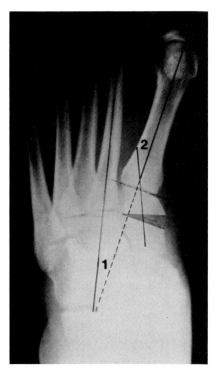

**Fig. 15-28.** Dorsoplantar radiograph demonstrating excessive obliquity of the first metatarsocuneiform joint. Notice the increase in the angle between the medial cuneiform and first metatarsal bone. An increase in the intermetatarsal angle is also identified. Opening medial cuneiform osteotomy would be an appropriate procedure for correction of this deformity, assuming normal motion to be present at the metatarsophalangeal joint.

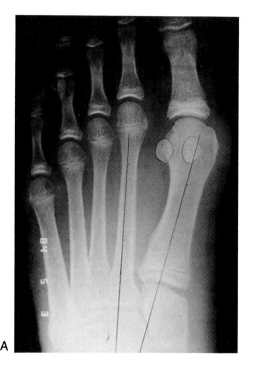

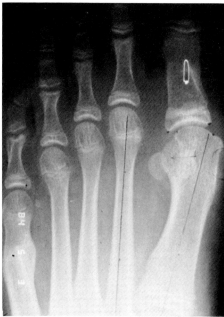

**Fig. 15-29.** Preoperative (**A**) and postoperative (**B**) dorsoplantar radiographs 2 months following inappropriate use of an Akin osteotomy for correction of a juvenile bunion deformity.

may be more common than has been previously recognized. The presence of a long first metatarsal on the dorsoplantar radiograph suggests the need for further evaluation to rule out an underlying metatarsus adductus component. In cases in which the deformity is severe and would prevent adequate correction of the hallux abducto valgus deformity, structural correction of the metatarsus adductus is recommended. The procedures most commonly employed include the modified Berman-Gartland type of osteotomy and the more recently described Lepird procedure[55-57] (Fig. 15-32).

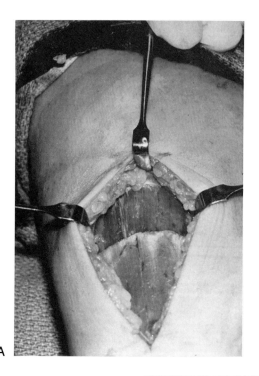

A

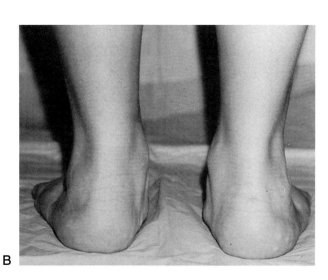

B

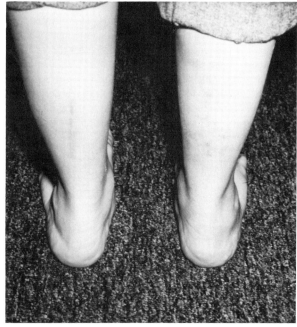

C

**Fig. 15-30.** (A) Intraoperative photograph showing an approximately 2-inch lengthening performed by a Strayer gastrocnemius recession procedure for equinus deformity in conjunction with correction of adolescent hallux abducto valgus deformity. (B) Preoperative and (C) postoperative clinical appearance from a posterior view following gastrocnemius recession, Evans calcaneal osteotomy, and base wedge osteotomy for correction of an adolescent bunion deformity.

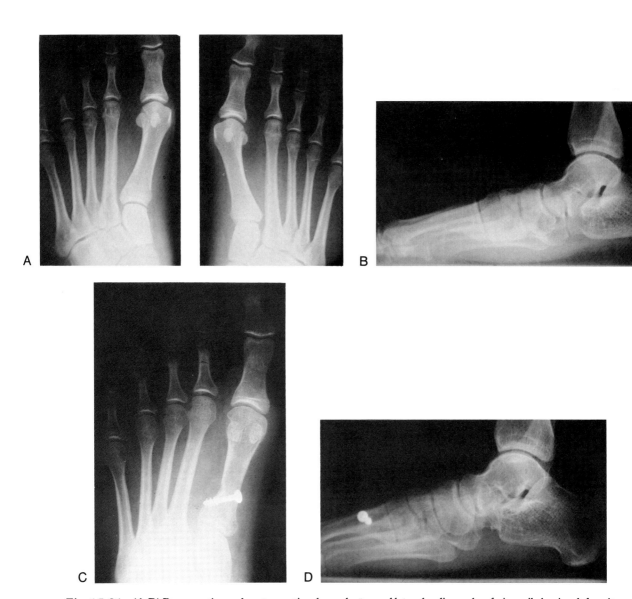

**Fig. 15-31.** **(A-D)** Preoperative and postoperative dorsoplantar and lateral radiographs of a juvenile bunion deformity with concomitant flatfoot deformity. The flatfoot component has been corrected by a posterior lengthening in conjunction with an Evans calcaneal osteotomy. Notice excellent restoration of the medial longitudinal arch. Excellent structural correction has been achieved in the first ray.

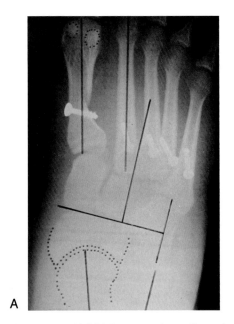
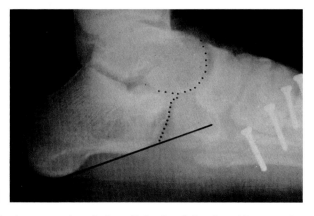

**Fig. 15-32. (A&B)** Postoperative radiographs following correction of a juvenile bunion deformity with concomitant metatarsus adductus. A modified Lepird procedure has been performed, as well as an Evans calcaneal osteotomy for the transverse plane flatfoot deformity. Fig. 15-7 shows the preoperative lateral radiograph of the same patient.

## SUMMARY AND CONCLUSIONS

Treatment of the juvenile or adolescent patient with a hallux abducto valgus deformity presents particular challenges to the physician. Emphasis should be placed on the identification of underlying structural deformities likely to compromise any surgical procedures. Great caution should be exercised in patients treated conservatively and they should be monitored closely with periodic radiographs to chart progression of the deformity. When surgery is necessary, it should include the correction not only of the first ray deformity but also of other deformities that are considered etiologic in nature and cannot be controlled or corrected by conservative modalities. Such underlying deformities may include equinus, metatarsus adductus, or collapsing pes plano valgus deformity. Failure to correct these conditions may result in less than optimal correction of the bunion deformity. Both the patient and the parents should be well advised concerning the nature of the deformity, the proposed surgical procedures, potential complications, and postoperative recovery and convalescence, as well as anticipated results. When the juvenile or adolescent hallux abducto valgus deformity is managed with a comprehensive approach, excellent results can be expected.

## ACKNOWLEDGMENT

Special acknowledgments and appreciation are extended to the Medical Photography Department of Meridia Huron Hospital and to Pauli Jaffe, medical photographer, for photography and the preparation of prints used in this chapter.

## REFERENCES

1. Goldner JL, Gaines RW: Adult and juvenile hallux valgus: analysis and treatment. Orthop Clin North Am 7:863, 1976
2. Carr CR, Boyd BM: Correctional osteotomy for metatarsus primus varus and hallux valgus. J Bone Joint Surg [Am] 50:1353, 1968
3. Halebian JD, Gaines SS: Juvenile hallux valgus. J Foot Surg 22:290, 1983

4. Helal B: Surgery for adolescent hallux valgus. Clin. Orthop 157:50, 1981
5. Piggott H: The natural history of hallux valgus in adolescence and early life. J Bone Joint Surg [Br] 42:749, 1960
6. Dorland's Illustrated Medical Dictionary. 26th Ed. WB Saunders, Philadelphia, 1981
7. Ruch JA, Bernbach M, DiNapoli DR, et al: Juvenile hallux abducto valgus. p. 227. In McGlamry ED(ed): Comprehensive Textbook of Foot Surgery. Williams & Wilkins, Baltimore, 1987
8. Scranton PE, Zuckerman JD: Bunion surgery in adolescents: results of surgical treatment. J Pediatr Orthop 4:39, 1984
9. Richardson EG: The foot in adolescents and adults. p. 829. In Crenshaw AH (ed): Campbell's Operative Orthopaedics. Vol. 2. 7th Ed. CV Mosby, St. Louis, 1987
10. Hardy RH, Clapham JC: Observations on hallux valgus. J Bone Joint Surg [Br] 33:376, 1951
11. Amarnek DL, Jacobs AM, Oloff LM: Adolescent hallux valgus: its etiology and surgical management. J Foot Surg 24:54, 1985
12. Cole S: Foot inspection of the school child. J Am Podiatr Med Assoc 49:446, 1959
13. Hardy RH, Clapham JC: Hallux valgus: predisposing anatomical causes. Lancet I:1180, 1952
14. McMurry TP: Treatment of hallux valgus and rigidus. Br Med J 2:218, 1936
15. Truslow W: Metatarsus primus varus or hallux valgus. J Bone Joint Surg 7:98, 1925
16. Jones AR: Hallux valgux in the adolescent. Proc R Soc Med 41:392, 1948
17. Ellis VH: A method of correcting metatarsus primus varus. J Bone Joint Surg [Br] 33:415, 1951
18. Lapidus PW: The operative correction of the metatarsus primus varus in hallux valgus. Surg Gynec Obstet 58:183, 1934
19. Ewald ET: Die Ätiologie des hallux valgus. Dtsch Z Chir 114:90, 1912
20. Inman VT: Hallux valgux: a review of etiologic factors. Orthop Clin North Am 5:59, 1974
21. Kalen V, Brecher A: Relationship between adolescent bunions and flatfeet. Foot Ankle 8:331, 1988
22. Hohmann G: Symptomatische oder physiologische Behandlung des Hallux valgus. Munch Med Wochenschr 33:1042, 1921
23. La Reaux RL, Lee BR: Metatarsus adductus and hallux abducto valgus: their correlation. J Foot Surg 26:304, 1987
24. Johnson O: Further studies of the inheritance of hand and foot anomalies. Clin Orthop 8:146, 1954
25. Sandelin T: Operative treatment of hallux valgus. JAMA 80:736, 1923

26. Trott AW: Children's foot problems. Orthop Clin North Am 13:641, 1982
27. Meier PJ, Kenzora JE: The risks and benefits of distal first metatarsal osteotomies. Foot Ankle 6:7, 1985
28. Glynn MK, Dunlop JB, Fitzpatrick D: The Mitchell distal metatarsal osteotomy for hallux valgux. J Bone Joint Surg [Br] 62:188, 1980
29. Engle ET, Morton DJ: Notes on foot disorders among natives of the Belgian Congo. J Bone Joint Surg 13:311, 1931
30. Barnicot NA, Hardy RH: The position of the hallux in West Africans. J Anat 89:355, 1955
31. Bonney G, Macnab I: Hallux valgus and hallux rigidus: a critical survey of operative results. J Bone Joint Surg [Br] 34:366, 1952
32. Shimazaki K, Takebea K: Investigations on the origin of hallux valgus by electrodynamic analysis. Kobe J Med Sci 27:139, 1981
33. Hoffman P: Conclusions drawn from a comparative study of the feet of barefooted and shoe wearing people. Am J Orthop Surg 3:105, 1905
34. Fook LS, Hodges AR: A comparison of foot forms among the non-shoe and shoe wearing Chinese population. J Bone Joint Surg [Am] 40:1058, 1958
35. Kato T, Watnabe S: The etiology of hallux valgus in Japan. Clin Orthop 157:78, 1981
36. Lapidus PW: The authors bunion operation from 1931 to 1959. Clin Orthop 16:119, 1960
37. Morton DJ: The Human Foot. Columbia Univ Press, New York, 1935
38. Mayo CH: The surgical treatment of bunions. Minn Med 3:326, 1920
39. Haines R, McDougall A: The anatomy of hallux valgus, J Bone Joint Surg [Br] 36B:272, 1954
40. Haas M: Radiographic and biomechanical considerations of bunion surgery. p. 23. In Gerbert J (ed): Textbook of Bunion Surgery. Futura, Mt. Kisco, NY, 1981
41. Kelikian H: Hallux Valgus, Allied Deformities of the Forefoot and Metatarsalgia. WB Saunders, Philadelphia, 1965
42. Mann RA, Coughlin MJ: Hallux valgus—etiology, anatomy, treatment and surgical considerations. Clin Orthop 157:31, 1981
43. Young JK: The etiology of hallux valgus or os intermetatarseum. Am J Orthop Surg 7:336, 1909
44. Wheeler PH: Os intermetatarseum and hallux valgus. Am J Surg 18:341, 1932
45. Jordan HH, Brodsky AE: Keller operation for hallux valgus and hallux rigidus. Arch Surg 62:586, 1951
46. Hiss JM: Hallux valgus, its causes and simplified treatment. Am J Surg 11:51, 1931
47. Grill F, Hetherington V, Steinbock G, Altenhuber J: Expe-

riences with the chevron (V) osteotomy on adolescent hallux valgus. Arch Orthop Trauma Surg 106:47, 1986

48. Scranton PE: Adolescent bunions; diagnosis and management. Pediatr Ann 11:518, 1982

49. Coughlin MJ, Mann RA: The physiology of juvenile bunions. Instr Course Lect 36:123, 1987

50. Trott AW: Hallux valgus in the adolescent. Instr Course Lect 21:262, 1972

51. Sgarlato TE: A Compendium of Podiatric Biomechanics California College of Podiatric Medicine, San Francisco, 1971, p. 221

52. Root ML, Orien WP, Weed JH: Normal and Abnormal Function of the Foot. Clinical Biomechanical Corp., Los Angeles, 1977, p. 377

53. Tax HR: Podopediatrics. 2nd Ed. Williams & Wilkins, Baltimore, 1985, p. 362

54. Trepal MJ: Hallux valgus and metatarsus adductus: the surgical dilemma. Clin Podiatr Med Surg 6:103, 1989

55. Yu GV, Wallace GF: Metatarsus Adductus. p. 324. In McGlamry ED (ed): Comprehensive Textbook of Foot Surgery. Williams & Wilkins, Baltimore, 1987

56. Yu GV, Johng B, Freireich R: Surgical management of metatarsus adductus deformity. Clin. Podiatr Med. Surg. 4(1):207, 1987

57. Yu GV, DiNapoli DR: Surgical management of hallux abducto valgus with concomitant metatarsus adductus. p. 262. In McGlamry ED (ed): Reconstructive Surgery of the Foot and Leg Update '89. Podiatry Institute Publishing Co., 1989

58. Ruch JA: First ray hallux abducto valgus and related deformities. p. 133. In McGlamry ED (ed): Comprehensive Textbook of Foot Surgery. Williams & Wilkins, Baltimore, 1987

59. Nelson JB: Mechanical arrest of bone growth in pedal deformities. J Foot Surg 20:16, 1981

60. Keats TE: An atlas of normal roentgen variants that may simulate disease. 3rd Ed. Year Book Medical Publishers, Chicago, 1984, p. 591

61. McCrea JD, Lichty TK: The first metatarsocuneiform articulation and its relationship to metatarsus primus adductus. J Am Podiatr Med Assoc 69:700, 1979

62. Stamm TT: The surgical treatment of hallux valgus. Guy's Hosp Rep 106:273, 1957

63. Cholmeley JA: Hallux valgus in adolescents. Proc R Soc Med 51:903, 1958

64. Mahan KT, Yu GV: Juvenile and adolescent hallux valgus. p. 61. In McGlamry Ed, McGlamry R (eds): Podiatry Institute Surgical Seminar Syllabus. Doctors Hospital Podiatric Education and Research Institute, Atlanta, 1985

65. Simmonds FA, Menelaus MB: Hallux valgus in adolescents. J Bone Joint Surg [Br] 42:761, 1960

66. De SD: Distal metatarsal osteotomy for adolescent hallux valgus. J Pediatr Orthop 4:32, 1984

67. Snijders JGN, Philippens MMGM: Biomechanics of hallux valgus in spread foot. Foot Ankle 7:26, 1986

68. Helal B, Gupta SK, Gojaseni P: Surgery for adolescent hallux valgux. Acta Orthop Scand 45:271, 1974

69. Coughlin MJ, Bordelon RL, Johnson K, Mann RA: Symposium: President's forum — evaluation and treatment of juvenile hallux valgus. Contemp Orthop 20:169, 1990

70. Ruch JA: Anatomic Dissection of Hallux Abducto Valgus. [film] Podiatry Institute, Atlanta, 1981

71. Auerbach AM: Review of distal metatarsal osteotomies for hallux valgus in the young. Clin Orthop 70:146, 1970

72. Ball J, Sullivan JA: Treatment of juvenile bunion by Mitchell osteotomy. Orthopedics 10:1249, 1985

73. Luba R, Rosman M: Bunions in children: treatment with a modified Mitchell osteotomy. J Pediatr Orthop 4:44, 1984

74. Dooley BJ, Berryman DB: Wilson's osteotomy of the first metatarsal for hallux valgus in the adolescent and young adult. Aust N Z J Surg 43:255, 1973

75. Allen TR, Gross M, Miller J et al: The assessment of adolescent hallux valgus before and after first metatarsal osteotomy. Int Orthop 5:111, 1981

76. Marcinko DE, Haden RA, Mandel E: Determination of the intermatatarsal ankle reduction following metatarsal head osteotomies. J Am Podiatr Med Assoc 74(2):65, 1984

77. Jahss MH, Troy AI, Kummer F: Radiographic and mathematical analysis of first metatarsal osteotomies for metatarsus primus varus: a comparitive study. Foot Ankle 5:280, 1985

78. Merkel KD, Katoh Y, Johnson EW, Edmund YS: Mitchell osteotomy for hallux valgus: long term follow up and gait analysis. Foot Ankle 3:189, 1982

79. Wanivenhaus A, Feldner-Busztin H: Basal osteotomy of the first metatarsal for the correction of metatarsus primus varus associated with hallux valgus. Foot Ankle 8:337, 1989

80. Golden GN: Hallux valgus — the osteotomy operation. Br Med J 1:1361, 1961

81. Geissele AE, Stanton RP: Surgical treatment of adolescent hallux valgus. J Pediatr Orthop 10:642, 1990

## SUGGESTED READINGS

Austin DW, Leventen EO: A new osteotomy for hallux valgus: a horizontally directed "V" displacement osteotomy of metatarsal head for hallux valgus and primus varus. Clin Orthop 157:25, 1981

Blais MM, Green WT, Anderson M: Lengths of the growing foot. J Bone Joint Surg [Am] 38:998, 1956

Cedell CA, Astrom, M: Proximal metatarsal osteotomy in hallux valgus. Acta Orthop Scand 53:1013, 1982

Craigmilie DA: Incidence, origin, and prevention of certain foot defects. Br Med J 2:749, 1953

DuVries HL: Acquired nontraumantic deformities of the foot. p. 206. In Inman VT (ed): DuVries' Surgery of the Foot. CV Mosby. St. Louis, 1973

Fox IM, Smith SD: Juvenile bunion correction by epiphysiodesis of the first metatarsal. J Am Podiatr Med Assoc 73:448, 1983

Giannestras N: Foot Disorders. 2nd Ed. Lea & Febiger, Philadelphia, 1973, p. 351

Gibson J, Piggott H: Osteotomy of the neck of the first metatarsal in the treatment of hallux valgus. J Bone Joint Surg [Br] 44:349, 1962

Gould N, Schneider W, Ashikaga T: Epidemiological survey of foot problems in the continental United States. Foot Ankle 1:8, 1980

Hawkins FB, Mitchell L, Hedrick DW: Correction of hallux valgus by metatarsal osteotomy. J Bone Joint Surg 27:387, 1954

Houghton GR, Dickson RA: Hallux valgus in the younger patient — the structural abnormality. J Bone Joint Surg [Br] 41:176, 1979

Kenzora JE: A rationale for the surgical treatment of bunions. Orthopedics 11:777, 1988

Lindgren U, Turan I: A new operation for hallux valgus. Clin Orthop 175:179, 1983

Mann RA: Hallux valgus. Instr Course Lect 35:135, 1986

Martin DE, Phillips AJ, Ruch JA: Intraoperative decision making in hallux valgus surgery. p. 1. In McGlamry ED (ed): Reconstructive Surgery of the Foot and Ankle. Update 1989. Doctors Hospital Podiatric Education and Research Institute, Atlanta, 1989

McBride ED: Hallux valgus, bunion deformity: its treatment in mild, moderate or severe stages. Int Surg 21:99, 1954

McKay DW: Dorsal bunions in children. J Bone Joint Surg [Am] 65:975, 1983

Mitchell CL, Fleming JL, Allen R. et al: Osteotomy/bunionectomy for hallux valgus. J Bone Joint Surg [Am] 49:41, 1958

Mygind HB: Some views on the surgical treatment of hallux valgus. Acta Orthop Scand 23:152, 1953

Resch S, Stensstrom A, Egund M: Proximal closing wedge osteotomy in adductor tenotomy for treatment of hallux valgus. Foot Ankle 9:270, 1989

Scranton PE, Rutkowski R: Anatomic variation in the first ray: Part I. Anatomic aspects related to bunion surgery. Clin Orthop 51:244, 1980

Wilson DW: Treatment of hallux valgus and bunions. Br J Hosp Med 20:548, 1980

# 16

# Common Pediatric Digital Deformities

MICHAEL S. DOWNEY
LAURENCE RUBIN

Digital deformities are common in the pediatric population. More often than not they are congenital in nature, with one or both of the parents having the same or a similar condition. These digital deformities are usually present at birth and can become worse with time. Rare instances of spontaneous resolution of some deformities have been reported; however, this is not the rule but rather the exception. One should not expect children to outgrow their deformities.

Digital malformations are usually asymptomatic in infancy and early childhood, when the most common presenting complaints are cosmetic in nature. However, as the child approaches skeletal maturity, the deformity often becomes more rigid and becomes progressively more symptomatic. It is recommended that the clinician examine the child while standing, walking, and sitting. The deformity may increase during weight-bearing or under the influence of muscle action. It is the responsibility of the clinician to determine if the malformation, even though asymptomatic at the time of examination, will eventually become a problem as the child matures.

Many of these deformities are unresponsive to conservative treatment. Conservative therapy should usually be attempted but may require an extended course with minimal gain. As the deformity becomes more fixed, surgery will most likely be required if correction is the goal. Digital surgery in the pediatric patient brings about its own special set of difficulties, most notably small anatomy and interference with growth. Often it may be advisable to delay surgery until later in childhood when larger anatomy is present.

## UNDERLAPPING TOES

Underlapping toes are a common deformity seen in the pediatric and adult population, most often involving the fourth and fifth toes. A special form of an underlapping toe is *clinodactyly* or *congenital curly toe*. This type of underlapping toe is a more complex deformity with a rotational component. Clinodactyly is common, follows a strong familial inheritance pattern, and is usually present at birth. One or more toes can be involved, with the toe or toes in a plantar-flexed and medially deviated position. A supinatus deformity is present at the distal interphalangeal joint, and in more severe cases the proximal interphalangeal joint can also be in varus. The presentation is frequently bilateral and symmetric, with toes three, four, and five most commonly affected (Fig. 16-1).

## Etiology

The exact etiology of clinodactyly is unclear. Trethowen[1] believed that the deformity was a congenital form of hammertoe. Sharrard[2,3] and Tachdjian[4-6] described it as secondary to a partial aplasia or a hypoplasia of the intrinsic muscles of the toe. Another possible etiology of clinodactyly is a weakness or hypoplasia of the quadratus plantae muscle, a muscle which acts on the flexor digitorum longus to give it a straighter pull. If the quadratus plantae is not functioning normally, the flexor digitorum longus will have a more medially displaced force vector, which can lead to clinodactyly of one or more toes. Addi-

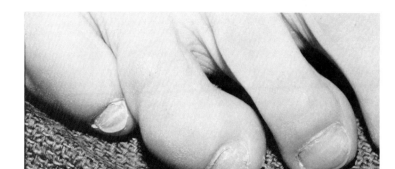

**Fig. 16-1.** Congenital curly toes (clinodactyly) of third, fourth, and fifth digits. Note that fourth digit demonstrates most severe deformity.

tionally, in the hypermobile foot with forefoot abductus, the flexor digitorum longus may contract early in an attempt to stabilize the forefoot. If this occurs, the long flexors will overpower the straightening pull of the quadratus plantae and a more medial adductory vector of force will again result. This abnormal force may result in a supinatory force being placed on the lateral digits, with resultant clinodactyly.

## Clinical Features

In children the deformity is often flexible and asymptomatic. As the child approaches skeletal maturity, the deformity tends to become more fixed and symptoms may develop. The distal aspect of the toe can under-ride the medially adjacent toe, thereby preventing the medial toe from weight-bearing and leading to increased pressure on the medially adjacent metatarsal head with subsequent pain or callus formation.[6] The curly toe can develop hyperkeratosis on the lateral aspect of the distal and proximal interphalangeal joints, along with calloused nail grooves from shoe irritation, especially in girls wearing pointed shoes. Clinodactyly is most easily identified when the child is weight-bearing and is accentuated with contraction of the flexor digitorum longus. Therefore the child should be examined in a weight-bearing position. Flexibility of the deformity can be determined by manually pulling the toe into a straight attitude. If the deformity cannot be reduced by this method, it is considered fixed.

## Treatment

Treatment is determined by the age of the patient, degree of deformity, and symptomatology. Conservative treatment usually consists of manipulation, orthodigital devices, and strapping. Trethowen[1] suggested that clinodactyly may be amenable to manipulation in infancy, but it was "expensive in time" and surgery was usually advised. Sweetnam[7] compared over- and understrapping with no treatment in 50 children and noted improvement in 25 percent of the treated and 27 percent of the untreated children. Turner[8] found that 68 percent of the toes improved with strapping but that a significant loss of correction occurred after the strapping was discontinued. He also reported that in a small population of untreated toes spontaneous improvement occurred in 33 percent of cases.

In children the deformity is often asymptomatic, and surgery is rarely indicated. Several authors have suggested that in severe deformities surgery may be necessary to improve the cosmetic appearance of the toe.[1,9] Furthermore, when the deformity is symptomatic and conservative treatment seems unsuccessful or unpromising, surgery is indicated. A plethora of surgical procedures has been suggested. Generally, flexible deformities are treated by soft tissue procedures and rigid deformities by more aggressive combined soft tissue and osseous approaches.

In deformities that can be corrected passively, Tachdjian[4] relates very satisfactory results with tenotomy of both the short and long flexor tendons performed through a plantar longitudinal incision. Similarly, Greenberg[10] advocated a small plantar incision with tenotomy of the short and long flexor tendons. Ross and Menelaus[9] performed flexor tenotomies on 188 toes of 62 children to correct either hammertoe or curly toes. The results were good or fair in 95 percent of the patients. Although none of the patients were aware of any loss of function, 43 had no flexor digitorum longus function. Plantar-flexory scar contracture across the interphalangeal joint was the only complication noted. Sharrard[2] and Tachdjian[4-6] advocated transferring the flexor digitorum longus tendon into the dorsolateral aspect of the extensor expansion. Sharrard stated that this would provide "immediate and permanent correction of the deformity in all but the most severe cases."

Pollard and Morrison[11] compared the flexor tenotomy with the flexor-to-extensor transfer. The flexor tenotomy was performed on 56 toes and the flexor transfer on 63 toes, and the two procedures were compared with respect to appearance and function. The appearance of the toe following the flexor tenotomy was good in 77 percent and fair in 23 percent of the cases, and the flexor transfer was rated good in appearance in 34 percent of the toes, fair in 43 percent, and poor in 23 percent. The function of the flexor tenotomy was rated fair in 100 percent of the toes, but that of the flexor transfer was rated good in only 8 percent of the toes, fair in 34 percent, and poor in 58 percent. The flexor tenotomy caused a decrease in active plantar-flexion of the interphalangeal joint but did not affect the passive range of motion. The flexor-to-extensor transfer created a stiff toe in 58 percent of cases, with very limited active or passive motion available at the interphalangeal joints. In yet another approach, Kelikian et al.[12] advised using a skin plasty and syndactylization of the adjacent toes in infants to correct flexible clinodactyly.

In more rigid deformities, combined soft tissue and osseous procedures are commonly employed. Although osseous deformity is most common in the middle phalanx, procedures have addressed both the middle and proximal phalanges. In the older child with more fixed deformity, Tachdjian[4] again suggested flexor tendon transfer to the dorsolateral extensor hood but advised combining this procedure with a middle phalangeal greenstick osteotomy stabilized with a Kirschner wire. Friend[13] found that the head of the middle phalanx was deviated in a medial direction. His procedure of choice was a middle phalangectomy, which corrected for the elongated bone and eliminated the deviated middle phalanx. Korn[14] described the lazy S incision for an underlapping fifth toe, which provides exposure to the dorsal, plantar, and lateral aspects of the toe. His approach involved an arthroplasty of the head of the proximal phalanx and a hemiphalangectomy of the middle and distal phalanges. For deformities that are fixed and present after skeletal maturity, Kelikian et al.[12] advocated skin plasty and syndactylization in combination with partial or complete proximal phalangectomy. Finally, Trethowen[1] suggested arthrodesis of the proximal or distal interphalangeal joint, depending on where the deformity was greatest. He combined this with a skin ellipse to help correct the adduction and rotation of the toe.

## Authors' Preferred Technique

When considering surgery for the correction of an underlapping toe, we recommend that the toe be evaluated for a flexible versus a fixed deformity. To correct flexible deformities in the younger patient, a derotation skin plasty combined with tenotomies of the long and short flexors can be used. The skin wedge must be perpendicular to the axis of deformity of the toe. Use of a skin marker to assist in planning the skin incision is advised. The incision, which is lenticular in shape, is placed over the proximal or distal interphalangeal joint, depending on where the deformity is greatest. The long axis of the incision is dorsal-proximal-lateral to dorsal-distal-medial (Fig. 16-2). The incision is carried down through the dermis, and the wedge of skin is resected (Fig. 16-3). When the edges are reapproximated with suture, the toe should be in a corrected position. If desired, the flexor tendons may also be sectioned, which is achieved through a separate transverse plantar incision at the level of the proximal interphalangeal joint. The transverse approach is preferred over the longitudinal approach as the incision falls within relaxed skin tension lines. With healing, this minimizes plantar-flexory scar contracture.

In patients with a fixed deformity, the same incisional approach is utilized. Most commonly, osseous deformity is noted in the middle phalanx, in which case the skin plasty is placed over the distal portion of the phalanx. If the deformity is within the middle phalangeal base or proximal phalangeal head area, the skin plasty is placed more proximally at that level. The next step is a midline linear incision through the superficial fascia; this will help

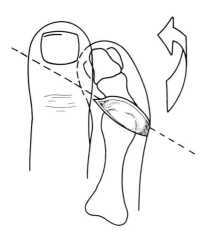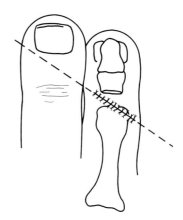

**Fig. 16-2.** A lenticular surgical incision consisting of two semielliptical incisions may be utilized to help derotate the supinatus component in the surgical approach to the congenital curly toe.

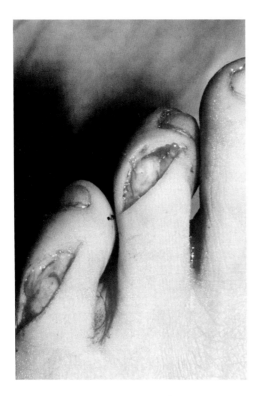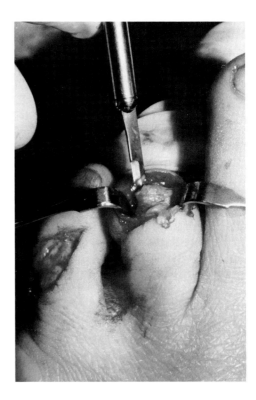

**Fig. 16-3.** Surgical demonstration of lenticular skin ellipses removed from fourth and fifth toes. In rigid deformities, osseous procedures may be performed through the same incision.

**Fig. 16-4.** A #67 blade is utilized to section the collateral ligaments of the distal interphalangeal joint.

to preserve the neurovascular structures. The conjoined extensor tendon is transversely transected, and the distal interphalangeal joint is entered. In the younger patient with small digital anatomy, a #67 Beaver blade may be used to section the tendon and collateral ligaments (Fig. 16-4). The head of the middle phalanx is resected with an oscillating saw or hand instrumentation. The tendon is reapproximated and the wound is sutured (Fig. 16-5). In some instances a Kirschner wire may also be used to splint the toe in its corrected position for the first 3 to 4 weeks. If the clinodactyly is secondary to a deformed base of the middle phalanx, the base rather than the head of the middle phalanx should be resected (Fig. 16-2). Similarly, if the deformity is within the proximal phalanx, an arthroplasty of the head of the proximal phalanx should be performed. Again, surgical release of the short and long flexor tendons may be performed if desired. This may be achieved through the dorsal surgical incision or through a separate plantar transverse incision

at the level of the proximal interphalangeal joint. The postoperative dressing should be used to hold the toe or toes in their corrected position.

## OVERLAPPING TOES

In congenital overlapping toe deformity one toe lies on the dorsal aspect of an adjacent toe. Such overlapping toes vary significantly in magnitude of deformity. Involvement of the second, third, or fourth digit is usually less severe than fifth digit involvement.

### Overlapping Central Digits

When one of the central digits is involved, the second toe is more commonly affected than the third or fourth toes. Tax[15] believed that the second digit tends to overlap the third digit in a large percentage of infants. Early in life

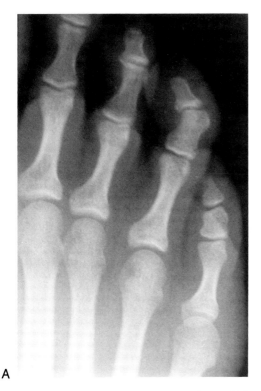
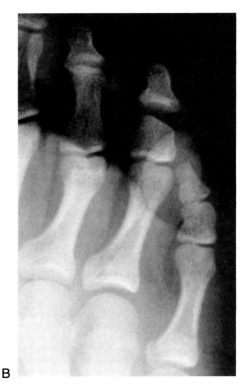

**Fig. 16-5.** **(A)** Preoperative radiograph in patient with fixed clinodactyly of the fourth toe. Note osseous deformity of the middle phalanx. **(B)** Postoperative radiograph of same patient following arthroplasty of the head of the middle phalanx.

this condition is symptom-free, but eventually it leads to discomfort at the dorsal aspect of the overriding toe. Suppan[16] suggested taping the toe by use of a cradle dressing for 6 months in children up to the age of 3 years. For older children he suggested a tenotomy with a capsulotomy if needed followed by splinting of the toe for 4 to 8 weeks. Kelikian et al.[12] suggested the use of syndactylization to correct this deformity.

We believe that extensor tendon lengthening or extensor tenotomy and metatarsophalangeal joint capsulotomy, with the concurrent use of skin plasties, will correct mild overlapping of the second, third, or fourth digit. If concurrent fixed contracture is present, this is also addressed, as will be discussed in connection with digital deformities. The corrected digital position is maintained with the dressing or with a Kirschner wire for at least 4 weeks. When more severe deformity is present, the overlapping central digit is treated more aggressively in a fashion similar to that used for the severely overlapping fifth toe.

## Overlapping Fifth Toe

The most common form of congenital overlapping deformity is the overlapping fifth toe. There are three components to the overlapping fifth toe; adduction contracture, dorsiflexion, and external rotation contracture along the longitudinal axis are present at the fifth metatarsophalangeal joint directing the toe into a varus attitude. The deformity has concomitant shortening of the medial collateral ligament and the medial aspect of the metatarsophalangeal joint capsule. There is usually a contracture of the extensor digitorum longus tendon and frequently the skin at the dorsomedial aspect of the web space is contracted. With time, there can also be adaptive deformation of the proximal phalanx. The toe will often appear smaller and flattened losing its cylindrical shape and taking on a paddle-like appearance. The nail is also smaller and flatter than usual (Fig. 16-6). The deformity is generally bilateral with a strong family inheritance and equal sex distribution.

### Etiology

Lantzounis[17] suggested that this deformity may be secondary to prolonged malposture of the fifth toe during intrauterine life, rather than a true congenital anomaly. Some authors feel the deformity, like underlapping toes, is secondary to an osseous abnormality with emphasis placed on the proximal phalanx. Dobbs[18] suggests that there may be a biomechanical role as well. He describes a lateral displacement of the flexor digitorum longus insertion when the forefoot abducts on the rearfoot. This will result in an abnormal medial force on the distal phalanx. Due to its most lateral position, the fifth toe is the most greatly effected by this medial force. This leads to an inversion of the toe with the middle and distal phalanges becoming more adducted than the proximal phalanx.

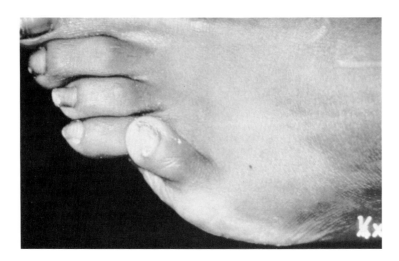

**Fig. 16-6.** Classic paddle-like appearance of congenital overlapping fifth toe deformity.

## Clinical Features

Patients are usually symptom-free in infancy and early childhood, but as the child approaches skeletal maturity, the condition can become symtomatic. Of patients with an overlapping fifth toe, 50 percent will develop symptoms related to a heloma durum on the dorsal aspect of the fifth toe, a heloma molle between the fourth and fifth toes, or a calloused lateral nail groove. Additionally, many patients or their parents will have concerns over the cosmetic appearance of this deformity.

## Treatment

Effective conservative treatment depends upon early diagnosis. In infancy, passive stretching and adhesive strapping are most often utilized. Jordan and Caselli[19] suggested splinting the digit for 4 to 6 weeks to achieve improved alignment and maintaining the alignment for an additional 2 to 8 weeks to accomplish full correction.

Surgical correction consists of soft tissue correction, bony correction, or a combination of both. Recurrence of deformity is the major postoperative complication associated with virtually all surgical approaches. For this reason an abundance of approaches have been described.

In view of the risk of recurrence, amputation has been described in the older literature. Amputation of the fifth toe was performed regularly when an overlapping fifth toe deformity was listed as a physical impairment precluding employment as a civil service worker. Fortunately, this very aggressive approach is rarely practiced today. The mechanical sequelae to fifth toe amputation are numerous, including lateral lesser digital drift, lesser metatarsalgia, and digital deformation of the remaining toes. Despite these drawbacks, however, one will occasionally still see a patient who has had a toe amputated for a congenital overlapping deformity (Fig. 16-7).

Soft tissue approaches to the overlapping fifth toe involve various combined approaches of lengthening dorsal skin contracture, releasing and rebalancing dorsal extensor and metatarsophalangeal joint contracture, tightening plantar skin redundancy, and tightening and rebalancing plantar flexor and metatarsophalangeal joint structures.

In one of the most unique approaches, Cockin[20] described Butler's operation for an overriding fifth toe. A dorsal racquet incision with a plantar handle (i.e., double racquet incision) is created at the metatarsophalangeal joint of the fifth toe. The plantar handle is longer than the

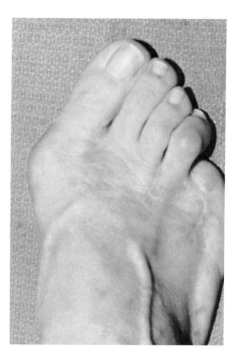

**Fig. 16-7.** This 51-year-old patient underwent amputation of the fifth toe as a teenager for congenital overlapping deformity. The patient now has lateral drift of all digits and transfer metatarsalgia of the fourth submetatarsal.

dorsal incision and angled in a lateral direction. A metatarsophalangeal joint capsulotomy is performed along with an extensor tenotomy. The toe is then swung down into the plantar handle of the incision and the wound is sutured, with the toe held in its new position in the suture line (Fig. 16-8). Of 70 operations performed by Cockin over 10 years, 91 percent afforded good results and 6 percent a fair result, while 3 percent were failures. Black et al.[21] reported on 36 operations, with excellent results in 78 percent of their cases and good results in 17 percent, and 5 percent being classified as failures. Although one of the major criticisms and concerns of this operation is potential vascular compromise, none of the failures in either of these studies were vascular in nature.

Another dorsal skin approach involves a V-Y skin plasty of the dorsomedial skin fold for correction of the overlapping fifth toe. This is done in conjunction with a dorsal metatarsophalangeal joint capsulotomy and an extensor tenotomy (Fig. 16-9). Wilson[22] stated that all seven of his patients had "very satisfactory" results,

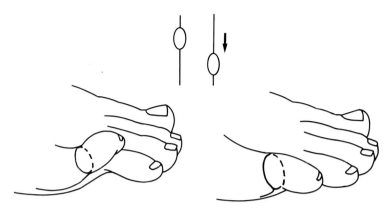

**Fig. 16-8.** Butler operation for the correction of congenital overlapping fifth toe. Note that a double racquet incision is used and extends circumferentially around the toe. The toe is moved plantarly in the incision and sutured in place.

with one having a slight recurrence. Paton[23] performed a V-Y skin plasty on 20 patients; in his early postoperative assessment he found 14 of these patients had good results, 3 had acceptable results, and 3 had poor results. However, an additional, longer retrospective analysis with a mean postoperative follow-up time of 2 years and 1 month showed that his results had deteriorated, with only 6 patients still having good, 2 having acceptable, and 12 having poor results. In similar fashion, Goodwin and Swisher[24] recommended a modified V-Y-shaped incision at the metatarsophalangeal joint. Their incision begins as a Y with the stem of the Y extending proximally over the extensor tendon. The dissection is carried down to the

tendon, where an open Z-plasty of the extensor tendon is achieved, along with a dorsal capsulotomy extending at least 108 degrees around the joint. The toe is placed into its corrected position and the tendon is repaired. Suturing of the skin incision is begun proximally and continued distally, with the toe in its newly extended position. The incision is then closed as a Y, but with a longer proximal stem (Fig. 16-9). In this sense their incision is closed in typical V-Y fashion. Goodwin and Swisher suggested maintaining the correction with casting followed by adhesive strapping. They reported 100 percent successful results in 20 cases.

Alternatively, surgical syndactylization has been sug-

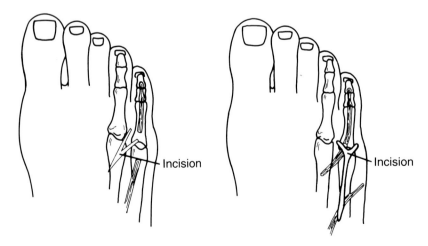

**Fig. 16-9.** **(A)** V-Y skin plasty approach as described by Wilson.[22] **(B)** Y-Y skin plasty approach as described by Goodwin and Swisher.[24]

gested by several authors. In infancy and early childhood syndactylization alone is used to correct the overlapping fifth toe. As the deformity becomes more fixed later in life, the syndactylization will need to be combined with either a partial or a complete phalangectomy.[12] Leonard and Rising[25] performed eight syndactylizations for overlapping fifth toes, obtaining a satisfactory result in seven (88 percent). Their follow-up was up to 5 years without recurrence. Scrase[26] operated on 42 digits, obtaining good results in 39 (93 percent) and fair results in the remaining three cases (7 percent). Thus, syndactylization would appear to be an alternative but has the disadvantage of permanent disfigurement.

Suppan[16] suggested an extensor tenotomy, a dorsal capsulotomy, and two transverse semielliptical incisions placed plantarly at the base of the toe. The skin wedge is removed, and the base of the toe is sewn to the ball of the foot. (Fig. 16-10). DuVries[27] similarly advocated an extensor tenotomy and a dorsal capsulotomy but added a dorsal skin plasty to his operation.

Lantzounis[17] described a modified Jones suspension. He drilled a hole through the distal end of the fifth metatarsal after cutting the extensor tendon distally, brought the extensor digitorum longus tendon through the hole and sutured it to itself. He combined this with a dorsal

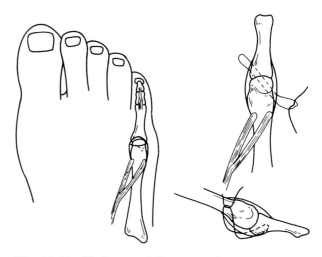

**Fig. 16-11.** The Lantzounis[17] procedure for the correction of a congenital overlapping fifth toe. Note that a modified Jones suspension of the extensor longus tendon to the fifth toe characterizes this procedure.

metatarsophalangeal joint capsulotomy and plantar metatarsophalangeal joint capsulorrhaphy ( Fig. 16-11). He performed this operation 25 times and was able to follow 23 of the patients. One patient who had the procedure bilaterally was lost to follow-up. He found excellent results in 16 cases (70 percent), good results in 4 (17 percent), and poor results in 3 (13 percent).

In yet another approach, Lapidus[28] described a procedure in which the long extensor is transected at the middle of the fifth metatarsal and the distal aspect of the tendon is pulled into a second incision over the fifth metatarsophalangeal joint. The tendon is then rerouted in a plantar, lateral, and proximal direction underneath the proximal phalanx and is sutured into the abductor digiti quinti and flexor digitorum brevis tendons where they insert into the lateral aspect of the fifth proximal phalangeal base (Fig. 16-12). A dorsal metatarsophalangeal joint capsulotomy is also performed. Lapidus believed that this procedure corrected the deformity and provided active maintenance of the correction by the insertion of the extensor tendon into the abductor and flexor digitorum brevis muscles.

Many surgeons believe that the deformity has a significant osseous component and have described approaches to either the proximal or middle phalanges. These bony procedures are usually combined with some form of soft tissue release, as already described. Rosner et al.[29] de-

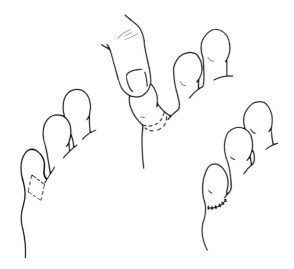

**Fig. 16-10.** Plantar skin wedge for the removal of redundant plantar skin. This wedge may be lenticular (i.e., two semielliptical incisions), oval, or diamond-shaped. The plantar wedge has been found to be instrumental in helping to prevent recurrent deformity.

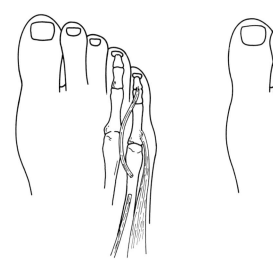
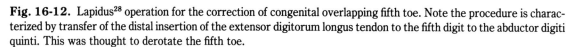

**Fig. 16-12.** Lapidus[28] operation for the correction of congenital overlapping fifth toe. Note the procedure is characterized by transfer of the distal insertion of the extensor digitorum longus tendon to the fifth digit to the abductor digiti quinti. This was thought to derotate the fifth toe.

scribed a procedure that incorporates an extensor tenotomy, a dorsal metatarsophalangeal joint capsulotomy, and an abductory wedge osteotomy of the proximal phalanx. They suggested that the osteotomy be executed at the phalangeal base and that a Kirschner wire be used for fixation. Kaplan[30] utilized an extensor tenotomy, an arthroplasty of the proximal phalanx, and a plantar elliptical excision of skin with approximation of the proximal aspect of the toe to the distal part of the ball of the foot. Kaplan claimed to have performed this operation in over 59 cases without any failures. Anderson[31] described what he referred to as *combination surgery*. This consisted of a fifth metatarsal head resection, a V-Y plasty of the dorsal skin, and excision of a transverse skin ellipse from the plantar aspect of the fifth toe with reapproximation of the plantar base of the fifth toe to the distal aspect of the ball of the foot. Dobbs[18] utilized a dorsal derotating skin ellipse as his incision, through which he performed an arthroplasty of the head of the proximal phalanx, with or without a hemiphalangectomy of the middle phalanx, or a middle phalangectomy with a lateral condylectomy of the head of the proximal phalanx. If necessary, this was done in conjunction with a flexor tenotomy or a Z-plasty of the dorsomedial skin.

Janecki and Wilde[32] reported on the Ruiz-Mora procedure, which consists of a total proximal phalangectomy through a plantar longitudinal skin ellipse. The toe is fused to the distal aspect of the ball of the foot at the end of the procedure. These authors reported 41 cases which were followed for 3.5 years. All patients had complete relief of symptoms and correction of the deformity of the fifth toe. However, on follow-up there were two significant secondary problems: 23 percent of the patients developed a prominent fifth metatarsal head or a bunionette, and 32 percent developed a hammertoe of the adjacent fourth toe. Thus, the Ruiz-Mora procedure entails problems similar to digital amputation. Kelikian et al.[12] and Tachdjian[4-6] also advocated a proximal phalangectomy but in conjunction with a syndactyly of the fourth and fifth toes. Sharrard[3] advocated an isolated proximal phalangectomy and cautioned that the procedure may affect growth of the toe in children.

All the above-mentioned procedures fail to correct at least one or more features of the deformity. Although the procedures will work in some cases or in the mildly overlapping fifth toe, they will not work universally or in cases of moderate to severe overlapping fifth toe deformity. Anderson[31] was correct in stating that a combined approach is necessary to prevent recurrence of the deformity. In order to surgically correct the toe, all aspects of the deformity must be addressed. The contracted dorsal and medial soft tissues, such as skin, capsule, ligaments, and tendon, must be either released or lengthened. Plantar redundant soft tissues, including skin and capsule, must usually be addressed, and any bone deformity must also be corrected at the time of operation. Failure to address all components of the deformity will lead to an increased chance of recurrence.

*Authors' Preferred Technique*

We believe that this complex deformity requires a thorough combined surgical approach. The first component addressed is the skin at the dorsomedial aspect of the web space. A dorsal Z-plasty approach is utilized, beginning with an oblique longitudinal incision placed in line with the skin tension. A second incision is made at the distal end of the first incision and is directed from distal-medial to proximal-lateral. This incision forms a 60-degree angle with the first incision and is the same length as the original incision. The third incision begins at the

proximal end of the original incision and runs from proximal-lateral to distal-medial; it also forms a 60-degree angle with the original incision and is the same length as the previous two incisions. The three incisions now form a Z (Fig. 16-13A). Dissection is carried through the subcutaneous tissues, with care taken not to damage the corners of the flaps (Fig. 16-13B). At the end of the procedure the flaps of the Z are transposed, so that the distal-lateral flap becomes proximal-medial and the proximal-medial flap becomes distal-lateral (Fig. 16-13I&J).

The extensor digitorum longus tendon is then addressed. If the deformity is flexible, an open Z-plasty lengthening is performed, but if the deformity is fixed, the tendon should be transected at the proximal interphalangeal joint and later transferred into the head of the fifth metatarsal. Additionally, if osseous adaption has occurred in the proximal phalanx, an arthroplasty of the proximal phalangeal head is performed. The head of the

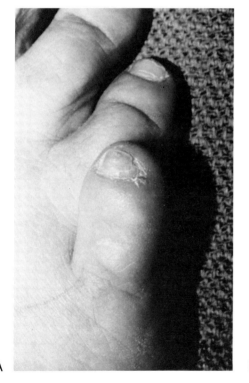

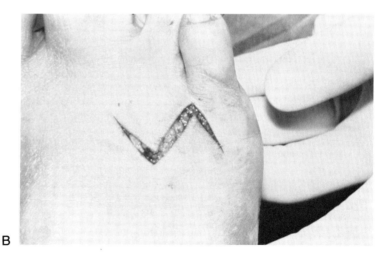

A                                                                B

**Fig. 16-13.** Combination surgical approach to the flexible overlapping fifth toe deformity. **(A)** Z-plasty skin incision oriented to release proximal-medial skin contracture. **(B)** Flaps are elevated, with subcutaneous tissue maintained intact to each flap. *(Figure continues.)*

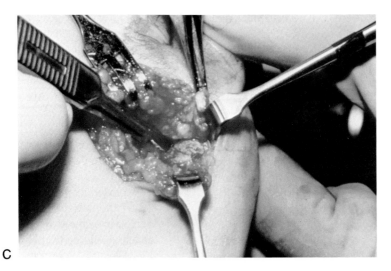

C

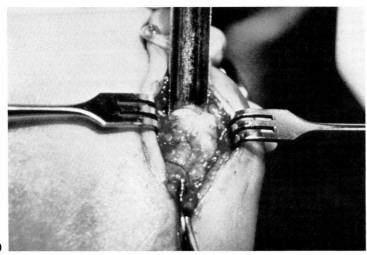

D

**Fig. 16-13** *(Continued).* **(C)** Dorsal metatarsophalangeal joint capsulotomy is performed after open Z-plasty of the extensor tendon. Note tendon retracted with forceps. **(D)** McGlamry metatarsal elevator used to free the plantar plate from the fifth metatarsal head. Elevator is passed plantarly through the dorsal capsulotomy between the metatarsal head and plantar plate. *(Figure continues.)*

proximal phalanx is exposed by carrying the incision longitudinally onto the dorsum of the fifth toe and entering the proximal interphalangeal joint. Once the head is exposed, the proximal phalanx is cut at the anatomic neck with a power saw or a bone-cutting forceps. A dorsal metatarsophalangeal joint capsulotomy is then performed (Fig. 16-13C), and if necessary, a plantar plate release is also performed (Fig. 16-13D). A skin wedge is

then removed from the plantar-proximal aspect of the toe and the distal aspect of the ball of the foot; this wedge is oval-shaped with the long axis extending from proximal to distal. The borders of the skin wedge are dissected down to and through the dermis, and the oval-shaped piece of skin is excised, leaving the subcutaneous layer intact (Fig. 16-13E). The toe is now plantar-flexed, and the distal half of the oval-shaped wound is sutured to the

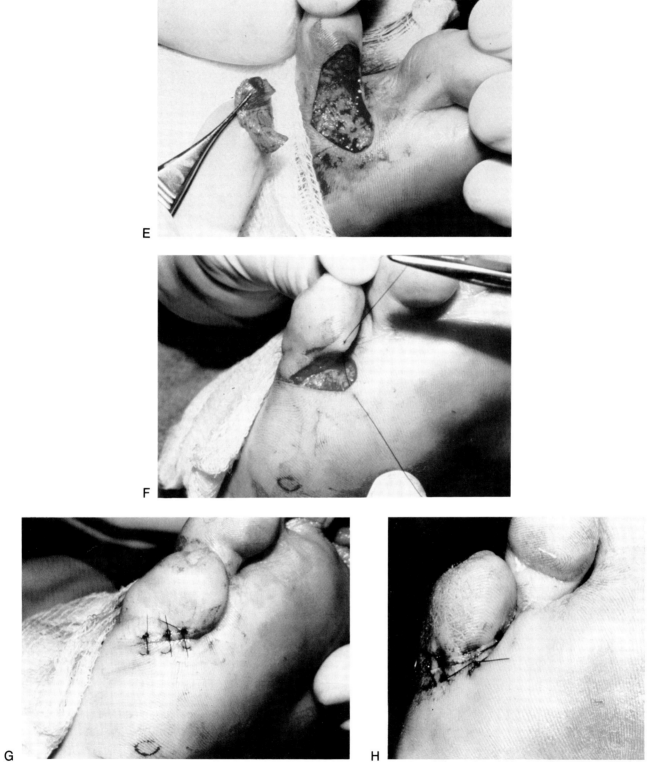

**Fig. 16-13** *(Continued).* **(E)** Oval-shaped skin wedge removed from plantar aspect of fifth toe. **(F–H)** Closure of plantar oval-shaped skin desmoplasty. *(Figure continues.)*

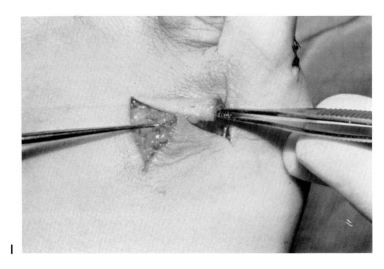

I

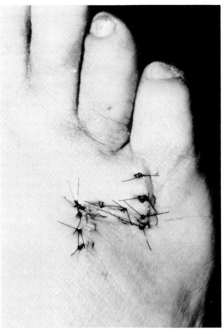

J

**Fig. 16-13** *(Continued).* **(I&J)** Transposition of dorsal Z-plasty skin flaps with closure. Note Z-plasty is now reoriented, with maximum tension created perpendicular to the direction of skin lengthening. Note overall improved alignment of the digit.

proximal half (Fig. 16-13F–H). Alternatively, the wedge may be diamond-shaped, with the four apices medial, lateral, proximal, and distal (Fig. 16-14). The open Z-plasty of the extensor tendon is reapproximated and sutured together in its lengthened position, and the flaps of the Z skin plasty are transposed and sutured (Fig. 16-13I&J). The toe should be splinted in its new position with bandaging or a Kirschner wire.

In fixed deformities we suggest a modified Jones suspension. The extensor digitorum longus tendon is dissected from the proximal interphalangeal joint at which it was previously transected and freed to the metatarsal

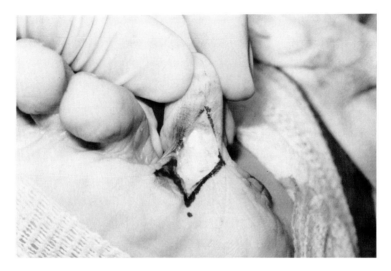

**Fig. 16-14.** (A) Plantar diamond-shaped skin wedge removed.

neck (Fig. 16-15A&B). A dorsal metatarsophalangeal capsulotomy and plantar plate release are then performed (Fig. 16-15C&D). Again, if osseous adaption has occurred in the proximal phalanx, an arthroplasty of the proximal phalangeal head is performed (Fig. 16-15E). After exposure of the head of the fifth metatarsal, a small trephine hole is placed through the center of the head from medial to lateral, with care taken not to enter the articular surface (Fig. 16-15F), and the tendon is passed through the hole and sutured to itself (Fig. 16-15G). The plug of bone from the trephine can now be placed back into the hole to hold the tendon more securely, after which closure is effected. Again, the toe should be splinted in its new position with the dressings or a Kirschner wire (Fig. 16-15H).

# DIGITAL CONTRACTURES

There are three basic digital contracture deformities: hammertoe, mallet toe, and claw toe. A hammertoe is characterized by dorsiflexion at the metatarsophalangeal joint, plantar-flexion at the proximal interphalangeal joint, and dorsiflexion at the distal interphalangeal joint. A mallet toe involves the distal interphalangeal joint, the distal phalanx being plantar-flexed on the middle phalanx. In claw toe the deformity consists of dorsiflexion at the metatarsophalangeal joint and plantarflexion at the proximal and distal interphalangeal joints.

## Hammertoe

### Etiology and Clinical Features

Hammertoe is one of the most common digital deformities, with the second toe most frequently affected. The deformity in its congenital form is usually seen bilaterally and symmetrically, with a high familial incidence. Hammertoe can also result from shoegear, abnormal biomechanics, trauma, and neurologic disorders. A congenital hammertoe is normally flexible and asymptomatic in infancy and early childhood, but as the child approaches adolescence, the deformity acquires a more fixed attitude. It is at this stage that a painful heloma durum can develop over the proximal interphalangeal joint. Severe deformities will eventually progress to a metatarsophalangeal joint dislocation. As the base of the proximal phalanx rides up onto the dorsal aspect of the metatarsal head, it forces it into a plantar-flexed position. This can create a callus on the plantar aspect of the foot beneath the metatarsal head. As the hammertoe progresses from a flexible to a fixed deformity, more aggressive corrective action will be needed.

### Treatment

Early on, conservative treatment should be attempted. This consists of passive stretching and strapping to maintain correction. Additionally, functional orthoses may be of benefit, especially in a patient with flexor

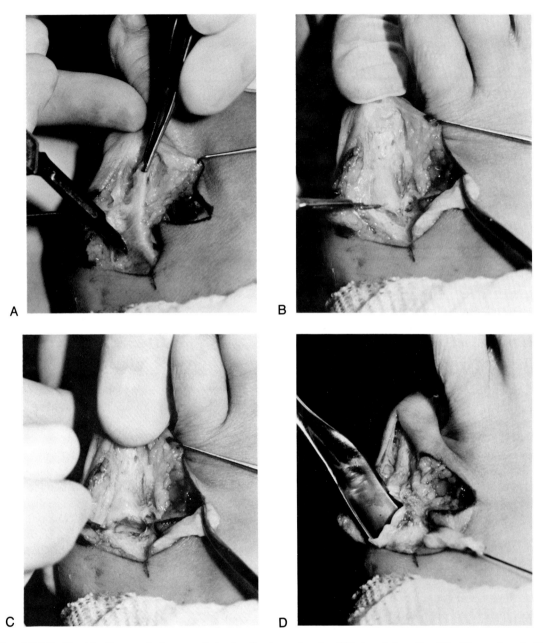

**Fig. 16-15.** Combination surgical approach to the fixed overlapping fifth toe deformity. **(A)** After a dorsal skin Z-plasty, the extensor tendon is identified. Note the extensor hood fibers extending plantarly from the extensor tendon and enveloping the base of the phalanx. **(B)** Extensor tendon released distally at the level of the proximal interphalangeal joint and dissected proximally to the metatarsal neck. The extensor hood apparatus is incised during this maneuver. **(C)** Dorsal metatarsophalangeal joint capsulotomy. **(D)** Release of plantar plate with McGlamry metatarsal elevator. *(Figure continues.)*

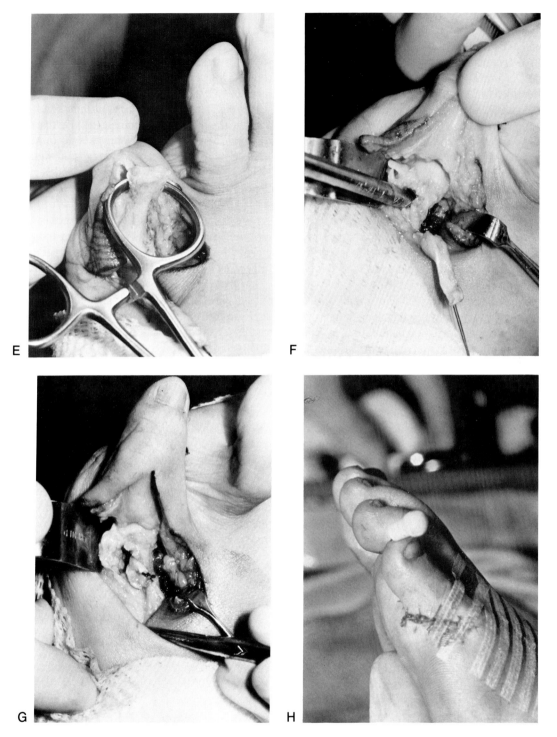

**Fig. 16-15** *(Continued).* **(E)** Exposure of proximal phalangeal head for resection at anatomic neck. **(F)** Trephine hole placed from lateral to medial in the distal neck of the fifth metatarsal. **(G)** The extensor tendon is passed through the trephine hole and sutured to itself. **(H)** Final digital position with Kirschner wire stabilization. Note oval-shaped plantar skin wedge.

stabilization or flexor substitution hammertoe. Although conservative treatment does not usually prove to be beneficial, it is worth an attempt, especially if the disorder is identified early. If symptomatology develops or if the hammertoe persists, surgical intervention will become necessary.

One of the earliest procedures described, as with all digital deformities, is amputation. However, this is antiquated, fraught with long-term negative sequelae, and no longer used. Soft tissue procedures can be attempted while the hammertoe is flexible. A simple tenotomy of the extensor tendon as an isolated procedure or in conjunction with a dorsal capsulotomy of the metatarsophalangeal joint is not indicated in the pediatric patient. The tendon will reanastomose or regenerate, and this will usually lead to a recurrent hammertoe.

Alternatively, Lapidus[33] suggested a dorsal capsulotomy at the metatarsophalangeal joint, along with plantar capsulotomies and dorsal capsulorrhaphy at the proximal and distal interphalangeal joints, and imbrication of the extensor tendons. He reported good or fair results in 27 of 30 toes (90 percent) and poor results in 3 toes (10 percent).

Ross and Menelaus[9] reported the results of tenotomies of the flexor digitorum longus and brevis in children with curly toes and hammertoes. Their results in 188 cases resulted in 179 of the procedures being rated as good or fair (95 percent), with only 9 found to be poor (5 percent). Although 43 patients had no function of the flexor digitorum longus, no patients reported any loss of toe function. Obviously, loss of flexor function and subsequent lack of digital purchase is not a desirable result in the pediatric patient.

Myerson and Shereff[34] described a procedure that entails a soft tissue release including a dorsal metatarsophalangeal joint capsulotomy, tenotomies of both extensor tendons, transection of the collateral ligaments, and incision of the interossei muscles. Release of the interossei would logically result in a floating toe deformity, an unwanted result in the young patient.

In a more unique approach, Taylor[35] described an operation, originally performed by G.R. Girdlestone, in which the flexor tendons are transferred into the extensor tendons. Taylor reviewed 68 patients with a follow-up of 1 to 12 years. The procedure resulted in good results in 50 patients (74 percent) and fair results in 11 patients (16 percent), while the remaining seven had poor results (10 percent). Tachdjian[5,6] advises against the procedure as described by Taylor because of the development of lateral rotation of the toes following the tendon transfer. Pyper[36] reviewed 45 feet in 1958 and concluded that good and poor results were almost equal. He found recurrence of the deformity in nearly 20 percent of the feet and recommended an arthrodesis of the proximal interphalangeal joint as a preferable alternative. Several authors have suggested detaching and splitting the flexor digitorum longus tendon and bringing both ends over the proximal phalanx in a sling-like fashion.[37-40] Sgarlato[38] found that the procedure alleviated painful dorsal lesions and repositioned the phalanx on the metatarsal head, Parrish[39] reported good or excellent results in 87 percent of feet operated on, and Marcinko et al.[40] claimed to have good to excellent results in over 400 cases. Barbari and Brevig[41] performed either Girdlestone's or Parrish's procedure in 39 feet and obtained satisfactory results in 35 of them (90 percent). The best cosmetic results were obtained in younger patients, although there were frequent complaints of stiffness. Elderly patients did not have the same difficulty with stiffness even though they often had decreased or absent passive motion. In a slight modification Kuwada and Dockery[42] described bringing the long flexor tendon dorsally through a drill hole in the proximal phalanx.

In a different approach, Frank and Johnson[43] advocated the extensor shift procedure, in which the long extensor tendons to all five toes are detached, the interphalangeal joint of the hallux is fused, and the extensor hallucis longus is placed through a drill hole in the first metatarsal. The long flexors to the lesser toes are also transected, and the second and third slips are placed into the third metatarsal and fourth and fifth slips into the fifth metatarsal. This was Frank and Johnson's standard procedure, but they described several variations. Of 22 cases, 9 showed excellent results (41 percent), 11 were satisfactory (50 percent), and 2 patients were unimproved (9 percent).

In reviewing these results, it is apparent that tendon transfer procedures in the pediatric population are quite difficult because of the small anatomy. The flexor tendon transfers universally affect toe purchase, and as shown by several authors, this is not usually well tolerated in the younger population. Correction of the hammertoe often requires more than a soft tissue procedure. Resection of bone provides a lengthening of the soft tissues and a reversal of the deformity. In view of this, Kelikian et al.[12]

suggest partial phalangectomy and syndactyly for hammertoe syndrome. For milder deformities they removed the base of the proximal phalanx, and for more fixed deformities they resected the entire proximal phalanx. When the second through fifth toes were involved, the second and third toes were syndactylized, as well as the fourth and fifth toes. Suppan[16] attempted to preserve the proximal interphalangeal joint with the cartilaginous articulation preservation CAP procedure, in which a metaphyseal osteotomy with resection of bone is performed but the collateral ligaments and the proximal interphalangeal joint are preserved. The capital fragment is held in place on the shaft of the proximal phalanx with tendon repair and soft tissue closure.

More direct osseous approaches include those of Post,[44] who in 1882 reported a procedure involving a head resection of the proximal phalanx; Soule,[45] who in 1910 described a fusion of the proximal interphalangeal joint; O'Neill[46] who in 1911 resected the head of the proximal phalanx and the base of the middle phalanx and interposed soft tissue between them; and Lambrinudi,[47] who in 1927 suggested fusion of both interphalangeal joints in order to create a single rigid beam. A peg-in-hole arthrodesis of the proximal interphalangeal joint was described by Higgs[48] and by Young.[49] Taylor[50] in 1940 introduced the use of a Kirschner wire for fixation of the proximal interphalangeal joint arthrodesis, and Selig,[51] who also utilized a Kirschner wire for fixation, advocated bending the end of the wire "to prevent the possibility of the wire wandering deeply into the tissues." Tachdjian[4-6] advocated a proximal interphalangeal joint arthrodesis in the adolescent patient, which is combined with a transfer of the extensor digitorum longus tendon into the metatarsal head if the metatarsal is plantar-flexed. Arthrodesis is not usually necessary in the pediatric patient; since this procedure will also interfere with growth, it is generally not indicated before skeletal maturity.

*Authors' Preferred Treatment*

We suggest a combination of soft tissue and bony procedures. A classic Post arthroplasty of the head of the proximal phalanx is performed, which relaxes contracture at both the proximal and the distal interphalangeal joints. Dorsiflexory contracture at the metatarsophalangeal joint is corrected by a stepwise approach. The Kelikian push-up test is used to determine if the toe will straighten out (i.e., if there is no dorsiflexory metatarso-

phalangeal joint contracture). This test is performed by placing a finger under the metatarsal head and pushing up, thereby effectively loading the metatarsal and the plantar plate and predicting whether the toe will become rectus with weight-bearing. If a dorsiflexed metatarsophalangeal joint reduces with the push-up test, no fixed contracture exists, and only a simple Post arthroplasty need be performed. However, if when the push-up test is performed a dorsiflexed position of the metatarsophalangeal joint remains, the contracture is fixed and must be addressed.

If an isolated Post arthroplasty is to be performed, it may be accomplished through a dorsolinear incision or two transverse semielliptical incisions. We prefer the transverse approach, as it excises any dorsal lesion, it falls within relaxed skin tension lines and thus gives a better cosmetic result, and the closure affords some stability in the plane of correction.

If the metatarsophalangeal joint must be addressed, this is accomplished in a stepwise fashion. A dorsolinear or combined dorsolinear-transverse approach is used for the incision. Dissection is carried down through the subcutaneous tissues to the conjoined extensor tendon, which is lengthened in open Z-plasty fashion (Fig. 16-16). The capsule of the proximal interphalangeal joint is entered, and the collateral ligaments are incised. The head of the proximal phalanx can now be delivered into the wound and resected at the anatomic neck (Fig. 16-15E). The push-up test is performed at this time to determine if the digit has corrected and is able to lie flat. If the metatarsophalangeal joint remains dorsally contracted with the push-up test, the surgeon should proceed to the next step, an extensor hood recession. This is accomplished by placing some tension on the extensor digitorum longus tendon and linearly incising the fibers that pass from the tendon enveloping the base of the proximal phalanx (Fig. 16-15A&B). The push-up test is repeated and metatarsophalangeal joint is again evaluated for continued dorsal contraction.

The next step is a dorsal metatarsophalangeal joint capsulotomy. The joint is distracted by placing distal tension on the proximal phalanx. With a #67 Beaver blade parallel to the joint surfaces, the dorsal, dorsomedial, and dorsolateral aspects of the joint capsule are incised (Fig. 16-13C and 16-15C). The push-up test is performed, and if dorsal metatarsophalangeal joint contracture persists, a flexor plate release is executed. We suggest the use of a McGlamry metatarsal elevator to

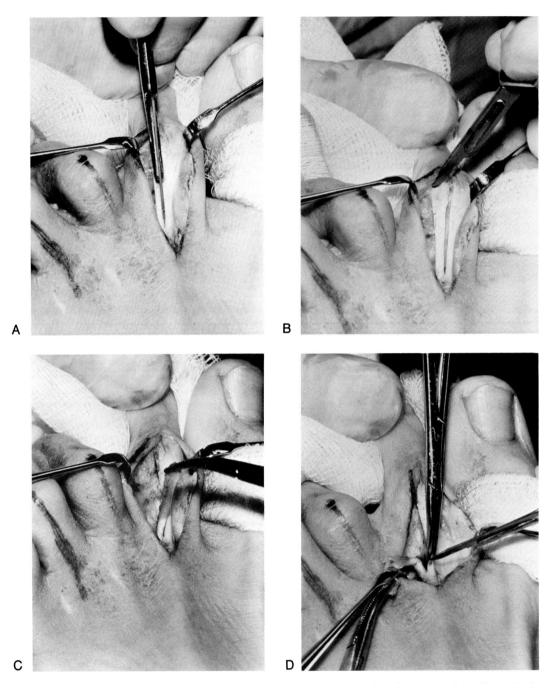

**Fig. 16-16.** Open Z-plasty of extensor tendon. **(A)** Initial longitudinal section of tendon into medial and lateral halves. **(B)** Distally, the lateral half of the tendon is sectioned. **(C)** The lateral half is then reflected proximally. **(D)** Proximally, the medial half of the tendon is sectioned. *(Figure continues.)*

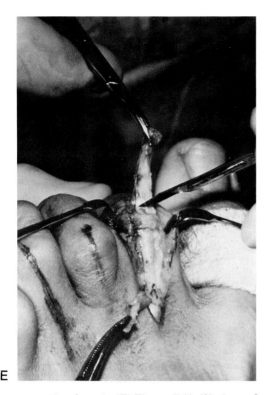 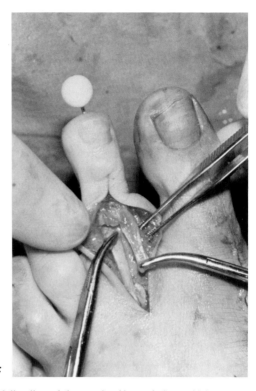

E                                    F

**Fig. 16-16** *(Continued).* **(E)** The medial half is then reflected distally and the proximal interphalangeal joint exposed. **(F)** During closure, the tendon is reapproximated in side-to-side fashion in a lengthened position.

accomplish this procedure (Figs.16-13D and 16-15D). Once the elevator can easily be passed along the plantar aspect of the metatarsal head and neck, the push-up test is repeated. If the toe remains dorsiflexed at the metatarsophalangeal joint, Kirschner wire fixation is used to help maintain a corrected position. A 0.045-inch Kirschner wire is driven in a retrograde fashion through the phalanges and seated into the base of the proximal phalanx. The push-up test is performed, and if dorsiflexion of the metatarsophalangeal joint still persists, the wire is driven into the metatarsal head with the metatarsophalangeal joint held in a straightened or slightly plantar-flexed position. The extensor is then reapproximated in its lengthened position (Fig. 16-16F). Closure is then completed.

When the Kirschner wire is driven across the metatarsophalangeal joint, the patient can bear weight in a wooden surgical shoe with a built-up sole ending distally to the metatarsal heads. This will allow the patient to ambulate without dorsiflexing the metatarsophalangeal

joint and placing stress on the Kirschner wire. Long-term management of the patient is supplemented with a functional orthosis.

## Claw Toe

Throughout the literature the terms *hammertoe* and *claw toe* are used interchangeably, but in actuality the terms define two distinct and separate deformities. The claw toe, as described previously, consists of dorsiflexion at the metatarsophalangeal joint and plantar flexion at the proximal and distal interphalangeal joints. In this deformity, which occurs less often than hammertoes, all the lesser digits are usually affected, and the hallux is also frequently involved. Claw toes are usually secondary to a pes cavus deformity or a neuromuscular condition, such as Charcot-Marie-Tooth disease, muscular dystrophy, Friedreich's ataxia, poliomyelitis, meningomyelocele, and cerebral palsy. Painful corns can develop over the proximal interphalangeal joint and at the end of the toe.

With time, metatarsalgia can occur, especially if the proximal phalanx is subluxated or dislocated onto the dorsal aspect of the metatarsal head.

Conservative treatment includes palliative care, padding, orthoses, and shoes with a large toe box. With time, these deformities almost always become rigid. When claw toe is semirigid or rigid, it seldom improves with conservative therapy alone.

The majority of surgical procedures performed on hammertoe are also suggested for claw toe. The Girdlestone-Taylor procedure and the several modifications mentioned above have been described for the correction of this deformity.[35,41,43] Similarly, fusion of the interphalangeal joints has also been advocated.[49,50]

For claw toes of non-neurologic etiology with dorsal metatarsophalangeal contracture, we use the same stepwise approach described for hammertoe. In cavus and neurologic claw toe deformities the surgeon must correct the underlying etiology either through osseous procedures or through the appropriate tendon transfers. Arthrodesis of the proximal interphalangeal joint is a viable alternative in the patient with rigid claw toes.

## Mallet Toes

Mallet toe deformity consists of a plantar-flexed distal interphalangeal joint. In the pediatric population it is often flexible and asymptomatic, but with time and skeletal maturity there is a continual loss of active and passive dorsiflexion at the distal interphalangeal joint, which can lead to a painful lesion at the most distal aspect of the toe. A heloma durum can also develop on the dorsal aspect of the head of the middle phalanx (Fig. 16-17A). The nail may also become involved, taking on a thickened appearance secondary to repetitive trauma. The deformity usually involves one or two toes, with the second toe most commonly affected. Mallet toes may have several etiologies. Longer toes that are forced against a short toe box in the shoe will, over time, develop a plantar-flexed attitude at the distal interphalangeal joint. This is the most likely reason that the second toe, which is the longest toe, is commonly involved. Diabetics with peripheral neuropathy may have a predisposition to mallet toe deformity.[52] In general, the mallet toe occurs when the flexor digitorum longus overpowers the conjoined extensor tendon.

Conservative treatment consists of splinting, padding, orthoses, manipulation, and palliative care. Conservative

treatment must be instituted early in the deformity in order to have any success. This treatment course may alleviate symptomatology but usually does not correct the deformity.

In the younger patient with a flexible deformity, a tenotomy of the flexor digitorum longus, along with a plantar capsulotomy of the distal interphalangeal joint, can be performed through a plantar stab incision in the flexion crease.

In more fixed deformities we suggest a resection of the head of the middle phalanx. A lenticular incision is placed over the distal interphalangeal joint, and the wedge of skin and dermis is removed (Fig. 16-17B). Care should be taken not to damage the nail matrix with this incision. The long extensor tendon is transversely transected, and the collateral ligaments of the distal interphalangeal joint are released (Fig. 16-17C&D). The head of the middle phalanx is exposed and resected with the use of an oscillating saw or hand instrumentation (Fig. 16-17E and F). If the distal phalanx remains plantar-flexed, tenotomy of the flexor digitorum longus is performed through the dorsal approach. In more severe deformities, we suggest holding the toe in proper alignment with a Kirschner wire, after which the extensor tendon is reattached and wound closure is performed (Fig. 16-17G). The lenticular skin incision will also assist in achieving correction.

Recalcitrant mallet toe deformities in skeletally mature patients can be corrected by distal interphalangeal joint fusion, in which the same incision and dissection as in the arthroplasty are used. Hand instrumentation is used to resect the cartilage from the head of the middle phalanx and the base of the distal phalanx. A Kirschner wire is placed into the remaining base of the distal phalanx and driven out through the end of the toe. It is then passed in a retrograded manner into the middle phalanx, accomplishing an end-to-end arthrodesis. Closure is performed as previously described.

## HALLUX ABDUCTUS INTERPHALANGEUS

Hallux abductus interphalangeus is defined as the angle created by the intersection of the longitudinal bisections of the proximal and distal phalanges of the hallux. The normal value for this angle is usually considered to be below 10 degrees, but some authors believe it to be as

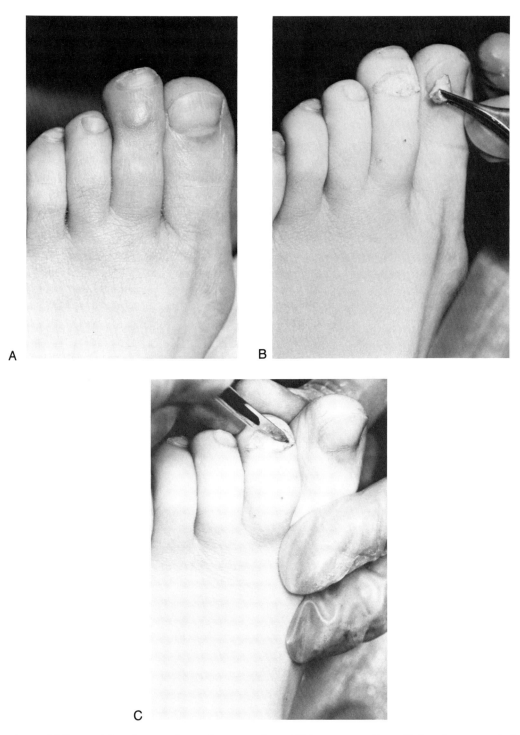

**Fig. 16-17.** Mallet toe deformity secondary to long second toe. **(A)** Appearance of toe with dorsal corn over the head of the middle phalanx. **(B)** Two transverse elliptical skin incisions used to excise the corn and expose deeper structures. **(C)** Transverse tenotomy of the conjoined extensor tendon. *(Figure continues.)*

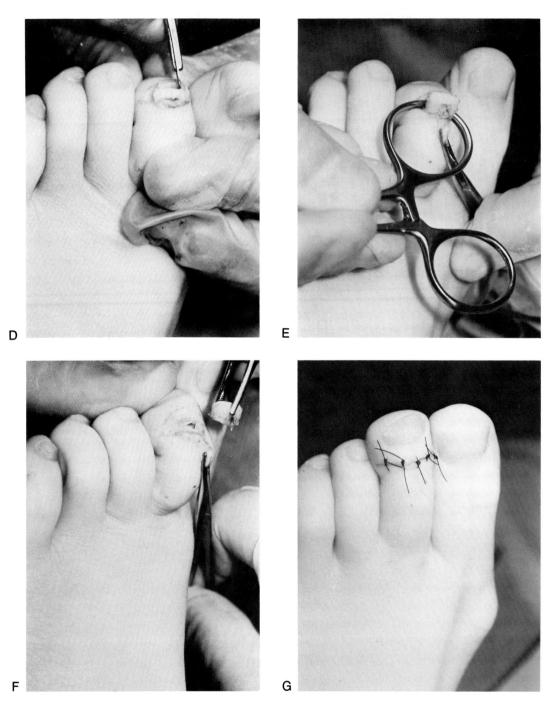

**Fig. 16-17** *(Continued).* **(D)** Release of the collateral ligaments of the distal interphalangeal joint. **(E)** The head of the middle phalanx is delivered into the wound. **(F)** The head of the middle phalanx is resected. **(G)** Closure of the tendon and skin is afforded.

high as 13.4 degrees.[53-55] Hallux abductus interphalangeus is determined by obliquity, the alignment of the articular surface of the head of the proximal phalanx with the longitudinal bisection of the proximal phalanx, asymmetry, the alignment of the articular surface of the base of the distal phalanx with the longitudinal bisection of the distal phalanx; and joint deviation, the angle created by the two articular surfaces of the interphalangeal joint. Abnormality in any one or any combination of these components can create an abnormally high hallux abductus interphalangeus angle. Most often the deformity is secondary to increased asymmetry of the distal phalanx.[53]

## Etiology and Clinical Features

Several etiologies have been described for excessive hallux abductus interphalangeus. Some authors believe that it can be acquired by hypoplasia of the lateral portion of the epiphysis of the distal phalanx.[53,56] This hypoplasia can be secondary to medial pressure on the hallux from shoes or, to placement of an infant in a prone position with knees drawn up and halluces pressed against the ground. Others believe the deformity can result from hyperplasia of the medial portion of the epiphysis of the distal phalanx.[5] Gillett[56] examined 752 feet of neonates 1.5 to 624 hours old, and found that only 8.9 percent had a hallux abductus interphalangeus angle greater than 10 degrees. In a smaller population examined at 14 to 56 days of age, the angle was greater than 10 degrees in 45.8 percent. Gillett believed these results to show that a small portion of this deformity is congenital in nature and that most cases of hallux abductus interphalangeus deformity are acquired early in life, most likely secondary to footwear. Wilkinson[57] found that histologic sections of fetuses had a hallux abductus interphalangeus comparable with that of adults.

Barnett[58] compared British adults, British children, and unshod New Guinea natives. Although the British adults had higher hallux abductus interphalangeus angles than the New Guinea natives, the difference was not statistically significant. Obviously, shoe pressure did not play a role in the hallux abductus interphalangeus of the natives. Additionally, when the children were compared with the adults, no appreciable difference was noted, and the angle did not increase with maturity. Finally, Barnett examined 59 fetuses and found a valgus deviation of the distal phalanx 90 percent of the time. On the basis of these findings he concluded that hallux abductus inter-

phalangeus is normal and congenitally present. The British adults and children both had a mean value of 13 to 14 degrees, and higher values were due to congenital variation.

Hallux abductus interphalangeus has been described in babies with myotonic dystrophy[59] and secondary to a delta phalanx.[60] Price[61] also found a significant relationship between the presence of an os tibiale externum and a high hallux abductus interphalangeus angle but could not explain why.

## Treatment

Younger patients rarely have symptoms associated with a high hallux abductus interphalangeus angle. However, with time irritation over the interphalangeal joint, blisters, and adventitious bursae can develop. Conservative treatment consists of palliative devices, but these may take up room in the shoe and worsen the condition. Surgical intervention will depend upon the age of the patient, the extent of the deformity, and the symptomatology. Tachdjian recommends excision of the medial protuberance and an arrest of the medial half of the epiphyseal plate.[5] If the child is skeletally mature with a severe deformity, he recommends excision of the medial protuberance and fusion of the interphalangeal joint.[5,6]

### Authors' Preferred Treatment

We suggest that the deformity should be identified at its proper level and addressed at that level. For a large angle of obliquity, a distal Akin osteotomy of the proximal phalanx should be performed. The skin incision can be a dorsomedial or a medial longitudinal approach. Dissection is carried through the superficial fascia, with care taken to preserve the neurovascular structures. The deep fascia and periosteum are incised and freed from the proximal phalanx by using a periosteal elevator. The dorsomedial aspect of the distal portion of the proximal phalanx is exposed. A transverse or oblique osteotomy can be performed with an oscillating or sagittal saw and should be placed in the distal aspect of the proximal phalanx, approximately 5 mm proximal to the interphalangeal joint. Care must be taken not to enter the joint, as this could lead to undesired postoperative complications and intra-articular arthritis. The osteotomy should be placed perpendicular to the weight-bearing surface, and if oblique it should run from proximal-medial to distal-lateral. If transverse, the osteotomy is made with the proximal cut perpendicular to the long axis of the proximal phalanx and the distal cut parallel to the joint surface (i.e., the joint surface on the proximal phalangeal head). In either case, the base of the wedge osteotomy should be placed medially, and a lateral apical hinge should be preserved. Once the osteotomy is apposed, it can be fixed with a Kirschner wire, small cortical screw, cerclage wire, or staple placed perpendicular to the osteotomy. The patient can be placed in a wooden shoe postoperatively, and if a percutaneous wire is used, it can be pulled at 4 weeks (Fig. 16-18).

If the deformity is due to asymmetry of the distal phalanx, a closing medially based wedge osteotomy should be performed at the base of the distal phalanx. If possible, it is prudent to wait until the child reaches skeletal maturity. The distal phalanx is a fairly small bone, and it may be difficult to perform the osteotomy and avoid the physis and the nail matrix. The incision is along the medial aspect of the distal hallux. Care is taken to avoid the medial proper digital branches of the medial plantar nerve and medial dorsocutaneous nerve. The deep fascia and periosteum are incised and freed by using a periosteal elevator. Again, care must be taken not to injure the nail matrix or the physis. An oblique or transverse osteotomy is accomplished by using an oscillating or sagittal saw. The osteotomy is placed at the base of the distal phalanx, beginning approximately 2 mm distal to the physeal plate. If oblique in nature, the osteotomy should be oriented from proximal-medial to distal-lateral. If it is transverse, the proximal arm of the osteotomy parallels the articular surface of the distal phalangeal base, and the distal arm is perpendicular to the long axis of the distal phalanx. The osteotomy can be fixed with a 0.045-inch Kirschner wire, small cortical screw, cerclage wire, or staple. With any fixation, care should be taken not to cross the interphalangeal joint. If a nonthreaded Kirschner wire is used, it its acceptable to cross the physis, but if possible this should be avoided.

Finally, in severe deformities, especially those involv-

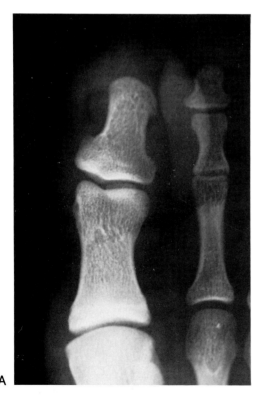
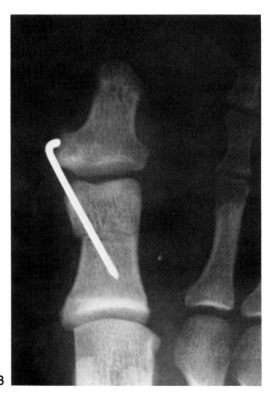

**Fig. 16-18.** Distal Akin osteotomy for congenital hallux abductus interphalangeus deformity. **(A)** Preoperative radiograph. Note the large angle of obliquity. **(B)** Postoperative radiograph. Single Kirschner wire fixation was utilized.

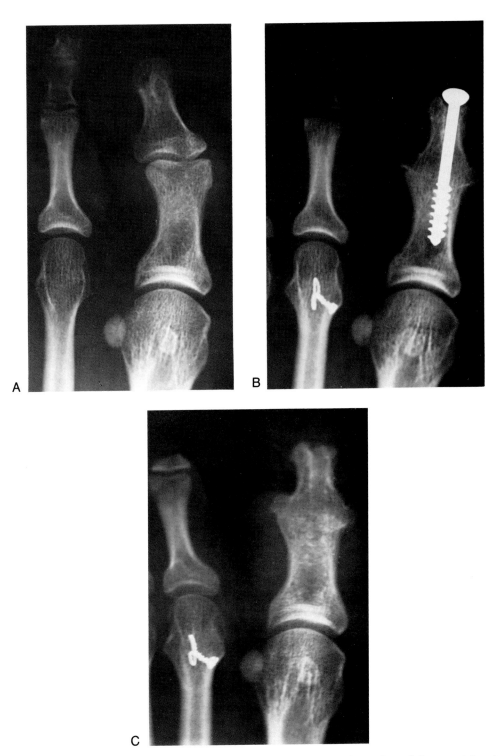

**Fig. 16-19.** Hallux interphalangeal joint arthrodesis for congenital hallux abductus interphalangeus deformity. **(A)** Preoperative radiograph. Note the increase in the angle of joint deviation. **(B)** Postoperative radiograph. Single screw fixation was utilized. **(C)** Long-term follow-up radiograph after screw removal. Patient now 2 years postoperative without recurrence of deformity.

ing an increase in the angle of joint deviation, we advise an arthrodesis of the interphalangeal joint with use of a partially threaded 4-mm screw. It is strongly recommended that the surgeon wait until the patient reaches skeletal maturity before performing this procedure. We use a linear incision over the interphalangeal joint. Dissection is carried down to the extensor hallucis longus; the tendon is transected transversely at the level of the interphalangeal joint; a linear transverse capsulotomy is performed; and the collateral ligaments are incised. The articular surfaces are resected, and the deformity is corrected by wedging the cuts in order to realign the distal and proximal phalanges. A 2-mm drill bit is placed in the base of the distal phalanx and driven distally. A transverse incision is placed at the distal aspect of the hallux where the skin is tented up by the drill bit. Care must be taken here to avoid damage to the nail plate. The 2-mm drill bit is placed in the distal hallux through the distal transverse incision and driven into the proximal phalanx with the two bones aligned. The drill bit should enter the subchondral bone of the base of the proximal phalanx without entering the metatarsophalangeal joint. We do not suggest countersinking the distal phalanx, but a depth gauge is used to determine the length of the screw. A 3.5-mm cancellous tap is placed in the distal aspect of the distal phalanx, and only a few turns are used in the proximal phalanx. A 4-mm partially threaded cancellous screw of appropriate length is driven from distal to proximal and tightened down to provide compression across the arthrodesis site (Fig. 16-19). Alternatively, two crossed Kirschner wires may be used for fixation. Tendon reapproximation and closure are done in a standard fashion.

# INGROWN NAILS
## Etiology

The ingrown nail is a painful deformity that can be seen at any age. The hallux is usually affected, and the medial nail border is most commonly involved. Some authors believed that ingrown nails in infancy could be secondary to a congenital malalignment of the hallux nail. Tax[15] expressed the view that some patients may demonstrate an inherited nail shape and deformity of the nail bed that will predispose the nail to become ingrown. Bailie and Evans[62] also suggested the possibility of an "inherited tendency" of the hallux nail to "grow inwards," which would require a secondary insult to create an ingrown

nail. Barth et al.[63] reported on two sets of monozygotic twins with a congenital malalignment of the hallux nails and stated that this malalignment can lead to an ingrown toenail. They believed these cases to demonstrate a genetic factor in this condition. Lathrop[64] believed that ingrown nails are primarily caused by an inherited abnormal shape of the distal phalanx; if the medial aspect of the distal phalanx is incurving, this could lead to an "unstable system," and an outside pressure, such as that caused by shoes, could then result in an ingrown nail. Hendricks[65] reported on a case that he believed was secondary to intrauterine position. Hammerton and Shrank[66] described a case of ingrown toenails in an infant that was caused by hypertrophy of the lateral nail folds. Ingrown nails can also be caused by outside influences such as tight-fitting shoes and socks and by sleeping prone in infancy.

Honig et al.[67] followed 41 newborns whose hallux nails appeared to be embedded in the distal aspect of the toe. The patients were followed for 12 months. All the nails were normal at 6 months of age, and none of the infants had any symptoms of an ingrown nail. These authors considered this to demonstrate that varying shapes of nails are commonly present at birth.

## Clinical Features

There are several stages to the ingrown nail. Stage 1 is the inflammatory stage, in which the patient will have erythema and edema and will be tender to palpation along the nail fold. This stage is usually treated conservatively with soaks and local topical methods. Stage 2 is the abscess stage, characterized by an increase in the erythema, edema, and dolor. Drainage is usually present and progresses from a serous to a purulent nature. The nail fold can be seen overhanging the nail plate. The patient can usually be managed conservatively, again with soaks, topical agents, and perhaps oral antibiotics; however, more severe cases will need surgical intervention. Stage 3 is the granulation stage, in which drainage is present and the nail fold is covered with granulation tissue. In this stage the patient will usually require some form of surgery to alleviate the symptoms.[52]

## Treatment

Connolly and Fitzgerald[68] treated 61 children for ingrown nails by placing chlorhexidine-soaked cotton wool pledgets underneath the nail edge. This method was successful in 72 percent of the cases. Brereton[69] followed 42 children with a total of 49 ingrown nails that had been treated by excising the nail fold and granulation tissue; he reported an 88 percent success rate. Lovell and Winter[70] advocated an elliptical excision of the nail fold as described in adults by DuVries. Sharrard[2] suggested Zadik's procedure if the deformity is on both sides of the nail. A flap of the posterior nail fold is raised, and the matrix is excised along with the nail.

We recommend a conservative approach when possible. The child should be prevented from sleeping prone and should be placed in open toe shoes. The toe should be soaked in a dilute, warm povidone-iodine or chlorhexidine solution several times a day. Local treatment with topical antibiotics or with chlorhexidine-soaked cotton wool pledgets is used. In the younger child (less than 3 years old), oral antibiotics are also used. If symptoms persist, a partial nail avulsion should be attempted. It should be noted that in young children, because of their small anatomy and inability to remain still, general anesthesia may be necessary. We suggest not attempting a matrixectomy unless there is a recurrence of the ingrown nail. In severe deformities with recurrence, a matrixectomy may become necessary; again, general anesthesia is advised. We further suggest removing only the portion of the matrix that is involved and preserving the nail if possible. In small children magnification loops may assist with the small anatomy. Caution must be used not to damage the matrix of the distal phalanx.

# REFERENCES

## Underlapping Toes

1. Trethowan WH: Treatment of hammertoe. Lancet I:1257, 1925
2. Sharrard WJW: Paediatric Orthopaedics and Fractures. 2nd Ed., Blackwell Scientific Publications, Oxford, 1971, pp. 295, 567, 1480
3. Sharrard WJW: The surgery of deformed toes in children. Br J Clin Pract 17:263, 1963
4. Tachdjian MO: Congenital deformities. p. 639. In Jahss MH (ed): Disorders of the Foot and Ankle. 2nd Ed. Vol. 1. WB Saunders, Philadelphia, 1991
5. Tachdjian MO: Pediatric Orthopedics. Vol 2. WB Saunders, Philadelphia, 1972, p. 1410
6. Tachdjian MO: The Child's Foot. WB Saunders, Philadelphia, 1985, p. 335
7. Sweetnam R: Congenital curly toes. Lancet 8:398, 1958
8. Turner P: Strapping of curly toes in children. Aust N Z J Surg 57:467, 1987
9. Ross E, Menelaus M: Open flexor tenotomy for hammer toes and curly toes in children. J Bone Joint Surg [Br] 66:770, 1984
10. Greenberg H: Plantar digital tenotomy for underlapping and contracted toes. J Am Podiatr Med Assoc 56:65, 1966
11. Pollard J, Morrison P: Flexor tenotomy in the treatment of curly toes. Proc R Soc Med 68:480, 1975
12. Kelikian H, Clayton L, Loseff H: Surgical syndactylia of the toes. Clin Orthop 19:208, 1961
13. Friend G: Correction of enlongated underlapping lesser toes by middle phalangectomy and skin plasty. J Foot Surg 23:470, 1984
14. Korn SH: The lazy S approach for correction of painful underlapping fifth digit. J Am Podiatr Med Assoc 70:30, 1980

## Overlapping Toes

15. Tax H: Podopediatrics. 2nd Ed. Williams & Wilkins, Baltimore, 1980, pp. 286, 306
16. Suppan R: Surgery for congenital deformities of the feet. Clin Podiatr Med Surg 1:667, 1984
17. Lantzounis LA: Congenital subluxation of the fifth toe and its correction by a periosteocapsuloplasty and tendon transplantation. J Bone Joint Surg 72:147, 1940
18. Dobbs B: Arthroplasty of the fifth digit. Clin Podiatr Med Surg 3:29, 1986
19. Jordan R, Caselli M: Overlapping deformity of the digits in the pediatric patient: a conservative approach to treatment. J Am Podiatr Med Assoc 68:503, 1978
20. Cockin J: Butler's operation for an over-riding fifth toe. J Bone Joint Surg 50[Br]:78, 1968
21. Black M, Grogan D, Bobechko W: Butler arthroplasty for correction of the adducted fifth toe: a retrospective study of 36 operations between 1968 and 1982. J Pediatr Orthop 5:439, 1985
22. Wilson JN: V-Y correction for varus deformity of the fifth toe. Br J Surg 41:133, 1953
23. Paton R: V-Y plasty for correction of varus fifth toe. J Pediatr Orthop 10:248, 1990
24. Goodwin F, Swisher F: The treatment of congenital hyperextension of the fifth toe. J Bone Joint Surg 25:193, 1943
25. Leonard M, Rising E: Syndactylization to maintain correction of overlapping fifth toe. Clin Orthop 43:241, 1965
26. Scrase WH: The treatment of dorsal adduction deformities of the fifth toe. J Bone Joint Surg [Br] 36:146, 1954
27. Coughlin MJ, Mann RA: Lesser toe deformities. p. 132. In Mann RA (ed): Surgery of the foot. 5th Ed. CV Mosby, St. Louis, 1986
28. Lapidus P: Transplantation of the extensor tendon for correction of the overlapping fifth toe. J Bone Joint Surg 24:555, 1942
29. Rosner M, Knudsen H, Sharon S: Overlapping fifth toe: a new surgical approach. J Foot Surg 17:67, 1978

30. Kaplan E: A new approach to the surgical correction of overlapping toes. J Foot Surg 3:24, 1964
31. Anderson B: Combination surgery for overlapping fifth digit. J Am Podiatr Med Assoc 61:137, 1971
32. Janecki C, Wilde A: Results of phalangectomy of the fifth toe for hammertoe. J Bone Joint Surg [Am] 58:1005, 1976

## Digital Contractures

33. Lapidus P: Operation for correction of hammertoe. J Bone Joint Surg 21:977, 1939
34. Myerson M, Shereff M: The pathological anatomy of claw and hammer toes. J Bone Joint Surg [Am] 71:45, 1989
35. Taylor RG: The treatment of claw toes by multiple transfers of flexor into extensor tendons. J Bone Joint Surg 33B:539, 1951
36. Pyper JB: The flexor-extensor transplant operation for claw toes. J Bone Joint Surg 40B:528, 1958
37. Bouchard JL: Congenital deformities of the forefoot. p. 590. In McGlamry ED (ed): Comprehensive Textbook of Foot Surgery. Williams and Wilkins, Baltimore, 1987
38. Sgarlato TE: Transplantation of the flexor digitorum longus muscle tendon in hammer toes. J Am Podiatr Med Assoc 60:383, 1970
39. Parrish TF: Dynamic correction of clawtoes. Orthop Clin North Am 4:97, 1973
40. Marcinko D, Lazerson A, Dollard M, Schwartz N: Flexor digitorum longus tendon transfer, a simplified technique. J Am Podiatr Med Assoc 74:380, 1984
41. Barbari SG, Brevig K: Correction of clawtoes by the Girdlestone-Taylor flexor-extensor transfer procedure. Foot Ankle 5:67, 1984
42. Kuwada GT, Dockery GL: Modification of the flexor tendon transfer procedure for the correction of flexible hammertoes. J Foot Surg 19:38, 1980
43. Frank G, Johnson W: The extensor shift procedure in the correction of claw toe deformities in children. South Med J 59:889, 1966
44. Post AC: Hallux valgus with displacement of the smaller toes. Med Rec 22:120, 1882
45. Soule RE: Operation for the cure of hammer toe. N Y State J Med 649, 1910
46. O'Neill BJ: Arthroplastic operation for hammer toe. JAMA 57:1207, 1911
47. Lambrinudi C: An operation for claw-toes. Proc R Soc Med 21:239, 1927
48. Higgs SL: Hammer-toe. Med Press 131:473, 1931
49. Young CS: An operation for the correction of hammer-toe and claw-toe. J Bone Joint Surg 20:715, 1938
50. Taylor RG: An operative procedure for the treatment of hammer-toe and claw-toe. J Bone Joint Surg 22:608, 1940
51. Selig S: Hammer-toe: a new procedure for its correction. Surg Gynecol Obstet 72:101, 1941

52. Crenshaw A (ed): Campbell's Operative Orthopaedics. 7th Ed. Vol. 2. CV Mosby, St. Louis, 1987, p. 923.

## Hallux Abductus Interphalangeus

53. Sorto L, Balding M, Weil L, Smith S: Hallux abductus interphalangeus: etiology, x-ray evaluation and treatment. J Am Podiatr Med Assoc 66:384, 1976
54. Palladino SJ: Inoperative evaluation of the bunion patient: etiology, biomechanics, clinical and radiographic assessment. p 1. In Gerbert J (ed): Textbook of Bunion Surgery. 2nd Ed. Futura Publishing Co., Mount Kisco, NY 1991
55. Weissman S: Radiology of the Foot. Williams & Wilkins, Baltimore, 1983, p. 55
56. Gillet H: Ungual phalanx valgus: survey of neonatal feet. J Am Podiatr Med Assoc 68:83, 1978
57. Wilkinson J: The terminal phalanx of the great toe. J Anat 88:537, 1954
58. Barnett C: Valgus deviation of the distal phalanx of the great toe. J Anat 96:171, 1962
59. Ray S, Bowen R, Marks H: Foot deformity in myotonic dystrophy. Foot Ankle 5:125, 1984
60. Neil M, Conacher C: Bilateral delta phalanx of the proximal phalanges of the great toes: a report on an affected family. J Bone Joint Surg [Br] 66:77, 1984
61. Price G: Metatarsus primus varus: including various clinicoradiologic features of the female foot. Clin Orthop 145:217, 1979

## Ingrown Nails

62. Bailie F, Evans D: Ingrowing toenails in infancy. Br Med J 9:737, 1978
63. Barth J, Dawber R, Ashton R, Baran R: Congenital malalignment of great toenails in two sets of monozygotic twins. Arch Dermatol 122:379, 1986
64. Lathrop R: Ingrowing toenails: causes and treatment. Cutis 20:119, 1977
65. Hendricks W: Congenital ingrown toenails. Cutis 24:393, 1979
66. Hammerton M, Shrank A: Congenital hypertrophy of the lateral nail folds of the hallux. Pediatr Dermatol 5:243, 1986
67. Honig P, Spitzer A, Bernstein R, Leyden J: Congenital ingrown toenails. Clin Pediatr (Phila) 21:424, 1982
68. Connolly B, Fitzgerald R: Pledgets in ingrowing toenails: clinical significance. Arch Dis Child 63:71, 1988
69. Brereton R: Simple old surgery for juvenile embedded toenails. Z Kinderchir 30:258, 1980
70. Lovell W, Winter R: Pediatric Orthopaedics. JB Lippincott, Philadelphia, 1986, pp. 967, 979

# SUGGESTED READINGS

Buggiani F, Biggs E: Mallet toe. J Am Podiatr Med Assoc 66:321, 1976

Burns A: Digital arthroplasty. Clin Podiatr Med Surg 3:11, 1986

Coughlin M: Lesser toe deformities. Orthopedics 10:63, 1987

Lloyd-Davies R, Brill G: The aetiology and out-patient management of ingrowing toenails. Br J Surg 50:592, 1963

Ely L: Hammertoe. Surg Clin North Am 6:433, 1926

Johnson C, Hugar D: A literature review of congenital digiti quinti varus: clinical description and treatment. J Foot Surg 22:116, 1983

Knecht JG: Pathomechanical deformities of the lesser toes. J Am Podiatr Med Assoc 64:941, 1974

Lapidus P: The ingrown toenail. Bull Hosp Jt Dis Orthop Inst Dis 33:181, 1972

Margo M: Surgical treatment of conditions of the fore part of the foot. J Bone Joint Surg [Am] 49:1665, 1967

Murray W: Onychocryptosis. Clin Orthop 142:96, 1979

Scott P: Ingrown toe-nails. Med J Aust 1:47, 1968

Sokoloff H: Soft tissue digital procedures. Clin Podiatr Med Surg 3:23, 1986

Sorto L: Surgical correction of hammertoes: a 5-year postoperative study. J Am Podiatr Med Assoc 64:930, 1974

Thompson T: Surgical treatment of disorders of the fore part of the foot. J Bone Joint Surg [Am] 46:1117, 1964

Turan I: Deformities of the smaller toes and surgical treatment. J Foot Surg 29:176, 1990

# 17

# Miscellaneous Developmental Disorders

*LOUIS J. CAPUTO*

## HAGLUND'S DISEASE

Posterior heel pain may have several etiologies. One frequently encountered in the adolescent population is the so-called pump-bump or Haglund's deformity (Fig. 17-1). The term *Haglund's deformity* or *disease* was first coined in 1948 by Hohman.[1] Patrick Haglund in 1928 was the first to describe the relationship between posterior heel discomfort associated with wearing tight, stiff shoe counters and the various shapes of the posterosuperior aspect of the calcaneus.[2] The entities of Achilles tendon bursitis and retrocalcaneal bursitis were also described in 1928 by Haglund as being associated with the prominent posterosuperior surface of the calcaneus. Today, some consider the triad of retrocalcaneal bursitis, superficial Achilles tendon bursitis, and Achilles tendon thickening in the presence of a prominent posterosuperior process of the calcaneus to be pathognomic of Haglund's disease.[3,4] This condition is seen most frequently in the adolescent; however, it may also be seen in the adult patient. Females are more commonly affected.[3,5,6]

It is apparent that certain anatomic configurations of the posterosuperior aspect of the calcaneus, or the entire foot in general, have a direct influence on the genesis of symptoms.[1-18] Root et al. have noted that compensated rearfoot varus, compensated forefoot valgus, and rigid plantar-flexed first rays are common foot types associated with Haglund's disease.[19] These entities frequently involve excessive frontal plane motion of the posterior calcaneus against the shoe counter, contributing to the irritation and inflammation. Posterior cavus, cavovarus, and calcaneal varus deformities also expose the posterosuperior portion of the calcaneus to the irritative influence of the shoe counter.[14,18,19]

Variations of the posterior aspect of the calcaneus are seen in Figure 17-2. Note the bone and soft tissue relationships of the Achilles tendon and the posterior portion of the calcaneus, known as the bursal projection. Figure 17-3 shows the relationships of the calcaneus to the surrounding anatomic soft tissue landmarks. The superficial Achilles tendon bursa, the retrocalcaneal bursa, and the Achilles tendon are the structures predominantly responsible for the symptoms associated with Haglund's disease. Some authors note that the superficial Achilles tendon bursa is observed in approximately 50 percent of the presenting cases and feel that it is adventitious in nature.[10,18]

Fowler and Philip categorized their patients into two groups: (1) those whose symptoms responded completely to excision of the superficial Achilles tendon bursa; and (2) those in which the superficial Achilles tendon bursa was not definable and therefore not excisable.[5] In the latter group dense, thickened tissue was noted superficially at the time of surgery. This group was not relieved by excision of this dense thickened tissue, and their symptoms would frequently return. Attention was directed toward the underlying bony structure in the latter group.

### Radiographic Evaluation

Fowler and Philip made an effort to identify and quantify the degree of osseous deformity of the calcaneus.[5] Cadaveric calcanei were measured, and specific angular

439

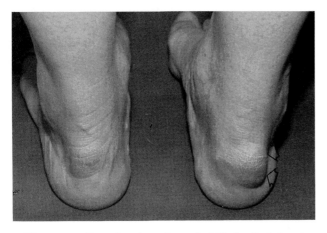

**Fig. 17-1.** Posterior view of a typical Haglund's deformity. Note the thickening of the Achilles tendon and the inverted attitude of the calcaneus.

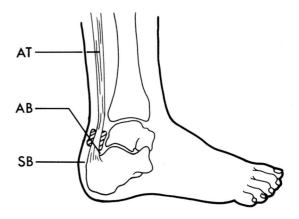

**Fig. 17-3.** Note the relationships of the calcaneus to the surrounding anatomic landmarks: Superficial Achilles tendon bursa, (SB); Retrocalcaneal Achilles bursa, (AB); Achilles tendon (AT). These are the structures predominantly responsible for the symptoms associated with Haglund's disease.

relationships were assessed and considered to be essential when evaluating Haglund's deformity. This is widely known as Fowler and Philip's angle (Fig. 17-4), formed by the intersection of a line drawn parallel to the plantar calcaneus with a line drawn parallel to the most posterior portion of the posterior surface of the calcaneus. Fowler and Philip identified a normal range of 44 to 69 degrees based upon examination of 45 specimens. Specimens with angles measuring more than 69 degrees were considered clinically significant. Notari and Mittler have measured radiographs of patients and concluded that 65 degrees is the upper limit of normal.[12] Fowler and Philip believe that when this angle exceeds 75 degrees in the clinically symptomatic patient, then surgical intervention is indicated. Fuglsang and Torup identified 29 patients with Haglund's deformity, 25 of whom had angles smaller than or equal to 75 degrees.[9]

Pavlov et al. noted the relationship between the osseous plantar projections of the calcaneus and the prominence of the calcaneal bursal projection.[4] They used a system of parallel pitch lines (PPLs) to evaluate the prominence of the bursal projection (Fig. 17-5). These lines are constructed by drawing a line from the anterior tuberosity of the calcaneus tangent to the medial posterior tuberosity, which is similar to drawing the

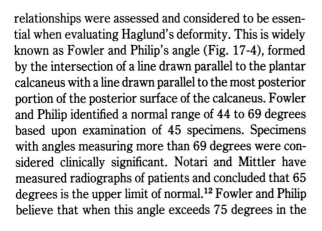

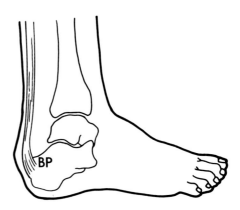

**Fig. 17-2.** Note the bone and soft tissue relationships of the Achilles tendon and the posterior portion of the calcaneus, known as the bursal projection (BP).

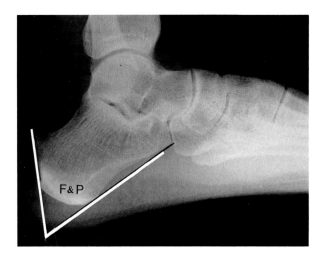

**Fig. 17-4.** Fowler and Philip's angle formed by the intersection of a line drawn parallel to the plantar calcaneus with a line drawn parallel to the most posterior portion of the posterior surface of the calcaneus. Fowler and Philip identified a normal range of 44 to 69 degrees in 45 specimens.

superior axis of the calcaneal inclination angle. A line is then drawn perpendicular to the most posterior portion of the talar articular facet. From this point an additional

line is drawn parallel to the first in a posterior direction. Osseous bursal projections above this line are considered positive (PPL-positive), and those below it are considered negative (PPL-negative). Pavlov et al. then characterized Haglund's syndrome radiographically as follows: (1) retrocalcaneal bursitis, seen as the loss of lucency of the retrocalcaneal recess between the Achilles tendon and the bursal projection; (2) Achilles tendonitis, seen in a lateral radiographic view as a greater than 9-mm anteroposterior width of the Achilles tendon at a point 2 cm above the bursal projection; (3) superficial Achilles tendon bursitis, seen as a convexity of the soft tissue posterior to the Achilles tendon insertion; (4) a cortically intact but prominent bursal projection (PPL-positive).

Vega et al. suggested that a total value of the Fowler and Philip angle and the calcaneal inclination angle that is greater than 90 degrees is clinically significant.[20] They also pointed out that the "total angle gives a better indication of the severity of deformity." Vega et al. correctly stated that the clinical severity depends upon the type of footwear worn in combination with the anatomic abnormality. Ruch also pointed to the additive influence of the calcaneal inclination angle upon the overall evaluation of Haglund's deformity.[14]

Burhenne and Connell in 1986 suggested a role for xeroradiography in the diagnostic evaluation of Hag-

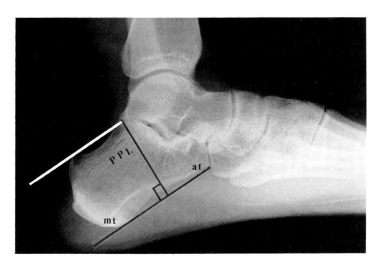

**Fig. 17-5.** Representation of the parallel pitch line (PPL) method of radiographic interpretation of Haglund's deformity, proposed by Pavlov and Henegan. Bursal projections identified as "B" on this radiograph that fall below the superior parallel pitch line are considered negative, as in this case. Bursal projections extending above the superior PPL are considered positive and characteristic of Haglund's syndrome. at, anterior tuberosity calcaneus; mt, medial posterior tuberosity calcaneus.

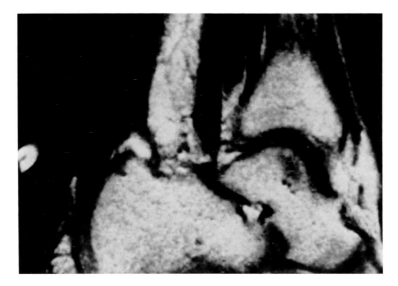

**Fig. 17-6.** MRI can be helpful in distinguishing between chronic Achilles tendonitis and bursitis. (Courtesy of Joan Oloff, D.P.M.)

lund's deformity.[8] Magnetic resonance imaging (MRI) also may be of considerable value in evaluating the degree of soft tissue inflammation of the posterior heel structures (Fig. 17-6).

## Clinical Features

The clinical diagnosis of Haglund's disease generally presents little difficulty. Palpable tenderness in the region of the posterosuperior process of the calcaneus, localized edema, localized erythema, inability to tolerate hard-countered enclosed shoes, and blistering and induration of the skin with bouts of Achilles tendonitis or peritendonitis are common findings (Fig. 17-1). An enlarged posterosuperior process of the calcaneus is easily palpated. Plantar flexion or dorsiflexion of the ankle may exacerbate symptoms when the condition is acute. Dorsiflexion of the ankle with inversion of the subtalar joint facilitates observation of the bursal projection of the calcaneus. Some authors have noted a seasonal incidence; in particular, colder climates are more likely to promote symptoms.[5] This appears to be related to the likelihood that irritation from enclosed shoes and boots is increasing the cumulative mechanical trauma rather than to any direct environmental or temperature effect.[20]

Although diagnosis usually presents little difficulty, the differential diagnoses should include primary Achilles tendonitis, retrocalcaneal traction exostosis (Fig. 17-7), and systemic arthropathies, (e.g., juvenile rheumatoid arthritis or Reiter's syndrome).[4] Pavlov et al. have noted that the pump bump is more diffuse and is more posterior to the Achilles tendon insertion when associated with systemic inflammatory disorders. The cortex of the bursal projection can be eroded, and when erosion is present radiographically, it is diagnostic of a systemic inflammatory articular process rather than of a traumatic process.[15] Other differential diagnostic considerations include osteomyelitis of the calcaneus and localized bone lesions. Correlation with other systemic findings and appropriate use of diagnostic laboratory data will generally help distinguish any of these entities from Haglund's disease.

## Treatment

Nonoperative treatment of Haglund's deformity is directed at eliminating the irritating shear forces and reducing the inflammation associated with the bursitis or tendonitis. Forefoot and hindfoot biomechanical control can eliminate excessive frontal plane shearing forces on the heel counter.[19,20] Functional foot orthoses or appropriate shoe wedging can be helpful. Heel lifts or wedges can elevate the bony prominence away from the shoe counter.[3] Intermittent use of open-backed shoes may

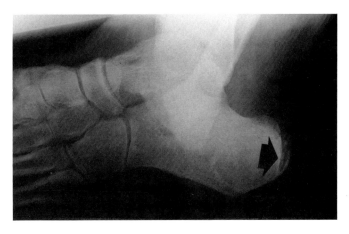

**Fig. 17-7.** The arrow points to the area of a traction exostosis of the calcaneus, which must not be confused with Haglund's syndrome.

help control symptoms. Heneghan and Pavlov have nicely shown the influence of the calcaneal inclination angle on the prominence of the bursal projection.[3] It was further shown that heel elevation decreases the functional calcaneal inclination angle and thereby reduces the prominence of the bursal projection and helps to control symptoms.[3,14] Acute symptoms may be controlled with local anti-inflammatory measures such as ice, elevation, and rest. Nonsteroidal anti-inflammatory medications provide a useful adjunct in symptom control. Local corticosteroid injection should be used judiciously and accurately to avoid steroid-induced tendon rupture. In severe cases immobilization may be necessary.

### Surgical Technique

Surgical treatment is indicated when symptoms are resistant to nonoperative treatment. As early as 1929 Saxl advised resection of the prominent posterosuperior portion of the calcaneus to eliminate the posterior shearing forces.[15] Retrocalcaneal ostectomy should not be performed prior to closure of the calcaneal apophysis since it may lead to regeneration of the deformity.[21,22]

Many approaches have been advocated.[15,18,20,22] A simple, time-honored approach is as follows. An approximately 5-cm linear incision is made parallel to the anterolateral border of the Achilles tendon directly over the lateral prominence of Haglund's bump. The incision is carried directly to bone without elevating skin flaps in order to preserve maximum blood supply to the skin and avoid skin slough. Posterior skin flap elevation superior to the Achilles tendon may be necessary if excision of a

superficial Achilles tendon bursa is performed. The posterosuperior portion of the calcaneus is exposed subperiosteally, and the retrocalcaneal bursa is excised if present. The Achilles tendon should be carefully retracted and protected from mechanical trauma in order to avoid postoperative Achilles tendonitis. A generous portion of the posterosuperior calcaneus is resected from lateral to medial with an osteotome or oscillating saw and smoothly remodeled with a power burr. Care should be taken to maintain as much hemostasis as possible. A small drain may be necessary. The wound is closed in two layers.

Postoperative care should involve an immediate period of rest and immobilization. In most cases partial reflection of the Achilles tendon is required for adequate exposure. It is therefore essential to limit excessive motion in this area to avoid inadvertent complete detachment. Achilles tendonitis is not infrequently seen postoperatively, but it can be substantially reduced as a postoperative complication if immobilization is used. Generally, 3 to 6 weeks' use of a short leg cast or posterior splint is required. Surgical approaches in this area of the foot are notorious for their tendency toward dehiscence. Immediate postoperative splinting reduces mechanical stress on the incision and further reduces the possibility of dehiscence. Postoperative sural neuritis is not infrequently encountered if tissue handling is aggressive or if sharp, self-retaining retractors are used without adequate protection of the sural nerve. Physical therapy may prove beneficial after the immediate immobilization period. Most patients will begin a graduated activity program after 6 to 8 weeks.

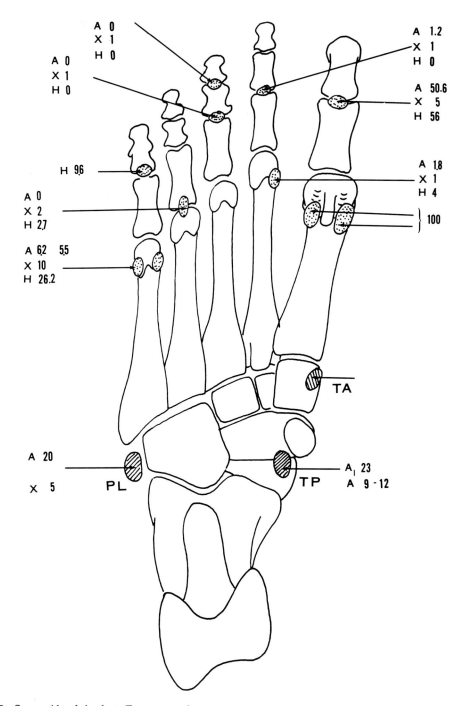

**Fig. 17-8.** Sesamoids of the foot. Frequency of occurrence as a percentage, based on anatomic investigation, A; radiographic investigation, X; histoembryologic investigation, H. TA, tibialis anterior; TP, tibialis posterior; PL, peroneus longus. (From Sarrafian,[23] with permission.)

## INFLAMMATORY DISORDERS AND INJURIES OF ACCESSORY AND SESAMOID BONES OF THE FOOT

The accessory bones, as compared with the sesamoid bones, of the foot represent true anomalous structures. Accessory bones are separations or subdivisions of ordinary bones, whereas the sesamoid bones, according to Sarrafian,[23] are always present in the same location. The distinction is that sesamoid bones are not separations or subdivisions of regularly recognized tarsal structures but develop as independent anatomic structures in utero.[23]

## The Sesamoid Bones

The sesamoid bones are small, oval, or round bones deriving their name from sesame seeds. They are usually found embedded within tendons. Some sesamoids always ossify whereas others remain cartilaginous or fibrocartilaginous for life. The radiolucency of the cartilaginous or fibrocartilaginous sesamoid bones accounts for the discrepancies encountered in studies reporting the frequency of occurrence of a given sesamoid.[24] Figure 17-8 shows various locations of a sesamoid bone on the foot, with frequency of occurrence (in percent) based upon anatomic, radiographic, and histioembryologic investigations.

### The Sesamoids of the Great Toe

Ossification of the sesamoids of the great toe generally takes place about the eighth or ninth year.[24] Congenital divisions or partitions are frequently seen (Fig. 17-9). Kewenter reported approximately 37 percent of males and 30 percent of females to have sesamoidal partitions.[25] The medial sesamoid of the first metatarsophalangeal joint is usually larger than the lateral.[23] From a clinical standpoint elicitation of pain directly inferior to the first metatarsophalangeal joint should alert the clinician to consider a set of unique clinical entities.[26-28] Os-

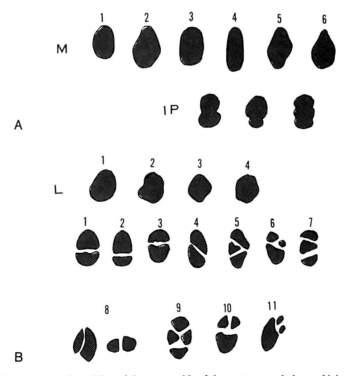

**Fig. 17-9.** Variations in contour and partition of the sesamoids of the metatarsophalangeal joint of the big toe. **(A)** M, medial sesamoid; L, lateral sesamoid. IP, intermediary partite; **(B)** Partite sesamoids. (Reprinted from Sarrafian,[23] with permission.)

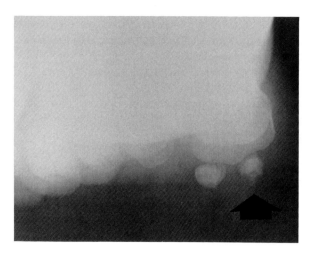

**Fig. 17-10.** The arrow indicates the area of typical sesamoidal fracture involving the medial sesamoid bone of the first metatarsophalangeal joint.

teochondritis of the sesamoid bones has been reported[28-30] and will be discussed in the section on the osteochondroses. It is important to delineate and rule out the normal congenital division often seen with the sesamoid bones of the first metatarsophalangeal joint when considering a diagnosis of osteochondrosis or fracture. Normal divisions can be oriented transversely or obliquely.[23,24] Generally, smooth contours remain be-

tween the fragments, in congenital divisions, helping to rule out fractures, which usually demonstrate rough irregular surfaces between divisions.

Fractures of the sesamoid bones may result from either direct trauma or chronic stress.[28,31] The former is most commonly seen. Falls directly onto the forefoot or other high-impact activities such as dancing or jogging may produce sesamoidal fractures of the great toe.[27] The medial sesamoid frequently has been described as being more susceptible to this type of injury; however, it has been my experience that either sesamoid bone is equally susceptible.[32] The symptoms are usually noted immediately, but occasionally they may be sufficiently low-grade to be ignored for weeks prior to professional attention. Diagnosis is usually aided by direct palpation of the injured bone. Dorsiflexion of the great toe accompanied by plantar palpation of the area usually reproduces symptoms. Standard radiographs should be supplemented with axial views to give the best visualization (Fig. 17-10). Occasionally, bone scans may be required, although specificity is lacking (Fig. 17-11).

Treatment should be directed toward immobilization and accommodation of the affected area.[28,33,34] Rigid immobilization is generally required for 3 to 6 weeks.[28] Follow-up radiographs may help identify callus development. Owing to the relative lack of vascular perfusion of these structures, lack of bone callus development in this region should not deter continued use of immobilization

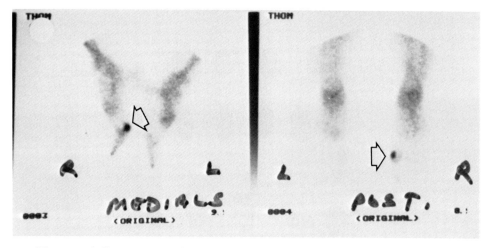

**Fig. 17-11.** The arrow indicates an area of increased radionuclide uptake consistent with a positive bone scan for sesamoidal fracture. A similar presentation may be seen in osteonecrosis of the sesamoid bones.

as a method of conservative treatment. Asymptomatic nonunion does occur in this region and should be considered a satisfactory result. Only in the most persistently symptomatic cases should excision be considered. In my opinion a 3- to 6-month trial of conservative care is not unreasonable.

### Interphalangeal Sesamoid Bone of the Great Toe

The interphalangeal sesamoid bone of the great toe is a small, generally innocuous structure located within the ligamentotendinous structures of the plantar aspect of the interphalangeal joint of the great toe. Generally solitary, its motion follows that of the distal phalanx. Radiographic studies have reported its occurrence as 5 percent, but anatomic dissection studies show a 50 percent occurrence rate.[35] This structure can cause significant discomfort when associated with hypertrophy and plantar callus development. Hyperextension deformities of the interphalangeal joint of the great toe may subject the plantar skin of the hallux to excessive shear force, as can seen in cases of hallux limitus with compensatory interphalangeal joint dorsiflexion.[36] In these cases effort

should be directed toward eliminating the compensatory extension in order to reduce the shearing stress. Functional orthoses or devices aimed at eliminating the etiology of the hallux limitus deformity may provide adequate conservative therapy.[33] In cases unresponsive to conservative care, excision of the interphalangeal sesamoid generally affords adequate control of symptoms. Surgical approaches may be either midline, medial, or lateral to the interphalangeal sesamoid bone. Excision is generally simple; however, caution is advised in order to avoid laceration of the flexor hallucis longus tendon, which may lie immediately adjacent to the interphalangeal sesamoid. Similarly, caution is advised when making medial or lateral approaches in order to avoid neurovascular injury. Postoperatively, recovery is generally uneventful with protected weight-bearing and surgical shoes required for approximately 1 to 3 weeks.

### Sesamoid Bones of the Lesser Metatarsophalangeal Joints

Sesamoid bones of the lesser metatarsophalangeal joints are rare; medial and lateral sesamoid bones being generally seen only at the fifth metatarsophalangeal joint (Fig.

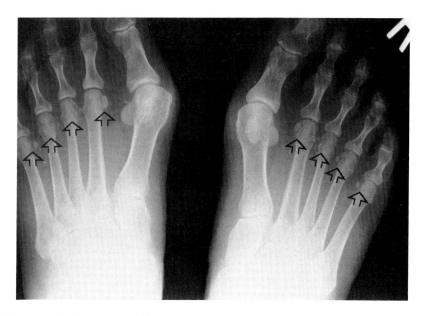

**Fig. 17-12.** The arrows indicate sesamoid bones of the lesser metatarsophalangeal joint. Note the solitary bones of the central metatarsophalangeal joints, with medial and lateral sesamoid bones accompanying the first and fifth metatarsophalangeal joints.

17-12). If these ossicles do occur at the central metatar-sophalangeal joints, generally only one is present. These sesamoid bones are of little clinical significance; however, isolated cases of avascular necrosis have been reported.[37]

### Sesamoid of the Peroneus Longus Tendon

The sesamoid of the peroneus longus tendon is sometimes referred to as the *os peroneum*. This structure is located in the substance of the peroneus longus tendon, usually at the level of the cuboid groove.[23,38] Some believe that this structure is always anatomically present[23] (Fig. 17-13), but radiographic indication of its presence is dependent upon its state of ossification (it is fully ossified in only approximately 5 percent of cases). This structure is usually round and solitary; however, segmental or fragmented ossicles have been described.[24] Fractures of this bone, with associated ruptures of the peroneus longus tendon, have been reported.[39,40] A supinatory force is generally responsible. Burman has speculated that this structure can be responsible for a pain syndrome seen in this region.[24] He describes patients with sharp pain at the lateral portion of the foot, which often radiates up along the peroneal musculature. Manipulation of the foot into varus will produce symptoms in the region of the ossicle. The acute stage is followed by a variably dull discomfort localized to the region of the ossicle. Foot strappings and physical ther-apy have been reported to provide relief. Japiot believed that an inflammation of the os peroneum may produce symptoms in the adolescent population.[41] Palpable pain in this region, with or without radiographic evidence of the os peroneum, should be treated conservatively in the adolescent population, but persistently painful traumatic injuries of this region may warrant excision of this structure.[38,42,43]

## Accessory Bones

Accessory bones are considered true developmental anomalies. Division or separation of the main ossification center is thought to be responsible for their appearance.[23] Some authors use the term "inconstant bones."[24] A detailed anatomic or ontologic discussion is beyond the scope of this text; however, it is interesting to note that many of these inconstant or accessory bones in humans are consistently found in comparative anatomic studies of lower mammals.

### Os Trigonum

The os trigonum is an osseous structure located at the posterolateral process of the talus (Fig. 17-14). The cartilaginous anlage is noted intrauterinely at 2 months.[23] It tends to ossify in about the eighth or ninth year.[24] Sarrafian reports its occurrence as 1.7 to 7.7 percent.[23] The os trigonum articulates with the posterolateral tubercle of

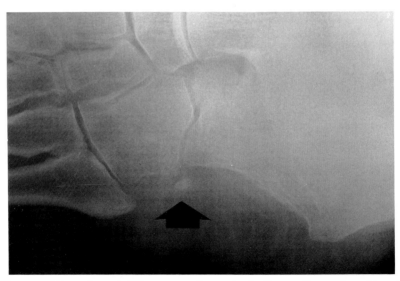

**Fig. 17-13.** This sesamoid bone (arrow) of the peroneus longus tendon is sometimes referred to as the *os peroneum*.

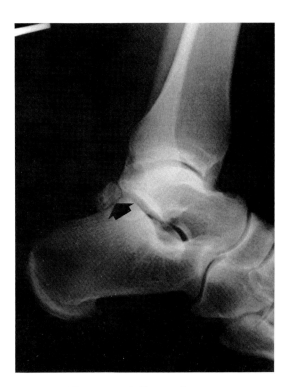

**Fig. 17-14.** The arrow indicates the osseous structure known as the *os trigonum*. It is present in 1.7 to 7.7 percent of cases, and the structure tends to ossify at about the eighth or ninth year.

the talus by fibrous, fibrocartilaginous, or cartilaginous tissue. When fused to the body of the talus, it is referred to as the *trigonal process*.[23] This bone is more often found bilaterally, but it is found unilaterally often enough to make asymmetry clinically unimportant. It is not unusual for a large os trigonum to abut on the posterior lip of the tibia.

Os trigonum fractures are rare; however, the fact that bipartite or multipartite os trigonum is rare is clinically important, and such a finding, along with a significant history of trauma, should raise one's index of suspicion of fracture. Fracture of the posterior process of the talus is a more commonly seen clinical entity. It is briefly discussed here in order to draw attention to its presence and to differentiate it from fracture of the free os trigonum. Injuries involving forced plantar flexion can lead to impingement of a large posterior talar process. Fractures of the corresponding posterior lip of the tibia are also seen. Forced dorsiflexion can also produce fracture of the posterolateral process of the talus.[44,45] This mech-

anism of injury can also detach a partially fused os trigonum. Torsional strain associated with dorsiflexion of the ankle stresses the attachment of the posterior talofibular ligament to the posterolateral process of the talus and produces the characteristic separation or fracture. Finally, crush injuries of the os calcis can literally pinch off the os trigonum between the tibia and the calcaneus.

*Clinical Features*

Clinically, fracture of the posterolateral process can be diagnosed by attempting to flex and extend the great toe. Flexion and extension of the great toe produces motion of the flexor hallucis longus tendon, which is located between the medial and lateral posterior tubercles of the talus and lies adjacent to the os trigonum. Local signs of palpable tenderness and/or crepitus directly over the os trigonum or the posterolateral process of the talus are also common. The position of comfort of the ankle is generally plantar flexion. Radiographic evidence of irregular edges of the bony fragments with reduction of Kager's space is also noted. Radionuclear studies can be valuable. Johnson et al. described three patients with posterolateral ankle pain in whom technetium 99 radionuclide studies showed focal uptake consistent with fracture of this region.[44] Excision of the fragment was ultimately required in two of the patients, with excellent outcomes. The third patient finally progressed to an asymptomatic nonunion with treatment by immobilization and local anti-inflammatory measures.

**Accessory Navicular Bone**

The accessory navicular bone is perhaps the accessory bone most likely to produce functional disturbances that are noted with any regularity in clinical practice.[24,29,36,46-56] A radiographic incidence ranging from 2 to 12 percent has been recorded.[23] The accessory navicular bone is also referred to in the literature as the *os tibialae externum* (Fig. 17-15).

Three types of accessory naviculars have been described.[48] Type I is the true sesamoid of the tibialis posterior. Type II is a true secondary ossification center, which ultimately forms a synchondrosis with the main body of the navicular bone. Type III, described as the *cornate navicular,* is thought to represent the end stage of the type II navicular. This may be considered a synostosis with a variably sized osseous bridge. Lawson notes that at skeletal maturity the accessory center of the type

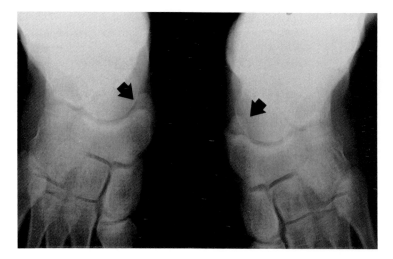

**Fig. 17-15.** The arrows indicate bilateral accessory navicular bones.

III navicular usually fuses with the navicular body to form a curvilinear bone.[49] This process is generally asymptomatic and is usually an incidental radiographic finding. Lawson points out that the type II pattern is generally the symptomatic pattern. The fibrocartilaginous bridging is generally the region of symptoms and this is usually seen in the active adolescent.[49]

### Clinical Features

Clinically, irritation of the overlying skin with adventitious bursa formation may be present. Tibialis posterior tendinitis is a frequent finding. Palpable tenderness may be noted over the medial fibers of the calcaneonavicular ligament and the tibialis posterior tendon. According to Sella and Lawson,[54]

> the degree of clinical pronation, the relationship of the accessory ossicle to the navicular body and the tension of the posterior tibial tendon are the factors which produce tension, shear, and/or compression forces on the synchondrosis of the type II accessory navicular and cause microscopic changes consistent with injury and repairs similar to those observed with a physeal fracture.

These authors further point out that standard radiographs are not reliable in identifying symptomatic accessory naviculars. Once again, radionuclide studies can provide useful clinical data, especially when accessory bones of this area are noted bilaterally. A positive bone scan is often obtained for the symptomatic side (Fig. 17-16).

Fractures of the navicular tuberosity are rare and are usually easily differentiated radiographically from the accessory navicular. Serration of the edges of the fragment and local findings of pain, ecchymosis, and edema with a significant history will usually make the diagnosis. Accessory naviculars are usually bilateral. Contralateral radiographs may help differentiate a navicular tuberosity fracture from a symptomatic accessory navicular. Various authors have stated that the insertion of the tibialis posterior is at a mechanical disadvantage in the presence of the accessory navicular, which contributes to the development of flatfoot. Kidner noted that alterations in the line of pull diminished the tibialis posterior tendon as a supinatory force.[47] It is apparent today that this theory is not generally accepted. In fact, Burman in 1930 stated, "We believe that flat foot is independent of the accessory scaphoid as a primary factor in its production, and that when the two exist together, the relationship is incidental and not causal." [24]

### Treatment

Treatment of the symptomatic accessory navicular should be initially directed nonsurgically. Cast immobilization, rest, physical therapy, and short courses of nonsteroidal anti-inflammatory drugs have proved useful. If midfoot pronatory changes are apparent, then orthoses may provide benefit.[36,48] When conservative measures fail, resection of the accessory ossicle is advised.[46-48,50-54,57] Care must be taken to maintain the integrity of the

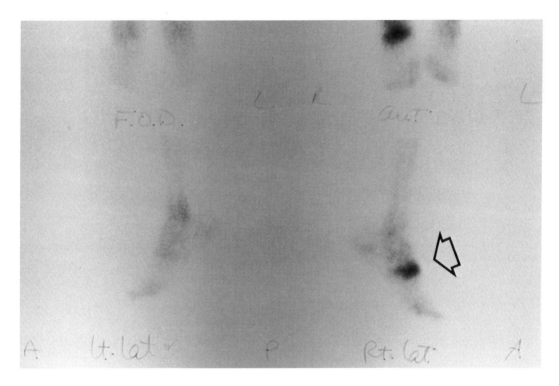

**Fig. 17-16.** Positive bone scan demonstrating a symptomatic accessory navicular bone. The asymmetric tracer uptake is characteristic and can help confirm diagnoses.

posterior tibialis tendon and the calcaneal navicular ligament. The technique is discussed in Chapter 14.

### Os Vesalianum

The os vesalianum is a rare accessory bone. Dameron reports its occurrence as 1 in 1,000 radiographically[23] (Fig. 17-17). There has been quite a bit of confusion about the identification of this bone. It is important to note that the styloid apophysis of the fifth metatarsal is not the os vesalianum. The styloid apophysis is present in children from ages 9 to 16, and fusion which is considered definite, reportedly takes place about the age of 16 years.[24] When present, the os vesalianum is oriented longitudinally to the shaft of the fifth metatarsal bone. It is adjacent to the styloid process of the fifth metatarsal and may demonstrate sclerotic borders.

Clinically, it is important to distinguish this accessory bone from styloid process fractures. Fractures of the styloid process of the fifth metatarsal are common and in general are oriented transversely to the shaft of this metatarsal. A history of inversion injury associated with pain, ecchymosis, and edema similarly should alert the clinician to fracture. Fractures are seen in the presence of an open apophysis of the fifth metatarsal (Fig. 17-18). Treatment in the adolescent is generally rest and immobilization for 2 to 6 weeks. I prefer short leg casting or splinting initially for 1 to 3 weeks, followed by use of a

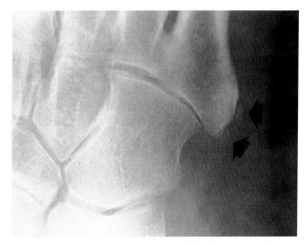

**Fig. 17-17.** The arrows indicate a bipartite os vesalianum.

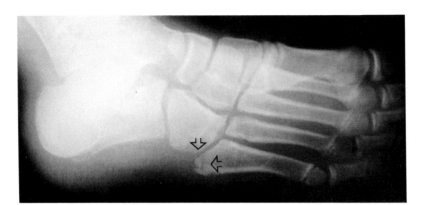

**Fig. 17-18.** Transverse fracture of the styloid process of the fifth metatarsal. Note that the apophysis is generally oriented in a longitudinal direction and parallel to the metatarsal shaft, whereas fractures of the styloid process of the fifth metatarsal will generally occur in the transverse direction.

wooden surgical shoe and elastic supports for the balance of the healing time. Healing is generally unremarkable in this young age group.

## OSTEOCHONDROSES OF THE FOOT

Osteochondroses of the foot are a poorly understood group of idiopathic diseases that are characterized by a disorder of enchondrial ossification. Atlases have been written detailing the many sites of occurrence throughout the body. Over 75 sites have been demonstrated, and some authors believe any bone is susceptible.[58] It has been theorized that disorders of enchondrial ossification are multifactorial.[59] Most authors believe that a vascular deficit in the subchondral region of the involved bone is responsible.[58-82] Direct trauma, metabolic disturbances, collagen vascular diseases, and genetic factors have all been presented as potential sources of vascular disruption associated with osteonecrosis. Primary osteochondrosis is considered idiopathic. Secondary osteochondrosis is associated with or attributable to other systemic diseases.[67]

Most patients complain of localized pain when the foot is involved. Limping is often seen. Occasionally, however, asymptomatic presentations are noted. Upon examination, guarding of the limb or retraction of the involved site may be all that is noted. Restriction of motion or effusion of the adjacent joints is not uncommon.

Radiographic evidence is subtle early in the course of the disease. Soft tissue swelling and patchy areas of altered radiodensity or nodularity are sometimes seen. Flattening of the involved bone is a classic finding and may be subtle in the early stages. Adjacent bony structures are generally not involved radiographically. In the early course of the disease radioisotope scanning reveals small filling defects of the involved osseous structure. In the later stages scanning generally shows uniform increases in radionuclide uptake throughout the involved area, which is consistent with regeneration and/or repair of the bone.[71] MRI characteristics compatible with the diagnosis of osteonecrosis of the tarsal navicular[67] have been described. Furthermore, it was determined that there were no differences in signal behavior characteristics between the primary and the secondary forms of this disease. It was also noted that combined CT and MRI studies proved more diagnostically reliable.

In the pediatric population it is important to have a high index of suspicion when dealing with the osteochrondroses. Differential diagnosis should include hematogenous osteomyelitis, bone tumors, infectious osteochrondritis, and fractures.[58] The osteochondroses have been associated with other clinically significant orthopedic entities. Kohler's disease of the tarsal navicular has been associated with cases of Legg-Calvé-Perthes and Osgood-Schlatter disease.[71] A careful history and complete physical examination of the patient are required. Laboratory studies are generally not helpful for direct diagnosis; however, they may prove helpful for indirect diagnosis by exclusion. Fortunately, in most cases the process is self-limiting and supportive care is all that is necessary. However, there are specific sites on the foot that require surgical intervention.

## Kohler's Disease

Spontaneous osteochondrosis of the navicular bone was first described by Kohler in 1908. In later years Kohler was also associated with another osteochondrosis of the foot known as *Freiberg's disease.* Some texts have referred to osteochondrosis of the navicular as Kohler's I

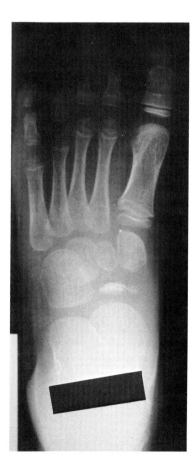

**Fig. 17-19.** This radiograph demonstrates the increased radiodensity and flattening typical of Kohler's disease.

and to osteochondrosis of the distal lesser metatarsals as Kohler's II. In addition, spontaneous osteochondrosis of the tarsal navicular in the adult is now generally referred to as the Muller-Weiss syndrome after the authors who described it in 1928 and 1929, respectively.[62] This entity presents quite a different clinical picture from that of Kohler's disease in children, and unlike the latter is frequently associated with prolonged disability. The most recent literature refers to Kohler's disease specifically as osteochondrosis of the tarsal navicular in children.

### Clinical Features and Treatment

Clinically, the presentation of Kohler's disease may be an incidental radiographic finding. Often, however, localized pain or an antalgic gait is noted. Occasionally mild swelling is seen. There is a male predominance, and most cases are unilateral. Radiographically, increased radiodensity and flattening of the tarsal navicular is pathognomic (Figs. 17-19 and 17-20). Fragmentation may also be seen. Lateral radiographs provide an excellent view. Biopsy of the navicular generally is unnecessary for diagnosis as with most of the osteochondroses. Complete recovery is almost always the rule; therefore, treatment efforts should be conservative. Cast immobilization provides satisfactory results. Reduced activities and arch supports or foot orthoses have also proved effective. Most cases respond within 8 months. Follow-up studies after 30 years have shown no residual degenerative changes in spite of severe fragmentation and flattening of the navicular. It is interesting to note that Kohler's disease has been reported to be associated with coalitions of this region.[61,78]

## Freiberg's Disease

In 1914 A.H. Freiberg described osteochondrosis of the distal lesser metatarsal heads. This condition, like other osteochondrosis, is thought to be a vascular disruption of the growth center of the involved bone and is felt by some to be mechanically induced.[59,63,67,79,81] Smillie felt that this was a dorsal trabecular stress injury of the metatarsal head.[74] Interference with the epiphyseal vessels may result in varying degrees of necrosis of the subarticular cartilage of the epiphysis and the subjacent bone. The effect is a disorderly proliferation of cartilage cells within the epiphysis. Appositional bone growth continues, however. Flattening and broadening of the

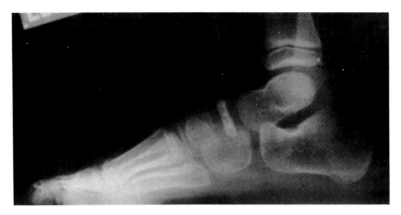

**Fig. 17-20.** Note the excellent visualization on the lateral radiograph, which is a typical finding of Kohler's disease.

metatarsal head are thought to occur because of failure of proliferation of the deeper cartilage cells, which are normally supplied by the epiphyseal vessels (Fig. 17-21). Fragmentation of the involved metatarsal head is frequently seen (Fig. 17-22), as well as widening of the shaft of the involved metatarsal in some patients. Because of the relative lack of mobility of the second and third metatarsals and their relatively increased length within the metatarsal parabola, Freiberg's disease affects these metatarsals most often.[67] The second metatarsal is involved 75 percent of the time, and the third metatarsal is involved in approximately 25 percent of the remaining cases. Fourth metatarsal involvement is rare. Freiberg's

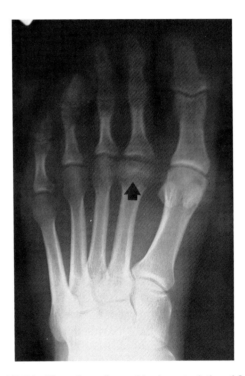

**Fig. 17-21.** Note the radiographic characteristics of flattening and broadening of the head of the lesser metatarsal, which are typical of Freiberg's disease.

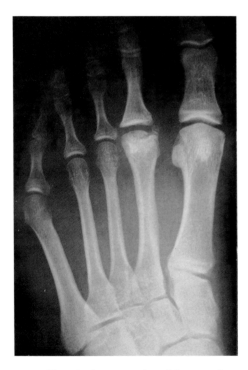

**Fig. 17-22.** Note the fragmentation of the second metatarsal head associated with Freiberg's disease.

disease is typically seen in children between the ages of 10 and 15, with a female to male ratio of 3 : 1. Approximately 10 percent of the cases are bilateral.[71]

### Clinical Features

Clinically, Freiberg's disease presents with dull or aching pain and swelling of the involved metatarsophalangeal joint without a history of trauma. Motion of the involved joint is painful, and crepitation may be elicited.

Radiographic examination in the early stages may reveal joint effusion only. More typically, rarefaction, sclerosis of the distal epiphysis, and flattening of the distal metatarsal head are seen (Fig. 17-22). In long-standing cases, a dorsal bony fragment may be seen on lateral radiographs. An articular step-off may also be seen. Smillie in 1957 developed a staging system for the disease, based on radiographic findings, as follows[74]: in stage I a fissure fracture of the ischemic epiphysis develops; in stage II the articular contour is altered from bone reabsorption without depression of the central fragment; in stage III a depression of the central core is formed, with lateral projections overhanging, but the plantar cortex remains intact (Fig. 17-23); in stage IV the plantar cortex gives way, producing a loose osteocartilaginous body, and the lateral projections break off; stage V is characterized by flattening and broadening of the joint with arthrosis.

### Treatment

Children who present during the early stages (I and II) of Freiberg's disease should be treated with cast immobilization for at least 6 weeks in order to prevent further trauma and articular collapse. Unfortunately, Freiberg's disease is frequently diagnosed in the later stages, and surgical intervention is frequently required. A variety of surgical procedures have been advocated. Most authors favor excision of loose fragments and remodeling of the involved metatarsal head.[63,79,81] Dorsal displacement or shortening osteotomies have been advocated when plantar prominences appear to be causing symptoms. Metatarsal head excisions have generally fallen out of favor because of the high incidence of transfer lesions and floating toe deformity. In severe cases metatarsal head replacement with Silastic implants has often proved successful. However, long-term follow-up is lacking, and implantation of Silastic joints in children or young adults should be avoided if possible.

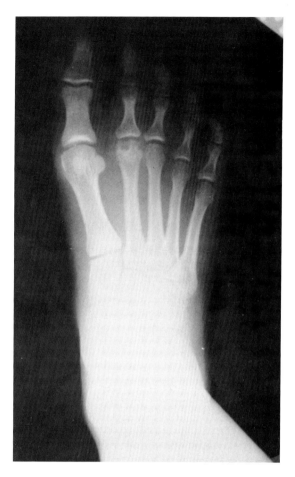

**Fig. 17-23.** This radiograph demonstrates stage III degeneration as described by Smillie.[74] Note the depression of the central core with lateral projections overhanging.

## Osteochondroses of the Hallucial Sesamoid Bones

Osteochondrosis of the small hallucial sesamoid bones can produce significant pain and disability. The sesamoid bones begin to ossify about the eighth or ninth year in girls and about the tenth to the eleventh year in boys.[60,72] They provide a fulcrum for the flexor tendons of the hallux and are subject to the repetitive trauma of direct weight-bearing.

### Clinical Features

Only rarely is there a history of a single episode of direct trauma. Repetitive vocational and avocational activities, rapid acceleration and deceleration sports, and dancing

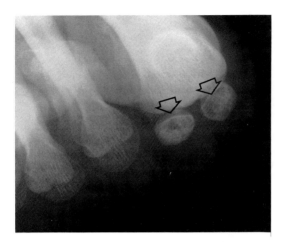

**Fig. 17-24.** The arrows indicate areas of rarefaction and mottling consistent with the early stages of osteochondrosis of the hallucial sesamoid bones. Later stages will show fragmentation and/or collapse.

are commonly associated.[72] Other overuse injuries of the forefoot should be ruled out. Point tenderness at the plantar aspect of the involved sesamoid is characteristic. Low-grade edema or joint effusion is sometimes noted. Active dorsiflexion and plantar-flexion of the first metatarsophalangeal joint reproduces symptoms. The differential diagnosis should include sesamoiditis, chondromalacia, degenerative joint disease of the metatarsosesamoidal articulation, fracture of the sesamoid, infectious osteochondritis, and systemic arthropathies such as psoriasis or ankylosing spondylitis.

Radiographic studies should include anteroposterior oblique, lateral, and axial sesamoid views of the foot (Fig. 17-24). Fragmentation, rarefaction, mottling, or collapse may be seen in later stages. Technetium bone scans will generally be positive prior to the appearance of the distinctive standard radiographic features[77] (Fig. 17-11).

### Treatment

Treatment required in the early stages is protected weight-bearing or immobilization with a short leg cast. Further conservative treatment may consist of accommodative orthoses, anti-inflammatory medications, metatarsal bars, injectable short-acting corticosteroids, and physical therapy modalities such as ultrasound and short-wave diathermy.[72,77] Conservative treatment for longer than 6 months or in the presence of degenerative radiographic changes is generally unsuccessful.

Excision of the affected sesamoid is considered the treatment of choice in chronic cases. Care must be taken to re-establish the capsuloligamentous stability of the first metatarsophalangeal joint in order to prevent iatrogenic complications such as hallux abductovalgus or a hallux hammertoe deformity.[83,84] Medial and plantar approaches for the extraction of the tibial sesamoid and plantar or dorsal direct approaches for lateral sesamoid extractions have been described. Each has its advantages and disadvantages. I prefer a medial approach to the tibial sesamoid. In the case of lateral sesamoid involvement, a plantar approach is used for patients with low intermetatarsal angles and a dorsal approach may be used for patients with higher intermetatarsal angles. Low intermetatarsal angles make a dorsal approach difficult without significant soft tissue disruption.

### Surgical Treatment

The plantar approach to the first metatarsophalangeal joint is made through a curvilinear incision beginning just lateral to and extending proximally and medially to the weight-bearing pad of the great toe joint, following natural skin lines, with the patient in the prone position. The fat pad is sharply dissected with a knife until the skin flap can be reflected medially. Extreme care should be taken to identify and avoid injuring the prominent plantar medial hallux nerve branch of the medial plantar nerve, which usually lies directly over or near the deep fascia of the fibular sesamoid. The deep fascia, capsule, and periosteum over the metatarsal sesamoid can be incised linearly, and the sesamoid bone can be "shelled out" without disrupting the integrity of the flexor hallucis brevis muscle attachment to the base of the proximal phalanx. The plantar first metatarsophalangeal joint can then be inspected, and the capsule and flexor brevis tendon can be tightly repaired. The skin incision is closed with interrupted fine nylon suture, and a non-weight-bearing posterior splint is applied. The patient should be kept non-weight-bearing for 3 weeks. This technique results in a very satisfactory plantar scar and has the advantage of ease of approach and preservation of the integrity of the flexor hallucis brevis muscle attachment.

## Osteochondritis of the Proximal Epiphysis of the Hallux

Ossification of the proximal epiphysis of the hallux usually appears after the second year. The epiphysis frequently multipartite.[76] Epiphyseal abnormalities of the toes were described by Thiemann in 1909 as part of a generalized disease if the small epiphyses of the fingers and the toes.[75] Thiemann considered these abnormalities examples of osteochondritis. His study was based upon radiographic and histologic evidence. Lyritis studied radiographs of 1,500 proximal epiphyses of the great toe and concluded that 3.5 percent of the children had evidence of fragmentation, sclerosis, and cone-shaped epiphyses.[70] Furthermore, one-quarter of the 3.5 percent group were found to have hallux rigidus deformities. The fragmentation noted at the epiphysis of the base of the great toe was considered to be a manifestation of Thiemann's disease at that site. An unexpectedly high incidence of other orthopedic problems was also noted in these children. Among them were Osgood-Schlatter disease, Freiberg's disease, and trichorhinoepiphyseal syndrome. The latter syndrome is characterized by short stature, brachydactylism, sparse, thin scalp, bulky nose, and high philtrum.

Clinically, these epiphyseal abnormalities of the great toe need to be differentiated from traumatic conditions. Generally a good history will help make the differentiation. Conservative care has been advised when the condition is identified early. Again, as with the other osteochondroses, immobilization, protected weight-bearing, and anti-inflammatory measures are advised. In advanced cases in which hallux rigidus or limitus is encountered, standard approaches to this deformity are recommended. These are beyond the scope of this discussion.

## Osteochondroses of the Midfoot

Osteochondroses of the bones of the midfoot, namely, the cuneiforms, navicular, and cuboid, have been reported. In general the presentation is similar to the osteochondroses previously mentioned. The diagnosis is established by careful history taking and physical examination of the area. Standard radiographs, careful evaluation of radionuclide bone scans or magnetic resonance imaging (MRI) scans and a high index of suspicion generally will consolidate the diagnosis. Early treatment with soft or rigid immobilization, anti-inflammatory medications, and physical therapy has proved helpful. In cases of severe fragmentation, degeneration, and/or persistence of clinical symptoms beyond 3 to 6 months in spite of aggressive conservative efforts, surgical debridement is advised. Loose fragments should be excised, and bone grafts should be used when possible with or without appropriate fusions to ensure adequate mid-

foot stability. A graduated rehabilitation program instituted in the postoperative period and follow-up treatment with orthoses or pressure-reducing devices are also advisable.

## Apophyseal Osteochondroses of the Foot

Apophyseal osteochondroses represent the nonarticular manifestations of osteochondroses of the foot.[59] A frequent site of irritation is the calcaneal apophysis, which usually appears between the ages of 5 and 12 (Fig. 17-25). Osteochondrosis of this structure is commonly referred to as *Sever's disease*. Prolonged or repetitive trauma to the calcaneal apophysis and the aggravating influence of the tension imposed by the Achilles tendon superiorly and the plantar fascia inferiorly are thought to induce calcaneal apophysitis.[59] The so-called Islin's disease, or osteochondrosis of the apophysis of the fifth metatarsal base is a similar example of apophyseal osteochondrosis.[59,60] Fragmentation or avulsion of the cartilage at the point of attachment, disruption of chondrogenesis, fibrosis, and ossification account for the radiographic and clinical features of pain and swelling. This can follow inversion injuries and may occur until the fifth metatarsal apophysis completely ossifies, which in most patients will occur in the thirteenth year.

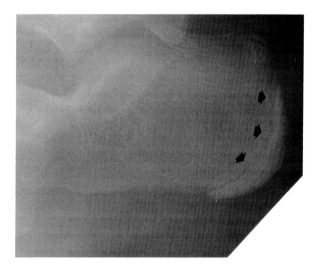

**Fig. 17-25.** Radiograph typical of Sever's disease. Note the increased density of the calcaneal apophysis, with irregular apophyseocortical junction.

Conservative treatment is generally successful. Radiographic recovery is generally not the rule, and apophyseal irregularities are frequently seen but are usually asymptomatic. Treatment should be symptomatic. Rest is paramount. Apophyseal osteochondroses are self-limiting conditions, relief of symptoms occuring coincidently with maturation of the apophysis.

# REFERENCES

## Haglund's Disease

1. Hohmann KG: Fuss und Bein, ihre Erkrankungen und deren Behandlung. 4th Ed. Munich, 1948, JF Bergmann,
2. Haglund P: Beitrag zur Klinik der Achillessehne. Z Orthop 49:49, 1928
3. Heneghan MA, Pavlov H: The Haglund painful heel syndrome. Experimental investigation of cause and therapeutic implications. Clin Orthop 187:228,
4. Pavlov H, Heneghan M, Hersh A et al: The Haglund syndrome: initial and differential diagnosis. Diagn Radiol 144:83, 1982
5. Fowler A, Philip J: Abnormality of the calcaneus as the cause of painful heel. Its diagnosis and operative treatment. Br J Surg 32:494, 1945
6. Rzonca EC, Shapiro P, D'Amico JC: Haglund's deformity. An electrodynographic approach to analysis. J Am Podiatr Med Assoc 74:482, 1984
7. Ayeres MJ, Bakst RH, Baskwill DF et al: Dwyer osteotomy, a retrospective study. J Foot Surg 26:322, 1987
8. Burhenne LJ, Connell DG: Xeroradiography in the diagnosis of the Haglund's syndrome. Can Assoc Radiol J 37:157, 1986
9. Fuglsang F, Torup D: Bursitis retrocalcanearis. Acta Orthop Scand 30:315, 1961
10. Hartman HO: The tendon sheaths and synovial bursa of the foot. Gustav Schwalb 1896. Foot Ankle 1:246, 1981
11. Miller AE, Vogel TA: Haglund's deformity and the Keck and Kelly osteotomy: a retrospective analysis. J Foot Surg 28:23, 1989
12. Notari MA, Mittler BE: An investigation of Fowler-Philip's angle in diagnosing Haglund's deformity. J Am Podiatr Med Assoc 74:486, 1984
13. Rossi F, La Cava F, Amato F et al: The Haglund syndrome (H.s.): clinical and radiological features and sports medicine aspects. J Sports Med Phys Fitness 27:258, 1987
14. Ruch JA: Haglund's disease. J Am Podiatr Med Assoc 64:1000, 1974
15. Saxl A: Die Schuhgeschwulst der Ferse. Z Orthop 51:312, 1929
16. Sebes JI: The significance of calcaneal spurs in rheumatic diseases. Arthritis Rheum 32:338, 1989
17. Smith LS, Tillo TH: Haglund's deformity in long distance runners. Nine surgical cases. J Am Podiatr Med Assoc 78:419, 1988
18. Torg JS, Pavlov H, Torg E: Overuse injuries in sport: the foot. Clin Sports Med 6:291, 1987
19. Root ML, Orien WP, Weed JH: Normal and Abnormal Function of the Foot. Clinical Biomechanics Corp., Los Angeles, 1977
20. Vega MR, Cavolo DJ, Green RM et al: Haglund's deformity. J Am Podiatr Med Assoc 74:129, 1984
21. Abend L, Bernstein DA, Wagreich C: Post-traumatic heel deformity. J Foot Surg 25:146, 1986
22. Giannestras NJ: Foot Disorders: Medical and Surgical Management. Lea & Febiger, Philadelphia, 1973

## Accessory and Sesamoid Bones

23. Sarrafian S: Anatomy of the Foot and Ankle. JB Lippincott, Philadelphia, 1983
24. Burman M: The functional disturbances caused by the inconstant bones and sesamoids of the foot. Arch Surg:936, 1930
25. Kewenter U: Die Sesambeine des I Metatarso-phalangealgelenks des Menschen. Acta Orthop Scand 2:43, 1936
26. Chioros PG, Frankel SL, Sidlow CJ: Sesamoid pain secondary to a plantar neuroma. J Foot Surg 26:296, 1987
27. Scranton PE Jr: Pathologic anatomic variations in the sesamoids. Foot Ankle 1:321, 1981
28. Richardson E: Injuries to the hallucial sesamoids in the athlete. Foot Ankle 7: 1987
29. Keating S, Fisher D, Keating D: Avascular necrosis of an accessory sesamoid of the foot. A case report. J Am Podiatr Med Assoc 77:612, 1987
30. Thomas AP: Osteochondral defects of the first metatarsal head in adolescence: a stage in the development of hallux rigidus. J Pediatr Orthop 9:236, 1989
31. McCarthy DJ, Herzberg AJ, Saunders MM: The morphogenesis of common pedal lesions. I: Scanning electron microscopic analysis. J Am Podiatr Med Assoc 73:497, 1983
32. McBryde AM Jr, Anderson RB: Sesamoid foot problems in the athlete. Clin Sports Med 7:51, 1988
33. Axe MJ, Ray RL: Orthotic treatment of sesamoid pain. Am J Sports Med 16:411, 1988
34. Velkes S: Osteochondral defects of the first metatarsal sesamoids. Arch Orthop Trauma Surg 107:369, 1988
35. Turner RS: Dynamic post-surgical hallux varus after lateral sesamoidectomy: treatment and prevention. Orthopedics 9:963, 1986
36. Root ML, Orien WP, Weed JH: Normal and Abnormal Function of the Foot. Clinical Biomechanics Corp., Los Angeles, 1977
37. Keating S: Avascular necrosis of an accessory sesamoid of the foot. J Am Podiatr Med Assoc 77:612, 1987

38. Le Minor JM: Comparative anatomy and significance of the sesamoid bone of the peroneus longus muscle (os peroneum). J Anat 151: 1987

39. Peacock KC, Resnick SJ, Thoder JJ: Fracture of the os peroneum with rupture of the peroneus longus tendon. A case report and review of literature. Clin Orthop 202:223, 1986

40. Tehranzadeh J, Stoll DA, Gabriele OM: Posterior migration of the os peroneum of the left foot, indicating a tear of the peroneal tendon. Skeletal Radiol 12:44, 1984

41. Japiot P: Os accessoires du tarse. Radiographies. Lyon Med 123:185, 1914

42. Burton SK, Altman MI: Degenerative arthritis of the os peroneum. A case report. J Am Podiatr Med Assoc 76:343, 1986

43. Wilson RC, Moyles BG: Surgical treatment of the symptomatic os peroneum. J Foot Surg 26:156, 1987

44. Johnson RP, Collier BD, Carrera GF: The os trigonum syndrome: use of bone scan in the diagnosis. J Trauma 24:761, 1984

45. McGlamry E: Comprehensive Textbook of Foot Surgery. Williams & Wilkins, Baltimore, 1987

46. Giannestras NJ: Foot Disorders: Medical and Surgical Management. Lea & Febiger, Philadelphia, 1973

47. Kidner FC: The prehallux (accessory scaphoid) in its relation to flat feet. J Bone Joint Surg 11:831, 1929

48. Lawson JP, Ogden JA, Sella E et al: The painful accessory navicular. Skeletal Radiol 12:250, 1984

49. Lawson JP: Symptomatic radiographic variants in extremities. Radiology 157:625, 1985

50. Macnicol MF: Surgical treatment of the symptomatic accessory navicular. J Bone Joint Surg [Br] 68:218, 1984

51. Macnicol MF, Voutsinas S: Surgical treatment of the symptomatic accessory navicular. J Bone Joint Surg [Br] 66A:218, 1984

52. Maffucci N: Traumatic lesion of some accessory bones of the foot in sports activity. J Am Podiatr Med Assoc 80: 1990

53. Sella EJ, Lawson JP, Ogden JA: The accessory navicular synchondrosis. Clin Orthop 209:280, 1986

54. Sella EJ, Lawson JP: Biomechanics of the accessory navicular synchondrosis. Foot Ankle 8:156, 1987

55. Haller J: Spontaneous osteonecrosis of the tarsal navicular in adults: imaging findings. AJIP 151:355, 1988

56. Viladot A: Necrosis of the navicular bone. Bull Hosp Jt Dis Orthop Inst 47: ,1987

57. Lawson JP: The painful accessory navicular. Skeletal Radiol 12:250, 1984

## Osteochondroses

58. Browler A: The osteochondroses. Orthop Clin North Am 14:99, 1983

59. Siffert R: Classification of the osteochondroses. Clin Orthop 158:10, 1981

60. Burman M: The functional disturbances caused by the inconstant bones and sesamoids of the foot. Arch Surg :936, 1930

61. Ertel AN: Talonavicular coalition following avascular necrosis of tarsal navicular. J Pediatr Orthop 4:482, 1984

62. Haller J: Spontaneous osteonecrosis of the tarsal navicular in adults: imaging findings. AJR 151:355, 1988

63. Helal B: Freiberg's disease: a suggested pattern of management. Foot Ankle 8: 1987

64. Ippolito E: Kohler's disease of the tarsal navicular: long-term follow up of 12 cases. J Pediatr Orthop 4:416, 1984

65. Japiot : Os accessoires du tarse. Radiographies. Lyons Med 123:185, 1914

66. Keating S: Avascular necrosis of an accessory sesamoid of the foot. J Am Podiatr Med Assoc 77: 1987

67. Kinnard P: Dorsiflexion osteotomy in Freiberg's disease. Foot Ankle 9: 1989

68. Lawson JP: The painful accessory navicular. Skeletal Radiol 12:250, 1984

69. Lehman R: Osteochondritis dissecans of the midfoot. Foot Ankle. 7: 1986

70. Lyritis G: Developmental disorders of the proximal Epiphysis of the hallux. Skeletal Radiol 10:250, 1983

71. Mandel G: Scintigraphic manifestations of infraction of the second metatarsal (Freiberg's disease). J Nucl Med 28: 1987

72. Richardson E: Injuries to the hallucial sesamoids in the athlete. Foot Ankle 7: 1987

73. Sella E: The accessory navicular synchondrosis. Clin Orthop 209: 1986

74. Smillie IS: Freiberg's infarction. J Bone Joint Surg [Br] 39:580, 1957

75. Thiemann H: Juvenile Epiphysenstörungen. ROFO 14:79, 1909

76. Thomas AP: Osteochondral defects of first metatarsal head in adolescence: a stage in the development of hallux rigidus. J Pediatr Orthop 9:236, 1989

77. Velkes S: Osteochondritis of the first metatarsal sesamoids. Arch Orthop Trauma Surg 107:369, 1988

78. Viladot A: Necrosis of the navicular bone. Bull Hospl J Dis Orthop Inst 47: 1987

79. Walsh HP: Etiology of Freiberg's disease? Trauma. J Foot Surg 27: 1988

80. Wiles S: Naviculocuneiform coalition. J Am Podiatr Med Assoc 78: , 1988

81. Young C.: Osteochondral disruption of the second metatarsal: a variant of Freiberg's infraction. Foot Ankle 8: 1987

82. Zimberg J: Osteochondrosis of the medial cuneiform. J Am Podiatr Med Assoc 75: , 1985

83. Nayfa TM, Sorto LA Jr: The incidence of hallus abductus

following tibial sesamoidectomy. J Am Podiatr Med Assoc 72:617, 1982

84. Turner RS: Dynamic post-surgical hallux varus after lateral sesamoidectomy: treatment and prevention. Orthopedics 9:963, 1986

## SUGGESTED READINGS

### Haglund's Disease

Coughlin RR: Common injuries of the foot. Often more than 'just a sprain.' Postgrad Med 86:175, 1989

### Accessory and Sesamoid Bones

Bloom RA, Libson E, Lax E, et al: The assimilated os sustentaculi. Skeletal Radiol 15:455, 1986

Griffiths JD, Menelaus MB: Symptomatic ossicles of the lateral malleolus in children. J Bone Joint Surg [Br] 69:317, 1987

Nayfa TM, Sorto LA, Jr: The incidence of hallux abductus following tibial sesamoidectomy. J Am Podiatr Med Assoc 72:617, 1982

Ogata K, Sugioka Y, Urano Y et al: Idiopathic osteonecrosis of the first metatarsal sesamoid. Skeletal Radiol 15:141, 1986

# 18

# Neuromuscular Disorders

*THOMAS K. KOCH*

Disorders of the neuromuscular system are relatively common in children. Their clinical presentation and course are determined by the site and extent of neurologic involvement, as well as by the pathophysiologic process and the age of the child. These disorders are generally classified according to their anatomic localization within the motor pathway.

The motor pathway can be divided into two major constituents, an upper motor neuron unit (Fig. 18-1), and a lower motor neuron unit (Fig. 18-2). The upper motor neuron unit consists of central nervous system neurons and their associated descending pathways through the brain stem and spinal cord. Neurons from the motor cortex and the corresponding corticospinal tracts are essential components of this network. There are also several indirect polysynaptic pathways operating through the basal ganglia and related subcortical nuclei that influence motor activity on a central level. These polysynaptic pathways constitute portions of the extrapyramidal system, while the corticospinal tract constitutes the pyramidal system. The lower motor neuron unit (Fig. 18-2) consists of the anterior horn cell within the spinal cord, its axon, the neuromuscular junction, and the muscle fiber innervated by the axon. The lower motor neuron unit receives its direction from the upper motor neuron unit.

In the assessment of a patient with a potential neuromuscular disorder, it is of paramount importance to determine whether a patient's weakness and/or muscle tone abnormality results from involvement of the upper or the lower motor neuron unit. Upper motor neuron disease, predominantly of a pyramidal variety, is heralded by a spastic increase of muscle tone, weakness of the extensors in the upper extremities, and weakness of the flexors in the lower extremities. There are accentuated deep tendon reflexes, including clonus and a positive Babinski sign. Muscle atrophy is generally minimal, and no fasciculations are present. Extrapyramidal disease is characterized by a rigid increase in muscle tone with an involuntary movement disorder such as chorea, athetosis, or dystonia. While increased muscle tone is a hallmark of upper motor neuron disease, infants may present with hypotonia. Lower motor neuron disorders are characterized by hypotonia, weakness, muscle atrophy, and absent or diminished deep tendon reflexes. Table 18-1 summarizes the significant differential signs distinguishing upper and lower motor neuron disorders.

## DISORDERS OF UPPER MOTOR NEURON UNITS

### Cerebral Palsy

*Cerebral Palsy* is a descriptive term for a clinical syndrome characterized by a chronic, nonprogressive disorder of motor control, resulting in abnormalities of posture, muscle tone, and motor movement. It is of paramount importance that these static motor encephalopathies be distinguished from recognizable progressive disorders that at a given moment may appear clinically similar. Cerebral palsy results from the disruption of motor regions, pyramidal and/or extrapyramidal, in the infant brain. The definition assumes "injury" to have occurred in the prenatal, perinatal, or early neonatal period. Cerebral palsy, while frequently associated with other handicaps, does not imply mental retardation, learning disabilitites, or epilepsy.

461

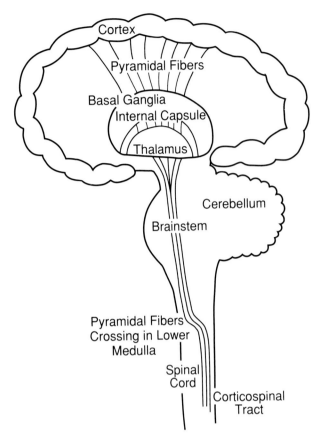

**Fig. 18-1.** The upper motor neuron pathway with both pyramidal and extrapyramidal components.

## Classification

Cerebral palsy is generally classified according to the most prominent upper motor neuron abnormality (Table 18-2). The most common form of cerbral palsy is the spastic variety. Spastic cerebral palsy may be subdivided into three major subgroups: in spastic diplegia, the most common subgroup, there is predominant lower extremity involvement with only modest upper extremity involvement; spastic hemiplegia involves the upper and lower extremities on one side; and quadriplegia involves all four limbs relatively symmetrically. On occasion the term *double hemiplegia* or *bilateral hemiplegia* is used to describe patients whose upper limbs are more severely affected than their lower limbs. An extrapyramidal form of cerebral palsy may manifest as either choreoathetosis or dystonia; mixed cerebral palsy can be seen in children who have combined extrapyramidal and spastic involvement. Other forms, including hypotonic

and ataxic cerebral palsy, are less common. The incidence of these forms of cerebral palsy varies widely among published reports. Clearly, the most common form is the spastic variety, with one study reporting an incidence of 91 percent.[1] Other studies generally indicate that spastic cerebral palsy accounts for approximately two-thirds of all patients, with extrapyramidal and mixed varieties accounting for the remainder.[2]

### Etiology

In 1861 Little reported 47 children with "a persistent spastic rigidity," which he concluded was the result of an abnormality of birth.[3] More recent studies have challenged this hypothesis, and it now appears that only in a minority of children with cerebral palsy is birth-related asphyxia the sole cause of their neurologic morbidity.[4-6] Currently, two of the most important risk factors for cerebral palsy are prematurity and low birth weight.[7] Affected infants typically present with a spastic diplegia, which is usually pathologically related to periventricular leukomalacia. Other significant factors resulting in cere-

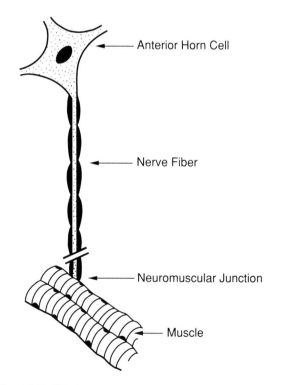

**Fig. 18-2.** The lower motor neuron pathway consisting of the anterior horn cell within the ventral horn of the spinal cord, nerve fiber, myoneural junction, and muscle.

Table 18-1. **Upper and Lower Motor Neuron Features**

| Feature | Upper Motor Neuron | | Lower Motor Neuron |
|---|---|---|---|
| | Pyramidal Type | Extrapyramidal Type | |
| Muscle bulk | Normal; decreasd late | Normal | Decreased |
| Fasciculations | Absent | Absent | Present |
| Muscle tone | Spastic[a] | Rigid[a] | Decreased |
| Strength | Decreased[b] | Normal or mild decrease | Decreased |
| Movement disorder | Absent | Present | Absent |
| Tendon reflexes | Increased | Normal or mild increase | Decreased |
| Babinski sign | Present | Absent | Absent |

[a] Decreased in infants.
[b] Decrease in upper extremity extensor strength and lower extremity flexor strength.

bral palsy include prenatal vascular accidents with cystic encephalomalacia; metabolic abnormalities such as hyperbilirubinemia and severe hypoglycemia; and congenital and perinatal infections such as cytomegalovirus (CMV), rubella, *Toxoplasma,* neonatal meningitis, and neonatal herpes (Table 18-3). With recent advances in nervous system imaging techniques, significant numbers of children with "idiopathic cerebral palsy" have been found to have cerebral malformations with neuronal migrational anomalies, including agenesis of the corpus callosum, cerebellar hypoplasia, and a variety of cortical abnormalities.[8]

### Clinical Features

The early diagnosis of cerebral palsy (during the first year of life) may be difficult. The signs and symptoms are dependent on the specific type of motor disability, its severity, and the age of the child. Infants often manifest early cerebral palsy with hypotonia, which later develops into spasticity or an extrapyramidal movement disorder. Patients commonly present with a history of gross motor delay. The more severe the involvement, the earlier is the age of presentation. On examination, persistence of primitive neonatal reflexes such as the tonic neck reflex and Moro's reflex, along with poor development of more mature reflexes such as neck righting, the Landau reaction, and the parachute reflex, indicate significant early

motor involvement. In less severe cases infants may present with an abnormal crawling pattern (combat crawl) or, in mild forms, toe walking. Hemiplegic cerebral palsy may present with a strong hand preference prior to 2 years of age.

In older children spastic cerebral palsy is manifest by increased muscle tone, characteristic weakness of the upper and lower limbs suggestive of an upper motor neuron process, accentuated deep tendon reflexes, clonus, and a Babinski sign. Children with spastic diplegia have predominant leg involvement, their gait being much more affected than their hand skills. Physical examination often discloses prominent scissoring of the lower extremities with tight adductors. Commonly, there will also be tightness of the heel cords, further impairing the child's stance and ambulatory abilities. Surgical intervention is almost always necessary in severe cases to achieve ambulation.

Children with spastic quadriplegia have involvement of all four extremities and usually are more severely neurologically disabled than children with spastic diplegia. A pseudobulbar palsy with weakness of the facial, lingual, and pharyngeal muscles, making speech and

Table 18-2. **Classification of Cerebral Palsy**

| Spastic | Hypotonic |
|---|---|
| Diplegia | Ataxic |
| Hemiplegia | Mixed |
| Quadriplegia | |
| Extrapyramidal | |
| Choreoathetosis | |
| Dystonia | |

Table 18-3. **Risk Factors Associated with Cerebral Palsy**

Prematurity
Low birth weight
Metabolic
    Anoxia
    Hypoglycemia
    Hyperbilirubinemia
Cerebrovascular accidents
    Stroke (pre- or perinatal)
    Intracranial hemorrhage
Infections
    Congenital (toxoplasma, CMV, herpes, rubella)
    Perinatal
Cerebral malformations

feeding very difficult, is frequently seen. These children have trouble handling their secretions, and recurring pneumonias are common. Ocular problems occur, especially strabismus. Additionally there is significant risk for associated mental retardation, seizures, and microcephaly.

Hemiplegic cerebral palsy presents with asymmetry of movement of the extremities. During infancy a strong hand preference, which persists, is noted. A hemiplegic gait develops with unilateral toe walking or circumduction of the affected leg. Often there is "paretic posturing" of the affected upper extremity, with flexion of the elbow, wrist, and fingers and a decrease in the natural arm swing. On physical examination the affected side demonstrates increased muscle tone, with accentuated deep tendon reflexes, and a unilateral Babinski sign. Most children with hemiplegic cerebral palsy learn to walk, although many require orthosis and careful orthopedic follow-up. Children are at risk for developing a focal seizure disorder and scoliosis.

Extrapyramidal cerebral palsy usually manifests either as choreoathetosis or dystonia. During infancy many of these children are hypotonic, but by 2 years of age a movement disorder develops. Choreoathetosis is manifest by abnormal dyskinetic movements of the face, tongue, and palate, with resulting facial grimacing and difficulties with speech and feeding. The limbs are dyskinetic, with constant erratic movement. Involvement is usually bilateral, but on occasion unilateral involvement may be seen. While choreoathetosis is the more common form of extrapyramidal cerebral palsy, a dystonic variety, with sustained twisted postures, also may be seen. Both these movement abnormalities dissipate during sleep. On physical examination children with extrapyramidal disorders may have accentuated reflexes and increased tone of a rigid quality. Clonus is not a common feature, nor is a positive Babinski sign. Because of the constant movement with choreoathetosis, contractures are less common than in spastic varieties of cerebral palsy. Dystonia may result in contractures and especially in deformities of the spine.

### Treatment

Treatment programs for children with cerebral palsy need to be specifically designed to the affected child's needs. Many disciplines are involved, including pediatrics, neurology, orthopedics, physical therapy, occupational therapy, speech therapy, psychology, and vocational counseling. The care of children with cerebral palsy extends over many years. Their problems are dynamic ones, changing with the growth and development of the central nervous system and the child. Goals need to be adjusted for associated problems, including mental retardation, learning difficulties, and epilepsy. For children with increased tone, physical therapy is often provided at a very early age. Children require careful orthopedic care, and when significant contractures develop, release procedures need to be performed. Alternative avenues of therapy for the treatment of spastic cerebral palsy are now available, the most notable of which is selective dorsal rhizotomy, which is being used with considerable success.[9,10] Initial reports suggest that dorsal rhizotomy is an effective method for reducing spasticity and improving ambulatory abilities. Its success is dependent upon the degree of spasticity and weakness manifest in the individual child as well as on compliance with an intense postoperative physical therapy program. Dorsal rhizotomy appears to work best in children who have pure spastic cerebral palsy with some preserved strength and who are free of contractures and have not undergone previous orthopedic procedures.[9,10]

## Spinal Dysraphism

The term *spinal dysraphism* refers to a heterogeneous group of congenital malformations of the spine. All the lesions within this group have incomplete midline closure of the osseous, mesenchymal, and neural tissues. These disorders may be classified as shown in Table 18-4.

*Spina bifida* is the incomplete closure of the bony elements of the spine, with or without extrusion of the contents of the spinal canal through the bony defect. *Spina bifida occulta* is an isolated defect of the fusion of the posterior vertebral arch without disruption of the underlying neuronal tissue. This defect is extremely common and is found in 10 percent of the general pediatric population. It usually involves the posterior arches of the L5 and S1 vertebrae and is frequently asymptomatic, being found incidentally on radiographic examination. The skin of the low midback may manifest a hairy tuft, dimple, or teratoma.[11] Occasionally, spina bifida occulta may be associated with other occult spinal dysraphisms

Table 18-4. **Spinal Dysraphism**

| | |
|---|---|
| Spina bifida | Occult spinal dysraphism |
|     Spina bifida occulta |     Dorsal dermal sinus |
|     Spina bifida aperta |     Tight filum terminale syndrome |
|         Meningoceles |     Spinal lipoma |
|         Myelomeningoceles |     Diastematomyelia |

and a tethering of the spinal cord. Children with this complication generally present with bowel and bladder dysfunction, scoliosis, gait abnormalities, lower extremity growth discrepancies, or foot deformities, especially a broad, shortened, or elevated arch.

In *spina bifida aperta (spina bifida cystica),* all or part of the contents of the spinal canal protrudes through a bony spina bifida, specifically in the form of meningoceles or myelomeningoceles. Myelomeningoceles constitute approximately 95 percent of spina bifida aperta cases. Although the defect may occur anywhere along the spinal cord, it is most common in the lumbar and lumbosacral areas corresponding to the site of the posterior neuropore closure. At birth the defect may have a variety of appearances, ranging from complete exposure of neural tissue to a partially epithelized membrane.

## Clinical Features

Clinical symptoms are dependent upon the corresponding anatomic level of involvement. Since the vast majority of myelomeningoceles occur caudally, the children exhibit varying degrees of a flaccid, areflexic paraplegia, with sensory deficits in the lower dermatomes. Bowel and bladder function are almost always compromised, with dribbling incontinence and poor rectal tone, which may result in rectal prolapse. With isolated sacral involvement, the patient may have saddle anesthesia and impaired bowel and bladder function, with normal motor integrity in the lower extremities. Since the pathology results in disruption of the spinal cord with anterior horn cell involvement, the majority of neurologic symptoms are referable to a lower motor neuron lesion. Upper motor neuron signs may be seen to variable extents as the child grows older and a tethered cord syndrome develops. Upper motor neuron signs may also occur as a result of an associated hydrocephalus secondary to a Chiari malformation of the brain stem, which is present in approximately 75 to 90 percent of patients with lumbosacral myelomeningoceles. Congenital joint deformities of the lower limbs may occur from denervation of in utero muscle. Infants may present with congenital contractures, valgus or varus deformities, hip dislocations, and/or lumbosacral scoliosis.

## Treatment

The treatment of spina bifida aperta requires early surgical repair of the spinal lesion and control of any associated hydrocephalus with ventriculoperitoneal shunting. The infant then requires a careful urologic evaluation and close orthopedic follow-up. Some controversy remains regarding aggressive treatment for infants who are severely affected with high spinal cord lesions and/or have severe hydrocephalus, since these infants generally have a poor prognosis. Unfortunately, assessment of the patient's future mental abilities remains a difficult task and is only poorly related to the thickness of the brain's cortical mantle as determined by nervous system imaging techniques. Lorber[12] established criteria that he felt tend to predict a poor prognosis despite modern operative, antibiotic, and rehabilitative techniques. These criteria included complete paralysis below the L1 vertebra, significant lumbar kyphosis or scoliosis, a head circumference larger than 2 cm above the ninetieth percentile, major associated congenital defects, and perinatal hypoxia. However, a number of children with several adverse criteria have been able to lead fulfilling lives.[13] Infants with untreated myelomeningocele have a 2-year survival rate of approximately 5 percent.[12]

## Occult Spinal Dysraphisms

Occult spinal dysraphisms include dorsal dermal sinuses, a tight filum terminale, spinal lipomas, and diastematomyelia (a sagittal division of the spinal cord into two hemicords around an associated bony or cartilaginous septum originating from the posterior vertebral arch). While pathologically these entities are distinct, clinically they frequently are associated with a cutaneous defect over the spine and may present during childhood with urologic, neurologic, or growth abnormalities. A common neurologic complication from these entities is the tethered cord syndrome. Anatomically this results from fixation of the spinal cord to surrounding structures, preventing its normal ascension within the spinal canal during the first year of life. A low conus medullaris extending below the L2 vertebra is the pathologic common denominator. While in the majority of situations a midline skin abnormality is discernible over the lumbosacral spine (Table 18-5), in approximately 30 percent of

Table 18-5. **Cutaneous Abnormalities Associated with Spinal Dysraphism**

| | |
|---|---|
| Hypertrichosis | Lipoma |
| Dimple | Hyperpigmentation |
| Hemangioma | Skin tag |

cases there may be no cutaneous abnormality. Orthopedic problems are common, with growth asymmetry of legs and feet secondary to chronic denervation resulting in cavus foot deformities, hammertoes, or scoliosis. Trophic ulceration may be a particular problem, especially in children with postural foot deformities. Gait abnormalities frequently occur, and disturbed bowel and bladder function is common. Patients may present with urinary incontinence, and occasionally low back pain may be present.

Formal neurologic examination discloses a combination of upper and lower motor neuron signs, depending on the specific site of anatomic disruption. Early diagnosis by magnetic resonance imaging (MRI) is necessary, followed by neurosurgical release of any tethering. Early diagnosis and surgical treatment are of paramount importance to prevent further progression of neurologic and urologic morbidity. While surgery appears to prevent the subsequent appearance of deficits, it may not reverse existing symptoms. It is therefore advised that any infant with a cutaneous abnormality directly over the lumbosacral spine should have a cystometrogram as well as spinal imaging. While previous recommendations have suggested spinal radiography as an initial screening study, there are reports of bony defects of the spine that are mild or poorly seen on radiography owing to immature calcification of the bony structures in infants which leads to erroneous interpretation of results. MRI scanning, while more costly, is clearly the most definitive and direct way of establishing whether or not a significant occult dysraphic state exists.

## DISORDERS OF LOWER MOTOR NEURON UNITS

Disorders of the lower motor neuron unit may be classified by anatomic localization to either the anterior horn cell (located within the ventral horn of the spinal cord), the nerve fiber, the myoneural junction, or the muscle (Fig. 18-2).

### Anterior Horn Cell Disease

#### Poliomyelitis

Poliomyelitis is a viral disease caused by three immunologically distinct polioviruses, which have their greatest effect on the central nervous system. Immunization with killed virus and attenuated live virus has ended the large-scale epidemics that previously occurred. Polio is still seen in nonimmunized children, and outbreaks have occurred in recent years among populations without immunizations. Transmission primarily occurs by human to human contact by secretions from the respiratory tract or by fecal contamination.

Clinically, infection with polio is heralded by headache, malaise, and myalgias. As the disease progresses, the patient develops fever, which may be low-grade, and nuchal rigidity. This is followed by muscle tightness, predominantly in the hamstrings, thighs, and neck. In children under 1 year of age, the characteristic clinical triad includes fever, nuchal rigidity, and spasms of the back muscles.[14] The more progressive the course of the disease, the more severe is the eventual involvement. Anterior horn cells of the brain stem and spinal cord are major targets for infection, and motor weakness is usually profound. The weakness is often asymmetric and scattered. Spinal involvement is more common than bulbar involvement in children under 1 year of age. Bulbar poliomyelitis presents with life-threatening compromise of respiratory and circulatory control centers in the brain stem as well as profound weakness of the respiratory muscles. Fulminant bulbar poliomyelitis has an extremely poor prognosis. Spinal fluid examination reveals a pleocytosis with mononuclear cells, a normal or mildly elevated protein concentration, and a normal glucose. A nonparalytic form of poliomyelitis exists, which is clinically indistinguishable from other forms of meningoencephalitis.

The acute management of poliomyelitis is dependent upon the severity. With the paralytic form of the disease, significant bulbar involvement requires mechanical ventilation and cardiovascular support. The initial flaccid weakness of the muscles may be replaced by gradual tightening and muscle spasms. Early and continued physical therapy is often required. Patients are eventually left with a strikingly asymmetric lower motor neuron paralysis, usually involving the lower extremities. Growth abnormalities, especially leg length discrepancies, are common sequelae from early poliomyelitis.

#### Progressive Spinomuscular Atrophy

Progressive spinomuscular atrophy is a hereditary degenerative disorder affecting the anterior horn cell of the spinal cord. A variety of classifications for these disorders have been described, each based on the age of onset of the disease. The earlier the onset, the poorer the prognosis, with short-term survival. Whether these disorders are variable expressions of one genetic disease or represent genetic heterogeneity is unclear. Clinically they may be divided into an acute variety, in which symptoms begin to appear prior to 6 months of age, and chronic varieties, with onset of symptomatology after 6 months of age. Infants with early onset of the disease generally do not survive past 12 to 24 months, while those with the chronic forms may survive to early adulthood.

Acute infantile spinomuscular atrophy (Werdnig-Hoffmann disease) may present at birth, the infant being profoundly hypotonic and weak. Approximately one-third of mothers may be able to relate a prenatal history of decreased fetal activity during the last few months of pregnancy. With onset after birth, the infant is noted to have a diminished cry and to develop difficulty with sucking and swallowing. As the disease progresses, there is a loss of major motor milestones. On physical examination infants are severely hypotonic and weak, with inability to oppose gravity. The cry is feeble and suck is poor. Tongue fasciculations may be seen, and there is complete areflexia. The thorax is commonly bell-shaped, with pectus excavatum, and paradoxical respirations are often seen. The disease progresses relentlessly, and patients have increasing difficulty handling secretions. They usually expire within the first 2 years of life from pneumonia or respiratory failure.

The chronic form of infantile spinomuscular atrophy begins its onset between 6 and 12 months of age. The progression of weakness is more insidious. Infants are normal until the onset, which is marked by delay in achieving further motor milestones. Although they are able to sit with support and on occasion to sit without support, they are never able to stand or walk. While the distribution of the weakness and the physical findings of hypotonia, weakness, fasciculations, and areflexia are similar to those in the acute infantile form, children with the chronic form of the disease have a slowly progressive course with longer survival. As a result, joint contractures of hips and knees may occur, as well as kyphoscoliosis, and equinovarus deformities. Recurring pulmonary infections remain a constant problem and increase with patient longevity.

Kugelberg-Welander disease is a juvenile variety of spinomuscular atrophy, with onset of symptoms be-

tween the ages of 5 and 15 years. The pelvic girdle is first affected, and patients present with gait abnormalities and difficulty in climbing stairs. Weakness gradually progresses, with eventual arm and shoulder involvement. An unusual lordosis appears, and there is significant loss of bulk of the thigh muscles. Atrophy of the forearm muscles appears later, with atrophy of the hands and fingers occurring late in the disease. On physical examination the deep tendon reflexes are depressed and later absent. This form of spinomuscular atrophy is relatively mild, patients maintaining the ability to walk for 20 years or more after diagnosis. At presentation it may be confused with muscular dystrophy on the basis of the distribution of early muscle weakness, but the lack of pseudohypertrophy and slower progression should distinguish it from dystrophy.

## Peripheral Nerve Disorders

### Hereditary Polyneuropathies

Hereditary polyneuropathies may be divided into those with primary sensory involvement — hereditary sensory neuropathies (HSN) — and those with motor and sensory involvement — hereditary motor and sensory neuropathies (HMSN).

#### Charcot-Marie-Tooth Disease

Type I HMSN, known as Charcot-Marie-Tooth disease is a relatively common hereditary neuropathy, accounting for approximately 50 percent of all cases of hereditary neuropathies in children.[15] It is usually an autosomal dominant disorder, which pathologically is characterized by degeneration of the posterior columns of the spinal cord, loss of anterior horn cells, and degeneration of the spinocerebellar tracts as well as the anterior and posterior nerve roots. Peripheral nerve pathology discloses a hypertrophic neuropathy with significant segmental demyelination of nerve fibers.

Clinically, symptoms begin during childhood, with peroneal muscle involvement presenting as a foot-slapping gait. With progression, the intrinsic foot muscles are affected, leading to development of a pes cavus deformity. Weakness and atrophy involving the intrinsic hand muscles follows, which later spreads to the forearm. The face, trunk, and proximal muscles are usually spared. Contractures of the wrist and fingers may develop, producing a claw-like hand. Patients have striking atrophy and weakness of the distal lower extremities, which gives them a stork-like appearance. Vibration and position sense are mildly diminished distally. Vasomotor signs, with flushing, cyanosis, and marbling of the skin, are common. Deep tendon reflexes are absent at the ankles and may be diminished elsewhere. Palpation of the nerves may reveal hypertrophy. Laboratory studies reveal an elevated cerebrospinal fluid (CSF) protein in 50 percent of patients. Reduced motor and sensory nerve conduction velocities constitute the hallmark of the disease. Progression is slow, and the patient may reach a plateau; there is no apparent shortening of the life span. No specific therapy is available aside from physical therapy to the affected extremities to maintain strength and range of motion. Orthopedic measures are designed to prevent disabilities.

### Peroneal Muscle Atrophy

Type II HMSN is peroneal muscular atrophy, a condition characterized by axonal degeneration of the peripheral nerve. Clinically, it is similar to Charcot-Marie-Tooth disease (Type I HMSN), with peroneal muscle weakness and atrophy. This entity at times has been referred to as the neuronal form of Charcot-Marie-Tooth disease. While it also is inherited in an autosomal dominant fashion, the onset of disease occurs later in life. On physical examination there is no palpable enlargement of the peripheral nerves. Weakness of hand muscles seems less severe, while involvement of the plantar flexor muscles of the foot is greater. Sensory loss is mild and usually involves the distal lower extremities. Nerve conduction velocities are often normal or near normal, which distinguish this disorder from type I HMSN. Electromyography reveals denervation. Nerve biopsy fails to show any histologic evidence of hypertrophic neuropathy or segmental demyelination, which are characteristic of type I HMSN.

### Dejerine-Sottas Disease

Type III HMSN, known as hypertrophic interstitial neuropathy of infancy or Dejerine-Sottas disease, is an autosomal recessive disorder, pathologically similar to Charcot-Marie-Tooth disease. Clinically, onset of symptoms occurs early in childhood, with cases reported at birth.[15] In infants and young children there is a delay in early motor development, with a disturbance of gait and weakness of the hands, as well as distal muscle atrophy and absent deep tendon reflexes. Sensation is impaired distally, particularly as it affects vibration and position. Some patients have been reported to be ataxic. Pupillary abnormalities are common, including pupillary miosis and decreased response to light. Peripheral nerves are hypertrophic and easily palpable. Deafness may occur. Approximately 35 percent of patients develop kyphoscoliosis and foot deformities. Laboratory studies disclose an elevated cerebrospinal fluid (CSF) protein content in 75 percent of patients and severely reduced motor and sensory nerve conduction velocities. Nerve biopsy discloses a markedly enlarged nerve, with decreased myelinated nerve fibers and evidence of segmental demyelination with an "onion bulb" formation. No specific treatment is available aside from physical therapy and orthopedic measures.

### Refsum's Disease

Type IV HMSN, known as Refsum's disease, is an autosomal recessive disorder with an insidious onset occurring at any time from early childhood to the third decade. It is characterized by anorexia, gait abnormalities, progressive ichthyosis, night blindness, retinitis pigmentosa, anosmia, a sensorineural hearing deficit, and a polyneuropathy with distal weakness, muscular atrophy, and loss of deep tendon reflexes. There is a mild impairment of touch, and a pes cavus foot deformity is frequently noted. On laboratory examination the CSF protein is elevated. The pathophysiologic basis of the disorder appears to be a peroxisomal deficiency in fatty acid metabolism with an inability to oxidize phytanic acid. Treatment is directed at reducing the serum phytanic acid level by dietary restriction of phytanic acid.

### Hereditary Sensory Neuropathies

There are several inherited clinical syndromes (HSNs) of which the outstanding feature is failure to respond in a normal manner to painful stimuli. Patients with these conditions have sensory impairment without muscular weakness. The deep tendon reflexes are diminished or absent. Trophic changes involving the digits of the upper and lower extremities are seen, as well as chronic perforating ulcerations of the feet with eventual destruction of the underlying bones.

The most notable disorder within this group is the Riley-Day syndrome (type III HSN, or familial dysautonomia). This is a multisystem autosomal recessive disorder, which is seen predominantly in Jewish children of eastern European descent. Clinical onset occurs during infancy and is characterized by feeding difficulties, vomiting, and pulmonary infections. Autonomic dysfunction is heralded by decreased or absent tearing, abnormal temperature regulation with increased sweating, skin blotching, and labile blood pressure. Neurologic examination discloses absent corneal reflexes, poor motor coordination, hypotonia, diminished or absent deep tendon reflexes, relative indifference to pain, and absence of the fungiform papillae on the tongue. Emotional lability and mental retardation have been reported. Scoliosis is commonly seen and becomes more marked with age. Patients often succumb during infancy or early childhood from cardiopulmonary arrest secondary to pneumonia or an episode of hypotension. Some may survive to young adulthood. Treatment has been symptomatic. Feeding and swallowing difficulties in the infant may necessitate gavage feeding, and hypertensive crises are treated with sedation and chlorpromazine. Pathologically, there is a decrease in unmyelinated fibers of the cutaneous nerves, as well as decreased myelination in the dorsal root and posterior columns of the spinal cord. The sympathetic ganglia are hypoplastic, and some patients have shown a lack of myelination and neuronal depletion in the pons and medulla.

## Friedreich's Ataxia

Friedreich's ataxia is a hereditary degenerative disease characterized by progressive ataxia. While it is best classified as a spinocerebellar degenerative disease, there is significant involvement of the peripheral nerves and the posterior columns of the spinal cord. The disorder is generally inherited as an autosomal recessive trait. Clinical manifestations usually begin during childhood, with a mean age of onset of 10 years.[16] Commonly, children present with gait instability and frequent falling, and occasionally they may be slow in learning to walk. With progression there is incoordination of the hands and frequently disturbed speech. Skeletal deformities are common, 75 percent of patients having pes cavus, hammertoes, and wasting of the intrinsic foot muscles; occasionally, foot abnormalities may be noted at birth. Kyphoscoliosis frequently develops. The most prominent neurologic sign is limb, truncal, and speech ataxia, and with progression there is weakness of the lower limbs and wasting of the small muscles of the hands and

feet. There is a gradual loss of vibration and proprioception, as well as complaints of pain, cramps, and paresthesias. Deep tendon reflexes are diminished or absent.

The disorder generally progresses slowly. Patients with advanced Friedreich's ataxia are bedridden and have difficulty in swallowing. Myocarditis is seen in the majority of patients, and electrocardiographic changes and congenital heart block are common. Death usually results from myocarditis, with intractable congestive heart failure. Patients with Friedreich's ataxia also may develop deafness, have an unusually high incidence of diabetes, and frequently have difficulty with bowel and bladder control. These patients should remain active for as long as possible and should participate in physical therapy. Owing to the progressive nature of the disorder as well as the cardiac involvement, orthopedic surgery for skeletal deformities is generally not advised.

## Toxic Neuropathies

Exposure to a variety of exogenous substances may result in an acquired toxic neuropathy. Major categories include antibiotic-induced neuropathies, antimetabolite neuropathies, heavy metal neuropathies, and glue sniffing neuropathy. In general these neuropathies cause weakness of the lower extremities, with foot drop and reduced deep tendon reflexes. Antibiotics associated with a peripheral neuropathy include isoniazid for tuberculosis,[17] kanamycin,[18] nitrofurantoin,[19] and high-dose chloramphenicol.[20]

The most notable neuropathic antimetabolite is vincristine, used in the treatment of leukemia and neuroblastoma.[21] Vincristine neuropathy is dose-related and commonly manifests with weakness of the extensor muscles of the fingers and wrists, as well as bilateral foot drop. Patients may be unable to walk or stand without support in severe cases. The neuropathy improves when the drug is stopped or the dose is reduced. Although the weakness subsides rapidly, the deep tendon reflexes may never return to normal.

A heavy metal neuropathy may be seen with lead, arsenic, or thallium exposure. Lead intoxication in children under 5 years of age generally produces an encephalopathy characterized by seizures, ataxia, and headache, with increased intracranial pressure. In older children and adults, a motor neuropathy with only mild sensory involvement may result. Children with lead intoxication commonly present with bilateral foot drop, while adults present with a wrist drop. The diagnosis is usually suggested by a history of lead exposure in the presence of anemia and basophilic stippling of red blood cells. Radiographic studies of the patient's long bones may disclose dense metaphyseal bands.

A sciatic neuropathy may result from the injection of a variety of substances into the buttocks and presumably the sciatic nerve of neonates and small children. Drugs clinically implicated include antibiotics (penicillin, streptomycin, sulfisoxazole), vitamins B and K, and tetanus antitoxin. Paralysis is usually apparent within days after the injection. The prognosis for recovery is usually poor, with only one-third of patients fully recovering. Physical therapy should be directed toward restoring function and preventing contractures. Orthopedic reconstruction may be necessary. Long-term sequelae from such an injury include limb growth retardation with plantar flexion and inversion deformities of the foot, as well as trophic ulcerations.

### Neuropathies Associated with Metabolic Disease

A number of metabolic diseases may be associated with a neuropathy; they include diabetes mellitus, uremia, acute intermittent porphyria, and vitamin deficiency states. The most notable of these is the diabetic neuropathy.[22] While this is an extremely important cause of chronic neuropathy in adults, it rarely occurs in children. There are several different forms of diabetic neuropathy, the most common being a slowly progressive, symmetric distal sensory polyneuropathy involving the lower extremities. There are often complaints of dysesthesia and distal pain. Autonomic involvement may develop and may be problematic. Less common are a mononeuropathy and multiple mononeuropathies with isolated cranial nerve and peripheral nerve lesions. In these the onset tends to be more rapid, and motor involvement is more severe than sensory involvement.

### Idiopathic Polyneuritis (Guillain-Barré Syndrome)

Guillain-Barré syndrome may occur at any age. Approximately 75 percent of children have a preceding nonspecific viral illness. Associations with infectious mononucleosis, mumps, rubella, and rubeola have been reported. The onset of the illness usually begins with distal weakness in the lower extremities but may be preceded or accompanied by paresthesias. Approximately 50 percent of patients may have cranial nerve involvement. With progression of the disease the weakness ascends, and if there is respiratory compromise, mechanical ventilation will be required for supportive care. Weakness of the affected extremities may be profound, and deep tendon reflexes are absent, but sensory deficits are minimal. Autonomic dysfunction may occur, as manifest by facial flushing, labile blood pressure, and occasionally cardiac arrhythmias. Laboratory evaluation discloses an elevated CSF protein level with little pleocytosis. Nerve conduction velocities are slow.

Treatment is generally supportive, with careful attention directed to the patient's pulmonary function. Plasmapheresis early in the course of the disease appears to be of benefit in adults as well as children.[23] While near complete recovery tends to occur in children, some patients may have mild residual deficits, and a few may have relapses over the course of months to years, with a more chronic course. The disorder appears to be immune-mediated. Early physical therapy should be instituted as soon as the patient is clinically stable.

## DISORDERS OF THE MYONEURAL JUNCTION

A number of disorders may cause peripheral nervous system dysfunction by disrupting transmission across the myoneural junction. These include myasthenia gravis, the myasthenic syndrome, botulism, and a variety of toxins. Of the various disorders the most important in children is myasthenia gravis.

Myasthenia gravis is a chronic disease characterized by variable and fluctuating weakness of skeletal muscles. True myasthenia gravis is an autoimmune-mediated disorder with antibodies against the acetylcholine receptor in muscle. Children with myasthenia gravis may present with one of three clinical forms, namely, neonatal, congenital, or juvenile.

The neonatal form of myasthenia gravis is seen in approximately 10 to 15 percent of infants born to mothers with myasthenia gravis and presumably occurs due to transfer of maternal acetylcholine receptor antibody across the placenta. At birth the infant is weak, with a feeble cry, ptosis, and poor suck. There is usually no pulmonary involvement. Since neonatal myasthenia is mediated by maternal antibody, it is a transient disorder, which resolves upon the disappearance of the maternal antibodies, within 3 to 5 weeks after birth.

The congenital form of myasthenia is quite uncommon, and the diagnosis is usually not made until the age of 1 or 2 years. At birth these infants are only mildly affected. There tend to be familial occurrences, and some of these patients may actually have a non-autoimmune-mediated hereditary problem of neuromuscular transmission. There have been reports of associated arthrogryposis at birth in some of these infants.

The juvenile form of myasthenia is the most common and is similar to the adult variety. Patients usually present with ptosis and extraocular muscle involvement. Symptoms tend to be worse at day's end, and fluctuating muscle weakness is a hallmark. Partial or complete remissions may occur. Muscle atrophy and joint contractures are generally not seen. There is an important association between juvenile myasthenia gravis and hyperthyroidism, necessitating a complete endocrinologic evaluation in any affected child.

# MUSCLE DISORDERS

The myopathies are primary diseases of skeletal muscle due to a variety of different causes. Muscular dystrophies are genetically determined diseases of muscle characterized by progressive muscle degeneration and weakness. Muscle diseases may be classified into three major groups, namely, muscular dystrophies, congenital myopathies, and inflammatory myopathies.

## Muscular Dystrophies

### Duchenne Muscular Dystrophy

Duchenne muscular dystrophy is clearly the most important myopathy affecting children. This disorder is an X-linked recessive disease primarily affecting young boys. Significant advances in the understanding of the molecular basis of this disorder have occurred in recent years. Duchenne muscular dystrophy and a variant known as Becker dystrophy are now known to result from abnormalities of the structural muscle protein dystrophin.[24] Clinically, patients with Duchenne muscular dystrophy appear normal until they begin to walk or run. While there may be some delay in unassisted walking, the parents usually become aware of a clumsy gait and a

tendency toward falling. The patient has difficulty climbing stairs and when rising from the floor will use the upper extremities to "climb up" his legs (Gowers sign). The child may complain of leg pain at the end of the day and often demonstrates a waddling gait, with toe walking and an accentuated lumbar lordosis. Physical examination reveals weakness of the proximal muscles of the extremity and frequently enlargement of the posterior compartment of the calf (pseudohypertrophy). Other muscles that may undergo pseudohypertrophy include the quadriceps, deltoid, and infraspinatus. The muscles are firm to palpation. Deep tendon reflexes are diminished.

The disorder progresses relentlessly, with loss of muscle bulk and strength such that most patients are confined to a wheelchair by early adolescence. Periods of immobilization appear to hasten the patient's inability to walk. Severe contractures and kyphoscoliosis are late complications. Progressive chest deformities impair pulmonary function, with resultant recurrent pulmonary infections. Cardiac involvement is common, and arrhythmias may be noted. Few patients survive to the third decade. Laboratory studies disclose a marked elevation of serum creatinine kinase (CK), which often occurs before there is clinical evidence of weakness. As the disease progresses, there is a slow decline in the CK level, paralleling the loss of muscle bulk. Biochemical testing for the dystrophin content of affected muscle discloses a deficiency, which is well documented and completely disease-specific.[24] There is no specific treatment for Duchenne dystrophy other than supportive care and careful attention to pulmonary function. Physical therapy early in the disease should be directed at prevention of contractures. Orthopedic procedures are frequently performed to maintain independent ambulation as long as possible.

### Becker Muscular Dystrophy

Becker muscular dystrophy is similar to Duchenne's dystrophy. It, too, is an X-linked disorder due to a dystrophin abnormality, and it has a similar clinical presentation. The most significant difference is that progression is slower and patients remain ambulatory for several decades. It is common for patients to survive into mid-adult life. Joint contractures and severe kyphoscoliosis are less common. Biochemically, the Becker type of muscular dystrophy appears to be related to a qualitative abnormality involving dystrophin and not to a quantitative deficiency as in Duchenne dystrophy.[24]

## Facioscapulohumeral Muscular Dystrophy

Facioscapulohumeral muscular dystrophy is an autosomal dominant disorder with onset of symptoms commonly beginning in the second decade. Clinically, patients first notice facial weakness, with difficulty in whistling and sipping. On examination there is wasting and weakness of the facial muscles, shoulder girdle weakness with scapular winging, and proximal arm muscle involvement. Ultimately there may be weakness in the anterolateral compartment of the lower limbs, with an associated foot drop. A significant lumbar lordosis may develop. Progression is usually slow, but if symptoms present early in childhood, the clinical course may be more severe. Laboratory studies reveal an elevated serum creatine kinase (CK).

## Limb-Girdle Muscular Dystrophy

Limb-girdle muscular dystrophy is a autosomal recessive disorder in approximately 60 percent of cases. Weakness usually begins in the proximal lower extremities during the second or third decade of life. Shoulder girdle involvement is noted, with sagging of the shoulders and weakness of neck flexors and extensors. The proximal arms are also weak, while facial involvement is minimal. Approximately 30 percent of patients may develop pseudohypertrophy, usually of the calves. As in the other dystrophies, the serum CK is elevated.

## Myotonic Dystrophy

Myotonic dystrophy is an autosomal dominant disorder characterized by muscle wasting, weakness, and myotonia. The disease usually appears in late adolescence or early adulthood, but congenital and juvenile forms may be seen. The degree of myotonia and weakness is variable in each patient.[25] Muscle wasting and weakness are most notable in the face, sternocleidomastoid, and limb girdle musculature. Eventually muscles of the forearm and hand and the anterolateral muscles of the lower extremity are affected. Distal weakness may be greater than proximal weakness. Weakness of the palatal and pharyngeal muscles may result in a nasal voice and a high-arched palate. Clinical myotonia is absent prior to 1 year of age and is present in only 12 percent of children less than 5 years of age.[25]

Myotonic dystrophy is a systemic disorder with a variety of associated abnormalities. Arthrogryposis may be noted at birth, and mental retardation is seen in 80 percent of patients with myotonic dystrophy. Cardiac conduction abnormalities with arrhythmias may be seen in 50 percent of patients, and posterior cataracts are present in adults. A variety of endocrine abnormalities have been reported, including diabetes mellitus, frontal baldness, loss of body hair, and testicular atrophy. The clinical course is one of gradual debilitation, with full development of the systemic features during adult years. Eventually cardiac involvement with conduction defects and ultimately congestive heart failure are the most serious complications. The serum CK is usually normal, but electromyography discloses prolonged trains of high frequency discharges arising from single fibers or groups of muscle fibers in response to electrode insertion or movement. Over a loudspeaker their sound is highly characteristic, like that of a "dive bomber." While the exact pathogenesis of the disorder remains unknown, it now appears that myotonic dystrophy is linked to chromosome 19.[26]

# Congenital Myopathies

The congenital myopathies are a group of disorders characterized by structural changes within the muscle cell. These conditions are apparent at or shortly after birth and are characterized by hypotonia and variable degrees of weakness. They are generally, nonprogressive or only slowly progressive. Frequently they are associated with skeletal abnormalities, including elongated facial features, a narrow high palate, hip dislocation, lordosis, kyphoscoliosis, and pes cavus deformities. While the serum CK is usually normal, electromyography frequently demonstrates mild myopathic findings. Microscopic examination of muscle reveals the characteristic pathologic changes for which the diseases have been named. While numerous congenital myopathies have been identified, the most important disorders include nemaline myopathy, central core disease, myotubular myopathy, and mitochondrial myopathy. Although these disorders were previously termed "benign congenital hypotonias," it is apparent that some of them may have severe involvements in early infancy, with profound respiratory and bulbar muscle weakness resulting in early death. There is an important association with malignant hyperthermia, especially in the case of central core disease.

## Inflammatory Myopathies

### Dermatomyositis

Dermatomyositis is the most common inflammatory muscle disorder of childhood. It is a systemic disease that is characterized by low-grade fever, fatigue, anorexia, a typical skin rash, muscle pain, and weakness. The initial symptoms usually are weakness and fatiguability. The skin rash frequently begins with an erythematous/violaceous discoloration of the upper eyelids and periorbital edema. There may also be erythematous scaly involvement of the extensor surfaces of the joints, particularly the knuckles, elbows, and knees. Muscle weakness is most marked proximally, with significant involvement of the flexor muscles of the neck and limb girdle. Early contractures at the ankles may produce a toe-walking gait. In children with an acute onset, the weakness may advance rapidly and involve the bulbar musculature, which indicates a poor prognosis and frequently a fatal outcome. Perforation of the gastrointestinal tract is another common sequela of fulminant dermatomyositis. Significant chronic sequelae also may result, including irreversible weakness, contractures, and subcutaneous calcium deposits.[27] Routine laboratory studies reveal an elevated erythrocyte sedimentation rate, as well as an elevated serum CK, and electromyography often reveals myopathic changes. A muscle biopsy reveals a vasculitis with endothelial cell degeneration and regeneration, muscle infarction, and denervation atrophy.

Untreated dermatomyositis has a poor prognosis. Early aggressive therapy with prednisone and immunosuppressive agents such as methotrexate, cyclophosphamide, and azothiaprine should be begun and continued for 1 to 2 years.[28] A structured program of physical therapy is also essential to the overall treatment and eventual prognosis. Of children who receive early intervention 80 percent have a favorable outcome.

### Other Inflammatory Diseases

A variety of disorders, including rheumatic fever, rheumatoid arthritis, and collagen vascular disease, may be associated with an inflammatory myopathy.[29] Chronic tuberculosis and sarcoidosis as well as parasitic infections such as trichinosis and toxoplasmosis may all produce a myositis. The treatment of these various inflammatory myopathies is dependent upon the specific etiology. A characteristic laboratory feature of most of these disorders is an elevated serum CK.

## REFERENCES

1. Franco S, Andrews BF: Reduction of cerebral palsy with neonatal intensive care. Clin Res 24:66a, 1975
2. Crothers B, Paine RS: The Natural History of Cerebral Palsy. Harvard University Press, Cambridge, 1959
3. Little WJ: On the influence of abnormal parturition, difficult labor, premature birth, and asphyxia neonatorum on the mental and physical condition of the child especially in relation to deformities. Lancet II:378, 1861
4. Nelson KB, Ellenberg JH: Antecedents of cerebral palsy: multivariate analysis of risk. N Engl J Med 315:81, 1986
5. Nelson KB: What proportion of cerebral palsy is related to birth asphyxia? J Pediatr 112:572, 1988
6. Paneth N: Birth and the origins of cerebral palsy. N Engl J Med 315:124, 1986
7. Ellenberg J, Nelson KB: Birthweight and gestational age in children with cerebral palsy or seizure disorders. Am J Dis Child 133:1044, 1979
8. Hagberg B, Hagberg G: Prenatal and perinatal risk factors in a survey of 681 Swedish cases. Clin Dev Med 57:116, 1984
9. Peacock WJ, Arens LJ, Berman B: Cerebral palsy spasticity: selective posterior rhizotomy. Pediatr Neurosci 13:61, 1987
10. Vaughan CL, Berman B, Staudt LA, Peacock WJ: Gait analysis of cerebral palsy children before and after rhizotomy. Pediatr Neurosci 14:299, 1988
11. Anderson FM: Occult spinal dysraphism: a series of 73 cases. Pediatrics 55:826, 1975
12. Lorber J: Spina bifida cystica: results of treatment of 270 consecutive cases with criteria for selection for the future. Arch Dis Child 47:854, 1972
13. Stein SC, Schut L, Ames MD: Selection for early treatment in myelomeningocele. Pediatrics 54:553, 1974
14. Abramson H, Greenburg M: Acute poliomyelitis in infants under one year of age: epidemiological and clinical features. Pediatrics 16:478, 1955
15. Hagberg B, Lyon G: Pooled European series of hereditary peripheral neuropathies in infancy and childhood. Neuropediatrics 12:9, 1981
16. Barbeau A: Friedreich's ataxia 1987 — an overview. Can J Neurol Sci 5:161, 1978

17. Jones WA, Jones GP: Peripheral neuropathy due to isoniazid. Lancet I:1073, 1973
18. Freemon FR, Parker RL Jr, Greer M: Unusual neurotoxicity of kanamycin. JAMA 200:410, 1967
19. Collings H: Polyneuropathy associated with nitrofuran therapy. Arch Neurol 3:656, 1960
20. Joy RJT, Scalettar R, Sodee DB: Optic and peripheral neuritis: probable effect of chloramphenicol therapy. JAMA 173:1731, 1960
21. Casey EB, Jellife AM, Le Quesne PM, Millett YL: Vincristine neuropathy: clinical and electrophysiological observation. Brain 96:69, 1973
22. Henson RA, Urich H: Metabolic neuropathies. p.l. In Vinken PJ, Bruyn GE (eds): Handbook of Clinical Neurology. Vol. 8. North Holland, Amsterdam, 1970
23. The Guillain-Barré Study Group: Plasmapheresis and acute Guillain-Barré syndrome. Neurology 35:1096, 1985
24. Hoffman EP, Fischbeck KH, Brown RH et al: Dystrophin characterization in muscle biopsies from Duchenne and Becker muscular dystrophy patients. N Engl J Med 318:1363, 1988
25. Harper PS: Myotonic dystrophy. WB Saunders, Philadelphia, 1979
26. Davies KE, Forrest S, Smith T et al: Molecular analysis of human muscular dystrophies. Muscle Nerve 10:191, 1987
27. Wedgewood RJ, Cook C, Cohen J: Dermatomyositis: report of 26 cases in children with a discussion of endocrine therapy in 13. Pediatrics 12:447, 1953
28. Fischer TJ, Rachelefsky GS, Klein RB et al: Childhood dermatomyositis and polymyositis: treatment with methotrexate and prednisone. Am J Dis Child 133:386, 1979
29. Mastaglia FL, Ojeda VJ: Inflammatory myopathies: Part 1 and Part 2. Ann Neurol 17:215, 317, 1985

# 19

# Operative Treatment of Neurogenic Foot Deformities

*SHLOMO PORAT*
*GERSHON CHAIMSKY*

Neurogenic foot deformities can be defined as developmental deformities caused by muscle imbalance secondary to disease of the central or peripheral nervous system. The foot deformity may be congenital when the neurologic deficit occurs prenatally; however, the vast majority of neurogenic foot deformities develop postnatally. The type of deformity that occurs is determined primarily by the specific etiology and pattern of the neurologic deficit and by the age of the child at the time that the deficit occurs. Classic examples of neurogenic foot deformity patterns that commonly occur as the result of specific neurologic disorders include pes equinovarus in poliomyelitis, pes calcaneus in spina bifida (myelomeningocele), pes cavovarus in hereditary motor and sensory neuropathy (type I Charcot-Marie-Tooth disease), and pes equinus in cerebral palsy.

Neurogenic foot deformities are usually progressive owing to the inherent lack of normal muscle balance. Treatment must include not only correction of the deformity but also muscle rebalancing and long-term maintenance of correction. The primary objective in the treatment of neurogenic foot deformity is to create a plantigrade foot, in which the distribution of forces during weight-bearing will be as normal as possible, through nonsurgical or surgical correction of any residual foot deformity, tendon transfers to produce appropriate muscle balance, and the use of braces and/or orthoses as needed.

## CLASSIFICATION OF NEUROGENIC FOOT DEFORMITIES

The classification of a neurogenic foot deformity is usually based upon its type and etiology. We divide neurogenic foot deformities into the following five categories according to the type of deformity present: (1) pes equinus or pes equinovarus; (2) pes calcaneus or pes calcaneovalgus; (3) pes cavus or supinatus; (4) pes valgus or pronated foot; and (5) congenital convex pes valgus. The surgical correction of these foot deformities described briefly below will be covered in this chapter.

### Classification by Type

#### Pes Equinus

In pes equinus (Fig. 19-1), plantar flexion of the forefoot and hindfoot usually develops secondary to weak anterior group dorsiflexors in the presence of normal or spastic plantar flexors of the posterior muscle group. Over time, contracture of the gastrosoleus and tibialis posterior muscles, long flexor tendons, and ligaments and joint capsule occurs in the varying combinations and severity. The calcaneus and talus assume fixed plantar-flexed positions. In the spastic child the equinus may be dynamic only, without true tissue contracture.

475

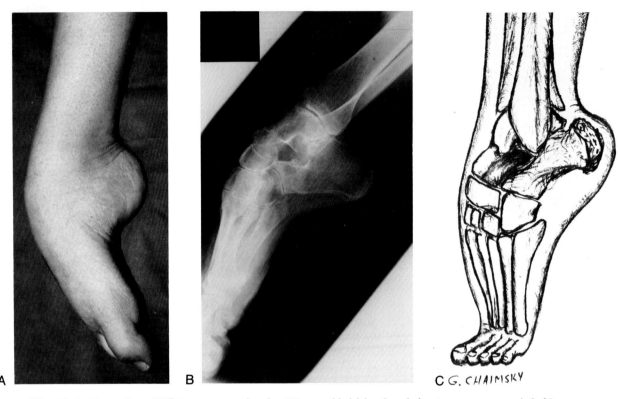

A      B      C G. CHAIMSKY

**Fig. 19-1.** Pes equinus. (**A**) Extreme pes equinus in a 17-year-old girl developed after trauma over a period of 2 years. (**B**) Radiograph of the same patient. (**C**) Graphic demonstration of pes equinus.

## Pes Equinovarus

In pes equinovarus (Fig. 19-2), the forefoot and hindfoot are in plantar flexion, with an associated hindfoot varus and forefoot supinatus. The deformity occurs as a result of weak dorsiflexion of the anterior muscle group and overpowering of the lateral muscle group evertors by normal or spastic plantar flexors and invertors of the posterior muscle group. Shortening and contracture of the gastrosoleus, tibialis posterior, long flexors, and posteromedial joint capsules and ligaments gradually develop. The pattern of weight-bearing depends upon the severity of the developing deformity. In extreme pes equinovarus most of the weight is born by the base and head of the fifth metatarsal, which often results in severe callus formation or ulceration (Fig. 19-2C).

## Pes Varus

Pes varus is a foot deformity in which both the hindfoot and forefoot are inverted, so that weight is borne on the lateral border of the foot. The forefoot may also be su-

pinated on the hindfoot. The most common etiology is the overpowering of weak evertors (peroneal muscle group) by normal or spastic invertor muscles.

## Pes Valgus

Pes valgus (Fig. 19-3) is a foot deformity in which both the lateral border of both hindfoot and forefoot is higher than the medial border. Weight is borne mainly by the medial part of the foot. Pes valgus occurs in feet with spastic peroneal muscles or in children with hypotonic muscle disorders.

## Pes Calcaneus

In pes calcaneus (Fig. 19-4) the hindfoot and forefoot are dorsiflexed so that most or all weight is borne by the heel, which often causes marked hypertrophy and callus formation of the heel pad. Fissures, scarring, and ulceration of the heel pad are common in older children. Pes calcaneus develops as a result of weakness or paralysis of posterior group muscles (gastrosoleus and long flexors), which are overpowered by normal or strong tibialis ante-

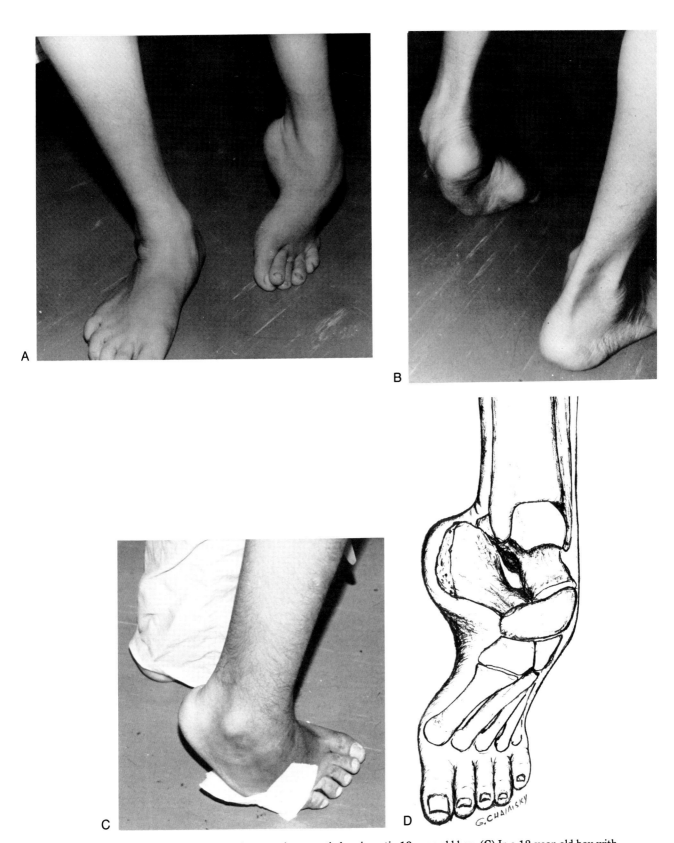

**Fig. 19-2.** (**A & B**) Spastic pes equinovarus in a spastic hemiparetic 13-year-old boy. (**C**) In a 12-year-old boy with myelomeningocele weight-bearing on the head of the fifth metatarsal results in a pressure sore. (**D**) Graphic representation of pes equinovarus.

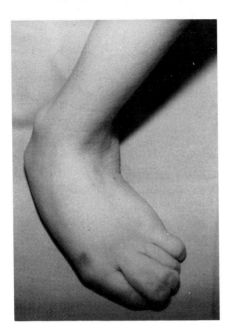

**Fig. 19-3.** Spastic pes valgus, with eversion of the forefoot.

rior, long extensors, and peroneals. Over time, contracture of the tibialis anterior, long extensors, and anterior joint capsule develops.

### Pes Calcaneovalgus

In pes calcaneovalgus the hindfoot is dorsiflexed at the ankle and the forefoot is everted or pronated relative to the hindfoot. Most of the weight-bearing occurs at the heel pad and along the plantar medial border of the foot. Pes calcaneovalgus is seen in myelomeningocele and spastic conditions.

### Pes Cavus

In pes cavus (Fig. 19-5) the os calcis is in the calcaneus position, whereas the forefoot is in equinus. Both the medial and lateral columns of the foot are accentuated. Calcaneus and/or varus deformity of the heel, equinus of the forefoot, a plantar-flexed first ray, and claw toes are often present. Weight-bearing occurs primarily at the heel pad and the ball of the foot. Severe callus formation and pain often occur at the heel pad and the plantar aspect of the metatarsophalangeal joints. Contracture of the plantar fascia is present.

### Pes Cavovarus

Pes cavovarus (Fig. 19-6) has all the characteristics of pes cavus in addition to a structural varus deformity of the calcaneus, which is demonstrated on axial radiographs of the heel.

### Congenital Convex Pes Valgus

Congenital convex pes valgus (Fig.19-7) is often called *congenital vertical talus* or *rocker-bottom foot*. The deformity has many elements of pes equinovarus but is more complex. The hindfoot is in equinus; the posterior tuberosity of the calcaneus is superiorly displaced, while the talar head is directed vertically toward the sole of the foot; and the forefoot is dorsiflexed on the hindfoot at the midtarsal joint. The uncorrected deformity in an ambulatory child results in a large callosity under the talar head.

## Classification by Etiology

Classification of neurogenic foot deformity by etiology is also essential to the development of an appropriate treatment plan and assessment of long-term prognosis. A brief classification of neurogenic foot deformity that is confined to the clinical material discussed in this chapter is presented in Table 19-1.

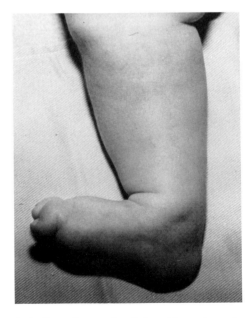

**Fig. 19-4.** Pes calcaneus in a baby with myelomeningocele.

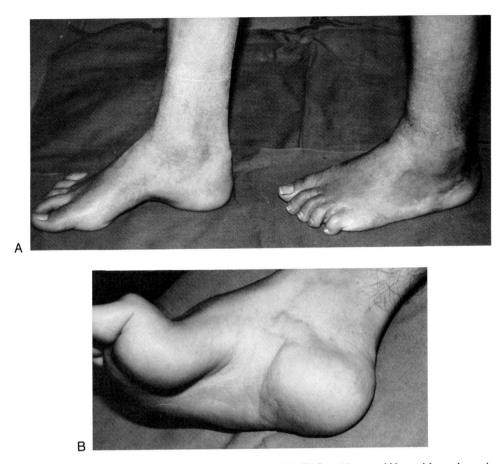

**Fig. 19-5.** Pes cavus. **(A)** Idiopathic pes cavus in a 15-year-old girl. **(B)** In a 17-year-old boy with myelomeningocele.

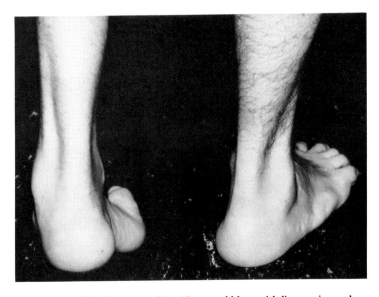

**Fig. 19-6.** Pes Cavovarus in a 17-year-old boy with lipomeningocele.

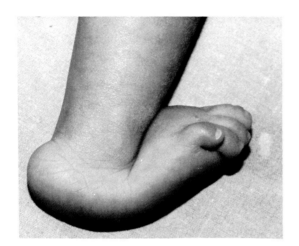

**Fig. 19-7.** Neurogenic vertical talus in a newborn with myelomeningocele.

## SURGICAL PROCEDURES

### Equinus

In our practice the most common cause of equinus deformity is cerebral palsy. Equinus usually develops as a result of the overpowering by spastic gastrosoleus and

Table 19-1. **Classification of Neurogenic Foot Deformities in Children by Etiology**

| Etiology | Type of Deformity |
| --- | --- |
| Central Nervous System Involvement | |
| Brain damage/cerebral palsy (includes perinatal brain damage, head injuries, and encephalitis) | Pes equinus<br>Pes equinovarus<br>Pes valgus<br>Pes calcaneovalgus |
| Myelodysplasia (includes meningocele, myelomeningocele, lipomeningocele, and spinal dysraphism with neurologic involvement) | Neurogenic pes equinovarus (clubfoot)<br>Pes calcaneus<br>Paralytic pes valgus<br>Combination |
| Anterior horn cell damage | Pes equinus<br>Pes equinovarus<br>Pes calcaneovalgus<br>Pes cavus<br>Pes cavovarus<br>Pes cavovalgus |
| Peripheral Nerve Disorders | |
| Hereditary motor and sensory neuropathies (type I Charcot-Marie-Tooth disease), Roussy-Levy syndrome[27] | Pes cavus<br>Pes cavovarus<br>Pes equinus<br>Pes equinovarus |
| Other neuromuscular diseases (includes arthogryposis multiplex congenita and spinal muscular atrophy) | Pes equinovarus<br>Pes equinus |

long flexors of weak anterior muscles. We do not recommend serial casting and cast wedging for treatment of equinus secondary to spasticity of the gastrosoleus muscle or contracture of the Achilles tendon. Experience with this technique has proved the end result to be poor and the amount of suffering imposed upon the child to be unjustified. Pressure sores are also common. We agree with Tachdjian, who condemns the use of wedged casts in the treatment of spastic equinus.[1] The most commonly employed treatment in our clinic in more recent years has been the Hoke technique for percutaneous lengthening of the Achilles tendon (Bowen R, personal communication).

The primary indication for Achilles tendon lengthening or gastrocnemius recession is either a fixed equinus due to a true contracture of the Achilles tendon or a dynamic equinus noted during ambulation secondary to a spastic gastrosoleus muscle group. One of the most important clinical signs to be aware of is a posterior thrust of the knee joint during gait, which indicates a short or spastic gastrosoleus muscle complex. The ground reaction force in a child with equinus often results in genu recurvatum with each step.[2] When the equinus is dynamic without true contracture of the Achilles tendon, a procedure to weaken the gastrosoleus muscle group should be considered. The preferred technique at our institution for recession of the gastrocnemius muscle complex, originally described by Vulpius, consists of one or two V-shaped incisions in the aponeurotic tendon of the gastrocnemius. The technique was also later modified by Baher (see Fig. 14-4). More recently, however, we have utilized the Hoke technique for most cases of spastic equinus. The final decision as to which procedure will be used sometimes cannot be made until the child is examined under anesthesia. Achilles tendon lengthening is the most common orthopedic surgical procedure performed at our institution for cerebral palsy.

### Hoke Techniques for Percutaneous Lengthening of the Achilles Tendon

The Hoke operation is performed under general anesthesia with the knee fully extended and the foot maximally dorsiflexed. The tendon is percutaneously partially sectioned at three sites, with a #15 surgical knife (Fig. 19-8). The knife is introduced distally at the midline of the tendon and turned medially, and half the width of the tendon is cut. The second cut is performed just distal to

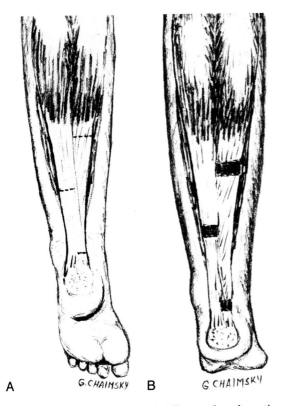

**Fig. 19-8.** Hoke technique for Achilles tendon elongation. (**A**) Three transverse cuttings. (**B**) After sliding, the tendon is longer, keeping its continuity.

the musculotendinous junction in the same manner as the first. The third cut is made from midline to lateral and equidistant from the proximal and distal cuts, and again half the width of the tendon is sectioned. The foot is then carefully dorsiflexed with the knee extended until the cut portions of the tendon give way and slide, enabling the foot to be positioned with 0 to 5 degrees of dorsiflexion. The dorsiflexion force must be well controlled in order to prevent complete separation of the tendon.

Postoperatively, the child is placed in a weight-bearing above-knee cast for 6 days for comfort only. After the cast is removed, a muscle stretching and strengthening physical therapy program is begun. A brace is not used postoperatively. Percutaneous Achilles tendon lengthening is most appropriate in younger children and is not recommended as a secondary procedure. Open Z-plasty lengthening of the Achilles tendon is preferred in older spastic children or in cases of recurrent equinus (prior operation).

# Pes Equinovarus

For purposes of this discussion we will include two conditions, spastic equinovarus and neurogenic equinovarus (clubfoot), within the neurogenic pes equinovarus deformity and will describe the evaluation and surgical management of each.

### Spastic Equinovarus

The primary pathologic elements of spastic equinovarus deformity are equinus of the entire foot, caused by spasticity and/or contracture of the gastrosoleus group, and varus of the hindfoot, caused primarily by spasticity or contracture of the posterior tibial muscle. In some cases the anterior tibial muscle may also contribute to development of the varus deformity. When surgical intervention is indicated, the Achilles tendon must always be lengthened. The decision as to whether to lengthen or to transfer the posterior tibial or anterior tibial tendon and which procedure to select is substantially more difficult. Although laboratory gait analysis is being used in some major centers,[3,4] the decision is based primarily on clinical evaluation in most clinics, including ours.[4-6]

In addition to Achilles tendon lengthening, the following three options are available for surgical management of spasticity or contracture of the posterior tibial muscle: (1) lengthening or recession (intramuscular tenotomy) of the tibialis posterior at its musculotendinous junction[7]; (2) complete transfer of the tendon to the dorsum of the foot[8]; and (3) split transfer of the tendon to the peroneus brevis.[9] If the deformity can be completely corrected passively and if the hindfoot varus appears mainly during the swing phase of gait and is mild, the deformity is dynamic and is caused by excessive activity of the posterior tibial muscle. We would prefer a posterior tibial recession procedure in a child under age 7 with such a dynamic spastic equinovarus deformity. The split posterior tibial tendon transfer is recommended for children aged 7 to adolescence with a persistent dynamic spastic equinovarus foot deformity. The split transfer provides a more even distribution of muscle balancing (inversion-eversion) forces than does the recession procedure. The third option, complete transfer of the posterior tibial tendon through the interosseous membrane to the middle cuneiform, is preferred in older or heavier children. It is important to place the transferred tendon at the midline of the foot, since transfer lateral to midline may cause a pes valgus deformity. Of course, any soft tissue procedure alone is contraindicated in a deformity that is fixed or not passively correctable.

### Technique of Posterior Tibial Transfer with Achilles Tendon Lengthening

The operation is performed under general anesthesia with use of a pneumatic thigh tourniquet and with the patient supine. The initial incision is made over the posterior tibial insertion. The tendon is detached from its multiple expansion insertion at the plantar aspect of the navicular, and a 1-0 Dexon suture is placed in the tendon.

The second incision is made proximal to the medial malleolus along the medial edge of the Achilles tendon. The posterior tibial neurovascular bundle is identified and protected, and the posterior tibial tendon is found, retracted from the proximal wound, and wrapped in moist gauze (Fig. 19-9). An intermediate incision may be necessary if the tendon cannot be freed. The Achilles tendon is then lengthened by Z-plasty technique under direct vision. The deep long flexor muscles and neurovascular bundle are retracted to expose the tibiofibular interosseous membrane, where a large enough longitudinal window is made to allow free excursion of the transferred tendon. A tunnel extending from the posterior wound to the dorsum of the foot is then created with a long, curved tendon passer or sponge holder, which is left in place.

The third incision, approximately 3 cm in length, is made directly over the middle cuneiform and over the top of the tendon passer, and a 4.5-mm drill hole is made in the middle cuneiform. Another tendon passer is then introduced through the distal wound, exiting proximally, the suture in the posterior tibial tendon is attached to this tendon passer, and the tendon is pulled through the wound (Fig. 19-9B). The suture attached to the distal end of the posterior tibial tendon is passed through the drill hole in the middle cuneiform with two straight needles, exiting the plantar aspect of the foot, and is tied over felt or sponges with the foot held at 90 degrees. Additional sutures are placed in the tendon at the inlet to the osseous tunnel in order to further secure the tendon.

A short leg cast is applied postoperatively and changed at 2 weeks, at which time sutures are removed. The cast is removed at 5 weeks postsurgery, and a weight-bearing ankle-foot orthosis (AFO) is used for 6 months, during which time a muscle strengthening and retraining physical therapy program is instituted.

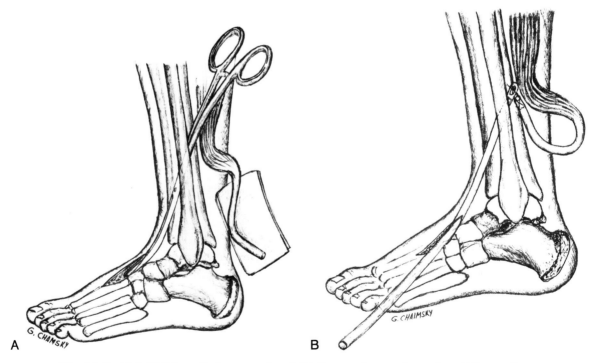

A                                                    B

**Fig. 19-9. (A & B)** Schematic demonstration of tibialis posterior transfer to the middle cuneiform.

*Technique of Split Anterior Tibial*
*Tendon Transfer*

The split anterior tibial tendon transfer was described by Hoffer et al. in 1974 for treatment of spastic varus hindfoot deformity.[10,11] We have used this procedure for varus foot deformity secondary to both spasticity and myelomeningocele. It is essential to carefully assess posterior tibial muscle activity when considering split anterior tibial tendon transfer. For example, if the posterior tibial muscle is overactive during the swing phase of gait, a posterior tibial recession procedure must also be performed in order to adequately reduce the hindfoot inversion force that contributes to the overall varus deformity.[11] However, the posterior tibial muscle may be weak in myelomeningocele, which would make complete transfer of the anterior tibial tendon unwise.

The initial incision for split anterior tibial tendon transfer is made at the tendon insertion at the medial cuneiform and the base of the first metatarsal. The tendon insertion is identified and sharply divided into medial and lateral halves by distracting the tendon as far distally in the wound as possible. A second incision is made above the ankle just lateral to the anterior tibial crest. The anterior tibial tendon is identified and again split distally until the two tendon incisions meet. An intermediate incision to facilitate splitting of the tendon may sometimes be needed. The lateral half of the tendon is then pulled out through the proximal wound and passed subcutaneously to the dorsum of the foot. We do not place the transferred portion of the tendon to the cuboid, as originally recommended by Hoffer, but instead suture it to the peroneus brevis tendon with 3-0 Vicryl® suture. Care should be taken to apply equal tension to both halves of the tendon, with the foot neutrally positioned. A short leg cast is used for 6 weeks, followed by an AFO for 6 months, during which time an anterior tibial muscle strengthening program is carried out.

## Talipes Equinovarus (Neurogenic Clubfoot)

The deformity seen in neurogenic clubfoot is similar to that seen in the idiopathic form, which is discussed in Chapter 6. The forefoot and hindfoot are in equinus, the hindfoot is in varus, and the forefoot is adducted and supinated. The pathoetiology in paralytic clubfoot is obvious, namely weakness or paralysis of both the dorsiflexors and evertors, associated with powerful flexors and invertors. This muscle imbalance explains the more severe deformities seen in this entity as compared with idiopathic clubfoot. The most common etiology of neurogenic clubfoot today is myelomeningocele. Neurogenic clubfoot is also often associated with poliomyelitis, arthrogryposis multiplex congenita, and a variety of other rare neuromuscular diseases.

Initial treatment is similar to that of idiopathic clubfoot. Manipulation and serial casting are begun immediately after birth. The objective is to stretch the contracted tissues as well as to correct the abnormal anatomic relationships between the various parts of the foot and leg. The cast maintains the corrected position, which is achieved through manipulation. Correction of the forefoot precedes that of the hindfoot in order to prevent iatrogenic rocker-bottom foot deformity. When a neurogenic clubfoot is resistant to manipulative treatment, it is usually quite obvious by 2 months of age.

The indication for surgical soft tissue release and reconstruction of neurogenic clubfoot is failure of manipulative therapy. The procedure is usually performed between 4 and 6 months of age, depending on the individual infant's development and foot size. The choice of surgical approach largely depends upon the surgeon's training and point of view regarding the nature of the procedure. There are two main surgical approaches: the "conservative" approach, in which the release is done mainly posteriorly, and the "radical" approach, in which a complete peritalar release is performed. We favor the radical approach and use the Norris Carroll[12,13] or Cincinnati incision.[14]

### Norris Carroll Technique

The child is positioned prone, with raised pelvis on the contralateral side of the operated foot. A thigh tourniquet is used. A medial incision is made from the base of the first metatarsal to the anterior border of the heel (Fig. 19-10). Dissection of the superior and inferior skin flaps is carried deep to the fascia, preserving the blood supply to the skin. The abductor hallucis muscle is dissected free from its origin and completely excised. Longitudinal dissection along the neurovascular bundle exposes the posterior tibial nerve and its medial and lateral plantar nerve branches. The lateral plantar branch is traced along its course to the plantar aspect of the hindfoot, deep to the plantar fascia.

Plantar fasciotomy is then performed if indicated. The plantar nerves and blood vessels are mobilized and re-

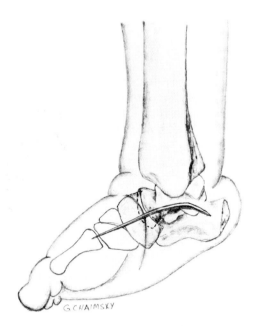

**Fig. 19-10.** The medial incision in clubfoot release, Norris Carroll method.

extends proximally to the midline of the calf. Its length depends upon the severity of the equinus deformity (Fig. 19-11). The sural nerve and vein are identified, mobilized, and protected, and the Achilles tendon is isolated and elongated via a sliding technique. The posterior tibial neurovascular bundle is freed by undermining the periosteum and protected by introducing a straight angle retractor from the posterior wound toward the medial wound, retracting the bundle away from the medial capsule. A portion of the peroneal tendon sheath is sectioned to allow retraction of the peroneal tendon away from the lateral subtalar joint capsule. The posterior, medial, and lateral capsules of the subtalar and ankle joints are sectioned. Care is taken not to section the flexor hallucis longus or the deep portion of the deltoid ligament. The lateral subtalar joint capsule is sectioned to the level of the calcaneocuboid joint, which includes sectioning of the posterior talofibular and calcaneofibular ligaments. A Kirschner wire is introduced at the central portion of the posterior talar body, pointed toward the central talar head and used as a lever to reduce the deformity. If

tracted plantarly. The attachment of the flexor hallucis and flexor digitorum longus to the plantar aspect of the navicular and lesser tarsus (Henry's knot) is released, and the plantar skeleton of the midtarsus is exposed by blunt dissection of the overlying soft tissues. The peroneus longus tendon sheath is incised and the tendon retracted to expose the calcaneocuboid joint, where a dorsomedial and plantar capsulotomy is performed. The lateral calcaneocuboid joint capsule is left intact to act as a hinge upon which the forefoot will be abducted. The tibialis posterior tendon is then sectioned or lengthened, depending upon the individual pathology. The talonavicular joint is identified and exposed by tracing the stump of the posterior tibial tendon to its insertion at the inferior aspect of the navicular tuberosity.

A medial, plantar, and dorsal talonavicular joint capsulotomy is performed. The thick mass of fibrous connective tissue between the talonavicular and calcaneocuboid joints is resected, which results in an apparently continuous midtarsal joint space. At this point the forefoot is easily mobilized, which allows anatomic reduction of the forefoot upon the hindfoot at the midtarsal joint.

The second incision starts from a point halfway between the lateral malleolus and the Achilles tendon and

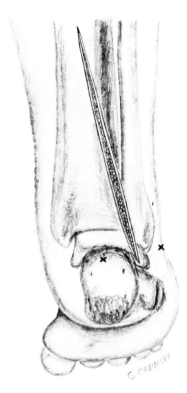

**Fig. 19-11.** Posterolateral incision in clubfoot release, Norris Carroll method.

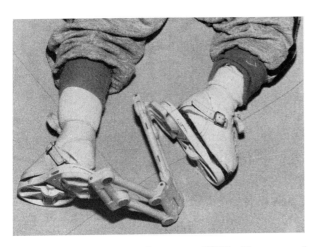

**Fig. 19-12.** Counter-rotation system (CRS) of Langer used in the postoperative management of clubfoot.

resistance occurs, the interosseous talocalcaneal ligament, starting with the posterior lateral portion, is progressively sectioned.

A triplane reduction of the clubfoot deformity, which is critical to long-term success of the procedure, can now be carried out. The calcaneus and foot must be rotated laterally upon the talus, and the posterior calcaneus must move inferiorly while the anterior calcaneus moves superiorly in order to reduce the equinus portion of the deformity. The reduced position is held by two buried Kirschner wires (one talonavicular and one a vertical talocalcaneal pin). We have more recently also used a third Kirschner wire, which is introduced from the posterior aspect of the calcaneus across the calcaneocuboid joint, in more severe clubfoot cases. The Achilles and posterior tibial tendons are repaired with the foot in neutral position. A soft, mildly compressive dressing is applied for 1 week, at which time a cast is applied under sedation. The sutures are removed 2 weeks postoperatively, and a new cast is applied. The Kirschner wires are removed under local anesthesia and a third cast is applied 6 weeks postoperatively. This cast is removed in 4 weeks, after which a Langer counter-rotation splint (CRS) is used (Fig. 19-12).

## The Cincinnati Approach

The Cincinnati approach is characterized by a different skin incision, the circumferential incision, which also provides an extensive exposure (Fig. 19-13). This approach was described by Crawford et al.[14] after many years of experience with this transverse incision, originally credited to Giannestras, who used it for one-stage correction of congenital vertical talus.

The skin incision begins at the naviculocuneiform joint; it is straight at first and then curves posteriorly, aiming under the tip of the medial malleolus. From there it is carried laterally at the level of the ankle joint, parallel to the skin folds. It crosses over the lateral malleolus and continues toward the sinus tarsi (Fig. 19-13B). The length of the anterior part of the incision on both the medial and the lateral aspects of the foot depends on the individual needs of each patient.

The dissection of the flaps must be developed deeply in order to preserve the blood supply of the skin flaps. The order of the different steps during surgical release of a clubfoot varies with the individual surgeon. The following description represents our own approach, as Crawford et al.'s description of the Cincinnati technique[14] refers only to the skin incision.

The Achilles tendon is isolated and lengthened by the sliding technique. The next step is isolation and mobilization of the neurovascular bundle and the flexor hallucis longus, which are retracted by a Penrose drain or a vessel loop. The sheaths of the flexor digitorum longus and tibialis posterior are partially opened, with release of Henry's knot. The peroneal tendons are identified and mobilized. At this stage enough clearance has been achieved to perform capsulotomies; usually the subtalar capsulotomy is done first, posteriorly, medially, and laterally. The release of the subtalar joint must extend distally enough to permit mobilization of the talus on the calcaneus. The interroseous ligament is not cut at this stage. By longitudinal dissection the ankle joint is identified, after which posterior, lateral, and medial capsulotomies are performed. Special care must be taken to avoid cutting the deep part of the deltoid ligament.

On the lateral aspect of the foot, the two main tethering structures, namely, the calcaneofibular and talofibular ligaments, are cut, which facilitates the most significant descent of the calcaneus (Fig. 19-13C). The incision over the medial aspect of the foot is then elongated and medial release is begun. The tibialis posterior is identified, its sheath is opened, and Z-plasty elongation is performed. By pulling the distal stump of the tibialis posterior tendon, identification of the talonavicular joint is facilitated and capsulotomy of this joint in its dorsal medial and plantar aspects is performed. In addition, the spring ligament and part of the bifurcate ligaments are cut. The lateral part of the incision is also distally ex-

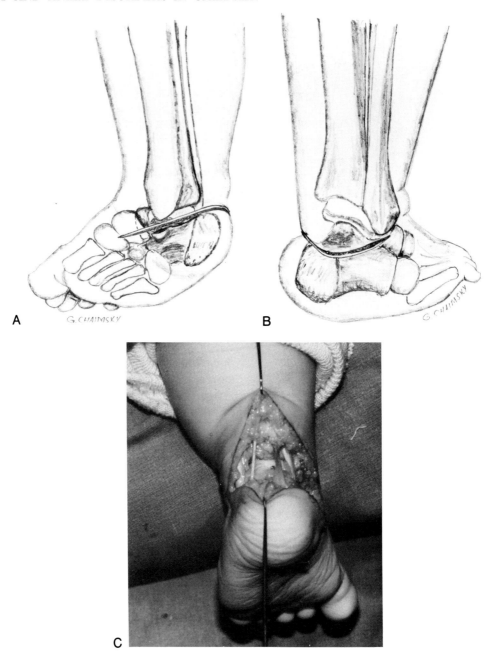

**Fig. 19-13.** Schematic demonstration of the Cincinnati incision in clubfoot. **(A)** Posteromedial view. **(B)** Posterolateral view. **(C)** The posterior release in the Cincinnati incision in clubfoot. The heel is now down.

tended for capsulotomy of the calcaneocuboid joint. More attention is given to the medial aspect of the ankle: the thick fibrous tissue, connecting the tuberosity of the navicular bone to the medial malleolus and constituting the medial tether, is cut. At this stage the forefoot has been released sufficiently to be aligned on the hindfoot anatomically. Anatomic reconstruction and Kirschner wire fixation as well as the postoperative treatment are the same as described previously for the Norris Caroll technique.

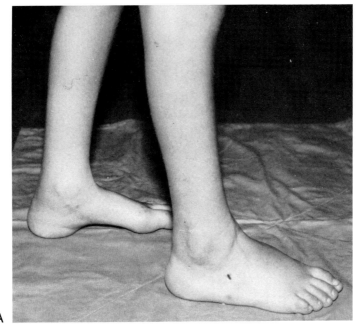

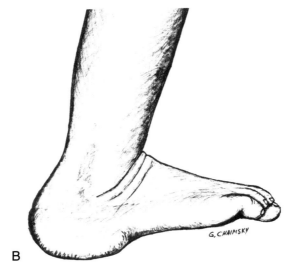

**Fig. 19-14.** Pes calcaneus in boy with myelomeningocele. (**A**) Clinical photograph. (**B**) Schematic drawing.

## Pes Calcaneus

Calcaneus deformity may be isolated or may be associated with a valgus (calcaneovalgus) or varus (calcaneovarus) condition. Weight-bearing occurs primarily through the hindfoot in all three forms of pes calcaneus.

The deformity results from weak or paralyzed plantar flexors, including the gastrosoleus muscle group. Pes calcaneus is typically seen in myelomeningocele with neurosegmental paralysis at the L4 level (muscles innervated by nerve roots distal to L4 are paralyzed) (Fig.19-14). Pes calcaneus also may occur secondary to polio-

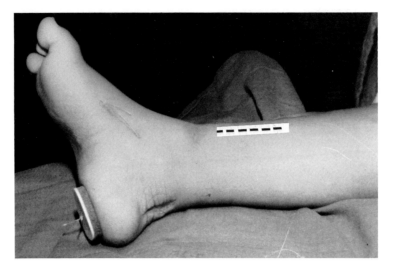

**Fig. 19-15.** Transfer of tibialis anterior tendon to calcaneus utilizing a three-incision approach. The broken line denotes the location of the proximal incision which is placed lateral to the anterior tibial crest.

myelitis but is relatively rare in spastic paralysis. Pes calcaneus deformity occurring with myelomeningocele is usually associated with an insensate heel pad. The combination of plantar insensitivity and increased weight-bearing concentrated in such a small area of plantar skin frequently results in pressure sores, ascending infections, and osteomyelitis. These complications often eventually require below-knee amputation.

Treatment should begin in early infancy, with the goal of creating a plantigrade foot. In cases of severe soft tissue contracture, in which the dorsum of the foot contacts the anterior aspect of the distal leg, percutaneous tenotomy of the tibialis anterior should be performed prior to manipulation and serial casting of the foot to neutral position. Definitive treatment of paralytic calcaneus deformity usually requires posterior transfer of the tibialis anterior to the calcaneus.[15] This operation is usually performed at age 3, since before this age ossification of the calcaneus is not complete enough to allow successful hosting of the transferred tendon.

An alternative surgical procedure is tenodesis of the Achilles tendon to the calcaneus.[16] This operation is performed alone only when the tibialis anterior is weak or is the only functioning dorsiflexor of the foot; it is often combined with posterior transfer of the tibialis anterior in cases of calcaneovarus or of the more common calcaneovalgus.[1,16] The various recommended combinations of tendon transfer in pes calcaneus, calcaneovalgus, and calcaneovarus have been described in detail by Menelaus.[17] Although a neutral foot is the goal, a mild equinus is preferable to calcaneus deformity.

## Technique of Transfer of the Tibialis Anterior to the Calcaneus

Transfer of the tibialis anterior tendon to the calcaneus is performed under general anesthesia, using a midthigh tourniquet, with the child in the supine position. Three incisions are required to transfer the tibialis anterior tendon through the interosseus membrane to the posterior calcaneus (Fig. 19-15). The technique is similar to that used for anterior transfer of the tibialis posterior tendon. The initial incision is a short longitudinal incision over the insertion of the tendon at the medial cuneiform and the base of the first metatarsal. The tendon is freed as far proximally as possible and detached.

A second 5- to 6-cm longitudinal incision is made just lateral to the anterior tibial crest at the middle third of the leg. Through this incision the proximal portion of the tendon is freed, distracted from the wound, and wrapped in moist gauze. The anterior tibial neurovascular bundle is retracted, which exposes the interosseous membrane. A full width 3-cm long "window" is opened in the membrane, with care taken to avoid the vessels just posterior to the interosseous ligament. A tunnel is then created by passing an awl or tendon passer from anteroproximal to posteroinferior through the window, aiming for the posterosuperior calcaneus. A third 3- to 4-cm longitudinal incision is made at the superior portion of the calcaneus just lateral to the Achilles tendon. A 4- to 5-mm drill hole is made from superior, penetrating the skin and exiting the plantar heel. A tendon passer is introduced through the posterior heel wound, transferring the tendon through the previously created tunnel. Care is taken to pass the tendon deep to the extensor hallucis longus muscle and to make the interosseous membrane window as large as is necessary to allow unrestricted excursion of the tendon. The tendon is then passed through the drill hole and anchored over a buttress pad at the plantar heel with the foot in 10 degrees of plantar flexion. A well padded cast is applied with the foot in 10 degrees of equinus and maintained for 6 weeks, after which an AFO is used for 5 months. Physical therapy is recommended in older children.

## Pes Cavus and Pes Cavovarus

Pes cavus may be divided into two categories by etiology: (1) developmental neurogenic pes cavus, which occurs secondary to some neurologic disturbance and (2) idiopathic pes cavus, which is not associated with any neurologic disorder and is often familial. Some studies have shown about 50 percent of all patients presenting with pes cavus deformities to have abnormal neurologic findings after careful evaluation. A large spectrum of neuromuscular diseases have been associated with pes cavus, including myopathies such as progressive muscular dystrophy, peripheral neuropathies such as Charcot-Marie-Tooth disease, and central lesions such as poliomyelitis (spinal level) and cerebral palsy (cerebral level). Pes cavus is also commonly associated with neurologic disorders of the extrapyramidal system and spinocerebellar tracts, such as Friedreich's ataxia. All patients presenting with pes cavus deformity should be thoroughly evaluated for possible neurologic etiologies before a treatment plan is formulated.

Soft tissue releases may be adequate in early flexible deformities. Clinical examination combined with comparison of weight-bearing and non-weight-bearing radiographs will determine whether the deformity is flexible or rigid. Rigid deformities require a combination of soft tissue and osseous procedures. Any surgical correction must be individualized for the specific deformity and must address both primary and secondary deformities.

Procedures will vary with the child's age and state of ossification and physeal development. For example, a simple, flexible pes cavus foot with reducible claw toe deformities may respond to plantar release and transfer of the long extensor tendons to the metatarsal necks.[18,19] However, a rigid cavus deformity may also require dorsally based closing wedge osteotomies of the tarsal or metatarsal bones, and rigid, cavovarus, or cavovalgus deformity will, in addition, require appropriate calcaneal osteotomy.

The typical adolescent cavovarus deformity is usually typified by a combination of heel varus and forefoot equinus, with progressive osseous deformity associated with soft tissue contracture. The surgical plan should address three main components of the deformity: (1) contracture of the plantar fascia and intrinsic plantar musculature; (2) plantar flexion of the first metatarsal (plantar-flexed first ray) and claw toe deformity; and (3) heel varus. Surgical correction in such a case (Figs. 19-5B and 19-6) requires three procedures: (1) Steindler release of the plantar fascia and intrinsic plantar muscles; (2) dorsally based closing wedge osteotomy of the first metatarsal; and (3) laterally based closing wedge osteotomy of the calcaneus.[18,20,21]

### Technique of Combined Osseous and Soft Tissue Correction of Pes Cavovarus

The operation is performed under general anesthesia with use of a midthigh tourniquet with the child supine. The plantar release is performed through a 4-cm incision at the junction of the medial hindfoot and plantar skin (Fig. 19-16). The plantar fascia is identified by palpation and direct vision and, along with the short intrinsic plantar muscles, is completely released from its calcaneal origin. Adequate dissection is necessary to avoid injury to the lateral plantar nerve and vessels. The height of the arch will not be altered dramatically after plantar release alone, but the plantar release is necessary to allow successful reduction of the other two osseous components of the deformity.

The second stage of the operation consists of a dorsally based closing wedge osteotomy of the first metatarsal, which is performed subperiosteally with a small power saw through a dorsal 4-cm incision, leaving the plantar cortex and periosteum intact as a hinge (Figs. 19-16 and 19-17A). When the first metatarsal physis is open, the osteotomy is performed just distal to the phy-

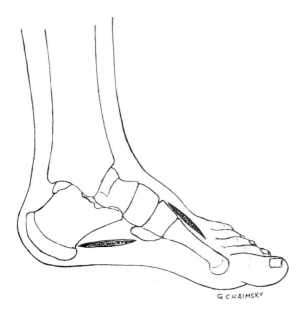

**Fig. 19-16.** Incisions in pes cavus for Steindler operation and osteotomy of base of first metatarsal.

seal plate. The osteotomy is held closed with two dorsally placed staples, introduced with a power staple gun (Fig. 19-17B).

A laterally based closing wedge osteotomy of the calcaneus is then performed to complete the procedure. The skin incision is parallel to and about 1 cm distal from the peroneal tendons (Fig. 19-18A). The skin incision is carried deep to the periosteum, excessive dissection or undermining of the skin being avoided in order to preserve the cutaneous blood supply. The peroneal tendons are mobilized and the osteotomy is performed parallel to the course of these peroneal tendons and the plane of the posterior subtalar joint (Fig. 19-18B). The base width of the excised wedge of bone is usually 0.7 to 1 cm. One should attempt to preserve the integrity of the medial periosteum and cortex. The osteotomy is held closed with two laterally placed staples.

The patient is kept in a short leg non-weight-bearing cast for 6 weeks. If adequate bone healing is demonstrated radiographically, the patient is then placed in a walking cast for an additional month. Preoperative clinical photographs and radiographs of a 16-year-old girl with idiopathic bilateral cavus feet are shown in Figures 19-5A and 19-19, and postoperative photographs and radiographs of the same girl 1 year after surgical reduction are presented in Figure 19-20.

## Neurogenic Convex Pes Valgus (Vertical Talus)

Neurogenic convex pes valgus is due to a muscle imbalance, which results in hindfoot equinus, dorsiflexion and eversion of the forefoot, and dorsal dislocation of the talonavicular joint.[22,23] The pathology of convex pes valgus is thoroughly discussed in Chapter 7. The result is a severe rocker-bottom flatfoot deformity (Figs. 19-7

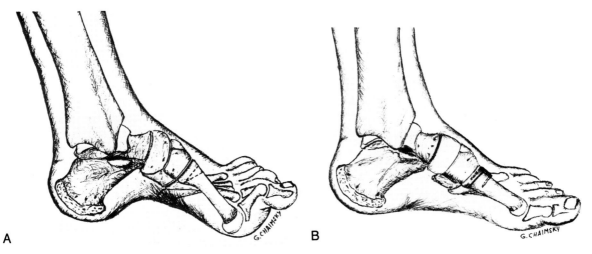

A                                                                    B

**Fig. 19-17.** Schematic drawing of pes cavus, with plantar flexion of the first ray and clawing of the toes. (**A**) Before osteotomy. (**B**) After closing wedge osteotomy.

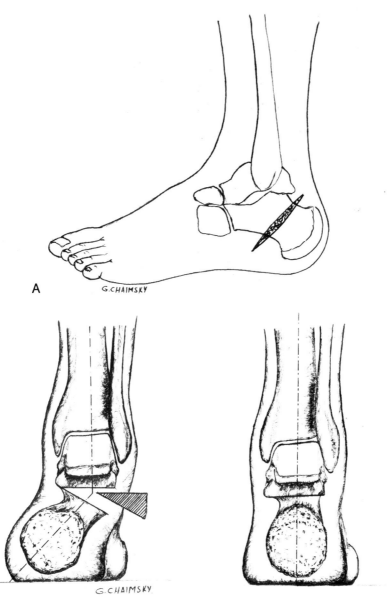

**Fig. 19-18.** Schematic drawings of Dwyer osteotomy for pes cavovarus. **(A)** Skin incision. **(B)** Laterally based removal of wedge, with closing wedge to lateral.

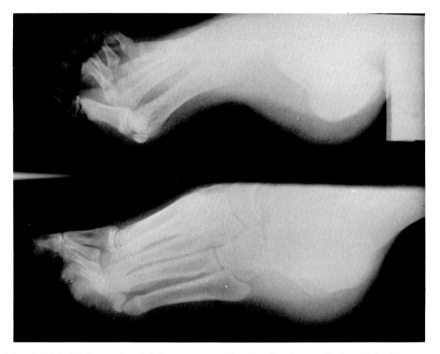

**Fig. 19-19.** Radiographs of right pes cavus, showing the plantar flexion of the first ray.

and 19-21). Congenital neurogenic vertical talus is often found in myelomeningocele, cerebral palsy, arthrygryposis multiplex congenita, and other, rarer neuromuscular disorders. Myelomeningocele is the most common cause of neurogenic convex pes valgus. The deformity is usually firmly established at birth (Fig. 19-22), although Menelaus has also described a type that develops postnatally.[17] The muscle imbalance that produces the convex pes valgus deformity is characterized by weak gastrosoleus, plantar flexors, and tibialis posterior muscles combined with stronger dorsiflexors, evertors, and tibialis anterior muscles. Menelaus has stated that intrinsic muscle paralysis is the main component of the deformity.[17] Other authors have found a variable pattern of paralysis.[24,25,26]

Manipulation and frequent serial cast reduction of the deformity should be started at birth. Treatment is described in detail in Chapter 7. Rigid contracture of the anterior tibial tendon that prevents manipulative reduction may require percutaneous tenotomy. Most vertical talus feet are rigid and respond poorly to nonoperative treatment.[27] A one-stage surgical release and reduction of the deformity should be performed in rigid feet as soon as the child is old enough (usually 4 to 6 months of age)

and the foot large enough to allow easy technical completion of the procedure.

### Technique of Soft Tissue Release and Reconstruction of Neurogenic Convex Pes Valgus

We use a three-incision approach consisting of a medial and posterolateral incision identical to those used in the Norris-Carroll approach to clubfoot (Figs. 19-10 and 19-11) and an additional anterolateral incision (Fig. 19-23), which extends from just distal and anterior to the lateral malleolus to midline over the anterior ankle and is made with the child supine. The short extensors and the peroneus tertius are elongated, and the anterolateral ankle joint capsule is sectioned.

A capsulotomy of the calcaneocuboid joints is also performed through this incision if contracture is present. After completion of the anterolateral release, the child is turned to the prone position. The second incision is made over the medial aspect of the foot, as in the Norris Carroll approach[12] (Fig. 19-10). The dissection is also similar to that used in the approach to clubfoot. There is usually no need to release the plantar fascia or to lengthen the

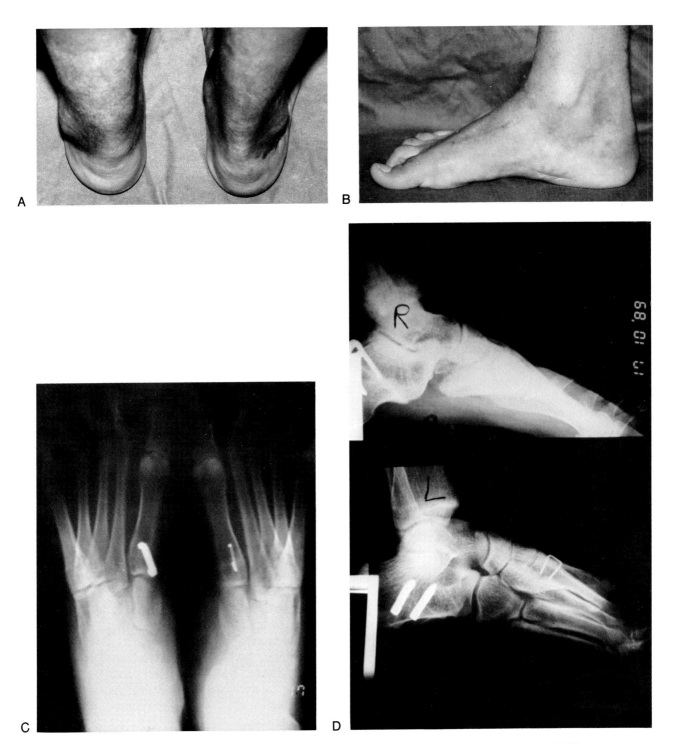

**Fig. 19-20.** Postoperative clinical and radiologic views of the patient shown in Figs. 19-5A and 19-19. (**A**) The varus was corrected by Dwyer osteotomy. (**B**) The longitudinal arch is normal without plantar flexion of the first ray (after Steindler release and osteotomy of first ray). (**C & D**) Radiographs of both feet in lateral and anteroposterior views.

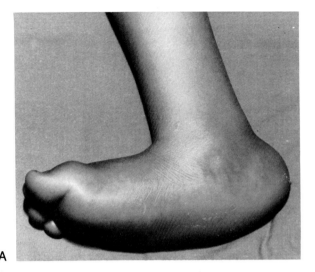

A

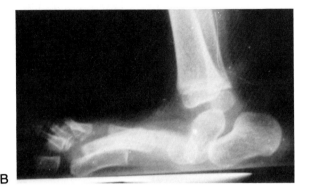

B

**Fig. 19-21.** Neurogenic vertical talus in young boy with myelomeningocele. (**A**) Clinical photograph of the rocker-bottom foot. (**B**) Radiograph shows the vertical talus, equinus of the hindfoot, and dorsiflexion of the forefoot.

posterior tibial tendon. The talar head is identified pointing directly plantar, and complete talonavicular joint capsulotomy is performed (Fig. 19-24). The pseudoarticulation of the underdeveloped navicular bone with the dorsal talar neck is identified, and the third and final posterolateral incision is now made (Fig. 19-11).

A complete posterolateral release similar to that used for clubfoot is performed. Both the talus and calcaneus are fixed in a position of rigid plantar flexion in convex pes valgus. The subtalar joint capsulotomy must be extended far anterior, both medially and laterally (to the calcaneocuboid joint), and the posterior talofibular and calcaneofibular ligaments are sectioned and the peroneal tendons and sheath mobilized to allow reduction of the

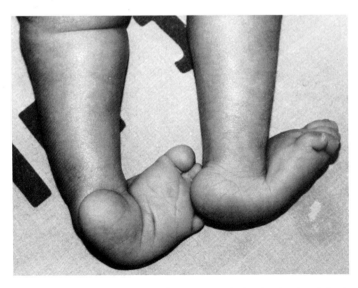

**Fig. 19-22.** Neurogenic talipes equinovarus in left foot and vertical talus in the right foot of a newborn with myelomeningocele.

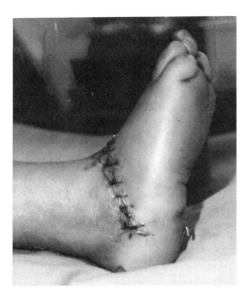

**Fig. 19-23.** Postoperative picture of vertical talus foot. The suture line is the anterolateral incision, one of the three incisions.

equinus position of the talus and calcaneus. Once a complete peritalar and ankle capsular release has been completed, longitudinal Kirschner wires are introduced at the posterior aspect of both the talus and the calcaneus to serve as levers for reduction of the talus and calcaneus.

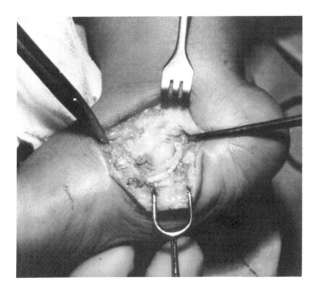

**Fig. 19-24.** Intraoperative picture of same patient as in Fig. 19-23 shows the head of the talus pointing to the dome of the reverse arch.

The navicular must be reduced upon the talar head, and the calcaneal tuberosity must be distracted inferiorly and rotated laterally.

The Kirschner wires are driven forward into the navicular and cuboid once anatomic reduction has been achieved, and a third Kirschner wire is placed vertically from the plantar heel through the subtalar joint (Fig. 19-23).

After radiographic verification of anatomic reduction of the deformity, the Achilles tendon is repaired and the wounds are closed in two layers. The cast is changed and the Kirschner wires are removed at 6 weeks. It is important to continue to mold the arch portion of the cast well at each cast change. Soft tissue release is effective up to the age of 1 year and may be considered up until 18 months of age. Thereafter, osseous adaptation may preclude soft tissue release alone. Naviculectomy is one surgical option that may facilitate reduction of rigid vertical talus deformity in the older child.

## REFERENCES

1. Tachdjian MO: The Child's Foot. WB Saunders, Philadelphia, 1985
2. Simon SR, Deutsch SD, Nuzzo RM et al: Genu recurvatum in spastic cerebral palsy. J Bone Joint Surg [Am] 60:882, 1978
3. Bleck EE: Orthopaedic Management in Cerebral Palsy. MacKeith Press, Oxford, 1987
4. Perry J, Hoffer MM: Preoperative and postoperative dynamic electromyography as an aid in planning tendon transfers in children with cerebral palsy. J Bone Joint Surg [Am] 59:535, 1977
5. Banks HH, Panagakos P: Orthopaedic evaluation in the lower extremity in cerebral palsy. Clin Orthop 47:117, 1966
6. Adler N, Bleck EE, Rinsdey LA: Decision making in surgical treatment of paralytic deformities of the foot with gait electromyograms. Orthop Trans 9:90, 1985
7. Ruda R, Frost HM: Cerebral palsy spastic varus and forefoot adductus treated by intramuscular posterior tibial tendon lengthening. Clin Orthop 79:61, 1971
8. Watkins MG, Jones TB, Ryder GT, Brown JH: Transplantation of the posterior tibial tendon. J Bone Joint Surg [Am] 36:1181, 1954
9. Green NE, Griffin PP, Shiavi P: Split posterior tibial tendon transfer in spastic cerebral palsy. J Bone Joint Surg [Am] 65:748, 1983
10. Hoffer MM, Reiswig J, Garrett A, Perry J: Split anterior

tibial tendon transfer in the treatment of spastic varus hindfoot of childhood. Orthop Clin North Am 5:31, 1974

11. Hoffer MM, Barakat G, Koffman M: 10 year follow-up of split anterior tibial tendon transfer in cerebral palsied patients with spastic equinovarus deformity. J Pediatr Orthop 5:432, 1985

12. Carroll N, McMarty R, Leete SF: The pathoanatomy of congenital clubfoot. Orthop Clin North Am 9:225, 1978

13. Porat S, Kaplan L: Critical analysis of results in clubfeet treated surgically along the Norris Carroll approach. Seven years of experience. J Pediatr Orthop 9:137, 1989

14. Crawford AH, Maryen JL, Osterfeld DL: The Cincinnati incision: a comprehensive approach for surgical procedures of the foot and ankle in childhood. J Bone Joint Surg [Am] 64:1355, 1982

15. Peabody CW: Tendon transplantation in the lower extremities. Instr Course Lect 6:178, 1949

16. Banta JV, Sutherland DH, Wyatt M: Anterior tibial transfer to the os calcis with Achilles tendon for calcaneus deformity in myelomeningocele. J Pediatr Orthop 1:125, 1981

17. Menelaus MB: The Orthopaedic Management of Spina Bifida Cystica. 2nd Ed. Churchill Livingstone, Edinburgh, 1980

18. Steindler A: Operative treatment of pes cavus. Surg Gynecol Obstet 24:612, 1917

19. Chuinard EG, Baskin M: Claw toes deformity. Treatment by transferring the long extensors into the metatarsals and fusion of the interphalangeal joints. J Bone Joint Surg [Am] 55:351, 1973

20. Dwyer FC: Osteotomy of the calcaneum for pes cavus. J Bone Joint Surg [Br] 41:80, 1959

21. Dwyer FC: The present status of the problem of pes cavus. Clin Orthop 106:254, 1975

22. Lamy L, Weissman L: Congenital convex pes valgus. J Bone Joint Surg 21:79, 1939

23. Osmond-Clarke H: Congenital vertical talus. J Bone Joint Surg [Br] 38:334, 1956

24. Drennen JC, Sharrard NJW: The pathological anatomy of convex pes valgus. J Bone Joint Surg [Br] 53:455, 1971

25. Specht EE: Congenital paralytic vertical talus. J Bone Joint Surg [Am] 57:842, 1975

26. Dyck PT: Inherited neuronal degeneration and atrophy affecting peripheral motor, sensory, and autonomic neurons. p. 1609. In Peripheral Neuropathy. Vol. 2. 2nd Ed. WB Saunders, Philadelphia, 1984

27. Colton CL: The surgical management of congenital vertical talus. J Bone Joint Surg [Br] 55:566, 1973

# 20

# Principles of Fracture Management in Children

*STEVEN J. DeVALENTINE*

The characteristics, distribution, and treatment of fractures in children and in adults are often quite different. The child's bone has different structural characteristics, which make it more malleable and capable of absorbing higher energy loads before failure. Plastic deformation may occur instead of complete disruption. The periosteum of pediatric bone is also much thicker than that of adult bone and often remains intact after fracture; this undoubtedly contributes to a much lower incidence of fracture displacement and provides an anatomic hinge that allows relatively easy reduction of many displaced fractures. The rich blood supply and growth capability of pediatric bone contribute to more rapid healing and much greater remodeling potential than can be expected of adult bone. These and other unique characteristics of fractures in children have historically resulted in a very low incidence of open reduction as compared with adult fractures. Shaft fractures of long bones or tubular bones rarely require open reduction. Nonunion is not a major concern in children; it almost never occurs, and when it does, it is usually associated with a pathologic condition.

Blount established general guidelines on the treatment of long bone fractures in children based upon the child's age, fracture location, and degree of angulation.[1] Greater angulation is acceptable in a younger child with a fracture nearer the end of the long bone, especially if the angulation occurs in the plane of joint motion. Near anatomic reduction is necessary in an older child with less growth and remodeling potential and also if angulation or rotational deformity is present. Slight valgus angulation of a lower extremity bone is better tolerated than varus angulation.

In addition to the different structural and biomechanical characteristics of growing bones in children, the ends of long bones and tubular bones have physes (growth plates) that are not present in adults. The physis tends to be the weakest part of the bone-ligament complex and is often the site of failure. The differential strength characteristics of the epiphysis, physis, and metaphysis create unusual fracture patterns not seen in mature bone. Unfortunately, the weakest point of the child's bone, the physis, which is a common site of injury, is also the area in which anatomic reduction is most essential to attempt to prevent growth disturbance or angulation deformity.

Thus, management of fractures in children can be considerably different from management in adults, and the management of a long or tubular bone fracture in a child may be very different from treatment of a physeal or an intra-articular fracture in the same child. Also, the treatment of a particular type of ankle fracture in a 5-year-old child with many years of remaining growth may vary significantly from the management of that same fracture in a 12-year-old, who is almost a skeletally mature adolescent. In choosing a specific treatment approach, one must consider the child's age, sex, fracture type, and blood supply, the presence of angular or rotational deformity, and local and systemic factors that affect growth. A functional knowledge of the anatomy and physiology of growing bone is essential to proper management of these injuries. Only time will determine whether the outcome is a success or failure.

497

# FUNCTIONAL ANATOMY AND PHYSIOLOGY OF GROWING BONE

## Limb Development and Bone Formation

### Prenatal Development of Limbs and Long Bones

The extremities of the human fetus are first identifiable as limb buds at about the fifth week of gestation. The embryonal ectodermal layer forms a budding growth at the origin of each of the four extremities. Between the ectodermal and endodermal layers there is an undifferentiated layer of mesenchyme, which has the capability of forming such varied connective tissue structures as muscle, bone, cartilage, and fascia. This mesenchymal tissue migrates into the central portion of the ectodermal limb bud. A dense concentration of these mesenchymal cells in the very center of the limb bud then differentiates into hyaline cartilage and the cartilaginous precursor of bone. The latter enlarges by central multiplication of cartilage cells and by peripheral laying down of cartilage by the perichondrium. Inorganic salts are deposited with resulting calcification of the cartilage.

Ossification of this calcified cartilaginous precursor of bone first appears about the seventh week of gestation and is stimulated by an increase in tissue oxygen pressure brought about by invasion of the central nutrient artery. The calcified cartilage is destroyed and replaced by bone produced by osteoblasts. The axial and appendicular skeletons are formed through this process of endochondral ossification, in which a cartilaginous precursor of bone is first formed and then replaced by true bone. In contrast, cranial and facial bones are ossified directly from the primitive fibrous mesenchymal precursor without the intermediate formation of cartilage. This process of direct ossification is referred to as *membranous bone formation;* both this term and the term *endochondral ossification* refer only to primary bone development. Once primary bone formation has occurred, both endochondral ossification and membranous bone formation contribute to continuing bone growth. Long bones grow in length through endochondral ossification of physeal cartilage and in diameter through metaphyseal remodeling of this endochondral bone. The diaphyseal portion of long bones also grows in diameter through direct periosteal conversion of fibrous tissue to bone, which is really a type of membranous bone formation.

The central portion of the long bone is the first area to exhibit endochondral ossification and is referred to as the *primary ossification center.* Endochondral ossification of the end of the long bone, which occurs in response to invasion of the epiphyseal arteries, produces the secondary ossification center of the epiphysis. The primary ossification center of all long bones is present at birth.

### Long Bone Development in Childhood and Adolescence

Secondary ossification centers may or may not be present at birth depending upon the bone and individual variations (see Figs. 1-1 and 1-2). The distal femoral epiphysis and the proximal tibial epiphysis are usually present at birth, but the distal tibial and fibular epiphyses are not radiographically visible until the age of 6 months to 1 year. The diaphysis and epiphysis continue to enlarge through endochondral and periosteal bone formation during growth and are separated by the physis, which is made up of various layers of cartilage cells within a matrix ground substance. These physeal cartilage cells multiply, producing long bone growth and are gradually converted through endochondral ossification to bone on the metaphyseal side of the physis. Complete ossification of the physis occurs during adolescence, when vascular channels within the metaphysis finally invade the physeal proliferating cartilage, with a resulting increase in oxygen tension, which promotes ossification, resulting in bone union between the metaphysis and epiphysis and cessation of growth at skeletal maturity. The sequence of events that results in growth plate closure is an orderly and fairly predictable process, although the initiation of the process may vary from child to child. Radiographic measurement of a child's skeletal age may be compared with chronologic age to better predict the outcome of physeal injuries.

### Development of the Small Bones of the Foot

Formation of the small bones of the foot occurs in a manner similar to long bone formation. A primary ossification center develops in the center of the cartilaginous precursor of the irregular cancellous bones that make up the greater and lesser tarsus in response to the invasion of a nutrient artery. The primary ossification centers of the calcaneus, talus, and cuboid are present at birth. The primary ossification center of the lateral cuneiform appears at about 1 year of age and those of the navicular and medial cuneiforms between 3 and 4 years of age. Gradual ossification of the cartilaginous precursor of the tarsal bones proceeds outward from the center in a circumferential manner, following the pre-existing cartilage template. The primary ossification centers of the small tubular metatarsals and phalanges are present at birth. A physis is initially present at both ends of the metatarsals and phalanges. A secondary ossification center develops only at one end, however; the physis at the other end degenerates into a small, spherical wafer of cartilage between the primary ossification center and the articular hyaline cartilage.

Occasionally, a secondary ossification center may occur in association with the cartilaginous remnant of a pseudoepiphysis. This is most common at the distal end of the first metatarsal and could be easily mistaken for a fracture. No growth occurs at pseudoepiphyses. A true secondary ossification center (epiphysis), which contributes to longitudinal growth, does form at the proximal ends of the phalanges and first metatarsal and at the distal ends of the lesser metatarsals and is usually radiographically visible at about 3 years of age. Secondary ossification centers also develop in other areas of the foot and can easily be mistaken for avulsion fractures if the clinician is not familiar with their location and the time when they first become radiographically apparent. The epiphysis at the base of the fifth metatarsal becomes evident between about 9 and 14 years of age. The calcaneal apophysis usually appears between ages 6 and 10. A secondary ossification center may also form at the navicular tuberosity (os tibiale externum) or at the posterior aspect of the talus (os trigonum), first becoming radiographically visible between the ages of 8 and 12. These may or may not fuse to their primary ossification centers (navicular and talus).

Although avulsion, slipping, or fracture of any of these secondary centers can occur, careful clinical correlation is necessary to avoid overdiagnosis of these injuries. When injuries to traction epiphyses (apophyses) of the foot occur, displacement is usually minimal and reduction is usually not necessary since these growth plates do not contribute to overall foot length. In the rare event of complete avulsion, reduction and pinning should be performed since these traction epiphyses are sites of tendon insertions (i.e., Achilles and peroneus brevis tendons).

## Joint Development

Joints develop from the same multipotential mesenchymal cells that produce bone. The joint cavity forms from a cleft in the mesenchymal tissue, the outer lining of which forms the joint capsule and is continuous with the periosteum. The inner lining of the joint capsule forms a false epithelium of synovial membrane, which provides the lubricating joint fluid and nutrition for hyaline cartilage. Hyaline cartilage is formed from the same cartilage that undergoes endochondral ossification to form bone, but once differentiation occurs, hyaline cartilage will not undergo ossification. This partially explains the failure of rotated or inverted osteochondral fracture fragments to become incorporated and ossified.

# The Physis

The physeal plate (physis) is made up of layers of chondrocytes differentiated from the same cartilaginous anlage that forms the limb bone. Because the physis is radiolucent and is not well defined radiographically in the younger child, its shape and location must be inferred from the distal end of the ossified metaphyseal contour. As the child grows and the secondary ossification center enlarges, the physis becomes visible as a distinct narrow, radiolucent band, which is usually transversely oriented to the long axis of the bone. Since the greater part of the loading in most long bones is usually applied in an axial manner, the transverse orientation of the physis allows the greatest resistance to applied stresses. The physis also assumes an irregular, wavy contour characteristic of each location. Small cartilaginous interdigitations called *mammillary processes* extend from the physis into metaphyseal bone. The contoured, irregular shape of the physis and mammillary processes greatly increases the surface area of the physis and increases its resistance to shear stresses. Furthermore, the physeal portion of the metaphysis of a long bone is usually about twice the diameter of the diaphysis. This greater cross-sectional area also increases resistance to shear stresses at the physis and to load failure of the bone and helps to compensate for the inherently weaker stress resistance of the loosely woven spongiosa bone of the metaphysis and

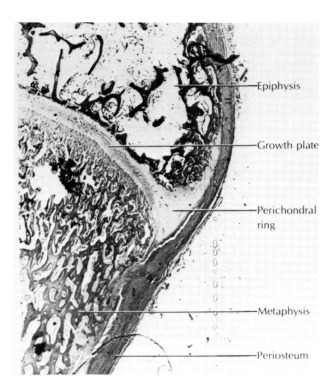

Fig. 20-1. The peripheral edge of a rodent long bone. (From Rockwood,[33] with permission.)

epiphysis as compared with the dense cortical bone of the diaphysis.

The chondrocytes of the physis are arranged in microscopically identifiable layers and are embedded in a ground substance composed of collagen fibers in chondroitin sulfate (Fig. 20-1). Salter likened this matrix of ground substance to reinforcement rods in concrete.[2] The layer of cells nearest the epiphysis is embedded in an abundant amount of strong matrix and is referred to as the *germinal* (or resting) cell layer or zone. The next layer is composed of cells undergoing rapid mitosis and is referred to as the *zone of proliferation;* these cells ap-

pear to be stacked in columns with their long axes parallel to the long axis of the bone. The mitotic activity of the cells in the zone of proliferation is largely responsible for longitudinal growth of the bone.

The third layer, termed the *zone of maturation,* is composed of chondrocytes, which hypertrophy to as much as five times their normal size. These cells gradually grow larger, accumulating glycogen and alkaline phosphatase while retaining their columnar orientation. Because of the greater size and number of chondrocytes in the zone of maturation, there is a corresponding decrease in the amount of cementing ground substance. The hypertrophic cells of this zone of maturation gradually "disintegrate," forming a very thin layer of calcified, necrotic cells adjacent to the metaphyseal bone *(zone of calcification).* Metaphyseal blood vessels and osteoblasts invade the tunnels that result from degeneration of the chondrocytes, raising the oxygen pressure and stimulating endochondral ossification which follows the template of the calcified chondrocytes in the zone of calcification.

The area between the zone of maturing cells and the zone of calcification is the weakest part of the physis because of the reduced concentration of cementing ground substance, and this is the area in which cleavage is most likely to occur[2] (Table 20-1). In a classical type of physeal disruption the germinal, proliferating, and hypertrophic layers would be expected to remain intact, attached to the epiphyseal fragment. With near anatomic reduction, one would not expect growth arrest to occur as long as these layers remain undisturbed.

## Vascular Supply

There are three primary sources of blood supply to long bones (Fig. 20-2A). The nutrient artery is the major source of blood supply to the diaphysis and the metaphyseal sinusoids supplying the metaphyseal side of the physis (area of endochondral ossification). Epiphyseal

Table 20-1. **Applied Histology of the Physis**

|  | Zone | Cell Activity | Strength |
|---|---|---|---|
| Epiphysis | Resting | Germinal | } Matrix abundant, plate strong |
|  | Proliferation | Mitotic | } Matrix scanty, plate weak |
|  | Maturation | Hypertrophic |  |
|  | Calcification | Calcified necrotic | } Matrix calcified, plate stronger |
| Metaphysis | Endochondral ossification | Osteoid | } Metaphyseal bone |

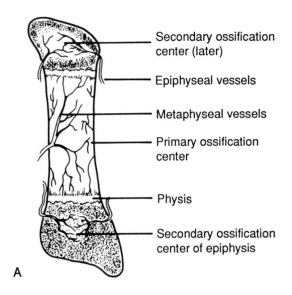

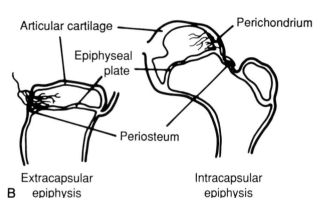

**Fig. 20-2.** (A) The primary sources of blood supply to the ends of long bones. (Adapted from Rockwood,[33] with permission.) (B) The two basic patterns of blood supply to the epiphysis. With disruption of the intracapsular epiphysis (femoral or radial head), epiphyseal vessels are frequently sheared off with resulting loss of vascular supply to the epiphysis and germinal cell layers, which may cause avascular necrosis. (Adapted from Salter,[2] with permission.)

vessels, which enter the bone through the joint capsules, supply the majority of the germinal and proliferative layers of chondrocytes found responsible for growth. Periosteal and perichondral vessels supply the periphery of the diaphysis and epiphysis. Perichondral vessels also supply the perichondral ring that forms the lateral portion of the growth plate; this ring adds lateral growth to the plate and increases its strength. Because the peri-

chondral ring has a separate blood supply, injuries can occur that will cause central but not peripheral growth arrest or vice versa. Rang felt that blunt trauma to the periphery of the physis may damage the blood supply to the perichondral ring, resulting in the development of a peripheral osseous bridge that would cause an angular deformity.[3]

Most epiphyses, including all in the foot and ankle, are extra-articular. When physeal disruption occurs, the joint capsule and therefore also the epiphyseal vascular supply to the germinal and proliferating portion of the physis usually remain intact. In classical types of physeal separation, in which the growing chondrocytes and their blood supply are relatively undisturbed, the prognosis for undisturbed growth should be good. When open reduction of physeal injuries is performed, it is extremely important to avoid stripping perichondrium, periosteum, or joint capsule from the epiphysis. Stripping or sectioning of soft tissue attachments to the epiphysis will impair physeal blood supply and could lead to growth arrest.

Some epiphyses, such as the femoral and radial heads, are intra-articular. The epiphyseal vessels must enter through the joint capsule on the metaphyseal side of the physis, from which they traverse the surface of the physis to enter the epiphysis (Fig. 20-2B). When separation of intra-articular epiphyses occurs, epiphyseal vessels are very easily damaged. This explains the high incidence of avascular necrosis that occurs in intracapsular epiphyses, such as the capital femoral epiphysis.

## Growth

A thorough understanding of the normal physeal growth process as well as the effect of local and distant factors on physeal growth is essential for any clinician who treats extremity injuries. A number of local and systemic factors that affect physeal growth are listed in Table 20-2. The most important of the systemic factors is probably genetic, and the most important nongenetic factor is probably nutrition. Nutritional differences are generally thought to be responsible for increases in height in the general population over the last few hundred years.

The exact mechanism that induces "growth spurts" in children or is responsible for differential growth rates among different epiphyses remains a mystery. Although increases in circulating growth hormone, androgens, estrogens, and other hormones can stimulate growth, it is known that increases in circulating hormones alone are

Table 20-2. **Factors Affecting Epiphyseal Growth**

| Systemic Factors | Effect on Growth |
|---|---|
| Genetic Factors | ↑ ↓ |
| Nutrition | ↑ ↓ |
| Growth hormone (GH) | ↑ GH → gigantism<br>↓ GH → dwarfism |
| Thyroid hormone (TH) | ↑ TH ↑ rapidity<br>↓ TH → cretinism |
| Androgens | ↑ growth → eventual closure |
| Estrogens | ↑ growth → early closure |
| Local Factors | |
| Compression | slight ↑ → ↑ growth<br>large ↑ → ↓ growth |
| Nearby fracture | ↑ growth |
| Infection | ↓ |
| Injury | ↓ |
| Interference with circulation | ↓ |

(From DeValentine,[32] with permission.)

not responsible for growth spurts. Perhaps the most intriguing question is how different epiphyses (including different epiphyses in the same bone) can respond to circulating hormones with different growth rates. Increases in growth rates do correlate with physeal thickness. Small, slow-growing bones such as the phalanges have very thin physes, whereas larger, faster-growing bones such as the femur and tibia have very thick physes. The thickness of the physis also increases during adolescent growth spurts. This may be an important factor in the increased incidence of physeal fractures during adolescence, since the probability of mechanical physeal failure has been shown to increase in proportion to physeal thickness. Proximal epiphyses are usually responsible for a much greater percentage of extremity growth than distal epiphyses. This becomes important in dealing with potential limb length discrepancies from epiphyseal injuries. Injuries about the ankle, for example, are of much less consequence in determining overall limb length than injuries about the knee joint. The distal femur and proximal tibia are thought to contribute about two-thirds of lower extremity length (40 and 27 percent, respectively), while the proximal femur and distal tibia contribute the remaining one-third (15 and 18 percent, respectively).[4] Specific charts are available to calculate anticipated remaining extremity growth based on skeletal age as defined by comparison of hand films for bone age. These charts are based on sample populations of normal children and are not necessarily completely reliable in any individual case.

A potential also exists for a differential growth rate within any individual epiphysis. A primary local factor affecting such differential growth is compression; a slight increase in compression stimulates physeal growth, whereas a larger increase in compression may retard it. Bright et al. have pointed out that physiologic tibia vara and genu varum undergo spontaneous correction as a result of differential physeal growth stimulated by slight increases in compression from angular deformity[5] (Fig. 1-7). The typical child with physiologic tibia vara or genu varum in infancy responds to slightly increased compression of the medial epiphyses about the knee by increasing the growth rate of the medial physis as compared with that of the lateral physis, which reduces the physiologic varus deformity. The same type of spontaneous correction of physiologic genu valgum in the slightly older child usually occurs. An understanding of this concept becomes extremely important in evaluating the ability of an individual epiphyseal injury to undergo spontaneous correction.

Angular deformities of less than 15 degrees in younger children with substantial remaining growth can usually be expected to undergo spontaneous correction. The rate of correction can be expected to be proportional to the rate of growth of the involved epiphysis, with modification for local or systemic factors that may affect physeal growth. In some cases in younger children, it may be more prudent to accept a slight deformity, which will probably correct itself spontaneously, than to risk growth plate damage from manipulation that is too forcible. Spontaneous correction is more likely when the distal part is angulated in the plane of joint motion and the degree of malalignment is relatively minimal. Spontaneous correction is less likely in a child over age 10, who has little remaining growth in the physes of the distal leg and foot. One should also remember that spontaneous correction of angular deformity may be substantially less with varus or valgus deformities and that rotational deformities will not spontaneously reduce and always require anatomic realignment.

## BIOMECHANICAL PROPERTIES OF GROWING BONE

A basic knowledge of the normal biodynamics of bone as well as the differences between adult and pediatric bone is essential for appropriate clinical management of skeletal injuries. The components of the skeletal system (bone, cartilage, ligaments) are dynamic living tissues which are constantly undergoing microstructural and

macrostructural changes that reflect the primary functions of protection, support, and motion. As in nature in general, form follows function.

Cortical bone is dense lamellar bone, which is more rigid than metaphyseal bone and has a greater strength-to-size ratio than metaphyseal bone. Metaphyseal and epiphyseal bone is trabecular woven bone, which is more porous (less dense) than cortical bone but has a more rapid ability to remodel in response to variable applied loads. The greater porosity of metaphyseal and epiphyseal bone makes it a very effective shock absorber in transmitting loads from articular surfaces to diaphyseal bone. Both cortical and trabecular bone are in a constant state of remodeling in adults and children, the result of bone resorption and bone deposition. Trabecular bone is remodeled as the osteoclasts traverse the surface of the trabeculae and are replaced by osteoblasts. In cortical bone the osteoclasts create longitudinal canals referred to as *cutting cones*. The osteoblasts then follow, laying down new bone and forming new osteons. The overall effect of this process of bone resorption and production is to allow bone to change in response to applied stresses in accordance with Wolff's law.

Immature (pediatric) bone is in a much more dynamic state than mature (adult) bone, which results in a more rapid healing rate. A greater variability of fracture pattern also occurs, owing to constantly changing bone microstructure. Immature cortical and trabecular bone is also more porous (less dense) than mature bone. Pediatric bone is not less ossified than adult bone, merely less in volume. The greater porosity and lower density of im-

mature bone results in greater elasticity than is seen in mature trabecular or cortical bone; this, in turn, allows greater flexibility and greater shock and energy absorption capability.

The response of bone to an applied load is the sum of a number of intrinsic and extrinsic factors. Intrinsic factors characteristic of immature bone, such as greater porosity (lower density), remodeling potential, elasticity, and energy-absorbing capacity, change with growth, and failure (or fracture) patterns vary accordingly. Extrinsic factors that determine a bone's response to applied loads include the magnitude, direction, duration, and rate of application of force. In children these extrinsic factors are constantly changing with growth and with increase in body weight and size, as well as with increasing physical activity with age.

External loading of bone produces force concentrations referred to as *stresses,* which can be measured as force per unit area. The response to stress (applied force) is termed *strain,* which can be measured as stretch per unit of length. The strain produced by constant or repetitive low-grade stresses results in normal remodeling in accordance with Wolff's law. When stress forces applied to bone increase beyond the bone's inherent strain point, microfractures develop. If the force continues, these microscopic deformations coalesce to form macroscopic fractures and the bone fails.

Different types of stresses occur when loads are applied from different directions. Stresses that culminate in longitudinal strains of bone are referred to as *compression, tension, or elongation* stresses. Forces applied to

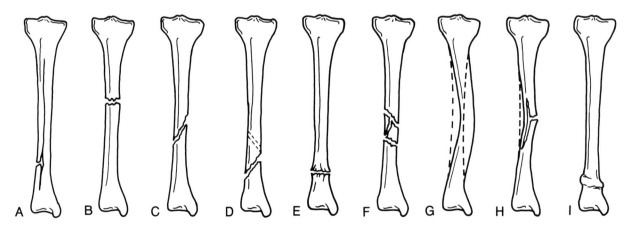

**Fig. 20-3.** Various typical fracture patterns in pediatric long bones. (A) Longitudinal; (B) transverse; (C) oblique; (D) spiral; (E) compression; (F) comminuted; (G) plastic deformation; (H) greenstick; (I) torus.

bone at oblique angles result in shear stress, and rotational forces produce torsional stress. Each type of stress tends to cause certain types of strain failure (Fig. 20-3). Stresses that are applied to bone in other than longitudinal directions tend to produce *transverse* or *oblique* fractures through areas of bone with the least strain resistance (i.e., metaphysis, physis, and epiphysis). These fracture patterns may vary significantly with the changing structure of these dynamic areas of pediatric bone. Torsional stresses result in *spiral* fractures, which usually involve the diaphysis of long bones (e.g., tibia, fibula) or occasionally short tubular bones (e.g., metatarsals, phalanges). *Compression* or crush fractures occur as a result of a direct compression stress, most commonly in the metaphyseal area. *Comminuted* fractures result from stresses applied in several directions. The younger the child, the less common is fracture comminution owing to the greater capability of immature porous bone to absorb energy.

Although the location and frequency of the preceding types of fractures vary considerably more in children than in adults, the mechanism and mode of failure are basically the same. The strain response of immature bone to longitudinal compression force is much different from that of mature bone. When a longitudinal compression force is applied to the more elastic, tubular, naturally curved long bone of a child, a slight bending occurs. A compression strain occurs on the concave side and tensile strain occurs on the convex side. Below a certain stress point the bone responds by bending and then, after removal of the stress, returns to its prior shape. The greater elasticity of immature bone allows greater deformation than would be possible in mature bone. Beyond that stress point immature bone may undergo a permanent bowing without returning to its prestress shape. This is called *plastic deformation* and has been demonstrated in the long bones of children. Plastic deformation is rarely seen in the foot. In the lower extremity, bowing of the fibula is usually seen in combination with a tibial fracture and may make reduction of the tibial fracture difficult.

With an increasing compression load, failure will occur on the tensile side of the bone, causing a *greenstick fracture* (Fig. 20-4). A portion of the periosteum and cortex is left intact on the compression side of the bone and aids in reduction. Greenstick fractures become less common as children approach adolescence and bone density increases and elasticity decreases. Another type of

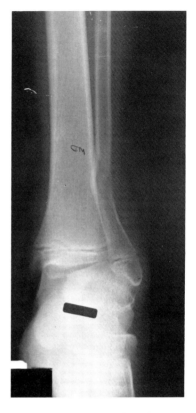

**Fig. 20-4.** A greenstick fracture of the fibula associated with a Salter-Harris type III medial malleolar fracture and lateral ankle dislocation in a pronation–external rotation injury in an adolescent. (From DeValentine,[32] with permission.)

fracture that occurs only in children, primarily as a result of immature bone's ability to undergo plastic deformation, is the *torus* fracture (Fig. 20-5). This is a compression fracture of the metaphyseal bone in which the thinner cortical metaphyseal bone of a child fails on the compression side first, leaving the tensile side intact. Torus fractures are by nature very stable but do require protection, since one can assume that plastic deformation and probable microfracture have occurred even on the undisrupted tensile side of the metaphysis.

## Physeal Biomechanics

Bright et al. described the physis as a nonhomogeneous, anisotropic, visoelastic substance[5] — in other words, as a physical material that reacts differently to a given physical stress along different axes and whose ability to with-

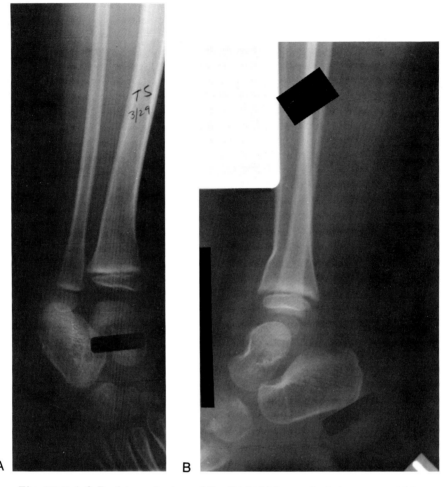

**Fig. 20-5 A & B.** A torus fracture of the distal tibial metaphysis in a young child.

stand strain increases proportionally with the rate at which the stress is applied. Simply put, the epiphysis, physis, and metaphysis of pediatric bone tolerate greater forces when those forces are applied at more rapid rates, which is of optimal benefit in most injury situations. The physis is routinely subjected to the same types of stresses as the remainder of the bone. It is most susceptible to disruption with torsional loading and least susceptible to disruption with axial loading, the effect of bending forces being intermediate.[5] The nonhomogeneous, viscolastic physical properties of the physis, as well as its irregular contour and interdigitating mamillary ridges and the porous, elastic quality of the surrounding spongiosa bone, combine to provide maxi-

mum resistance to injury to this delicate skeletal structure.

The physis is the second most rigid musculoskeletal structure, bone being the most rigid. Because of this, the physis is more likely to absorb force than surrounding soft tissue structures, and physeal disruption normally occurs before soft tissue injury. Once the physis slips, the surrounding soft tissue structures (periosteum, joint capsule, ligaments, etc.) undergo loading. Most researchers believe that physeal disruption can occur without displacement. Such injuries may be easily mistaken for sprain, and one should always maintain a high index of suspicion with injuries near epiphyses. Injuries that may cause ligament tears, tendon rupture, or joint

dislocation in adults may produce physeal injuries in children. The only signs of epiphyseal injury without disruption may be distinct local tenderness over the epiphysis or slight widening of the physis on radiographs as compared with the normal side. Follow-up radiographs in 2 to 3 weeks should demonstrate evidence of bone healing if disruption has occurred.

Salter and others, on the basis of their experimental work, stated that classical physeal disruption always occurs between the hypertrophying layer and the ossifying layer, leaving the germinal cell layer intact.[2] Bright et al., on the basis of their experimental work, suggested that physeal fractures may take a circuitous course through other layers of the physis, including the germinal cell layer, as often as 50 percent of the time.[5] Certain types of forces, such as loading in tension, were noted to have even a higher frequency of germinal layer disturbance. This indicates that the possibility of growth disturbance should be considered with any physeal injury. It is particularly important to discuss this with the child's parents even though the likelihood of growth disturbance may be very low.

## Fracture Healing

Fracture healing occurs in essentially the same sequence and via the same physiologic and cellular processes in children as it does in adults. Historically, this process has been somewhat arbitrarily divided into three overlapping phases on the basis of morphologic and histologic appearance: (1) inflammatory phase, (2) reparative phase, and (3) remodeling phase.[6]

The inflammatory phase begins with the traumatic injury to the bone and surrounding soft tissue and the formation of fracture hematoma.[7] Initial pain and swelling result in physiologic immobilization of the injured part. Invasion of fracture hematoma by surrounding blood vessels and inflammatory cells is followed by phagocytosis of any necrotic soft tissue and bone that may be present as a result of injury and by the development of granulation tissue within the fracture hematoma within a few days of injury.[8]

The reparative phase, which begins within a few days of injury, is mainly characterized by osteoblast proliferation. Osteoblasts are thought to develop from primitive multipotential mesenchymal cells, fibroblasts, or chondroblasts. The two tissues most responsible for bone

formation and thus fracture healing are periosteum and endosteum. Endosteal bone formation normally plays the major role in bone healing but usually occurs slightly more slowly than periosteal bone formation. Periosteal bone formation is responsible for laying down an early peripheral ring of bone callus within the first few weeks postinjury and plays a significantly greater role in stabilization and early healing of displaced fractures.[8-10] Patches of osteoid bone form within the granulation tissue through endochondral ossification within a few weeks. Mineralized osteoid bone may be radiographically apparent in children as early as 1 ½ weeks post injury but usually not before least 3 weeks or more in adults.

The major distinguishing features of fracture healing in children are the accelerated rate of healing and the remodeling potential (Fig. 20-6). The abundant blood supply of pediatric bone results in the formation of a rich hematoma, which bridges the fracture gap; rapid development of granulation tissue; and accelerated osteoblastic proliferation.[11] The peripheral bone callus that is characteristic of so-called secondary bone healing develops rapidly in response to even minimal motion at the fracture site and serves to immobilize the fracture. More motion at the fracture site results in greater peripheral callus formation.

During the remodeling phase, which begins after initial bone callus is fully ossified and may last for several years, osteoclasts and osteoblasts work together to rebuild the bone's normal shape, size, and strength. Remodeling capability is greatest near the epiphyseal end of the bone in children who have at least 2 years of remaining skeletal growth. The greatest degree of remodeling can be expected in younger children and at the most rapidly growing physes. For example, the proximal tibia has greater remodeling capability than the distal tibia, and the distal tibia has greater remodeling capability than a metatarsal. Fractures occurring closer to the end of a long bone or epiphysis also have greater remodeling capability than midshaft fractures. In fact, although bone callus formed at midshaft fractures will undergo extensive remodeling, significant alteration of overall bone alignment is unlikely.

Angulation deformity remodels best and is better tolerated if displacement occurs in the same plane as joint motion, but only limited remodeling can be expected when angulation occurs at right angles to the plane of

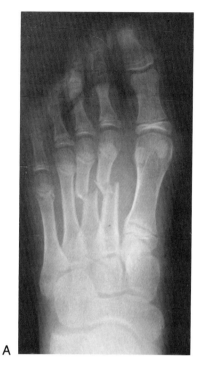 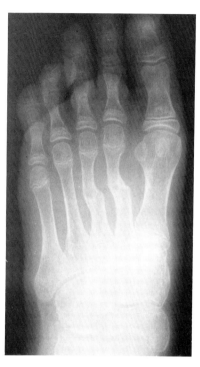

**Fig. 20-6.** (A) Displaced diaphyseal fractures of the second and third metatarsals from a skateboard injury in a 9-year-old boy. Note that metatarsal head alignment is reasonably good. (B) Fractures 1 year later, showing substantial remodeling at the fracture site. Further remodeling can be expected. Note that diaphyseal remodeling will not compensate for rotational malalignment. (From DeValentine,[32] with permission.)

joint movement. Valgus and especially varus angulations of the ankle of more than a few degrees are not well tolerated. Although some correction of angulational deformity can be expected, no spontaneous reduction of rotational malalignment will occur with growth. Therefore care must be taken to adequately assess and to reduce any rotational malalignment at the time of injury. Overgrowth of long bones in children after fracture is commonly recognized; this is most often associated with femur fractures in the lower extremity and is the reason that some shortening is accepted or even preferred with these injuries. Overgrowth is probably due to a post-injury hypervascularity of the physis.[12] Although overgrowth of the tibia, fibula, or metatarsal is possible, it is far less likely in paired bones or in bones with limited growth potential.[13]

The remarkable healing response and remodeling ability of pediatric bone, although an important addition to the pediatric surgeon's armamentarium, should not serve as justification for acceptance of a substandard fracture position.

## INCIDENCE OF PEDIATRIC FOOT AND ANKLE FRACTURES

Although pediatric musculoskeletal injuries are known to be quite common, the incidence of all types of injury in the general population is not well documented. The resilience of the child's skeleton to failure is commonly cited, and this is theoretically supported by the documented greater plasticity of pediatric bone. Hanlon and Estes estimated the incidence of fractures or dislocations in children at about 14 percent of all pediatric injuries.[14] This estimate was derived by comparing a calculated estimate of the total annual number of pediatric fractures in the general population of Bethlehem, Pennsylvania with a calculated estimate of the total number of pediatric injuries in the same geographic area. Hanlon and Estes's estimate is comparable with those of other studies.[15,16] These authors also found that about two-thirds (65 percent) of all fractures in 698 pediatric patients occurred in the upper extremity, with slightly less than one-third (31 percent) affecting the lower extremity and the remaining 4 percent involving the trunk and skull. Peterson and Peterson, who considered only physeal fractures, found a similar distribution, with 61 percent of 330 physeal fractures involving the upper and 39 percent the lower extremity.[17] These statistics are generally comparable with those of other studies.

Less information is available concerning the epidemiology of ankle fractures in children and even less concerning fractures of the foot. Peterson and Peterson[17] and Hanlon and Estes[14] both found the incidence of metatarsal and phalangeal fractures of the foot to be between 5 and 6 percent of total fractures in children. In my clinic over a 1-year period from March 1986 through February 1987, fractures of the foot occurred in 22 (10 percent) of 222 pediatric musculoskeletal injuries that were referred for follow-up care. The distribution of these fractures can be seen in Table 20-3. The vast majority of foot fractures (86 percent) involved the metatarsals and phalanges, with nonphyseal fractures predominating (91 percent). No fractures of the talus or calcaneus were seen in this group, which confirms the rarity of literature reports of fracture of these bones in children. Both lower axial loading (less body weight) and the greater shock-absorbing capacity of pediatric cancellous bone are probably major factors in preventing fracture of the mid- and rearfoot bones in children.

Canale and Kelly, in a review of 71 talar neck fractures seen at the University of Tennessee over a 32-year period, from 1942 to 1974, found only 12 cases involving patients under age 17, and 6 of those patients were 15 or 16 years old at the time of injury.[18] Only four patients were under 10 years of age, and the causes of the injuries tended to be violent in nature (e.g., falls from extreme heights or motor vehicle accidents). Similarly, Marti found only three calcaneal fractures in his large Amsterdam clinic over a 10-year period (all 3 patients were 12 or 13 years of age and had fallen from extreme heights).[19] Only one intra-articular calcaneal fracture in a child under age 10 has been seen in my clinic over a 5-year period.

Landin and Danielsson found that ankle fractures accounted for 373 (4 percent) of 8,682 pediatric fractures in a large study conducted in Malmo, Sweden from 1950 to 1972.[20] Similarly, of 222 pediatric musculoskeletal injuries seen in my clinic over a 1-year period, 4 percent involved the ankle, but all were physeal injuries. When only physeal fractures are considered, however, the ankle ranks second only to the distal radius as the most frequent site of physeal fracture. Peterson and Peterson found that injuries to the distal tibial and fibular physes accounted for 24 percent of 330 physeal injuries in their study.[17] Rogers also found that 25 percent of 118 physeal injuries involved the ankle.[21] Karrholm et al. found the following distribution in 251 pediatric physeal ankle fractures: 136 (54 percent) distal tibia; 85 (34 percent) distal fibula; and 30 (12 percent) distal tibia and fibula.[22] Their study evaluated a geographically defined Swedish population, which received all its medical care through the university hospital. These investigators found the overall incidence of pediatric ankle fractures in the general population to be as follows: distal tibia 0.5 to 1 percent; distal fibula 3 to 4 percent; and distal tibia and distal fibula 1 percent.

Both Landin and Danielsson and Karrholm et al. preferred modifications of the Dias-Tachdjian and Gerner-Smidt classification systems for pediatric ankle fractures. Of the 373 ankle fractures in Landin and Danielsson's study, 23 percent were of the Dias-Tachdjian supination-adduction type, which makes this the single most common type of physeal ankle fracture (Table 20-4). Surprisingly, the second and third most common

Table 20-3. **Distribution of 22 Foot Injuries**[a]

| Site | Nonphyseal No. | Nonphyseal % of total | Physeal No. | Physeal % of Total |
|---|---|---|---|---|
| Digital | 5 | 23 | 2 | 8 |
| Fifth metatarsal base | 6 | 27 | | |
| Lesser metatarsal | 5 | 23 | | |
| First metatarsal | 1 | 5 | | |
| Midfoot | 3 | 14 | | |
| Talus | 0 | 0 | | |
| Calcaneus | 0 | 0 | | |
| Total | 20 | | 2 | |

[a] These injuries were among a total of 222 pediatric musculoskeletal injuries seen in the follow-up clinic over a 1-year period from March 1986 through February 1987.

Patients seen in this clinic were initially evaluated by a primary care or emergency room physician, and the injury was considered significant enough to require follow-up care. Minor injuries not requiring follow-up care are not included.

Table 20-4. **Distribution of 373 Pediatric Ankle Fractures According to Fracture Type**

| Fracture Type | % |
|---|---|
| Supination–adduction (I, 16%; II, 6%; I & II, 1%) | 23 |
| Supination–plantar flexion | 3 |
| Supination–external rotation | 3 |
| Pronation–external rotation | 3 |
| Juvenile Tillaux | 6 |
| Triplane | 8 |
| Avulsion of a small portion of tip of malleolus | 35 |
| Adult fracture patterns | 11 |
| Unclassifiable | 3 |

(From Landin and Danielsson,[20] with permission.)

injuries were the triplane and juvenile Tillaux fractures (8 and 6 percent, respectively). Avulsion type fractures of the tips of the malleoli were the most common of all types of injuries (35 percent). This seems a rather high number in my experience, and one would wonder if some accessory ossicles were included in this group. Another interesting group in Landin and Danielsson's study are those children whose fractures exhibited an adult-type fracture pattern (8 percent). All children in the study were age 16 or under, but those exhibiting adult fracture patterns had partially or completely fused growth plates. Landin and Danielsson also found the right ankle to be involved 1.7 times more frequently than the left ankle

but did not speculate as to cause and did not correlate this finding with right- or left-sided dominance.

The incidence of all types of fractures in children varies with age and sex. Fractures in those under age 1 are extremely rare. Most studies show a small increase in the frequency of fractures between ages 2 and 5, followed by a gradually increasing risk of fracture, which peaks during adolescence. This is followed by a declining risk of fracture after physeal closure through the last half of the second decade and through the third decade. The peak incidence of physeal fractures in adolescents corresponds to a rapid increase in growth and body weight together with thickening of the physeal plate and an increase in physical activity. Studies have shown that thicker physes are more susceptible to mechanical failure. Also, as the child nears skeletal maturity, the perichondrium and periosteum become much thinner and provide less stability. Once the physis closes, the risk declines.

Peterson and Peterson found that the peak incidence of physeal fractures in girls occurred between ages 8 and 13 and in boys between ages 12 and 16 (Fig. 20-7). Although the peak incidence of fractures occurs approximately 2 years earlier in girls, the risk of injury is not significantly different until after the age of 13 to 14, when the risk of fracture in general, including ankle frac-

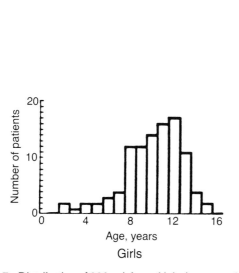
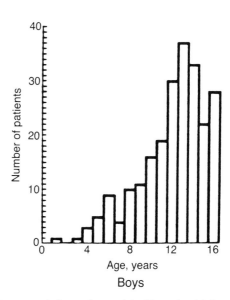

**Fig. 20-7.** Distribution of 330 epiphyseal injuries over a 20-year period reveals a peak incidence in girls between the ages of 8 and 13 and in boys between the ages of 12 and 16. (From Peterson and Peterson,[17] with permission.)

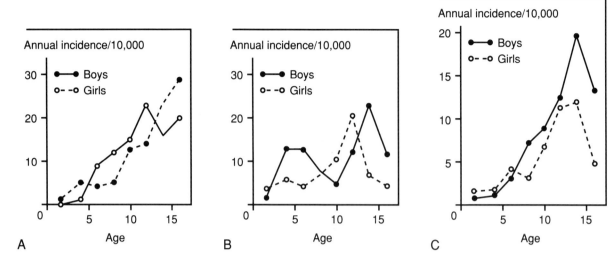

**Fig. 20-8.** (A) Annual incidence of pediatric ankle fractures per 10,000 population in Sweden. (B) Annual incidence of tarsometatarsal fractures per 10,000. (C) Annual incidence of toe fractures per 10,000. (From Landin,[34] with permission.)

tures, in boys increases to twice that of girls. This trend continues into the next two decades of life.[22] Peterson and Peterson stated that the increased incidence of fracture in boys starting at age 13 to 14 was probably because the physes of boys remain open longer and because of greater exposure to trauma rather than because of any intrinsic physical difference between boys and girls.[17]

Most injuries in Landin and Danielsson and Karrholm et al.'s studies of ankle fractures in children resulted from low-energy trauma (Fig. 20-8). Both groups found bicycle accidents in children under age 7 to be one of the most common causes of injury. Falling from a height was also common in this age group. Karrholm et al. found motor vehicle accidents and sports injuries to be the most common cause of ankle fracture in older children. Winter sports were most often implicated in Karrholm et al.'s Swedish study. In contrast, Hanlon, in an earlier study of all types of pediatric fractures in Philadelphia, found that the largest number of cases, without regard for age, were sustained as a result of athletic activity (30.9 percent), with football as the most common single cause; falling was second (25.6 percent) and motor vehicle accidents third (12.9 percent). Landin and Danielsson found a threefold increase in the incidence of pediatric ankle fractures over the 30-year period recorded in their study. They attributed this striking increase to increased participation in organized athletic programs.

## CLASSIFICATION OF PHYSEAL FRACTURES

Categorization of physeal injuries is the first and most important step in the determination of an appropriate course of treatment. A useful classification system allows one to subdivide a general category of problems to identify individual variations and then, through observation and adequate follow-up, to determine more individually appropriate types of treatment and prognoses. A universal classification also improves communication between physicians and therefore facilitates knowledge-sharing and fosters better overall patient care. In addition, a useful classification system should be simple enough to allow widespread use but detailed enough to adequately subdivide problems into categories. Obviously, many of the desired criteria mentioned above are diametrically opposed to one another. Classification systems for physeal fractures have been proposed that are based on fracture pattern, radiographic appearance, treatment and prognosis, and mechanism of injury.[3,23-28]

The first popular classification system for physeal fractures was proposed by Poland in 1898 on the basis of anatomic fracture patterns. Salter in 1963 and Aitken in 1965 both proposed modifications of Poland's classification system based on radiographic appearance of the fracture. The five-type classification system proposed by

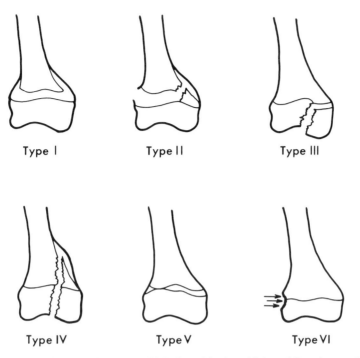

Type I    Type II    Type III

Type IV    Type V    Type VI

**Fig. 20-9.** Salter-Harris classification of epiphyseal injuries with the addition of Rang's type VI perichondral ring injury.

Salter and Harris is the most widely used in the United States (Fig. 20-9). Although this system is based solely on the static radiographic appearance of the fracture and does not provide any information about the mechanism of the fracture, it is simple to apply and widely known and provides useful information concerning treatment and prognosis. In 1969 Rang modified the Salter-Harris classification system to include a sixth type of growth plate injury. All clinicians who treat pediatric musculoskeletal injuries should be familiar with the six physeal fractures types.

## Salter-Harris System

### Salter-Harris Types I and II Fractures

Types I and II fractures are extra-articular fractures and in general carry the best prognosis. A type I injury is a simple transverse slippage of the growth plate. The fracture occurs through physeal cartilage and does not penetrate metaphyseal or epiphyseal bone. Type I fractures are more common in younger children and constitute the most common injury of the distal fibular physis. These fractures have been noted to occur with increased frequency in some pathologic conditions, such as rickets or scurvy.

Type II fractures involve a metaphyseal fracture on the compression side of the bone, which is continuous with a separation of the remaining physis. The radiographic appearance of the proximal triangular wedge of displaced metaphyseal bone attached to the displaced epiphysis is referred to as the *Thurston-Holland sign* and is pathognomonic for a type II injury. Type II fractures are the most common type of physeal injury and are more common in older children, especially those over 10 years of age). Both type I and type II injuries usually have an intact periosteal hinge on the compression side of the injury, which facilitates closed reduction and helps to prevent over-reduction. The vast majority of type I and II fractures can be satisfactorily treated by closed reduction, and slightly less than anatomic reduction may be acceptable. Since types I and II fractures involve primarily cartilaginous tissues, healing usually occurs in approximately half the time required for type III or type IV injuries.

## Salter-Harris Types III and IV Fractures

Types III and IV fractures are intra-articular fractures combined with physeal separation. These are high-risk fractures, which most often require open reduction with even minimal displacement. Restoration of a congruent articular surface and prevention of vertical epiphyseal displacement are of paramount importance to prevent late joint arthroses and partial growth arrest. Vertical physeal displacement tends to promote fusion of the metaphysis on one side of the vertical fracture with the epiphysis on the other side of the fracture, which causes an angular deformity to develop. In contrast, transverse displacement of the physis alone may result in growth arrest but is less likely to cause angular deformity. Types III and IV fractures of the foot and ankle are most often seen in the medial malleolus. They may be seen to a lesser extent at the metatarsophalangeal joints.

## Salter-Harris Type V Injury

Salter and Harris described the type V injury as a relatively uncommon injury resulting from application of a crushing force to the physis through the epiphysis. Since there is usually no visible fracture and no displacement, this injury may be difficult or even impossible to diagnose at the time of injury. It also may coexist with another Salter-Harris type of fracture and not be recognized. One must have a high index of suspicion for this type of injury with significant axial loading types of mechanisms, some of which will only be identified through careful follow-up. Type V injuries have also been described that are due to nontraumatic etiologies such as metaphyseal osteomyelitis or epiphyseal aseptic necrosis, both of which usually cause central growth arrest.

## Rang's Type VI Injury

In 1969 Rang proposed a sixth growth plate injury class, which is often used in conjunction with the Salter-Harris system.[3] Typically this injury is characterized by gradual development of angular deformity following blunt trauma without evidence of fracture at the time of injury. It has been described following a blow to the extremity or a burn injury or after an extremity has been run over by a motor vehicle.[29] Angular deformity following type VI injury is thought to occur as a result of injury to the perichondral ring at the periphery of the physis. Either the injury or the reparative process following blunt trauma causes the formation of a peripheral osseous bridge, which can be detected on radiography.

## Additional Classification Systems

In 1980 Weber proposed a variation of the Salter-Harris classification which is widely used in Europe.[26] The main feature of the Weber system is its distinction between type A extra-articular physeal injuries (Salter-Harris I and II which are labeled types A1 and A2) and type B intra-articular physeal injuries (Salter-Harris III and IV, which are labeled types B-1 and B-2). In 1981 Ogden proposed a more complex version of the Salter-Harris system, which included four more types of injury as well as numerous subtypes.[27] Although Ogden's system may be of some additional descriptive value, in my opinion it is too cumbersome to be clinically useful on a broad basis.

Additional classification systems have been proposed for physeal fractures in specific anatomic areas. Both Dias and Tachdjian[28] and Gerner-Smidt[30] have proposed mechanism-based classification systems for pediatric ankle fractures that are based on the Lauge-Hanson system for adult ankle fractures. Although somewhat more complex, these mechanism-based classification systems do offer some significant advantages over anatomy- or radiography-based systems. Since the ankle involves two bones with two physes, it is often difficult and confusing to attempt to describe the various combinations of injuries with the Salter-Harris system alone. A mechanism-based classification also provides more predictive information about the extent of injury and best method of closed reduction. Moreover, it is similar enough to the Lauge-Hanson classification to be easily learned and can be combined with the Salter-Harris system to provide maximal information. These classification systems for pediatric ankle fractures will be discussed further in Chapter 22.

# EVALUATION AND MANAGEMENT OF PEDIATRIC FOOT AND ANKLE FRACTURES

## Clinical Evaluation

Obviously displaced fractures offer little challenge in diagnosis. Minimally displaced or undisplaced fractures may be quite a bit more difficult to diagnose. The history, time elapsed since injury and, if possible, the mechanism of injury are often useful clues to potential injuries. Point tenderness and local swelling are among the earliest physical signs of musculoskeletal injury. Point tenderness may be the only distinguishing feature between lateral collateral ligament injury of the ankle and undisplaced physeal injury of the distal fibular physis. Manipulation of the distal portion of a fractured bone should also elicit indirect pain or crepitus at the suspected fracture site. Reluctance to bear weight on an injured extremity in a very young child should trigger a careful examination to rule out fracture or significant soft tissue injury.

The examining physician must also be careful to rule out other types of injuries, including other musculoskeletal trauma, through history and thorough examination. In extremity trauma it is important to carefully check and record the neurovascular status of the part distal to the injury. The child should be asked to move the foot and toes to evaluate tendon function. In the case of severe soft tissue trauma such as crush injury, bicycle spoke trauma, or motor vehicle trauma, the child should be carefully followed for potential compartment syndrome. Some or rarely, all of the classic clinical signs of pain, paresthesia, pallor, and diminished pulse may be present. Compartment pressures should be measured if there is any question of possible compartment syndrome. Fasciotomy of involved compartments should be considered if resting pressures rise to greater than 30 to 40 mmHg.[31]

It is important to attempt to classify physeal injuries and to discuss the potential for growth disturbance with parents. One should not frighten parents, but they must have a clear understanding that potential growth arrest is a consequence of injury, not treatment, and that close follow-up is necessary.

## Diagnostic Imaging Studies

Any child suspected of having a fracture of the foot or ankle on the basis of clinical examination should have a minimum of three plain radiographs, with at least two of the films taken at 90-degree angles to one another. Radiographic evaluation should not be considered a substitute for a careful clinical examination. A thorough physical examination should provide a differential diagnosis that will determine the most appropriate radiographic examination and will help to avoid missing other injuries. Anteroposterior, lateral, and mortise views of the ankle or anteroposterior, lateral, and oblique views of the foot

are recommended. Additional specialized views, such as additional obliques or axial views of the heel or metatarsals, may be obtained if necessary once initial films have been viewed. When a physeal injury is suspected, it is helpful to attempt to position the physis perpendicular to the radiograph film. In some cases individual variation or irregularity of the physeal plate contour may make comparison views of the uninjured extremity useful. The only radiographic sign of a Salter-Harris type I physeal injury may be a slight widening or irregularity of the peripheral portion of the physis.

Questionably displaced or slightly displaced physeal or intra-articular fractures may be difficult to evaluate on plain films. Although I prefer tomograms in some situations (e.g., for evaluation of nonunions or osteochondral fractures or when hardware is present) computed tomography (CT) may be more helpful in evaluating the degree of displacement of most intra-articular or physeal fractures of the foot and ankle.

## Treatment of Nondisplaced Fractures

Fortunately, most foot and ankle fractures in children are nondisplaced and fairly easily managed. Each fracture should be individually evaluated and classified if possible. The biomechanics and principles of fracture propagation and healing presented in this chapter should serve as a "template" of knowledge that the physician can use to individually assess the stability and healing potential of each fracture.

I treat almost all fractures (including those that are minor and inherently stable) and severe soft tissue injuries in children with cast immobilization. Children are generally more functional and more comfortable in a short leg walking cast for 3 to 4 weeks, and stiffness and osteopenia are rarely problems, as they can be in adults. Nonphyseal fractures that may be unstable to weight-bearing should be immobilized in a non-weight-bearing cast for 3 to 4 weeks, followed by a weight-bearing cast until radiographic union. Soft tissue healing and bone callus formation should be adequate to stabilize most fractures within 3 weeks. Absence of clinical tenderness, crepitus, and swelling on clinical examination is a good indicator of satisfactory stability even before radiographic evidence of callus mineralization. The younger the child and the more rapid the bone growth, the more rapidly the fracture can be expected to heal.

Radiographic evidence of bone union should always serve as the primary criterion for discontinuing immobilization, just as it does in adults. Although radiographic union cannot be adequately assessed in Salter-Harris type I physeal fractures, these injuries are primarily cartilaginous and often require cast immobilization for only about half the time required by fractures of ossified bone in children of the same age. Activity restriction is usually recommended for an additional 3 weeks. If a physeal injury is suspected on the basis of clinical examination but cannot be confirmed on radiography, I prefer to treat the child with 2 to 3 weeks in a short leg walking cast. Follow-up radiographs may demonstrate evidence of fracture healing.

## Treatment of Displaced Fractures

Closed reduction should be attempted as the first line of treatment for almost all nonphyseal and Salter-Harris type I and II physeal fractures of the foot and ankle. The thick periosteum of immature bone on the compression side of the injury serves as a hinge upon which the fracture can be reduced and helps to prevent over-reduction. Time elapsed from injury is of critical importance when considering closed reduction. Reduction can be most easily accomplished immediately after injury before the development of swelling, pain, muscle splinting, and hematoma consolidation, all of which make manipulation of the fracture more difficult. Soft tissue healing progresses so rapidly in children as to make closed reduction difficult to impossible within 3 to 5 days postinjury. Mineralized bone callus at the fracture site often makes open reduction difficult or impossible later than 10 days postfracture. Physeal fractures heal even more rapidly, and if early reduction cannot be performed, it may be more prudent to accept incomplete reduction than to risk more trauma to the growth plate through forcible manipulation or surgery.

If closed reduction is selected, one must choose between no sedation, parenteral sedation-analgesia, or general anesthesia. If the fracture is fresh and simple and if it is anticipated that the reduction can be performed quickly and easily, no sedation may be used in select cases (especially in infants or older adolescents). The starting of an intravenous line or intramuscular or local anesthetic injections may be more traumatic than a quick, well executed reduction of a simple fracture. A low-dose intramuscular injection of a centrally acting narcotic-sedative combination can sometimes be used in toddlers or very young children in whom it may be difficult to start an intravenous line.

Complex fractures or physeal fractures in young children usually require general anesthesia. Even if anesthesia could be accomplished by other methods, it is usually difficult to obtain adequate muscle relaxation and the complete cooperation of a frightened child without the use of a general anesthetic. Cooperative older children and adolescents may do well with a combination of intravenous sedation-analgesia and a local anesthetic. Careful titration of doses calculated by weight and continuous monitoring are essential in children. A narcotic antagonist (e.g., naloxone hydrochloride) as well as supportive therapy should always be immediately available before administering intravenous narcotics to children. Hematoma infiltration together with titrated intravenous sedation-analgesia often works well in fresh fractures. Adequate amounts of local anesthesia (maximum dosage is determined according to the child's age and weight) must be infiltrated directly into the fracture area or joint communicating with the fracture. In the case of forefoot or digital fractures, an ankle nerve block or digital block may be quite effective.

The most important part of closed reduction is distal traction and disengagement of the fracture. Disengagement is accomplished by slight accentuation of the mechanism of injury or movement of the distal part toward the compression side of the fracture. Once disengagement is accomplished the fracture is reduced by reversing the mechanism of injury. Most displaced fractures should reduce fairly easily. A finger trap or stockinette type of traction device is sometimes used alone or as a precursor to manual reduction to promote muscle relaxation through fatigue (Fig. 20-10).

If reduction has not been achieved after three attempts with nonphyseal fractures or two attempts with physeal fractures, one should strongly consider an alternative method of analgesia or reduction. For example, if closed reduction of a Salter-Harris type II fracture of the ankle cannot be accomplished on the second attempt with intravenous sedation, then closed reduction under general anesthesia should be tried for better relaxation. If reduction still is not achieved after one or two attempts under general anesthesia, then open reduction should be attempted. Particularly with physeal fractures, repeated forcible manipulation can do irreversible damage to the growth plate. Once the fracture has been reduced, the position should be held while an assistant applies an im-

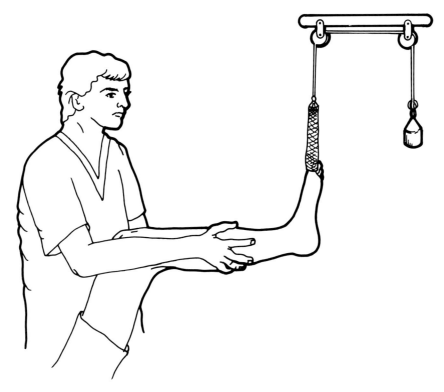

**Fig. 20-10.** Technique of finger trap reduction used to reduce a displaced metatarsal fracture.

mobilizing splint or cast and radiographs are taken to confirm adequate reduction.

Many fractures can be treated in an outpatient setting. It is especially important that parents have a clear understanding of what to expect, both during the procedure and at home afterward. Cast precautions should be explained to parents. Any fracture that requires reduction should be kept non-weight-bearing at least until soft tissue healing and preliminary callus formation provide satisfactory fracture stability (usually in about 3 weeks). In the case of very young or noncompliant children or fractures that are rotationally unstable (e.g., supination-external rotation or triplane fractures of the ankle), a long leg cast with the knee flexed at 15 to 45 degrees should be used initially.

## Open Reduction of Fractures in Children

In general, closed reduction is preferred for pediatric fractures. Nonunion and cast immobilization "disease" do not pose a problem as they can in adults, and healing ability and capacity for correction of some types of malalignment are considerable in children. Adequate realignment is also more easily achieved with closed reduction in children than in adults. Thus, operative treatment should only be selected when closed treatment would not be expected to produce a satisfactory outcome. Open reduction is rarely needed for diaphyseal fractures but would be expected to be needed more often for adequate reduction of physeal fractures. All intra-articular fractures must be anatomically reduced and therefore would be expected to have the highest frequency of operative treatment.

Some common situations in which closed reduction may fail are as follows: (1) a spike of bone on the compression side of the fracture may "buttonhole" through the periosteum; (2) a loose flap of periosteum or other soft tissue (including tendon) on the tension side of the fracture may fall into the fracture gap, thus preventing reduction; (3) loose fracture fragments may dislodge and fall into the fracture gap, impeding complete reduction; and (4) soft tissue or osseous support to maintain reduction may be lacking (e.g., in multiple metatarsal or tarsometatarsal fractures). If open reduction becomes necessary, it should be performed under general anesthesia. Furthermore, any time that closed reduction under general anesthesia is elected, permission for open reduction should be obtained at the same time.

It is sometimes possible to treat some reducible but inherently unstable fractures (e.g., multiple metatarsal neck fractures) with closed reduction and percutaneous pinning under image intensification control. There are also some physeal fractures for which open reduction is almost always obligatory (displaced Salter-Harris type III and IV, juvenile Tillaux, and triplane fractures of the distal tibia).

Once open reduction has been elected as the best course of action, adequate surgical exposure is the single most important consideration. Incisions should be no longer than necessary but long enough and optimally placed for unimpeded access to the interior of the entire fracture. Optimal incision placement requires thorough presurgical knowledge of the fracture type. One should avoid stripping any more periosteum or joint capsule than is absolutely necessary in order to prevent interruption of the blood supply to the physis and should also avoid forcible instrumentation of the physeal cartilage. Bright has recommended that if the periosteum must be reflected near or over the physis, it should be excised for 1 cm around the physis to avoid development of a peripheral osseous bridge.[29] Manipulation should be as gentle as possible, and fracture fixation should be the minimum amount that will secure a stable reduction.

Whereas rigid internal fixation is usually striven for in the adult, this is not as important in children. Pediatric bone is more honogenous and more compact than adult bone and can usually be adequately stabilized with minimal internal fixation. Kirschner wires are the most frequently used internal fixation devices. Lag screws are often useful, and plates are rarely indicated. If possible, transmetaphyseal or transepiphyseal fixation that does not cross the growth plate is preferred. Cannulated lag screws are very useful, since the position of the guide wire can be radiographically confirmed prior to screw insertion.

When fixation does cross the physis, only smooth, small-caliber Kirschner wires placed as perpendicular to the physis as possible should be used. One often encounters a dilemma when applying pin fixation through the physis, because although parallel pins placed perpendicular to the physis theoretically are least likely to impede growth, they also offer less stability in many situations than crossed pins. An individual judgment must be made in each case as to which type of fixation offers adequate stability with the least physeal trauma. In any event, Kirschner wires that cross the physis should be removed as soon as possible after fracture healing.

Intraoperative radiographs should always be obtained to ensure that reduction is anatomic and to check placement of hardware. Long leg casts are usually not necessary after open reduction unless reduction is tenuous or in the case of a very young or noncompliant child. Nonweight-bearing should be continued for a minimum of 3 weeks or until preliminary union is satisfactory to allow protected weight-bearing.

# REFERENCES

1. Blount WP: Fractures in children. Williams & Wilkins, Baltimore, 1955
2. Salter RB: Injuries involving the epiphyseal plate. J Bone Joint Surg [Am] 45:587, 1963
3. Rang M: The Growth Plate and Its Disorders. Williams & Wilkins, Baltimore, 1969
4. Digby KH: The measurement of diaphyseal growth in proximal and distal direction. J Anat 50:187, 1915
5. Bright RW, Burstein AH, Elmore SM: Epiphyseal plate cartilage. J Bone Joint Surg [Am] 56:688, 1974
6. Chapman MW, Woo SL-Y: Principles of fracture healing. p. 115. In Chapman MW (ed): Operative Orthopaedics. JB Lippincott, Philadelphia, 1988
7. Potts WJ: The role of the haematoma in fracture healing. Surg Gynecol Obstet 57:318, 1933
8. Rhinelander FW, Baragry RA: Microangiography in bone healing. I. Undisplaced closed fractures. J Bone Joint Surg [Am] 44:1273, 1962
9. Rhinelander FW: Tibial blood supply in relation to fracture healing. Clin Orthop 105:35, 1974
10. Rhinelander FW, Phillips RS, Steel WM, Beer JC: Microangiography in bone healing. II. Displaced closed fractures. J Bone Joint Surg [Am] 50:643, 1968
11. Trueta J: Blood supply and the rate of healing of tibial fractures. Clin Orthop 105:11, 1974
12. Bisgard JD: Longitudinal overgrowth of long bones with special reference to fractures. Surg Gynecol Obstet 62:823, 1936
13. Schuberth JM: Principles of fracture management in children. Clin Podiatr Med Surg 4:267, 1987
14. Hanlon CR, Estes WL: Fractures in childhood—a statistical analysis. Am J Surg 87:312, 1954

15. Beekman F, Sullivan JE: Some observations on fractures of long bones in children. Am J Surg 51:722, 1941

16. Steinert V, Bennek J: Unterschenkelfrakturen im Kindesalter. Zentralbl Chir 91:1387, 1966

17. Peterson CA, Peterson HA: Analysis of the incidence of injuries to the epiphyseal growth plate. J Trauma 12:275, 1972

18. Canale T, Kelly F: Fractures of the neck of the talus. J Bone Joint Surg [Am] 60:143, 1978

19. Marti R: Fracture of the talus and calcaneus, p. 373. In Weber BG, Brunner CH, Freuler F (eds): Treatment of Fractures in Children and Adolescents. Springer-Verlag, New York, 1980

20. Landin LA, Danielsson LG: Children's ankle fractures. Classification and epidemiology. Acta Orthop Scand 54:634, 1983

21. Rodgers LF: The radiography of epiphyseal injuries. Radiology 96:289, 1970

22. Karrholm J, Hansson LI, Svensson K: Incidence of tibiofibular shaft and ankle fractures in children. J Pediatr Orthop 2:386, 1982

23. Poland J: Traumatic Separation of the Epiphyses. Elder & Co., London, 1898

24. Aitken AP: Fractures of the epiphyses. Clin Orthop 41:19, 1965

25. Salter RB: Injuries of the ankle in children. Orthop Clin North Am 5:147, 1974

26. Weber BC: Treatment of Fractures in Children and Adolescents. Springer-Verlag, New York, 1980

27. Ogden JA: Skeletal Injury in the Child. Lea & Febiger, Philadelphia, 1982

28. Dias LS, Tachdjian MO: Physeal injuries of the ankle in children. Clin Orthop 136:230, 1978

29. Bright RW: Physeal injuries. p. 87. In Rockwood CA, Wilkins KE, King RE (eds): Fractures in Children. JB Lippincott, Philadelphia, 1984

30. Gerner-Smidt M: Anklebrud Hos Børn. Nordiskt Förlag, Copenhagen, 1963

31. Whitesides TE, Haney TC, Morimoto K, Harada H: Tissue pressure measurements as a determinant for the need of a fasciotomy. Clin Orthop 113:43, 1975

32. DeValentine SJ: Foot and ankle fractures in children. p. 473. In Scurran BL (ed): Foot and Ankle Trauma. Churchill Livingstone, New York, 1989

33. Rockwood C: Fractures in Children. JB Lippincott, Philadelphia, 1984

34. Landin LA: Fracture patterns in children. Acta Orthop Scand 54: suppl. 202, 1983

## SUGGESTED READINGS

Blais MM, Green WT, Anderson: Lengths of the growing foot. J Bone Joint Surg [Am] 38:998, 1956

Currey JD: Differences in tensile strength of bone of different histological types. J Anat 93:87, 1959

Currey JD, Butler G: The mechanical properties of bone tissue in children. J Bone Joint Surg [Am] 57:810, 1975

Daly PJ, Fitzgerald RH Jr, Melton LJ, Ilstrup DM: Epidemiology of ankle fractures in Rochester, Minnesota. Acta Orthop Scand 58:539, 1987

Figura MA: Metatarsal fractures. Clin Podiatr Med Surg 2:247, 1985

Garroway MW, Stauffer RN, Kurland LT, O'Fallon MW: Limb fractures in a defined population. I. Frequency and distribution. Mayo Clin Proc 54:701, 1979

Hert J, Kucera P, Vavra M et al: Comparison of the mechanical properties of both primary and haversian bone tissue. Acta Anat (Basel) 61:412, 1965

Hirsch C, Evans F: Studies on some physical properties of infant compact bone. Acta Orthop Scand 35:300, 1965

Light TR, Ogden DA, Ogden JA: The anatomy of metaphyseal torus fractures. Clin Orthop 188:103, 1984

MacNealy GA, Rogers LF, Hernandez R, Poznanski AK: Injuries of the distal tibial epiphysis: Systematic radiographic evaluation. Am J Radiol 138:683, 1982

Martin W, Riddervold HO: Acute plastic bowing fractures of the fibula. Diagn Radiol 131:639, 1979

Ogden JA: Injury to the growth mechanisms of the immature skeleton. Skeletal Radiol 6:237, 1981

Panjabi MM, White AA III, Southwick WO: Mechanical properties of bone as a function of the rate of deformation. J Bone Joint Surg [Am] 55:322, 1973

Sisk TD: General principles of fracture treatment. p. 1557. In Crenshaw AH (ed): Campbell's Operative Orthopaedics. Vol. 3. CV Mosby, St. Louis, 1987

Tachdjian MO: Pediatric Orthopedics. WB Saunders, Philadelphia, 1972

Tachdjian MO: The Child's Foot. WB Saunders, Philadelphia, 1985

# 21
# Fractures of the Foot

*JOHN M. SCHUBERTH*

Foot fractures in children are relatively uncommon owing to several physiologic and mechanical properties of the pediatric skeletal system. Although the specific reasons are discussed elsewhere in this text, it is primarily the plasticity of the pediatric skeleton that accounts for the paucity of injuries in this age group. Most of the fractures seen in the younger age group are the result of a direct mechanism such as the dropping of a heavy object on the foot. Indirect mechanisms are often of insufficient energy to cause the spiral or spiral-oblique type of fracture pattern in the younger patient. As the child grows older and the skeleton assumes adult-like properties, the incidence of foot fractures increases, as indirect mechanisms can now cause failure in the less resilient bone. Forces that would not produce fracture in the younger child can be expected to produce skeletal injury in the older child and adolescent, although the fracture pattern may be somewhat different than that observed in the adult patient.

Although the smaller bones of the foot have ossification centers that account for longitudinal growth, the significance of injuries to the physeal plate is diminished because the foot grows relatively quickly in comparison with the rest of the body. In fact, little longitudinal growth occurs after the age of 5 years.[1] By the age of 12 the average foot has attained 96 percent of its total length in girls and 88 percent in boys.[2] Therefore the susceptible period for growth disturbances is greatly diminished. However one should not accept mediocrity of treatment in younger children who sustain injuries to the growth plates. Functional deficits can result when significant growth arrest of the metatarsal physes has occurred. Cosmetic concerns can arise when the phalangeal physes are injured at an early age (Fig. 21-1).

In spite of these potential problem areas, fractures of the pediatric foot are relatively benign injuries in most cases. High-energy injuries involving open fractures may constitute exceptions, but as a rule there are few closed fractures of the foot that result in disabling deformity. Treatment of the majority of nonarticular, nonphyseal fractures is often symptomatic, especially in the younger child. The heightened healing potential of pediatric bone ensures bony union in the vast majority of cases. The heightened remodeling capabilities also account for the extremely low incidence of complications in these injuries. Treatment of specific pedal fractures will be discussed in the remainder of this chapter.

## FRACTURES OF THE TOES
### Hallux Fractures

Fractures of the great toe are infrequently encountered in the pediatric age group for reasons described above. When they do occur, the usual mechanism of injury is a direct blow to the foot, which is most frequently the result of dropping a heavy object on the foot. Midshaft or other nonarticular fractures of the proximal phalanx can be treated with closed reduction in the vast majority of cases unless there is significant residual rotational deformity. Comminuted fractures of the distal tuft can occur and are treated as in the adult, by immobilization and symptomatic therapy.

Articular fractures should be treated as they are in adults. Often open reduction and internal fixation are indicated. Physeal fractures of the proximal phalangeal base should be addressed with the guidelines of the particular Salter-Harris fracture type in mind. Those fractures that have an intra-articular component should be treated by anatomic reduction and internal fixation (Fig.

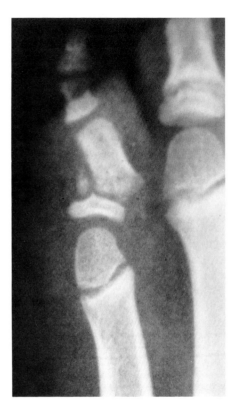

**Fig. 21-1.** Anteroposterior radiograph of a 9-year-old girl who kicked an unyielding object, sustaining this open fracture of the fifth proximal phalangeal base. It was treated in another hospital but was not reduced. Three days later the fracture was irreducible with conventional measures. The malposition and slight cosmetic deformity were then accepted. Further cosmetic changes can be expected if growth is compromised with regard to angulation or length of the digit.

21-2). Complications from these fractures may cause growth disturbances or early degenerative changes of the first metatarsophalangeal joint. In rare instances the physis of the distal phalanx may be involved. Open reduction may be indicated in isolated cases, particularly when there is extension into the interphalangeal joint.

Indirect mechanisms usually result in a fracture through the physis of the proximal phalanx. The distal segment can dislocate superiorly or inferiorly, depending on the moment of force. Closed reduction is almost always adequate for this particular injury because it is extremely rare that soft tissue interposition would necessitate surgical intervention. In addition, sagittal plane angular deformities would gradually correct in younger

children. In some cases the pull of the long extensors and flexor may serve to maintain the deformity. Closed pinning may be necessary to prevent further deformity in the unstable reduction.

## Lesser Digit Fractures

Fractures of the digits often occur from direct forces applied to the toes. The classical example is that of the bedpost fracture of the fifth toe. The injury can occur through the physis or through the shaft of the phalanx. Whatever the location, closed reduction is required to realign the toe under local anesthesia. The digit is best reduced by applying distal traction to the part and then reversing the mechanism of injury. Occasionally the mechanism must be accentuated to disengage the bony fragments. A pencil can be placed in the web space to enhance the lever arm while reducing the fracture (Fig. 21-3). Once the fracture is reduced, the toe can be taped to the adjacent toe and the child placed in a wooden shoe. The younger child or the child with a more unstable fracture should preferably be placed in a short leg walking cast for comfort and ease in management.[2] Immobilization is necessary for 3 to 4 weeks whether one chooses tape, a cast, or both. In the unstable fracture, periodic radiographs should be obtained early to ensure that displacement does not occur. After 2 to 3 weeks displacement is unlikely. If there is early displacement, Kirschner wire fixation may be indicated.

Articular fractures through the proximal phalangeal base once again should be managed as any adult intra-articular fracture. Open reduction is indicated in order to reduce the likelihood of degenerative joint disease of the metatarsophalangeal joint (Fig. 21-4). Significant growth disturbances can be expected only in the very young.

## FRACTURES OF THE METATARSALS

Fractures of the metatarsals are relatively uncommon. In most cases the injury is the result of a direct blow to the foot. As DeValentine[2] points out, most of the fractures are seen at the distal end of the metatarsal, either through the physis or slightly proximal to it. Fractures at the base of a metatarsal are less common and are likewise the result of direct trauma. Shaft fractures are un-

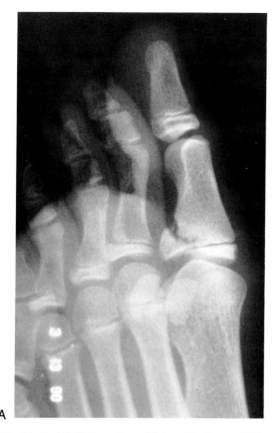 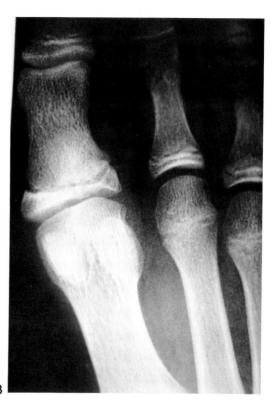

A B

**Fig. 21-2.** **(A)** Oblique view of Salter-Harris type III fracture of the proximal phalanx of the hallux. This was treated with open reduction and internal fixation. **(B)** Anteroposterior radiograph of the same patient 8 months later. Note the relative congruity of the first metatarsophalangeal joint.

common because of the resilience of pediatric bone, but when they do occur, they are the result of more significant trauma; they are often displaced and are likely to be unstable.

Solitary metatarsal fractures most often result from direct trauma and are relatively rare. They can usually be managed with closed reduction. In fact, many of the isolated injuries require no reduction at all because of the low probability of significant displacement. The integrity of the transverse metatarsal ligaments and the thick periosteal tissues helps to prevent dorsal or plantar migration. As with all metatarsal fractures, satisfactory dorsoplantar position is of paramount importance regardless of the treatment. The vast majority of isolated fractures can be managed with a short leg weight-bearing cast after closed reduction or acceptance of the injury position. Closed reduction is more likely to be necessary

in the more distal injury, in which there is an occasional loss of longitudinal apposition. When there is no longitudinal apposition, closed reduction is mandatory, since even though the fracture would probably unite, the resultant position would often not be acceptable. Remodeling would probably be insufficient even in the younger patient.

Finger traps applied to the involved digit will attain the necessary longitudinal traction. The surgeon should then achieve end-on-end alignment via reversal of the mechanism of the injury. In rare instances in which the reduction is grossly unstable, percutaneous or open, Kirschner wire fixation would be indicated.

Injuries to the first metatarsal may require more substantial stabilization than those involving the lesser metatarsals; since there are no medial stabilizing structures, displacement may be more significant and

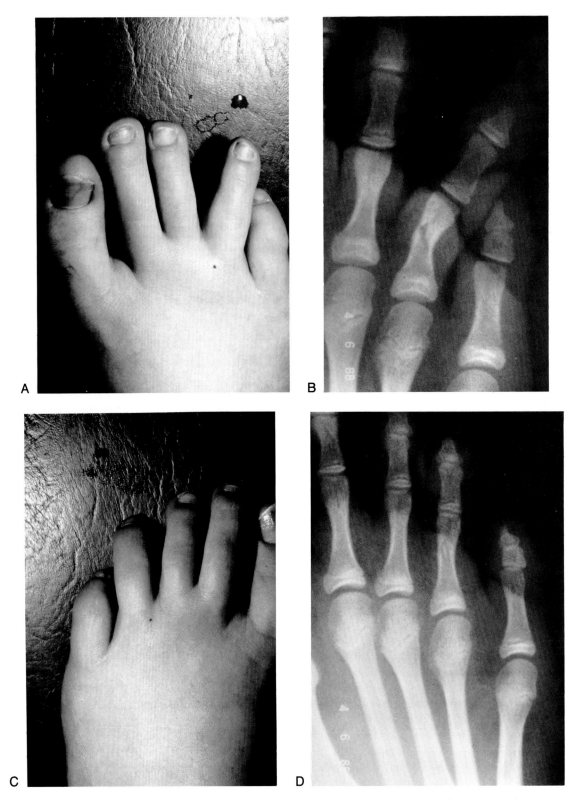

**Fig. 21-3. (A)** Photograph of 12-year-old girl who kicked a bedpost, sustaining an obvious deformity of the fourth toe. **(B)** Anteroposterior radiograph showing the lateral displacement of the digit. **(C)** Clinical appearance after closed reduction. Buddy taping to the third toe will help reduce the residual deviation. **(D)** Postreduction anteroposterior radiograph showing anatomic reduction.

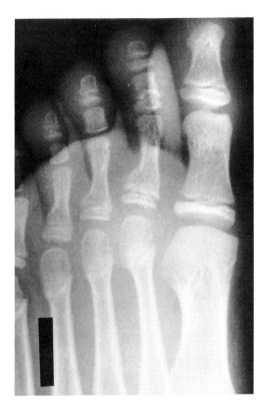

**Fig. 21-4.** Oblique radiograph of a minimally displaced Salter-Harris IV fracture of the proximal phalangeal base of the second toe in a 9-year-old girl. This was treated with strict non-weight-bearing and a short leg cast. The fracture healed uneventfully.

reductions less stable. Treatment may be as simple as a non-weight-bearing cast or as involved as an open reduction with internal fixation. Again, maintenance of the correct sagittal plane position is critical.

Multiple metatarsal fractures usually represent more severe injuries. They are also relatively unstable injuries because of the loss of intact adjacent soft tissue structures. The same principles apply to these fractures as to isolated metatarsal fracture. However, the threshold for closed pinning or open reduction should be lowered to ensure adequate alignment (Fig. 21-5). Often, fixation of the most unstable fracture is sufficient to provide stability to the adjacent metatarsals through the vassal phenomenon.

Torus fractures of the metatarsals are somewhat common. They usually occur at the distal ends of the lesser metatarsals and the proximal ends of the first

metatarsal (Fig. 21-6). Treatment is only symptomatic, usually requiring a short-leg walking cast.

## FRACTURES OF THE MIDFOOT

Midfoot fractures in children are extremely uncommon. As DeValentine[2] indicates, there have been no reports of midfoot fractures in children in the world literature. I have not encountered any fracture of the navicular, cuboid, or cuneiforms in children over an 8-year period. These bones are largely cancellous and extremely resilient to trauma. If individual fractures should occur, they should be managed with common sense and a high regard for the forgiving potential of the pediatric skeleton. Since there is no physis and these are not long bones, the remodeling potential is limited. The surgeon should be aware of subtle compression fractures that may influence proximal or distal alignment of the contiguous structures. Grossly displaced intra-articular fractures should be managed as any adult injury.

Tarsometatarsal fracture-dislocations are uncommon but not rare. Wiley[3] has provided a report of 18 cases of tarsometatarsal joint injuries in children, which also cites other reports of these injuries in the pediatric age group.[4-7] The earliest reported case was that described by Easton[8] in 1938, involving a 9-year-old who sustained a Lis-Franc injury. Wiley[3] reported the case of a 6-year-old in his series of 18 patients, and I have since reported the case of a 3-year-old girl who sustained complete dissociation of the Lis-Franc articulation when a garage door fell on top of her foot[9] (Fig. 21-7).

The most common mechanism of injury, according to Wiley,[7] is the acute forced plantar flexion of the forefoot. This is similar to that seen in the adult population. Wiley described three distinct situations in which the required combination of force and position can occur. The first results from striking the ground in the so-called tiptoe position. Significant axial load is required for fracture-dislocation to occur, but once the force of body weight is transmitted through the fixed forefoot, the path of least resistance is through the weaker dorsal ligamentous complex. Another possible mechanism producing acute forefoot flexion occurs when a heavy object anchors the forefoot to the ground and the child tries to escape the painful stimulus and pulls the foot away. This most commonly happens when the child's foot is run over by a car. The third mechanism described by Wiley[7] is that of heel-

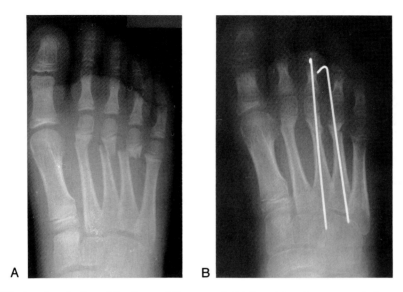

**Fig. 21-5. (A)** Displaced metaphyseal fractures of the second, third, and fourth metatarsals in an 8-year-old child. **(B)** Open reduction and internal fixation of this inherently unstable fracture. (Courtesy of S.J. DeValentine, D.P.M.)

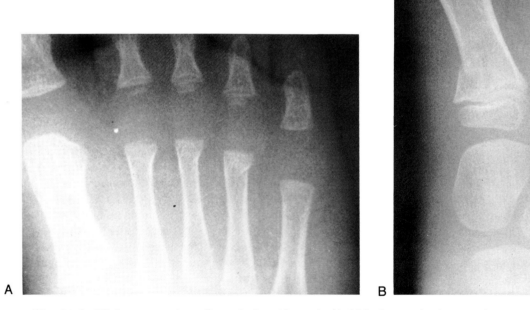

**Fig. 21-6. (A)** Anteroposterior radiograph of an 18-month-old child who sustained a torus fracture of the fourth metatarsal. This required a short-leg walking cast for approximately 10 days. **(B)** Anteroposterior radiograph of a 5-year-old child who sustained a torus fracture to the first metatarsal. Again this also required symptomatic treatment only, in this case a walking cast for 3 weeks.

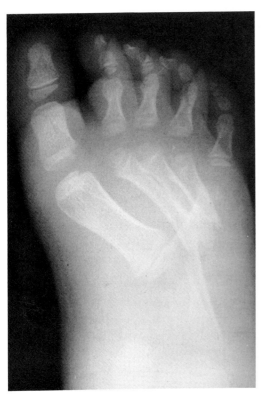

**Fig. 21-7.** Anteroposterior radiograph of a 3-year-old girl injured by a garage door dropping on her foot. There is a complete disruption of the medial Lis-Franc articulation. Only the fourth and fifth metatarsal base articulations with the cuboid remained intact, at the expense of middiaphyseal fractures of the fourth and fifth metatarsals. The first, second, and third metatarsals were completely dislocated from their respective cuneiforms. There was the expected soft tissue damage from the crush injury, with complete severance of the dorsalis pedis artery and vein. Open reduction followed unsuccessful closed attempts. Wound healing was compromised with full thickness skin loss over traumatized area. This was the same area supplied by the dorsalis pedis arterial tree.

to-toe compression, which occurs when the load strikes the heel of a kneeling victim. The direct mechanism of injury in the 3-year-old mentioned above can also occur, but predictable patterns of dislocation are not observed.[7]

Treatment of this entity should be based on the degree of displacement and the intra-articular involvement of the fractures. The traditional approach is closed reduction with or without percutaneous wire fixation. However, a more aggressive open approach to the management of these injuries[10] has been suggested. Although this concept has been described for adult victims, the principles can certainly be applied to children with the same sound logic. The long-term follow-up of adults seems to support the concept of aggressive intervention. Wiley's[3] longest follow-up in his study of 18 patients was only 8 months postinjury. Perhaps if a longer-term evaluation were made of adult patients who sustained Lis-Franc injuries as children that were treated by closed reduction, the results would not be so promising. Wiley[3] alludes to this possibility and speculates that poor results were probably due to incomplete reduction and the presence of intra-articular fractures.

I believe that most Lis-Franc injuries should be reduced anatomically under direct vision. This, of course, necessitates open reduction of the tarsometatarsal articulations, which is the same approach used for the adult patient with this injury. Because the Lis-Franc articulation is such a crucial weight-bearing joint, it seems not only logical but necessary to address dislocations of this joint as one would those of any other weight-bearing joint. This logic would be erroneous if there were enough evidence to support a paucity of symptoms in the long-term follow-up examination.

Three longitudinal incisions are usually sufficient to relocate all the metatarsal bases. The first incision is made over the medial aspect of the first metatarsal base, the second over the convergence of the second and third metatarsal bases, and the last over the fourth and fifth metatarsal bases. If there is less than complete dislocation of all the tarsometatarsal bases, the incisional pattern may be modified. The transverse incision can be used but is more likely to lead to vascular embarrassment.

Once anatomic reduction is attained, each respective metatarsal base is fixed to the corresponding tarsal bone with a smooth Kirschner wire. Wires of adequate caliber should be used in order to prevent migration secondary to bending of the wire. It is seldom sufficient to rely on perimeter fixation of the first and fifth metatarsals because the intermetatarsal basal ligaments are almost always disrupted. Here the central metatarsals may be unstable in spite of secure peripheral stabilization. Dorsal migration of the metatarsal base may occur. Intraoperative radiographs should be obtained in the anteroposterior, oblique, and lateral projections to ensure anatomic alignment prior to closure.

The skin should be observed closely for wound complications during the first 2 weeks. These can best be avoided by strict elevation postoperatively, prompt efforts at reduction, and careful handling of the soft tissues. The patient is treated with a non-weight-bearing cast for 6 to 8 weeks, followed by a short leg walking cast for 2 to 4 weeks, depending on the age of the patient. Wires are removed at 8 weeks, usually in an office setting.

## FRACTURES OF THE TALUS

Fractures of the talus are relatively rare in children. However, there are numerous reports in the literature on the small percentage of patients with talar fractures who are under 16 years of age.[11-15] As compared with adult bone, the pediatric talus is more resilient to the compressive forces involved in the vast majority of talar fractures because of the high percentage of the talar

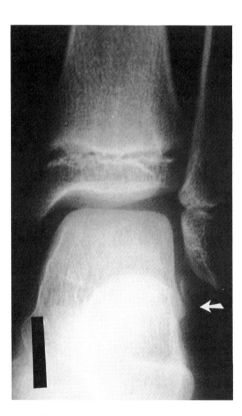

**Fig. 21-8.** Anteroposterior radiograph of the ankle in a 7-year-old girl showing an intra-articular flake (arrow) of bone that resulted after an inversion type of injury. Acute symptoms resolved after several weeks in a cast. Operative intervention in these relatively minor injuries is not indicated.

body that is composed of cartilage. In fact, significant fractures of the talus usually occur only with violent trauma such as falls from heights or high-speed motor vehicle accidents.

Fractures of the talus in children can be classified similarly to adult injuries. However, only the most significant injuries in the child require prudent and aggressive intervention. Fractures that involve the margins of the talus are most likely to be inconsequential and to require little if any attention other than recognition and symptomatic management (Fig. 21-8). The three most important categories of talar fractures in children are the talar neck fracture, the transchondral fracture, and the body or transcorporal fractures. The most familiar classification schemes are reviewed elsewhere in detail.

### Avascular Necrosis

As DeValentine[2] points out, the talus is quite vulnerable to vascular embarrassment because there is little surface area for the nutrient artery. Also, the talar body is covered primarily by cartilaginous surface. For these reasons any displaced fracture has some likelihood of disrupting one or more of the main arterial branches to the talus, but the probability of avascular necrosis in the pediatric patient is probably lower than the incidence reported in the adult. The reasons for this are not known but presumably are related to the cartilaginous composition of the talar body. If the blood supply were disrupted and the cartilaginous anlage were avascular, significant collapse would not occur. However, as the bone ossifies, as in the older child and adolescent, the resultant revascularization phase would demineralize the bone and allow for collapse. Therefore it would seem that avascular necrosis (AVN) in these injuries is an age-related phenomenon. Younger patients, in whom the talus is mostly cartilaginous, would be at minimal risk for the complication, whereas children in whom the talus is mostly ossified would probably be as prone to avascular necrosis as an adult patient. On the other hand, there is some evidence to support a higher incidence of avascular necrosis in children following a talar neck fracture[14,15] It is safe to say that the question of the relative incidence of avascular necrosis in children has not been resolved.

Nevertheless, avascular necrosis can have devastating consequences. Therefore it should be diligently sought in any talar fracture. One should remember that bone that does not have a blood supply cannot change its radiographic density, a fact that constitutes the basis of the so-called Hawkins sign. If the blood supply is intact from the onset, the period of immobilization and non-weight-bearing will cause a localized osteopenia. The cancellous bone will appear less dense than the surrounding subchondral cortex, resulting in the Hawkins sign. This is a favorable condition, as it indicates intact vascularization of the talus. It takes a minimum of 4 to 6 weeks for these radiographic changes to occur, but the absence of the Hawkins sign does not represent definite avascular necrosis. If there is any suspicion of avascular necrosis even 8 weeks after injury, the question can be resolved via magnetic resonance imaging (MRI) techniques or radionuclide imaging. The delivery of radioactive tracer to the talar body signifies an intact blood supply (Fig. 21-9). Plain film evidence of the Hawkins sign can be expected

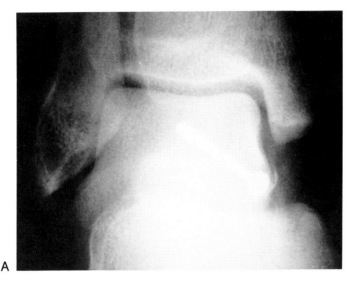

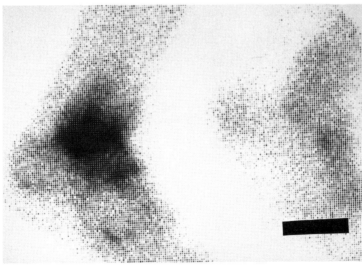

**Fig. 21-9.** **(A)** Anteroposterior view of the ankle 12 weeks after open reduction and internal fixation of a talar neck fracture. Note the absence of subcortical atrophy or Hawkins' sign. **(B)** Technetium bone scan showing increased uptake in the proximal portion of the talar body. This indicates an intact blood supply to the body of the talus. Avascular necrosis is highly unlikely in view of this finding in spite of the lack of Hawkins' sign.

to appear in the subsequent weeks. The absence of up-take of the marker is highly specific for avascular necrosis, and the patient should be managed appropriately.

## Talar Neck Fractures

### Hawkins Type I Fractures

Fractures of the talar neck are the result of hyperdorsiflexion of the talus against the anterior edge of the tibial plafond. The most commonly used classification scheme is that of Hawkins,[16] which is based upon the continuation of forces through the ankle joint area. With continued propagation of forces, the injury worsens, along with the prognosis. The Hawkins type I fracture is defined as a fracture of the talar neck. It can be displaced or nondisplaced. Because the blood supply of the talus is not usually disrupted, the probability of AVN is small. The fracture line is almost always posterior to the dorsal talar neck vessels from the dorsalis pedis supply, so that all the major nutrient branches are not compromised (Fig. 21-10).

If the fracture is not displaced or minimally displaced, treatment is conservative, with a long leg cast for 4 to 6 weeks followed by a short leg weight-bearing cast for 2 to 4 weeks. Careful interval radiographic analysis is important to assess interim positional changes. Closed reduction of displaced fractures should be attempted. If it is successful, the patient is managed in a plantar-flexed non-weight-bearing cast for 4 to 6 weeks. If closed reduction is unsatisfactory, open reduction is indicated. This is best performed with removable fixation in the skeletally immature child and with compression screw fixation in the more mature child. Surgical intervention reportedly adds to the likelihood of avascular necrosis, so that it is important to achieve rigid fixation regardless of the method. A decreased chance of avascular necrosis in patients treated by rigid fixation has been reported.[17]

### Hawkins Type II Fractures

Further propagation of the dorsiflexion moment of force will result in dislocation of the subtalar joint, the so-called Hawkins type II fracture (Fig. 21-11). The posterior portion of the body is extruded posteriorly to wedge behind the posterior facet of the subtalar joint. Interestingly, I have observed several cases in which the primary fracture line was well posterior to the normal anatomic depression on the dorsum of the talar neck, where the lip of the tibia usually impinges (Fig. 21-11). This finding suggests that the mechanism may be more of a shearing action than a direct mechanical wedge phenomenon and also may explain the variable occurrence of avascular necrosis. The nutrient foramina are located clearly within this depression on the talar neck. The sparing of this third arterial branch may account for the survival of many talar bodies after supposedly unequivocal avascular incidents.

This fracture is best treated with prompt closed reduction to reduce the morbidity associated with prolonged dislocation of any articulation. The patient is positioned with the knee bent 90 degrees. The surgeon's thumbs are placed on either side of the Achilles tendon to feel the talar body in the posterior triangle. With forced plantar flexion the surgeon pushes the talar body into its anatomic cavity. This maneuver becomes increasingly

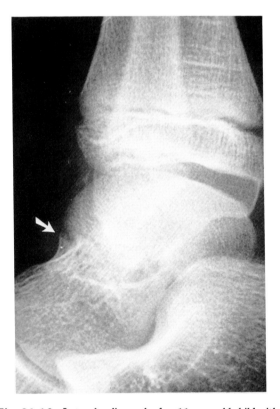

**Fig. 21-10.** Lateral radiograph of an 11-year-old child with a non-displaced Hawkins I fracture of the talar neck (arrow). This was sustained in an auto accident. The child also suffered an ipsilateral femur fracture.

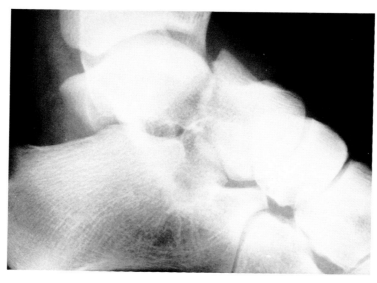

**Fig. 21-11.** Lateral radiograph of a 19-year-old man who fell off a ladder for a distance of about 10 feet. Note the dislocation of the subtalar joint. Also note that the location of the fracture line is well posterior to the depression on the talar neck where the nutrient vessels course into the neck.

more difficult as time passes because of the massive swelling that ensues. After the talar body has been relocated, postreduction radiographs are obtained. If the reduction is acceptable, the same principles used for treatment of a Hawkins type I fracture are followed. If closed reduction is unsuccessful, the patient should be taken to the operating room for another attempt and possible open reduction. If the closed reduction is still unacceptable, open reduction is indicated (Fig. 21-12).

Open reduction is accomplished through a medial incision between the anterior and posterior tibial tendons (Fig. 21-12). Extensive soft tissue stripping is avoided, especially in the area of the deltoid ligament and the tarsal sinus. Although the primary blood supply of the deltoid ligament is still intact, up to a 50 percent chance of avascular necrosis has been reported in the adult patient.

### Hawkins Type III and IV Fractures

The Hawkins type III fracture occurs when the talar body is dislocated from both the subtalar joint and the ankle joint. This fracture is virtually impossible to reduce in a closed manner. The patient should undergo prompt surgical reduction in order to reduce the vascular compromise that results from twisting of the talar body on its major vascular pedicles. The talar body almost always twists 90 degrees. If the posterior tibial or peroneal branches are intact, there is likely to be vascular compromise due to this rotation. An anteromedial approach allows reduction of the talar body into its proper location in the ankle mortise. Once reduction of the dislocations is accomplished, the fracture is reduced just as in the displaced type I injury. The incidence of avascular necrosis in this fracture can be as high as 100 percent owing to the disruption of both the major arterial supplies. However, it has been my experience that not all type III fractures result in avascular necrosis, which is consistent with other published reports.[14,17]

Type IV fractures are defined as talar neck fractures with dislocation of the subtalar, ankle, and talonavicular joints. This is very rare and, again, is usually treated with open reduction and internal fixation. AVN is seemingly imminent, but its occurrence is, surprisingly, not absolutely certain (Fig. 21-13).

## Fractures of the Body of the Talus

Fractures of the body of the talus result from violent trauma and may involve associated injuries. These injuries should be treated as any adult intra-articular injury. Open reduction is almost always indicated in the acute and immediate setting. Precautions to avoid avascular necrosis should be observed, but one must be persistent in establishing articular congruity except in the very

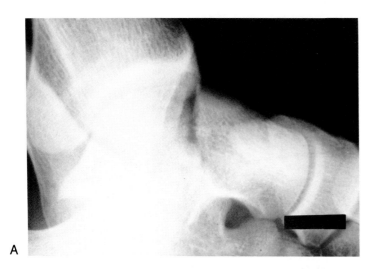

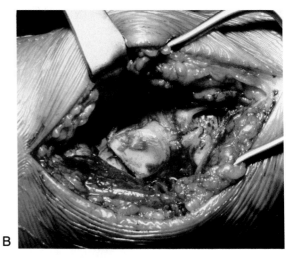

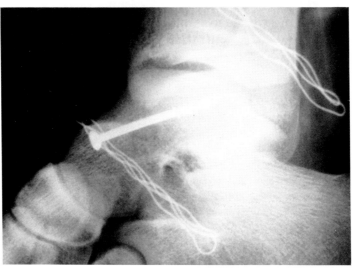

**Fig. 21-12.** **(A)** Closed reduction of the fracture of the patient in Fig. 21-11. There is still significant step-off of the main fragments, necessitating open reduction. **(B)** Intraoperative view of the fracture line from the medial approach. This is a left talus and the toes are to the right of the photograph. Note the posterior location of the fracture. **(C)** Intraoperative radiograph demonstrating anatomic reduction of the fracture.

young child. A medial or lateral malleolar-osteotomy may be indicated in order to facilitate exposure of the highly comminuted fractures (Fig. 21-14).

## Fractures of the Talar Dome

Fractures of the talar dome are encountered infrequently in the pediatric age group. Their incidence is probably much less than in the adult population, but the reasons for this remain speculative. Presumably many of the twisting type injuries to the ankle do not result in a cartilaginous defect because of the resilience of the cartilage, which is able to absorb both compressive and shearing forces. Many of the injuries are silent and do not manifest with symptoms until the patient is no longer classified as a child.

A frequent situation is represented by the adolescent patient who presents with symptoms within a year of

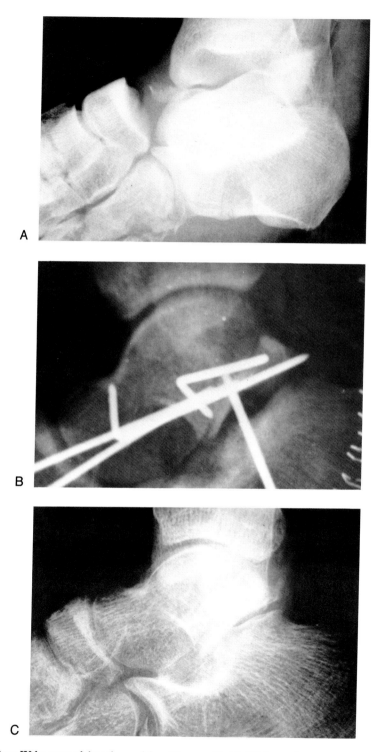

**Fig. 21-13.** (A) Type IV fracture of the talar neck in a 13-year-old girl. (B) Immediate postoperative radiograph. The talonavicular joint and the subtalar joint were stabilized with Steinmann pins. (C) Lateral radiograph showing normal bone density 18 months after the reduction. It is surprising that avascular necrosis did not develop in this patient.

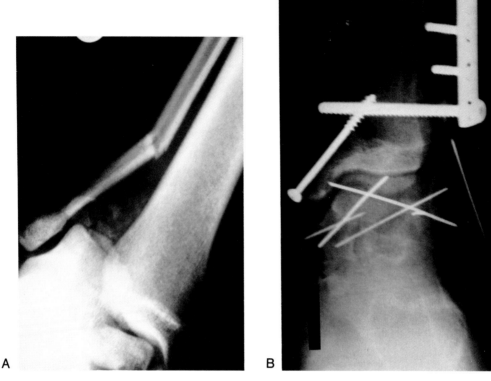

A                                    B

**Fig. 21-14. (A)** Immediate postinjury film of a 13-year-old boy who fell 30 feet. Note the comminution of the talar body and dislocation of the talus out of the mortise. **(B)** Postoperative radiograph showing adequate reduction using multiple Kirschner wires. Exposure was facilitated through a medial malleolar osteotomy.

sustaining a seemingly minor ankle injury. The symptoms may include pain, swelling, effusion, and instability. In some instances no specific, memorable history of trauma can be elicited even with vigorous verbal probing. One should be suspicious of a talar dome lesion when there are chronic symptoms not responsive to the usual measures of conservative care. Initial radiographic evaluation may not reveal the pathology, but follow-up radiographs may show the lesion. Although the entity of osteochondritis dissecans may actually be an entirely different entity from an osteochondral fracture, the defects in the talar dome will be treated as if they represented the same pathologic process.

There are few studies to document the efficacy of treatment of the talar dome fracture in the pediatric age group. Berndt and Harty[18] reported poor results in 73 percent of pediatric patients who were initially treated nonoperatively. Even though pediatric injuries have been presumed to have better cartilage healing potential, complete healing is probably unlikely even with prolonged immobilization. One of the problems of assessing results of treatment is the uncertain age of the injury. If the injury is treated acutely, results with conservative treatment may actually improve. Nevertheless the trend is toward more aggressive surgical treatment earlier in the course of the injury.[19]

A stage I fracture of the talar dome is defined as a small area of subchondral bone compression. A stage II lesion involves a partially detached osteochondral fragment, and a stage III injury consists of a complete detachment of an osteochondral fragment that remains within its crater. A stage IV lesion is differentiated from a stage III injury by the fact that the detached fragment is displaced or inverted in its crater.

## Stage I and II Lesions

Stage I talar dome lesions may be difficult to diagnose on the basis of acute radiographic findings. In fact, the subchondral compression may not be radiographically visible but may be demonstrable by direct arthroscopic or open surgical inspection or advanced imaging techniques such as MRI or computed tomography (CT). These procedures or tests may reveal the diagnosis when previous methods have failed. However, I feel that delay in diagnosis of type I lesions has little impact on long-term prognosis or, for that matter, on healing potential. Therefore I believe that these expensive imaging techniques and invasive procedures should be performed sparingly in the acute setting in order to confirm the diagnosis of a type I lesion. One may counter this idea with the argument that the subchondral depression may progress to a more advanced lesion with repetitive trauma. However, the yield of positive results with these modalities is probably too low to justify their use as routine diagnostic tests.

Acute stage I and II injuries should probably be treated with a non-weight-bearing cast for 6 to 8 weeks. Radiographic evidence of healing may not be present for months afterward, but careful monitoring of symptoms may dictate significantly shorter periods of immobilization. If symptoms dissipate, further casting is probably unnecessary. Long-term prognosis with regard to future arthrosis is unlikely to be affected even if the radiographs do not demonstrate healing.

Failure of conservative treatment is unlikely, but when symptoms warrant, the injury should be addressed as a type III or IV lesion, which requires surgical intervention. In the stage I fracture there may not be a specific fragment to excise, but there is usually a nonadherent piece of cartilage overlying the subchondral bony defect. The cartilage piece should be removed, the depressed subchondral bone should be excavated, and the underlying cancellous bone should be drilled to bleeding bone.

## Stage III and IV Lesions

A stage III lesion of the talar dome is unlikely to heal even in the acute phase of injury. However, a trial of conservative therapy to give the patient the benefit of the doubt may be indicated. If a period of casting fails to achieve healing or abate symptoms, surgical treatment is indicated.

If the diagnosis is made well after the acute traumatic episode, casting is unlikely to result in healing of the fracture fragment. If the child is symptomatic, surgical treatment is indicated. The surgical approach and technique are identical regardless of time between onset of injury and definitive treatment. The fragment is excised and the bed drilled through an anterolateral arthrotomy for the lateral lesions. In the medial lesions the surgeon must be prepared to perform a medial malleolar osteotomy because the fracture is more likely to be located in the central or posterior aspect of the talar dome, which precludes an anteromedial approach. Tomography or CT scans are indicated to map the exact location of the lesion. I also obtain a forced plantar flexion lateral radiograph to see if the fracture can be projected anterior to the medial malleolus. If it can, a malleolar osteotomy is not necessary. If the physis is still open, the osteotomy should be placed slightly lower to avoid injury to the physis. Fixation should be by smooth Kirschner wires placed across the physis. Screws or other fixation methods are acceptable in adolescent patient with mature growth plates.

Arthroscopic surgical intervention is also an alternative to open surgical treatment. Lateral lesions are approached arthroscopically without much difficulty. Usually the fragment can be drilled with a Kirschner wire

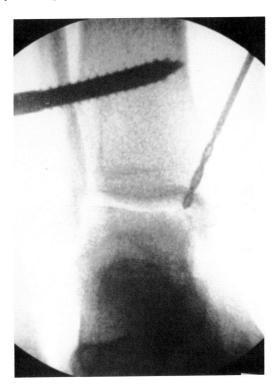

**Fig. 21-15.** Intraoperative fluoroscopic image of the drill directed through the medial malleolus directly at the medial talar dome lesion. In the case of open epiphyses, the drill can be placed below the growth plate.

with arthroscopic visualization. However, medial lesions are often more posterior, and application of instrumentation to the bed of the fragment is difficult. Even with the gouging techniques of Lundeen,[20] I still find it difficult to adequately drill the bed to good vascular bone. Therefore I prefer to drill directly through the medial malleolus, and aiming at the medial corner of the talus. The contact of the drill can be controlled by manipulating the position of the ankle in the mortise with dorsiflexion or plantar flexion. The arthroscope is used to visualize the dome and direct the position of the lesion to the drill or Kirschner wire point (Fig. 21-15).

Stage IV lesions have an extremely poor chance of healing, and one should proceed directly to surgery if the patient is symptomatic. The same principles and techniques apply as for stage III lesions.

### Internal Fixation of Fragments

In some cases of stage II, III, or IV lesions with large fracture fragments, internal fixation of the loose fragment may restore anatomic contour to the dome of the talus and lessen the chance of post-traumatic arthritis. The loose fracture fragment should be freed from any fibrous tissue by curettage. Fixation can be accomplished with Kirschner wires, screws, or even fibrin glue. The disadvantage of Kirschner wire fixation is that range of motion is impossible if the wire protrudes above the level of the cartilaginous surface. In addition, there is no appreciable compression across the fracture site. Screw fixation is ideal in the pediatric population because there is usually a thick layer of articular cartilage so that the screw head can be countersunk below the level of the articular surface (Fig. 21-16). Although I have had limited experience with fibrin glue, it is ideally suited for use with the small fragment or when a deep cavity remains after curettage of all necrotic bone. In these latter instances, it is preferable to fill up the cavity with autogenous cancellous bone and hold the graft in place with the glue. The usual and expectant fibrocartilage cap can then cover the graft and fill up the small cavity. In anticipation of this technique the patient should donate autogenous blood in advance for use in preparation of the fibrin mixture.

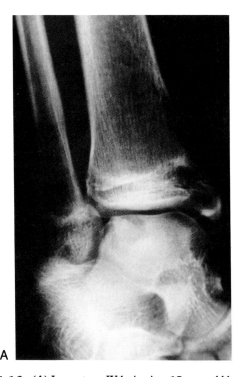
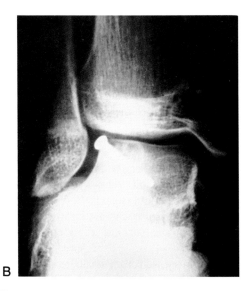

A          B

**Fig. 21-16. (A)** Large type IV lesion in a 15-year-old boy. The osteochondral fragment is detached but still located within its crater. **(B)** Postoperative radiograph showing replacement of the large fragment with a 2.7-mm cortical screw. The fracture was completely healed in 6 weeks.

# FRACTURES OF THE CALCANEUS

Calcaneal fractures in pediatric patients are uncommon. Matteri and Frymoyer[21] reported a 6 percent incidence of calcaneal fractures in children. However, they contend that the fracture is probably under-reported because the injury is often overlooked on initial radiographic evaluation. Joint involvement in childhood injuries is usually very subtle. Minor involvement of the posterior subtalar joint is usually identified by bursting of the lateral wall of the calcaneus, producing a longitudinal sliver of bone; this is seen only on the calcaneal axial view. This finding is supported by Wiley and Profitt.[22]

Extra-articular fractures may be more common than intra-articular fractures in children. Schmidt and Weiner[23] found a 63 percent incidence of extra-articular fractures in this age group. However in a study of 32 children with 34 calcaneal fractures, 28 had involvement of the posterior subtalar joint.[22] Some of these injuries produced only minor disturbances of subtalar joint congruity. Further analysis of these studies suggests that the discrepancy is probably more related to age than to anything else. Younger patients are less likely to have subtalar involvement than older children and adolescents, which corresponds to a gradual increase in the density of the bone and a decrease in its resilience with age. Regardless of the anatomic involvement, fractures in the pediatric age group are less severe than the adult counterparts because of the resilience of cartilage and bone, which tend to absorb impact from vertical compression loads.

Associated fractures of the extremities are more common in children than in adults, but axial skeleton injuries are only half as common. Extra-articular fractures can almost always be treated conservatively, as in the adult population. Significant displacement is uncommon, owing to the resilience of the bone and the periosteum. Fracture patterns that are only seldom seen in the pediatric age group include the pediatric counterpart of Rowe type II fractures involving the calcaneal apophysis.

In children with intra-articular fractures, the treatment of choice is conservative, particularly in the under 10 age group. Satisfactory results are related to the growth potential and remodeling of the osteocartilaginous bone in young children. Treatment usually is by a short leg cast for 3 to 4 weeks or until bony union occurs. Long-term follow-up studies are scarce, but most reports rate functional results as excellent even when there is intra-articular involvement. This observation is primarily due to the potential for remodeling in children and the fact that articular involvement is usually much less than in adults.

Adolescents with intra-articular calcaneal fractures should be treated as adults. At this age the injury produces pathology that can lead to significant morbidity, including articular incongruity and widening of the heel. In adolescents, unlike younger children, significant remodeling of the incongruity cannot be expected. Adolescents will likely have higher activity demands and a longer life span than most adult patients. Although I would treat many adult calcaneal fractures with open reduction and internal fixation, treatment should be decided upon by individual surgeons on the basis of their training, experience, and ability to treat these injuries.[24]

It does seem prudent to attempt anatomic reduction in those patients with significant articular displacement and widening of the heel. In fact, it is my feeling that adolescent patients with displaced fractures deserve open reduction even in those cases that might be treated by closed reduction if that patient were an adult. Closed reduction is difficult and seldom effective in restoration of proper calcaneal width and height. It may be sufficient in a few selected cases, but one should be prepared to open the fracture if the preoperative goals of treatment are not realized.

Open reduction is best accomplished through the extended lateral approach. Medial exposure can also be used when the medial sustentacular fragment is comminuted or cannot be repositioned from the lateral side. An L-shaped incision is made inferior to the peroneal tendons, and a single layer flap is elevated directly to the lateral aspect of the calcaneus. The peroneal tendons are elevated in the same flap and are never exposed from their sheath. The lateral wall is disimpacted, and the lateral aspect of the posterior facet is elevated and then fixed to the medial portion of the posterior facet, which is located on the medial fragment. Fixation is accomplished with small cannulated screws, conventional screws, or Kirschner wires (Fig. 21-17). The tuber or body portion is then reduced to the combined sustentacular and posterior facet fragments by manipulating the former fragment downward. This is best accomplished by insertion of a Shantz screw into the posterolateral aspect of the body fragment. Once the proper relationships are restored, temporary fixation is introduced. Large-caliber Kirschner wires are driven from the calcaneus into the talus to maintain anatomic positions. It is here that me-

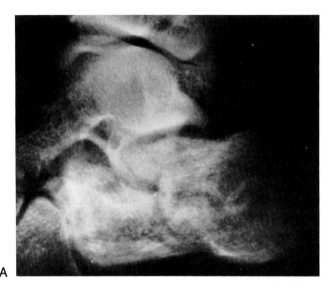

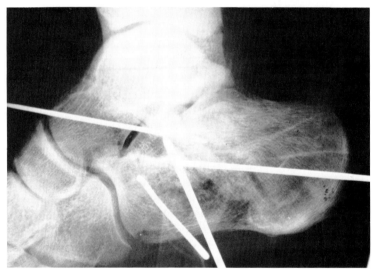

**Fig. 21-17.** **(A)** Preoperative lateral film of a 14-year-old boy who sustained a calcaneal fracture. Note the marked reduction in calcaneal height and the loss of Bohler's angle. **(B)** Postoperative radiograph showing restoration of Bohler's angle and anatomic reduction of the posterior facet. This was done through the extended lateral approach. Bone graft was not required. Additional fixation was not used, as the reduction was stable.

dial exposure may be necessary to disimpact the medial fragment.

If there is a calcaneocuboid joint component, it should be addressed next. Interfragmentary screw fixation is used after reduction of the joint under direct vision. The major fragments are then permanently fixed after intraoperative radiographs are checked. Several options are available — I favor the use of large, multiple-limbed H plates placed on the lateral aspect of the calcaneus. Other options include other types of plates and Kirschner wires. Bone graft is seldom necessary in this age group because of the excellent osteogenic potential of adolescent bone. If rigid fixation is attained, early range-of-motion exercises can be initiated; if this is not possible, the foot is immobilized in a short leg cast. In either case the patient is kept off weight-bearing for 6 weeks.

Weight-bearing in a cast is then allowed and continued for 2 to 4 additional weeks.

Long-term follow-up is important in assessing the results of treatment. Unfortunately, reports of the results of conservative treatment modalities are sparse and there is even less information on the results of operative reduction of calcaneal fractures in the pediatric age group.[25,26]

# REFERENCES

1. Blais MM, Green WT, Anderson M: Lengths of the growing foot. J Bone Joint Surg [Am] 38:998, 1956
2. DeValentine SJ: Foot and ankle fractures in children. p 485. In Scurran BL (ed): Foot and Ankle Trauma. Churchill Livingstone, New York, 1989
3. Wiley JJ: Tarso-metatarsal joint injuries in children. J Pediatr Orthop 1:255, 1981
4. Bonnel F, Barthelemy M: Traumatismes de l'articulation de Lisfranc; entorses graves, luxations, fractures. 3:573, J Chir (Paris) 1976
5. Collet HS, Hood TK, Andrews RE: Tarsometatarsal fracture dislocations. Surg Gynecol Obstet 106:623, 1958
6. Rainaut JJ, Cedard C, D'Hour JP: Les luxations tarsométatarsiennes. Rev Chir Orthop 62:685, 1976
7. Wiley JJ: The mechanism of tarso-metatarsal joint injuries. J Bone Joint Surg [Br] 53:474, 1971
8. Easton ER: Two rare dislocations of the metatarsals at Lis-Franc's joint. J Bone Joint Surg [Am] 20:1053, 1938
9. Schuberth JM: Principles of fracture management in children. Clin Podiatr Med Surg 4:267, 1987
10. Arntz CT, Veith RG, Hansen ST: Fractures and fracture-dislocations of the tarsometatarsal joint. J Bone Joint Surg [Am] 70:173, 1988
11. Stevens NA: Fracture dislocations of the talus in childhood: a report of two cases. Br J Surg 43:600, 1956
12. Spak I: Fractures of the talus in children. Acta Chir Scand 107:533, 1954
13. Kenwright J, Taylor RG: Major injuries of the talus. J Bone Joint Surg [Br] 52:36, 1970
14. Canale ST, Kelly FB: Fractures of the neck of the talus. J Bone Joint Surg [Am] 60:143, 1978
15. Letts RM, Gibeault D: Fractures of the neck of the talus in children. Foot Ankle 1:74, 1980
16. Hawkins LG: Fractures of the neck of the talus. J Bone Joint Surg [Am] 52:991, 1970
17. Peterson L, Romanus B, Oahlberg E: Fracture of the neck of the talus. Acta Orthop Scand 48:696, 1977
18. Berndt A, Harty M: Transchondral fractures (osteochondritis dissecans) of the talus. J Bone Joint Surg [Am] 41:988, 1959
19. Flick AB, Gould N: Osteochondritis dissecans of the talus (transchondral fractures of the talus): review of the literature and new surgical approach for medial dome lesions. Foot Ankle 5:165, 1985
20. Lundeen RO: Medial impingement lesions of the tibial plafond. J Foot Surg 26:37, 1987
21. Matteri RE, Frymoyer JW: Fracture of the calcaneus in young children. Report of three cases. J Bone Joint Surg [Am] 55:1091, 1973
22. Wiley JJ, Profitt A: Fractures of the os calcis in children. Clin Orthop 171:150, 1982
23. Schmidt TL, Weiner DS: Calcaneal fractures in children. An evaluation of the nature of the injury in 56 children. Clin Orthop 171:150, 1982
24. Schuberth JM, Karlin JM, Daly N: Calcaneal fractures. p 456. In Scurran BL (ed): Foot and Ankle Trauma. Churchill Livingstone, New York, 1989
25. Drvaric DM, Schmitt EW: Irreducible fracture of the calcaneus in a child. Case report. J Pediatr Orthop 2:154, 1988
26. Marti R: Fractures of the calcaneus. p 381. In Weber BG, Brunner C, Freuler F (eds): Treatment of Fractures in Children and Adolescents. Springer-Verlag, New York, 1980

# 22
# Ankle Injuries

*JOHN M. SCHUBERTH*
*STEVEN J. DeVALENTINE*

Ankle injuries in children are unique, challenging, and relatively common. Although pediatric ankle fractures account for only about 4 to 5 percent of all types of pediatric fractures and about the same percentage of all ankle fractures (adults and children), they represent about 25 percent of all physeal fractures[1-3] (see Ch. 20). The ankle is the second most common site of physeal fracture in children, only the distal radius being more frequently injured.[4,5] In addition, the ankle is by far the most common site of physeal fracture in the lower extremity.[2,5] When the hip joint is excluded, physeal fractures of the ankle have been reported to account for 70 to 90 percent of all lower extremity physeal injuries.[6-8]

The management of physeal fractures of the ankle is complicated by a significant potential for growth disturbance with some types of fractures and by the fact that two bones and thus two physes (tibia and fibula) are often involved. Intra-articular fractures add still another dimension to these injuries. Optimal treatment requires a thorough understanding of the evolution and physiology of these injuries and a classification system that is practical in terms of both treatment and prognostic value.

Unfortunately, in spite of the relatively high frequency of physeal ankle fractures, the English language literature on this subject has been relatively sparse until recent years, with much more attention being devoted to other anatomic areas. Terminology among different authors is often varied and confusing, and attempts to describe and categorize physeal ankle fractures in terms of the anatomic classification systems of Aitken or Salter and Harris alone have often been frustrating and somewhat inadequate. Different fracture patterns often occur in the tibia and fibula simultaneously and in varying combinations, and some fracture patterns (juvenile Til-

laux and triplane fractures) cannot be adequately described by the Salter-Harris anatomic classification system alone. This has led to the development of several mechanism-based classifications.

Ashhurst and Bromer in 1922 were the first authors to present a widely accepted mechanism-based classification for adult ankle fractures.[9] Much of their work was based on earlier anatomic studies by Dupuytren and others. They describe four basic mechanisms of injury: adduction, abduction, external rotation, and axial compression. External rotation was noted to be the most common mechanism of ankle fracture in adults. Ashhurst and Bromer's classic and relatively simple mechanistic classification system became the standard for description of ankle fractures in the English language literature and is still widely used by many surgeons. Bishop, who in 1932 reviewed physeal fractures in 32 children between 9 and 14 years of age according to Ashhurst's and Bromer's classification system,[10] found adduction (inversion) injuries to be most common (53 percent of his series).

Carothers and Crenshaw in 1955 reported 54 cases, seen over a period of 30 years, of physeal fractures of the ankle in children which they classified by the mechanism of injury.[2] They modified the Ashhurst-Bromer[9] and Bishop[10] mechanistic classifications to include adduction, abduction, plantar flexion, external rotation, and axial compression mechanisms. They found abduction and adduction injuries to be most common and noted, as have most subsequent authors, a higher incidence of growth disturbance following adduction injuries (Salter-Harris III and IV fractures of the tibia). Carothers and Crenshaw expressed the view that the medial talar dome exerts a compressive force against the medial tibial plafond as the

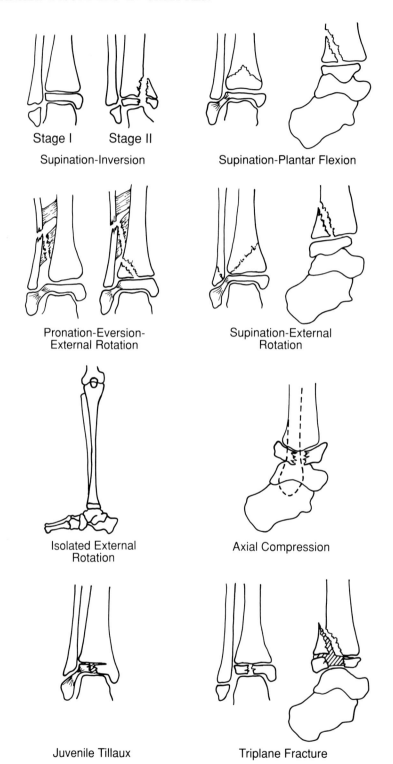

**Fig. 22-1.** Modified Dias-Tachdjian classification system for pediatric ankle fractures.

foot is forced into inversion and that this compression injury of the physis, together with vertical separation of the physis, is responsible for a higher incidence of growth disturbance in adduction injuries. They recommended accurate reduction (open if necessary) of adduction tibial fractures.[2,11] Although most authors during that period believed acceptance of minimal displacement of the distal tibial physis (especially anterio-posterior displacement) to be preferable to repeated forcible manipulation or open reduction, a gradual trend toward open anatomic reduction of adduction fractures (Salter-Harris III and IV tibia) has developed. Carothers and Crenshaw also believed that abduction and external rotation injuries are not as likely to cause distal tibial physeal compressive injuries because lateral movement of the fibula allows lateral displacement of the distal tibial epiphysis in most cases so that the physis is not impacted by the trailing edge of the distal tibial metaphysis.

In 1950 Lauge-Hansen proposed a mechanism-based classification system derived from experimental reproduction of fractures in cadaver limbs, which is now widely accepted as the standard in describing adult ankle fractures.[12] Danis[13] 1949 and Weber[14] in 1966 proposed similar dynamic, mechanism based classification systems for adult ankle fractures, which are widely used in Europe. Although physeal fractures of the ankle can probably be adequately managed in most cases without the use of a Lauge-Hansen type mechanistic classification, a thorough understanding of the mechanism of injury not only aids in elucidating the most effective technique of closed reduction, but also provides a useful framework for a more physiologic approach to discussion and treatment of these injuries.

Gerner-Smidt in 1963 and Dias and Tachdjian in 1978 separately described classification systems for pediatric ankle fractures based on the Lauge-Hansen system.[15,16] The Gerner-Smidt classification, which is the only classification system that has been derived from experimental reproduction of pediatric ankle fractures, includes five major types of injury as follows: supination-adduction, supination-inversion, supination-eversion, pronation-abduction, and pronation-eversion. Many of the major types of mechanisms are divided into subtypes. Although the Gerner-Smidt classification system is often widely referred to in the European literature and has some advantages, we find it too complex to be clinically useful on a widespread basis.

Dias and Tachdjian based their classification system on

Table 22-1. **Comparison of Classifications**

| Dias-Tachdjian | Gerner-Smidt, Karrholm | Ashhurst |
|---|---|---|
| Supination-external rotation (SER) | Supination-eversion | External rotation |
| Pronation-eversion-external rotation (PEER) | Pronation-abduction Pronation-eversion | Abduction |
| Supination-plantar flexion (SPF) | (? Supination-inversion, stage III) | |
| Supination-inversion (SI) | Supination-adduction Supination-inversion | Adduction |
| Axial compression | | Axial compression |
| Juvenile Tillaux | Supination-eversion, stage 1A | External rotation |
| Triplane | Supination-eversion, stage IV | — |
| Others | | |

the Salter-Harris as well as the Lauge-Hansen system. Although this complicates their classification system somewhat, it has the distinct advantage of allowing easy incorporation of prognostic data that have been reported in terms of the various Salter-Harris types. In addition, the Lauge-Hansen and Salter-Harris systems are very familiar to most English-speaking foot surgeons, allowing a more unified approach to the management of adult and pediatric ankle fractures. A modified Dias-Tachdjian classification system will therefore be used for the purpose of this discussion (Fig. 22-1). Gross has provided a useful comparison of the Gerner-Smidt, Dias-Tachdjian, and Ashhurst-Bromer classification systems for those who are interested in a more lengthy discussion of this subject[17] (Table 22-1).

## CLASSIFICATION OF PEDIATRIC ANKLE FRACTURES

The Dias-Tachdjian classification system for physeal ankle fractures, based on the Lauge-Hansen and the Salter-Harris systems, comprises six mechanistic classification types, which were derived from a retrospective review of 71 case studies and not from experimental reproduction of fractures, as was the case with the Lauge-Hansen and Gerner-Smidt systems. Of the 71 cases, 58 (82 percent) were identified as belonging to one of four fracture patterns: supination-inversion, supination – plantar flexion, pronation-eversion-external rotation, or supination-external rotation. Of the remaining 13 cases, 3 other (4 percent) were classified as juvenile Tillaux fractures and 6 (9 percent) were classified as triplane fractures. Thus, 95 percent of 71 physeal fractures could be classified in one of these six categories (supination-inversion, supination–plantar flexion, pronation-eversion-external rotation, supination-external rotation, juvenile Tillaux, and triplane).

As in the Lauge-Hansen system, each fracture type is described by two or three terms, of which the first describes the position of the foot at the time of injury and the second and third refer to the direction in which the talus is driven by the injuring force. Thus, in a supination-external rotation injury, the foot remains supinated at the time of injury while being forcibly externally rotated. Since the foot is usually fixed to the supporting surface, this movement is equivalent to internal rotation of the leg (Fig. 22-2). Individual stages of injury within each mechanism type are defined in terms of the Salter-Harris system. Thus, a stage I supination-inversion fracture is characterized by both a Salter-Harris I or II fracture of the fibula and a Salter-Harris III or IV fracture of the distal medial tibia. Dias and Tachdjian were unable to classify either the juvenile Tillaux or triplane fracture patterns using a Lauge-Hansen or Salter-Harris type of classification system alone. Although it is generally

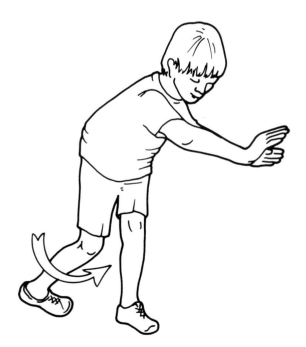

**Fig. 22-2.** Artist's rendering of a supination-external rotation type of injury mechanism.

agreed that these two transitional fractures result from an external rotation type of injury, they are usually classified separately from supination-external rotation or pronation-eversion-external rotation, owing to their rather specific and unusual characteristic fracture patterns.

In a later article Dias also included axial compression as a mechanism of injury.[18] The pure axial compression mechanism results in a Salter-Harris type V physeal injury of the distal tibial physis and would be expected to carry a very poor prognosis. This is a very rare injury, and no cases were reported by Dias. Of the 54 physeal fractures reviewed by Carothers and Crenshaw, only 2 (4 percent) were axial compression injuries.[2] One of these resulted from a motor vehicle accident and the other from a fall from a tree, and both occurred during early adolescence. One patient was lost to follow-up and the other had developed no deformity at age 16. Radiographic changes may be absent or difficult to detect at the time of injury, and the diagnosis may not be made until premature closure of the growth plate occurs.

Another rarely reported injury, the isolated rotational fracture of the distal tibial physis, was originally described in 1968 by Lovell[19] and was included by Dias in his stage I supination-external rotation fracture. However, this fracture appears to be the result of a primarily external rotational force (whether supination-external rotation or pronation-external rotation is undetermined) and will be categorized separately, as will the juvenile Tillaux and triplane fractures.

## Supination-Inversion Injuries

A supination-inversion injury occurs when an inversion force is applied while the foot is fixed in the supinated position. This is the same injury that results in ankle sprain, lateral collateral ligament rupture, or supination-adduction (inversion) ankle fracture in an adult. Supination-external rotation is known to be the most common mechanism of injury in adult ankle fractures, of which it accounts for about 60 percent,[20] and is also probably the most common mechanism of injury in pediatric ankle fractures (if juvenile Tillaux and triplane fractures are included in this category), with supination-inversion being very nearly as frequent. Dias found 39 percent of his 71 juvenile ankle fractures were of the supination-inversion type, making it the most common in his study.[16] Karrholm et al.[21] and Gerner-Smidt[15] found that supination-inversion fractures constituted about 35 to 37 percent of their series, which makes these injuries only slightly less common than supination–external rotation injuries (40 percent in Karrholm et al.'s series). Additional confusion exists because some authors have included juvenile Tillaux and triplane fractures within their supination–external rotation category. Most authors do agree that supination-inversion injuries are most commonly seen at slightly younger ages than supination–external rotation injuries.

Dias[18] divided supination-inversion injuries into two stages. Stage I is characterized by a lateral "pull-off" injury of the fibula and stage II by a "push-off" type injury of the medial malleolus. As in the Lauge-Hansen system, stage I is presumed to precede stage II, and the stage I injury can be inferred by the radiographic presence of stage II.

### Stage I Supination-Inversion Fractures

Stage I of the supination-inversion injury usually consists of a Salter-Harris I, II, or III fracture of the distal fibular physis (Fig. 22-3). The corresponding injury in an adult would be either a lateral rupture of a collateral ankle ligament or a distal fibular pull-off fracture. Although a lateral ligament tear may occur in a child, a physeal injury is much more likely, particularly in a younger child, whereas ligament injuries become more common as the child approaches skeletal maturity.

Of 103 patients with supination-inversion injuries identified by Karrholm et al., 69 (67 percent) had

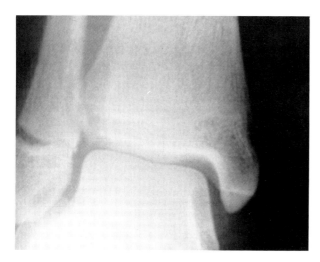

**Fig. 22-3.** Supination-inversion stage I ankle fracture. Note lateral separation of distal fibular physis. Physeal disruption may occur without displacement.

stage I injuries, of whom 44 (63 percent) had Salter-Harris I fractures, 15 (22 percent) Salter-Harris II fractures, and 10 (15 percent) Salter-Harris III fractures of the distal fibula.[21] Salter-Harris type I separation of the distal fibular physis is usually characterized by slight displacement (often not more than 3 to 5 mm) or by slight widening of the lateral portion of the physis. One should be aware that these injuries can occur without displacement and can be misdiagnosed as ankle sprains.[21,22] The only sign of injury may be localized tenderness and swelling about the physis with or without slight separation or notching of the physis on radiographs. In pediatric supination-inversion injuries, unlike adult ankle sprains, minimal or no tenderness is present directly over the lateral ankle ligaments. A younger child presenting with a history of supination-inversion injury and these physical findings should be treated with immobilization even if no displacement is observed on radiography. Repeat radiographs 3 weeks postinjury may show periosteal callus about the peripheral portion of the lateral physis, confirming a prior injury. The metaphyseal or epiphyseal fragment of a Salter-Harris II or III fracture of the distal fibula often consists of only a small sliver of bone; it may be medial or lateral. Occasionally, larger metaphyseal fragments may be seen with Salter-Harris II lesions.

Most stage I supination-inversion injuries do not require reduction, and growth disturbance is extremely unusual.[15,21,23] In fact, Karrholm et al. noted growth stimulation after Salter-Harris I distal fibular fractures on stereophotogrammetric analysis and believed that follow-up of these fractures was unnecessary.[24] If significant displacement is present, closed reduction can be performed by gentle eversion of the foot, with counterpressure against the fibula. Open reduction is virtually never necessary with distal fibular physeal fractures. Even in stage II injuries that require open reduction for tibial fractures, reduction of the fibular physeal component normally occurs as a by-product of reduction of the tibial fragment. Stage I lesions are usually treated with a short leg walking cast for 3 to 4 weeks.

### Stage II Supination-Inversion Fractures

As in the supination-adduction injury in the adult, a continuation of the inversion force results in a Salter-Harris III or IV push-off type of fracture of the medial tibial malleolus (Fig. 22-4A). Dias[18] stated that a Salter-Harris I or II distal tibial fracture with medial displacement may "rarely" occur with a supination-inversion injury, and

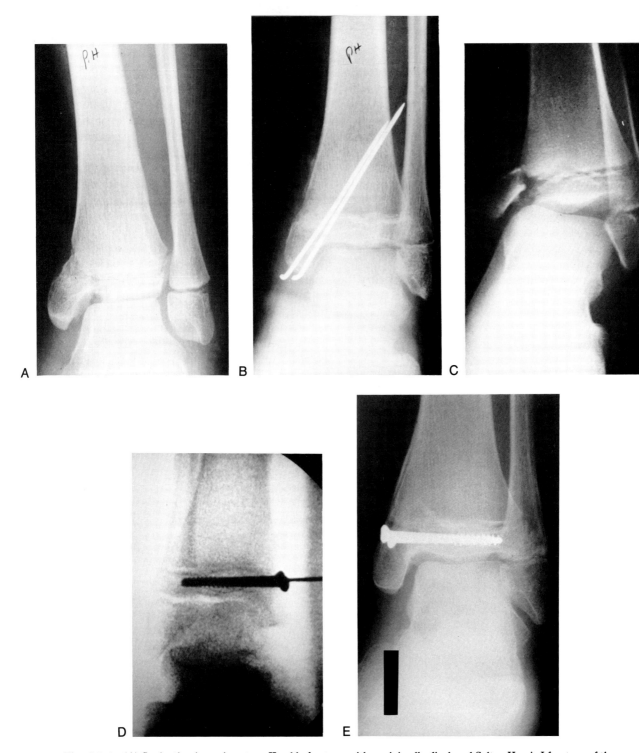

**Fig. 22-4.** (A) Supination-inversion stage II ankle fracture with a minimally displaced Salter-Harris I fracture of the distal fibular physis and a minimally displaced Salter-Harris IV fracture of the distal medial tibia. (B) Open reduction and internal fixation of the fracture in Fig. A. (C) Displaced supination-inversion stage II fracture. This fracture essentially always requires open reduction and internal fixation owing to its inherent instability and high risk of long-term complication without anatomic reduction. (D) Intraoperative image of open reduction and internal fixation of a Salter-Harris III fracture using a cannulated screw. The guide pin is introduced under fluoroscopic control, and the appropriate instrumentation is inserted over the pin. (E) Postoperative radiograph of fracture in Fig. D.

MacNealy et al. found only a single Salter-Harris type II tibial fracture (0.5 percent) resulting from adduction (inversion) injury among 194 distal tibial physeal fractures that they reviewed.[25] The average age at the time of injury for Salter-Harris III and IV tibial injuries has varied in different studies. Kling et al. found the average age for type III injuries to be 8 to 10 years, whereas type IV injuries were more frequently seen in children 10 to 13 years of age.[26] Other investigators have found the average age of patients with these injuries to be similar to or slightly older than in Kling's study.[5,22,25,27] Karrholm et al. found 34 (27 percent) of 128 physeal fractures to be supination-inversion stage II injuries,[21] of which 27 (79 percent) were classified as Salter-Harris type III and 7 (21 percent) as Salter-Harris type IV fractures.

While stage I fibular injury is fairly benign, stage II Salter-Harris type III or IV tibial injury can have serious consequences. Most authors have reported the highest incidence of growth disturbance with Salter-Harris type III and especially with Salter-Harris type IV fractures of the distal medial tibial epiphysis.[2,11,21,22,26-28] The medial malleolar fragment in type IV fractures tends to migrate proximally, resulting in vertical displacement of the physis, which seems to be more likely to cause growth disturbance. Loss of joint congruity is also a concern with type III and IV fractures. Both type III and IV fractures are difficult if not impossible to stabilize by closed reduction. Kling et al. reviewed 65 distal tibial physeal fractures (most of which were type III and IV) of which approximately half were treated by closed reduction and the other half by open reduction.[26] None of those fractures that were treated closed were found to be anatomic on follow-up review of postoperative radiographs. The authors found an 85 percent complication rate in the closed treatment group compared with only a 5 percent complication rate in those children whose fractures were treated by anatomic open reduction.

Spiegel et al., on the basis of a review of 184 distal tibial and fibular physeal fractures, included supination-inversion stage II Salter-Harris type III and IV fractures with more than 2 mm of displacement in their "high risk" group for growth disturbance.[27] They recommended open anatomic reduction for any of these fractures with more than 2 mm of displacement. Landin et al. following similar criteria, found no growth disturbance in 17 of 18 stage II type III and IV fractures (half of which were treated with open reduction) after an average 9-year follow-up.[29] Karrholm et al.[24] noted four patterns of

growth following stage II supination-inversion fractures using postfracture stereophotogrammetric analysis of distal tibial and fibular physeal growth. They measured the distance between implanted markers on either side of the growth plate in 10 cases. Postinjury growth patterns included the following: symmetric growth; temporary growth retardation; progressive growth retardation; and growth stimulation. Children younger than 11 years were most likely to exhibit progressive growth arrest.

Open reduction with internal fixation is recommended for stage II Salter-Harris type III or IV distal tibial fractures with more than 2 mm of displacement (Fig. 22-4). A medial incisional approach is used. Any loose soft tissue or periosteum that may fall into the fracture should be removed, but care should be taken not to strip periosteum from the epiphyseal fragment. Bright has recommended the removal of small metaphyseal fragments in Salter-Harris fractures in order to lessen the possibility of peripheral osseous bridge formation.[30] Transmetaphyseal or epiphyseal Kirschner wires or screws that do not cross the physis are preferable, but smooth, small-caliber Kirschner wires crossing the physis at close to 90 degrees are acceptable. Kirschner wires are usually preferred in younger children, in whom the smaller size of the epiphysis and the fracture makes it more difficult to use screws without penetrating the physis. Transepiphyseal or metaphyseal screws are more likely to be useful in older children or adolescents. Cannulated screws are ideal for this particular fracture because the passage of a guide pin under fluoroscopic control ensures accurate intraepiphyseal placement of the hardware without violation of the physeal plate (Fig. 22-4D&E). Following open reduction and internal fixation, a short leg non-weight-bearing cast is used for 3 to 4 weeks, followed by a short leg walking cast for an additional 3 to 4 weeks or until radiographic evidence of union.

Displaced stage II fractures clearly have the highest potential for growth distrubance, progressive varus angulation of the ankle joint being the most common angular deformity associated with the stage II injury. Although anatomic reduction of these fractures is imperative for best possible results, it is no guarantee that growth disturbance will not occur. Karrholm et al.[24] found growth disturbance in stage II fractures to be most highly correlated with fracture anatomy, degree of displacement, type of treatment (open versus closed), and level of skeletal maturity.

## Supination – Plantar Flexion Fractures

Both Carothers and Crenshaw[2] and Dias and Tachdjian[16] described supination-plantar flexion mechanisms of injury. Only 11 percent of Carothers and Crenshaw's 54 physeal ankle fractures and 8 percent of Dias and Tachdjian's 71 cases were classified as supination – plantar flexion fractures, which makes this one of the least common mechanisms of injury. Gerner-Smidt did not separately describe a supination-plantar flexion mechanism but probably included this type of fracture within his supination-inversion group.[15] The supination – plantar flexion injury is characterized by a Salter-Harris type II fracture of the distal tibial physis, with a posterior metaphyseal fragment and direct posterior displacement (Fig. 22-5). No fibular fracture is present, but the fibula does displace posteriorly with the distal tibial epiphysis. Less often (as in two of Dias' 56 cases and one of Carothers' and Crenshaw's 54 cases), a Salter-Harris type I distal tibial fracture may occur with direct posterior displacement.

As with most Salter-Harris type I or II fractures, closed reduction is usually adequate. Closed reduction is performed by first applying distal and posterior traction with the foot in plantar flexion to disengage the metaphyseal fragment and then gently pulling the foot anterior with countertraction against the anterior tibia. One must be careful not to damage the physis by impaction of the trailing edge of the distal tibial metaphysis during the reduction. If closed reduction cannot be easily achieved with intravenous sedation and/or ankle block, the patient should be scheduled for reduction under general anesthesia rather than being subjected to repeated forceful manipulations. Following closed reduction, a long leg cast is used for an additional 3 to 4 weeks. Although anatomic reduction is always superior, slight posterior displacement has been considered acceptable by most authors because displacement is in the plane of joint motion (which is easily compensated) and because transverse displacement of less than one-third of the metaphyseal cross-sectional area has been shown to remodel well in the younger child.[31,32]

## Pronation-Eversion-External Rotation Fractures

Dias and Tachdjian[16] described a one-stage pronation-eversion-external rotation injury involving both a distal tibial physeal fracture and a fibular fracture (Fig. 22-6).

The tibial fracture is characteristically of the Salter-Harris type I or II and occurs with a short oblique fracture of the fibula and lateral displacement. Most authors agree that the pronation-eversion-external rotation mechanism is the most common cause of the Salter-Harris type I distal tibial fracture.[15,33] Salter-Harris type I distal tibial fractures have rarely been reported to result from supination-inversion and are relatively rare as the result of supination-plantar flexion or supination-external rotation. However, a Salter-Harris type II distal tibial fracture with a lateral metaphyseal fragment is the most commonly seen tibial fracture in the pronation injury. Most pronation-eversion-external rotation fractures are the result of higher-energy types of injuries, and displacement is more common than with most other pediatric ankle fractures.

Dias and Tachdjian considered it difficult to separate pronation-eversion (abduction) injuries from pronation-external rotation injuries and stated that these fractures are usually produced by a combination of eversion and external rotational force. In their study pronation injuries were about half as common as supination-inversion or supination-external rotation fractures (including juvenile Tillaux and triplane fractures), constituting about 15 percent of 71 fractures.[16] Gerner-Smidt[15] and Karrholm et al.[33] divided pronation injuries into two or three types — namely, pronation-abduction (eversion), pronation-eversion (external rotation), and pronation-dorsiflexion — and expressed the view that each subtype has an individually identifiable fracture pattern. Pronation fractures accounted for 15 percent of fractures with open growth plates among 457 pediatric ankle fractures reviewed by Karrholm et al.[33]; this incidence is identical to that found by Dias and Tachdjian.[16] Karrholm et al. stated that in the pronation-abduction (pronation-eversion) mechanism, the metaphyseal fragment in the Salter-Harris type II fracture is located laterally or posterolaterally, whereas it is located anterolaterally in the pronation-eversion (pronation – external rotation) fracture type. Karrholm et al.[33] also found that an anterolateral displacement, rather than the posterolateral displacement described by Dias and Tachdjian, usually occurs in pronation-external rotation injuries. In order for lateral displacement of the distal tibial epiphysis to take place, either the interosseous membrane must rupture or a fibular fracture must occur. The most common mechanism is the one described by Dias and Tachdjian, in which a Salter-Harris type II fracture of the distal tibia with a lateral metaphyseal fragment is followed by a

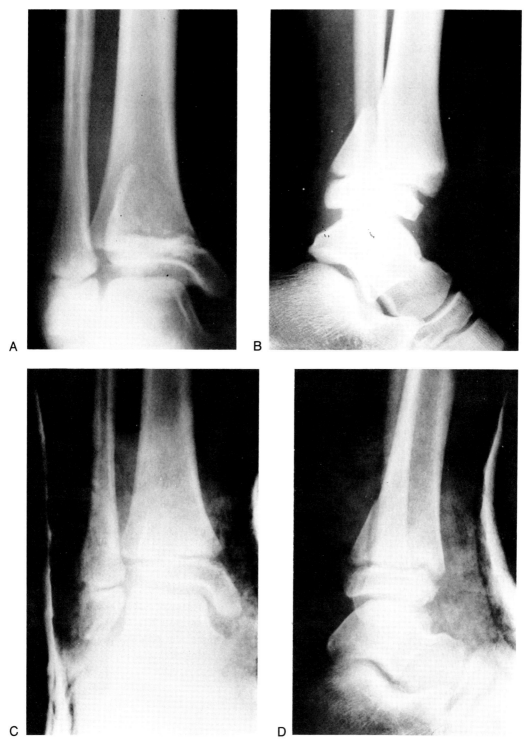

**Fig. 22-5.** (A) Anteroposterior radiograph of a displaced supination–plantar flexion ankle fracture in an 11-year-old boy, who fell off a fence, catching his foot in the fence. Note the absence of a fibular fracture. (B) Lateral view of the same fracture prior to reduction. (C&D) Postoperative radiographs after closed reduction of this fracture in the emergency room under a combination of intravenous analgesia/sedation and local anesthetic infiltration. Reduction is accomplished by first applying distal and posterior traction with the foot in plantar flexion to disengage the metaphyseal fragment and then gently pulling the foot anterior with countertraction against the anterior tibia.

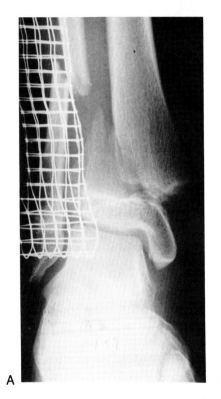
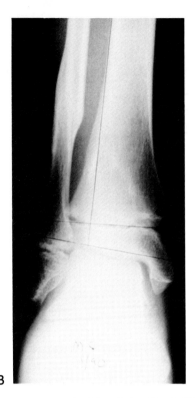

**Fig. 22-6.** **(A)** Pronation-eversion-external rotation ankle fracture characterized by a Salter-Harris II fracture of the distal tibia combined with a high transverse fibular fracture. **(B)** Postreduction anteroposterior view of the fracture, after healing has occurred.

relatively low transverse fracture or a higher oblique fracture of the fibula, depending upon whether the deforming force is primarily abduction or external rotation. Rupture of the interosseous membrane instead of fibular fracture is rare in children, but has been reported in association with a Salter-Harris type I distal tibial fracture.[34] This injury can occur with minimal displacement or with spontaneous reduction, so that no displacement is present on postinjury radiographs. Radiographs 3 to 4 weeks after injury may show calcification along the interosseous membrane.[34]

As with most Salter-Harris type I or II injuries, this fracture is usually amenable to closed reduction. (Fig. 22-7). After the deformity has been increased slightly by distal traction, the foot should be internally rotated and inverted. Restoration of fibular length, as with the adult pronation–external rotation injury, should be attempted; however, slight shortening and valgus angulation are acceptable in the younger child and should self-correct with growth. Valgus angulation in the older child

with limited growth potential requires anatomic reduction by closed or open means to prevent a residual valgus ankle deformity. Hindrance of closed reduction of the Salter-Harris type II fracture secondary to medial periosteal interposition has been reported.[35]

Open reduction is accomplished through an anterolateral incision (Fig. 22-8). The fracture site is exposed with minimal periosteal stripping, and clot or loose fragments are removed. Any loose periosteum about the peripheral portion of the physis should be excised in order to prevent peripheral osseous bridge formation. The fracture can then be reduced and fixed with transmetaphyseal pins or screws. In most cases fixation of the fibular fracture is not necessary, but occasionally stabilization of the fracture in anatomic alignment may not be possible without restoration of fibular length through internal fixation. This is especially true in the older adolescent.

Following closed reduction, a long leg cast should be used for 3 to 4 weeks to prevent rotation and weight-bearing, after which a short leg walking cast can be used

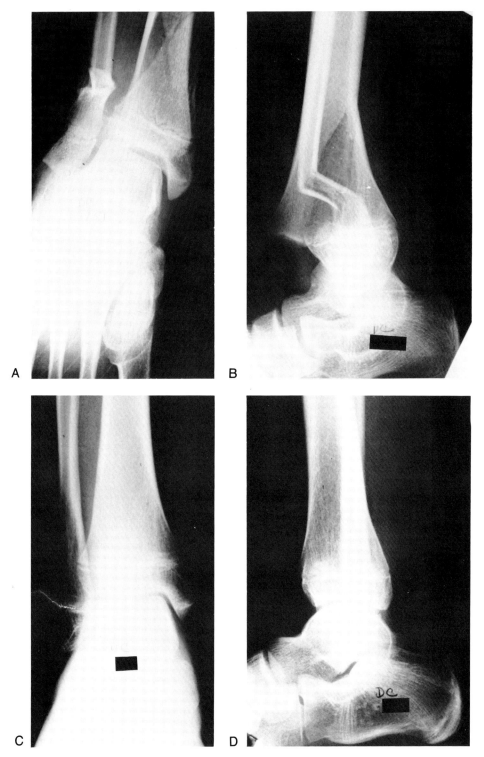

**Fig. 22-7. (A&B)** Pronation-eversion-external rotation "high-energy" fracture from a fall. **(C&D)** The fracture in Figs. A and B, 8 months after closed reduction.

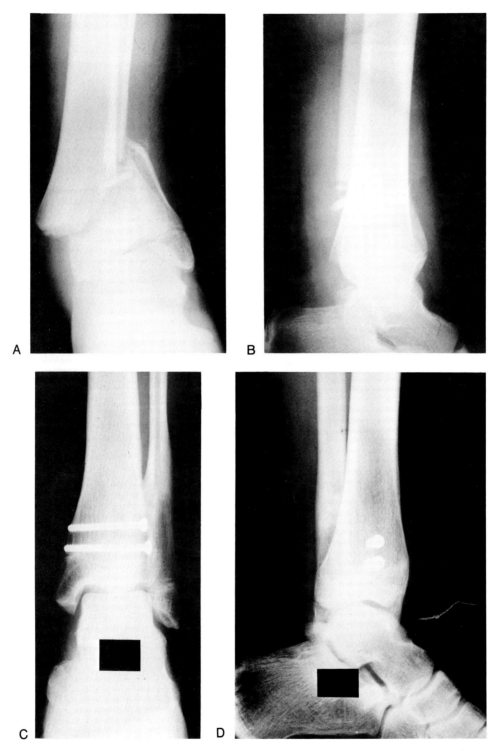

**Fig. 22-8. (A&B)** Attempted closed reduction of this pronation-eversion-external rotation ankle fracture under intravenous sedation and under general anesthesia failed, owing to interposed comminuted bone fragments and periosteum. **(C&D)** Postoperative radiographs after open reduction and internal fixation of the fracture in Figs. A and B with two transmetaphyseal lag screws.

for an additional 3 to 4 weeks or until radiographic evidence of fracture union. Following open reduction and rigid fixation, a short leg cast is acceptable. The most common growth disturbance following pronation-eversion-external rotation ankle fractures in children is a residual or progressive valgus angulation deformity of the ankle joint.

## Supination – External Rotation Fractures

Dias and Tachdjian[16] described a two-stage supination – external rotation ankle fracture characterized by a Salter-Harris II fracture of the distal tibia, which accounted for 18 percent of their 71 cases. They did not include juvenile Tillaux (4 percent) or triplane fractures (9 percent) in this category. Gerner-Smidt,[15] however, on the basis of experimental reproduction of the various fracture types, believed that juvenile Tillaux and triplane fractures simply represented a continuum of the supination – external rotation mechanism. Karrholm et al. found that these three fracture types (Dias-Tachdjian supination-external rotation Salter-Harris type II tibial, juvenile Tillaux, and triplane) comprised about 39 percent of 457 ankle fractures in children out of 919 lower leg fractures in their review.[36]

The best experimental evidence supports Gerner-Smidt's original view that these three very different fracture patterns are probably more the result of differential strength characteristics of the metaphysis, physis, and epiphysis during the transition to skeletal maturity than they are a function of the mechanism of injury. Hence the term *transitional fracture* is often used to refer to juvenile Tillaux or triplane fractures. Gerner-Smidt,[15] Lauge-Hansen,[37] and Thomasen[38] stated that supination-external rotation trauma will cause different fractures at different ages. Karrholm et al., on the basis of accumulated unpublished data, stated that the predominant fracture of the lower leg, including the ankle, in children under age 10 was a spiral diaphyseal fracture of the tibia.[36] The two-stage supination-external rotation Salter-Harris type II fracture described by Dias and Tachdjian[16] is most common in the preadolescent to early adolescent period. Once the medial distal tibial physis begins to fuse, the triplane fracture is more likely to occur (early to midadolescence). The juvenile Tillaux fracture only occurs just prior to complete closure of the

physis, when only the anterior lateral portion of the physis remains open.

### Stage I and II Supination – External Rotation Fractures

The supination-external rotation injury in children occurs via the same mechanism as in the adult injury but differs mainly in that stage I in the child involves a tibial fracture instead of a fibular fracture as in the adult (Fig. 22-9). As is characteristic of torsional physeal ankle fractures, the distal tibial physis fails before the fibular shaft. A Salter-Harris type II fracture with a large posterior metaphyseal fragment, similar to that which occurs in the supination-plantar flexion injury, can be seen on the lateral view. The metaphyseal fragment is usually posteromedial, and displacement is most commonly directly posterior. The distinguishing feature of the supination-external rotation stage I fracture, according to Dias and Tachdjian[16] is a long oblique fracture line, characteristic of a torsional force, which courses from distal-lateral-inferior to proximal-medial-superior on the anteroposterior radiograph.

The second stage of the supination-external rotation fracture involves a short oblique fibular fracture just above the distal fibular physis, which is secondary to progression of the external rotation force of the talus within the ankle mortise (Fig. 22-9). The distal tibial epiphysis and posterior metaphyseal fragment have a ligamentous attachment to the distal fibular fragment, and, as in the adult, displacement is usually posterolateral.

Anatomic alignment of supination external rotation stage I and II fractures can usually be achieved by closed reduction, which is usually fairly easily accomplished through reversal of the mechanism of injury (internal rotation) with application of distal traction. A thick, intact periosteal hinge on the compression side of the injury prevents over-reduction by providing a solid end point to the reduction. In a stage II fracture it is important to fully disengage the distal fibular fragment by slightly accentuating the deformity through external rotation and distal traction before reduction. Slight valgus angulation secondary to fibular shortening is acceptable in the younger child (less than 10 years old), in contrast to adults, because this angulation will generally reduce with growth. Occasionally, fracture comminution or soft

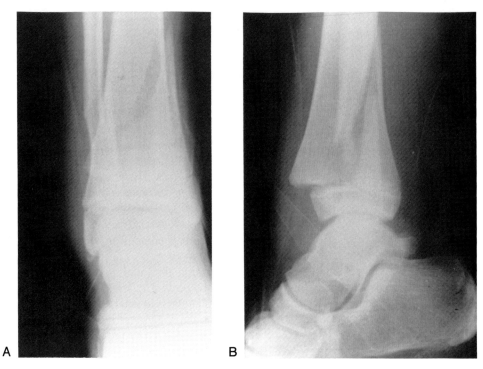

**Fig. 22-9. (A&B)** Displaced supination-external rotation stage II ankle fracture characterized by a Salter-Harris II fracture of the distal tibia with a posterior metaphyseal fragment. Note the oblique fracture line on anteroposterior view coursing in a distal lateral to proximal medial direction.

tissue interposition may prevent anatomic closed reduction. Open reduction can be performed through a posteromedial approach while anteroposterior transmetaphyseal pins or screws are inserted through small anterior stab incisions under image intensification fluoroscopic control. Because this is a rotationally induced injury, a long leg cast should always be used for the initial 3 to 4 weeks after closed reduction of displaced fractures. A short leg walking cast may be used after 3 to 4 weeks once stable fracture consolidation has been achieved.

Salter stated that the prognosis for subsequent undisturbed growth with Salter-Harris II fractures of the distal tibia is excellent, since the epiphyseal blood supply is undisturbed.[22] However, Spiegel et al. found a 16.7 percent complication rate among 66 Salter-Harris type II fractures of the distal tibia treated by closed reduction[27]; of these patients, 22 percent had associated fibular fractures. Spiegel et al.'s complication rate with Salter-Harris type II distal tibial fractures was actually higher than in minimally displaced type III or IV fractures. Of 11 patients who developed growth disturbance, 6 had angular deformities. Spiegel et al. attributed this for the most part to incomplete reduction and emphasized the importance of anatomic reduction in this somewhat "unpredictable" group of fractures. Karrholm et al. noted a higher tendency toward growth disturbance when a fibular fracture was present and speculated that fracture of the fibula allows greater displacement and greater exposure of the physis to damage.[34]

## Isolated External Rotation Fracture of the Distal Tibial Physis

The isolated external rotation fracture of the distal tibial physis is a fairly rare but unique fracture, which was first described in 1968 by Lovell[19] (Fig. 22-10). A total of five individual cases have been reported in the literature.[40-43] One of us (DeValentine) has also seen one case of this unusual fracture, and we suspect that a fair number of cases have been seen but not been reported in the literature. All six patients were between the ages of 7 and 14, with an average age of 11.8. The significance of this

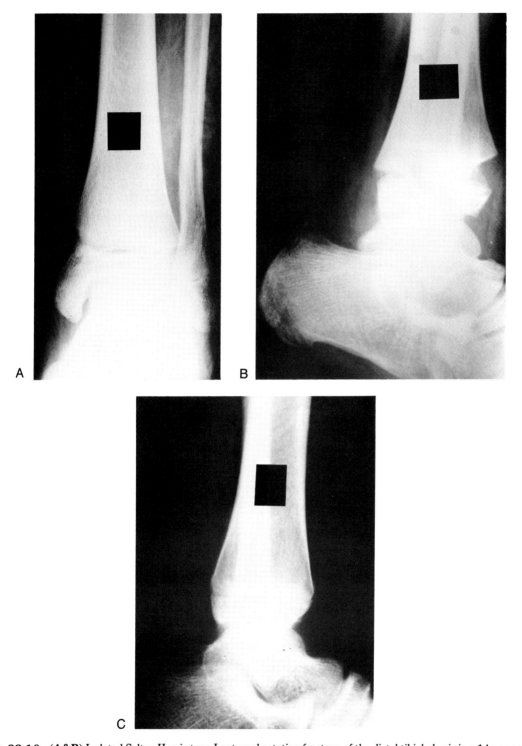

**Fig. 22-10.** **(A&B)** Isolated Salter-Harris type I external rotation fracture of the distal tibial physis in a 14-year-old high school football player whose leg was "trapped." Typical radiographic signs are apparent "widening" of the medial physis (which is actually a malalignment produced by rotation) and an unusually posterior appearance of the fibula. This latter finding is often falsely attributed to inadequate positioning. If full leg films are taken, the ankle joint will appear to be 60 to 90 degrees externally rotated with respect to the knee joint. **(C)** Lateral radiograph after closed reduction.

particular fracture is not its rarity but its unusual clinical and radiographic appearance. This fracture, characterized by a purely external rotational displacement of the distal tibial epiphysis without an associated fibular fracture, is essentially a Salter-Harris I variant. No metaphyseal or epiphyseal fracture is present. Typically, the child is brought to the emergency room following an indirect type of injury with the foot externally rotated 60 to 90 degrees. Little or no swelling is present, and no other deformity is observed. At first glance, radiographs are often interpreted as normal. Careful inspection of the radiographs will show slight widening of the medial distal tibial physis and an unusually posterior appearance of the fibula with respect to the tibia. Full leg radiographs that include the knee and ankle will show 45 to 60 degrees of external rotation of the ankle joint.

Broock and Greer were able to duplicate this injury in a freshly amputated limb by excising the periosteum and perichondrium about the physis.[40] No ligament injury or fracture was necessary. The interosseous ligament remains intact and allows at least 45 degrees of external rotation of the foot, distal tibial epiphysis, and fibula. Growth disturbance has been reported in one of the six cases reported by Nevalos and Colton.[41] Henke and Kiple speculated that growth disturbance might occur due to disruption of the perichondrial ring, leading to peripheral osseous bridge formation.[42] They recommended close follow-up of this fracture.

Closed reduction is easily performed in most cases under intravenous sedation and/or local block by internal rotation of the foot. A palpable "clunk" can be felt when the endpoint of reduction is reached, which some authors attribute to the relocation of the fibula within its tibial notch. A long leg cast is used for 3 to 4 weeks, followed by a short leg walking cast for an additional 3 to 4 weeks.

## Juvenile Tillaux Fractures

Most authors attribute the original description of the so-called juvenile Tillaux fracture to Sir Astley Cooper in 1822, but Kleiger and Mankin provided the first comprehensive description of this fracture in 1964 and referred to it as the *juvenile Tillaux fracture* because of its similarity to the adult injury of the same name.[44] Tillaux, the French surgeon for whom the fracture is named, performed experiments on adult cadaver limbs in the late 1800s, in which he demonstrated avulsion of a fragment of bone from the distal anterior tibia as the

result of an external rotational force through the distal tibiofibular ligament.[45] Anatomically the distal anterior tibiofibular ligament originates from the Tillaux-Chaput tubercle on the tibial epiphysis and inserts into the La-Fort-Wagstaff tubercle on the distal anterior fibula. The adolescent counterpart of the adult avulsion fracture described by Tillaux involves avulsion of a larger, roughly rectangular portion of the distal lateral tibial epiphysis rather than merely the small triangular Tillaux-Chaput tubercle (Fig 22-11). The juvenile Tillaux fracture appears radiographically on anteroposterior view as a Salter-Harris type III fracture of the lateral distal tibial epiphysis, which usually involves 20 to 50 percent of the

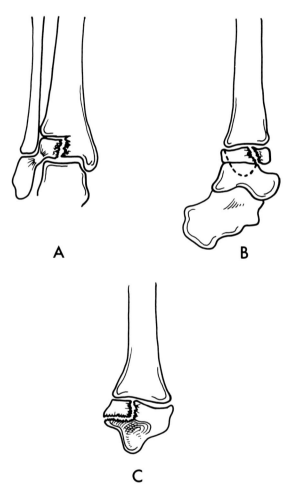

**Fig. 22-11.** Illustration of the juvenile Tillaux fracture. **(A)** Anteroposterior view. **(B)** Lateral view. **(C)** Inferior view of the tibial plafond showing the intra-articular nature of this fracture.

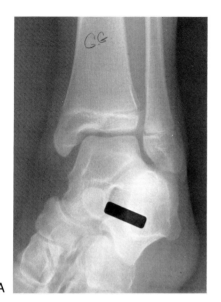
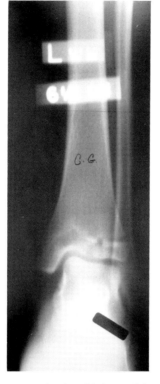
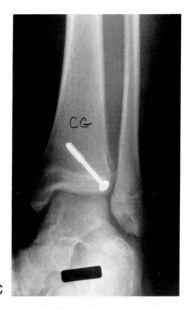

A          B          C

**Fig. 22-12.** **(A)** An oblique view of an adolescent patient's ankle is suspicious for a juvenile Tillaux fracture. **(B)** A tomogram of the same patient's ankle clearly shows the fracture line, with significant displacement of the anterolateral fragment. **(C)** Open reduction and internal fixation of the fracture with a single lag screw.

width of the epiphysis[46] (Fig.22-12). It differs from the Salter-Harris type III fracture, however, in that the vertical epiphyseal fracture line does not extend the full anteroposterior depth of the tibial epiphysis.

Kleiger and Mankin, on the basis of radiographic examination of 22 ankles that were beginning physeal closure, determined that the central portion of the physis closes first, followed by the medial portion, with fusion of the lateral physis taking place last.[44] They confirmed this pattern of physeal closure in two freshly amputated limbs and also noted that closure typically begins in an undulated area of the physis that they termed the *medial hump*. This consistent topographic pattern of physeal closure takes place over an approximately 18-month period, which usually begins between 12 and 14 years of age.[46,47] The juvenile Tillaux fracture normally occurs only during this period, after closure of the medial tibial physis but before closure of the lateral physis. The term *transitional fracture* is sometimes used to refer to both

juvenile Tillaux and triplane fractures because these injuries only occur during the transitional period between adolescence and skeletal maturity.[48] Although the triplane fracture usually occurs at a slightly earlier age, the juvenile Tillaux fracture will be discussed first because it will provide a better basis for understanding fracture propagation in the triplane injury.

Age at the time of injury varies in accordance with skeletal maturity. Spiegel et al. found the average age of six patients (three boys and three girls) with juvenile Tillaux fractures to be 13.5 years.[27] All nine patients in Dias' review of 71 physeal ankle fractures were between 12 and 14 years of age, but patients reported in the literature have ranged in age from 11 to 18 years. The injury definitely seems to be more common in girls. Of 78 reported cases that have been reviewed in the literature, 54 (69 percent) occurred in girls and 24 (31 percent) in boys.[1,27,36,44,46,49-52]

It has been well established that the juvenile Tillaux

fracture is an avulsion type of external rotation injury resulting from the pull of the intact distal anterior tibiofibular ligament. An intact distal anterior tibiofibular ligament, as well as reproduction of displacement with external rotation, has been confirmed at the time of surgery by numerous authors.[15,44,46,51,53] Spinella and Turco also found rupture of the distal tibiofibular interosseous ligament in two patients who underwent open reduction.[51] The anterior and posterior distal tibiofibular ligaments remained intact, and ankle diastasis was present; this finding would not be unexpected.

As the talus applies an external rotational force to the fibular malleolus in a child approaching skeletal maturity, the juvenile Tillaux fragment is first avulsed, since the biomechanical strength of the lateral physis is less than that of the distal anterior tibiofibular ligament or lateral malleolus. Once the juvenile Tillaux fracture occurs, tension is placed on the interosseous ligament, which is more likely to fail than the surrounding bone. This emphasizes the importance of considering the possibility of ankle diastasis in any adolescent with this injury. Although it is well established that the juvenile Tillaux fracture is produced by an external rotation mechanism, it has not been determined conclusively whether this can occur with the foot in either the supinated or pronated position. Dias and Giegerich[46] believed that either mechanism could produce these injuries, and Karrholm et al.[36] found that transitional fractures occurred with both the supination–external rotation and the pronation–external rotation mechanism. It is most probable that transitional and isolated rotational fractures of the distal tibial epiphysis occur as the result of both supination-external rotation and pronation–external rotation mechanisms (although supination-external rotation is about twice as common) and that these different fracture patterns are more a function of age-related differential biomechanical strength characteristics of the physis and surrounding bone than of the mechanism of injury.

The adolescent with the juvenile Tillaux fracture may present with minimal symptoms, which may easily be mistaken for those of an ankle sprain, and the only physical sign of this injury may be localized tenderness and swelling over the anterolateral portion of the ankle. If the fracture is nondisplaced or minimally displaced, the only radiographic sign may be a vertical fracture line through the epiphysis on the oblique view of the ankle because the fracture line is often obscured by the superimposed fibular malleolus on the anteroposterior view. Multiple oblique views are often helpful if this fracture is suspected. If displacement does occur, the fragment moves anterolaterally, and anterior displacement can often be identified on the lateral view. Although the displacement often appears to be only 1 to 3 mm on plain films, tomography often reveals greater displacement and is recommended whenever displacement, as observed on plain films, is questionable.[54]

The juvenile Tillaux fracture rarely causes growth arrest or angular deformity, since complete physeal closure must be imminent for this injury to occur, but significant long-term complications can occur as a result of joint incongruity, which can lead to ankle joint arthritis. Spiegel et al. included the juvenile Tillaux fracture in their high-risk category based upon a review of six cases, four of which were treated with closed reduction; in one of these four symptomatic articular incongruity developed. Fractures in Spiegel et al.'s high-risk group (Salter-Harris II and IV, juvenile Tillaux, and triplane) with less than 2 mm of displacement did not lead to articular incongruity in these authors' review of 184 distal tibial physeal fractures with an average follow-up of 26 months.[27] They recommended open reduction of any high-risk fracture with more than 2 mm of displacement.

Closed reduction can be effected by internal rotation of the foot while an extenal rotational torque is applied to the tibia. Nondisplaced fractures or fractures that have been nonsurgically reduced should be treated with a long leg cast for 3 to 4 weeks, followed by a short leg walking cast for 3 to 4 weeks. Closed reduction of displaced juvenile Tillaux fractures is often inadequate and may be unstable, and we prefer to surgically reduce and fix any displaced fracture. Most authors have reported excellent results with open reduction,[16,49,52] but several have found periosteum or other debris interposed at the fracture site, which had to be surgically removed before anatomic reduction could be accomplished.[36,49,50,55] Open reduction is performed through an anterolateral incision directly over the fracture site. The preferred method of fixation is insertion of a single lag screw from distal-lateral to proximal-medial. It is permissible for the screw to cross the physis, since growth is already complete, and the screw may be left in place permanently in most cases. Open reduction and internal fixation should be followed by a short leg non-weight-bearing cast for 3 to 4 weeks and then by a short leg walking cast for 3 to 4 more weeks.

## Triplane Fractures

The so-called triplane injury to the distal tibial epiphysis represents one of the most intriguing and complex fractures encountered in the pediatric age group. Lynn[56] was the first to use the term *triplane,* which is derived from the fact that fracture lines oriented to each of the three cardinal body planes are present.[57] Rang aptly points out that this is about the only point that is universally accepted by the various authors on the subject.[58] There is confusion and therefore disagreement on the mechanism of injury and the configuration of the fracture fragments, as well as on the most important aspect of treatment. As more becomes known on the subject and imaging techniques become more accurate, one may hope that some of the mystique of this fracture will disappear.

Although the specific configuration of the fracture fragments can vary, there is involvement of the epiphysis, physeal plate, and distal tibial metaphysis. The vertical fracture line cleaves the distal epiphysis in the sagittal plane, usually at the anterolateral aspect of the ankle joint. The fracture line then courses along the physis in the transverse plane and exits posteriorly through the distal tibial metaphysis. This frontal plane component of the fracture line completes the triplanar nature of the fracture (Fig. 22-13). Because of the epiphyseal disrup-

tion, the fracture is by definition an intra-articular fracture. This circuitous route of energy dissipation actually follows the path of least resistance. It is no accident that the degree of skeletal maturity of the distal tibial epiphysis largely dictates the actual configuration of the fracture fragments. As previously discussed, the anterolateral portion of the physis is the last to close; it thus constitutes a vulnerable area allowing the propagation of forces through the most logical pathway.

Although there are some discrepancies in the literature regarding the mechanism of injury, most authors agree that it involves external rotational forces to the foot. There is probably little if any frontal plane variance to the foot at the time of injury, although this aspect is disputed in the literature.[36,44,57,59,60] Some of the confusion arises from the different terminology used by the various authors. The fracture is similar to the juvenile Tillaux injury in that the anterior tibiofibular ligament initiates the avulsion of the anterolateral portion of the epiphysis. With continued external rotational force, the fracture exits through the weaker posterior metaphyseal bone. The various specific triplane fracture patterns produced by this type of mechanism depend on the degree of physeal closure and axial load at the time of injury. This latter parameter is influenced to a large degree by the sagittal plane positon of the ankle. Most authors contend that the ankle is usually plantar-flexed at the time of the rotatory moment.

Several fracture patterns can result from this mechanism. The most logical and consistent method of description is that based on the number of fragments, the patterns being classified as two-, three-, or four-part fractures. However, it should be remembered that the increasing number of pieces does not indicate that a higher force level was involved in their production — that is, the number of fragments does not correlate with progression of a universal mechanism. Rather, the number of pieces is determined by a combination of the various factors of axial load, plantar flexion, and specific physeal plate maturity.

### Patterns of Triplane Fractures

*Two-Part Triplane*

The two-part fracture represents the simplest form of the triplane injury. One fragment consists of the anterolateral and posterior portions of the epiphysis and the

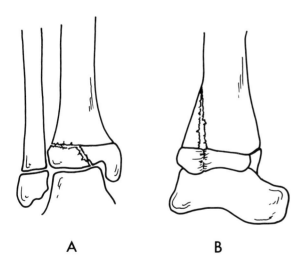

**Fig. 22-13.** **(A)** Illustration of the anterior aspect of the tibia, showing the transverse and sagittal plane components of the triplane fracture. **(B)** Lateral view of the distal tibia, showing the frontal plane component of the fracture.

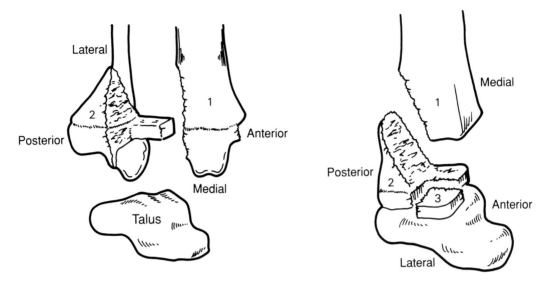

**Fig. 22-14. (A)** Diagram of the two-fragment triplane fracture as described by Cooperman et al.[60] One fragment consists of the tibial shaft (1) while the other fragment (2) remains attached to the fibula by virtue of an intact ligamentous complex. **(B)** Diagram of the three-part triplane fracture as described by Marmor.[57] The anterolateral (3) fragment is attached to the fibula but is different from that of the two-part fracture. The tibial shaft component (1) has no physeal or epiphyseal elements attached to the metaphysis; the posterior spike is attached to the large posteromedial epiphyseal fragment (2).

posterior part of the metaphysis, while the second fragment consists of the tibial shaft, the medial malleolus, and the remaining anteromedial aspect of the epiphysis (Fig. 22-14A). The first fragment usually remains attached to the fibula. Cooperman et al.[60] report that the majority of triplane fractures consist of these two fragments, although absolute certainty can only be obtained with computed tomography (CT). In the two-part fracture the detached portion of the epiphysis usually displaces posteriorly and laterally.

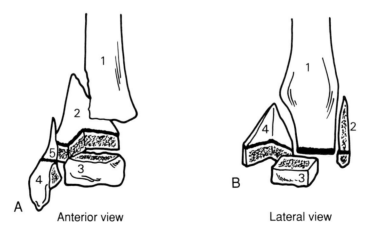

**Fig. 22-15.** Diagram of the four-part triplane fracture as described by Izant and Davidson.[61] The posteromedial epiphyseal portion (2) is attached to the supradjacent metaphysis, as is the anteromedial portion (4). The tibial shaft (1) is the fourth part. In the variant described by Kärrholm, the latter fragment is separated into epiphyseal (4) and metaphyseal sections (5). However, the metaphyseal fragment (5) is not separated from the main tibial shaft fragment (1).

## Three-Part Triplane

The three-part fracture has no components similar to those of the two-part fracture. The first fragment is the anterolateral portion of the epiphysis and is equivalent to the juvenile Tillaux fragment; the second fragment is the remainder of the epiphysis and the posterior metaphyseal spike; and the third fragment is the tibial shaft (Fig. 22-14B). In this pattern, first described by Marmor,[57] the free anterolateral epiphyseal portion often displaces anteriorly as it swings on its ligamentous hinge, while the remainder of the detached epiphysis displaces postero-laterally.

## Four-Part Triplane

The four-part fracture is extremely rare and has been only scantly reported.[15,59,61] It occurs in two variants (Fig. 22-15). The type described by Izant and Davidson[61] is similar to the three-part fracture of Gerner-Smidt[15]; the discrepancy in the number of fragments arises only from use of different classification schemes. This fracture is best described as a three-part fracture complicated by a coronal split of the medial metaphyseal-epiphyseal portion. Thus, the epiphysis is divided into three fragments, but two of these fragments are still attached to their respective metaphyseal portions. In the case reported by Kärrholm et al.[59] the pattern is also similar to the three-part fracture of Gerner-Smidt,[15] except that the anteromedial epiphysis is cleaved from its corresponding metaphyseal component. The posterior piece is attached to the metaphyseal spike, but the anteromedial piece is not. This latter finding can usually only be detected intraoperatively. One of us (Schuberth) has treated two cases of this four-part fracture.

## Medial Triplane

The medial triplane fracture represents another rare variant of the triplanar injury.[62,63] In this pattern the anterolateral epiphyseal fragment remains attached to the tibial metaphysis (Fig. 22-16), forming the first fragment. The second piece is the posteromedial portion of the epiphysis and a small posterior metaphyseal flag. The occurrence of this configuration is baffling because of the known pattern of epiphyseal plate closure. It is important to recognize this variant because of the large amount of articular surface involved in the injury.

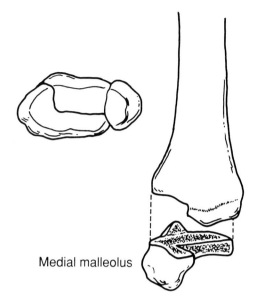

Medial malleolus

**Fig. 22-16.** Diagram of the medial triplane fracture from an anterior view. The vulnerable anterolateral epiphysis is not injured and remains attached to the second fragment or the tibial shaft. The second fragment is the posteromedial aspect of the epiphysis and its small metaphyseal flag.

## Radiographic Assessment of Triplane Fractures

Meaningful radiographic analysis of triplane injuries requires a thorough knowledge of the fracture and anticipation of the fragment patterns that can result. The triplane injury has always been described as a Salter III fracture on the anteroposterior view and a Salter II fracture on the lateral view. Although this fracture represents neither of these Salter classification types, it manifests their characteristics. The anteroposterior or mortise view shows the vertical fracture through the epiphysis (Fig. 22-17). As the age of the child increases, the fracture line generally appears more lateral, which corresponds with maturation of the physis.[48] In general, the fracture line is located near the center of the ankle joint surface. In some cases the posterior metaphyseal fragment may be evident on the anteroposterior view.

The contour of the medial aspect of the distal tibia should also be evaluated for incongruities of the metaphyseal and epiphyseal anatomy. Normally these two areas are represented by a smooth confluence without any offset to the epiphysis or metaphysis; irregularities may signify the presence of a medial triplane injury or

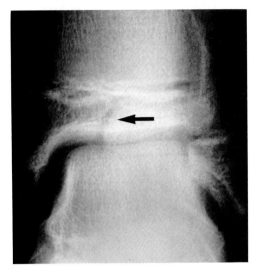

**Fig. 22-17.** Anteroposterior view of the ankle showing the vertical fracture line (arrow), which begins at the joint surface and proceeds proximally to the physis. This resembles a Salter-Harris III fracture pattern.

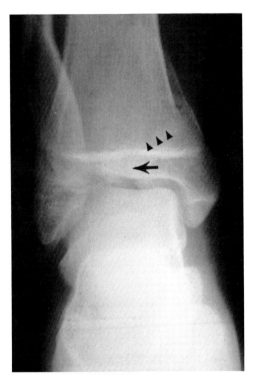

**Fig. 22-18.** Anteroposterior view of the ankle, showing disruption of the medial contour of the tibia (arrowheads). Note the vertical fracture line (arrow), which signifies a medial triplane injury.

other variants (Fig. 22-18). The amount of displacement of the anterolateral epiphysis from the rest of the epiphysis at the level of the joint should be carefully measured and evaluated. Displacements of 1 to 4 mm are quite common and will dictate treatment in most cases. Inspection of the fibula may reveal a distal fracture similar to that which occurs in adults by an external rotation mechanism. The fracture usually starts at the growth plate and is propagated from anteroinferior to posterosuperior. There is seldom radiographic evidence of tibiofibular syndesmotic disruption.

The lateral view elucidates the nature of the posterior metaphyseal fragment, the fibular fracture, if present, and the amount of displacement of the distal structures. It is rare for the extent of the sagittal fracture line to be identifiable on the lateral view, as it is usually obscured by overlap. The anterior aspect of the ankle joint may yield evidence as to whether the configuration is a Marmor[57] three-part fracture or a two-part fracture as described by Cooperman et al.[60] If the anterolateral epiphysis is displaced or visible anteriorly, a three-part fracture is likely; if the anterolateral epiphysis is not visible, this is probably because it was carried posteriorly by virtue of its attachment to the rest of the epiphysis, and thus a two-part fracture has occurred (Fig. 22-19).

Tomographic studies are indicated whenever there is any doubt as to the adequacy of closed reduction or the exact nature of the injury. CT is the procedure of choice when evaluating this parameter. The degree of initial displacement or adequacy of closed reduction can be easily calibrated from the tomograms. If CT scanning is unavailable, the same information can be obtained from both anteroposterior and lateral conventional tomograms. It is surprising that many patients have unacceptable amounts of displacement on the tomograms when the plain radiographs are relatively benign in appearance (Fig. 22-20). As will be discussed later, displacements of the epiphysis of more than 2 mm should be reduced through either closed or open methods. Sagittal or coronal reconstructions from the axial images will illustrate that this fracture fits best into a Salter IV pattern of injury. However, because of the complex and unique nature of this fracture it is seldom discussed in this manner (Fig. 22-21).

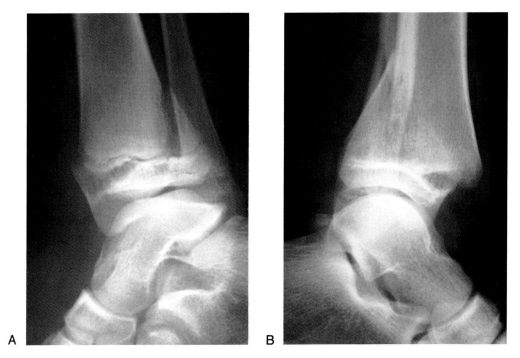

**Fig. 22-19. (A)** Lateral view of a three-part triplane fracture, showing overhang or anterior displacement of the anterolateral portion of the epiphysis. **(B)** Lateral view of another patient with a two-part fracture, showing only posterior displacement of the mobile fragment.

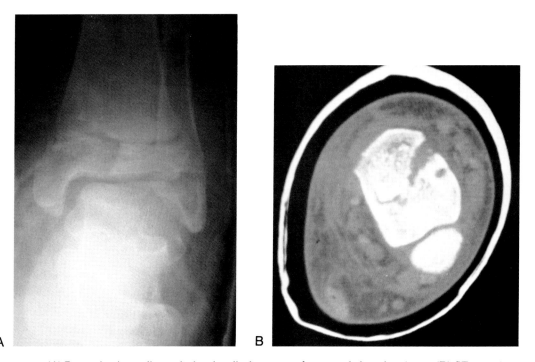

**Fig. 22-20. (A)** Postreduction radiograph showing displacement of apparently less than 2 mm. **(B)** CT scan showing actual displacement of 7 mm, necessitating open reduction.

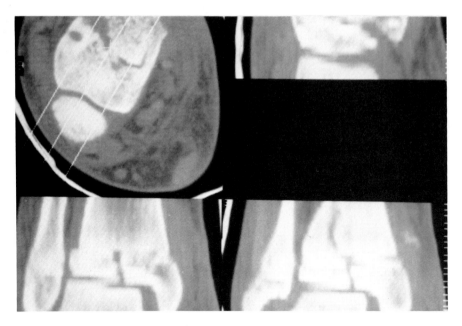

**Fig. 22-21.** Frontal plane reconstruction from CT scan demonstrating resemblance to a Salter IV type of fracture. Although not a classic Salter IV, the fracture line does cross both the epiphysis and the metaphysis.

### Treatment of Triplane Fractures

Treatment of the triplane fracture fortunately can be discussed in terms of a few basic tenets in spite of its complexity and many possible presentations. However, this does not imply that one can take a cavalier approach to the diagnosis and classification of this injury. The first principle that must be understood is that the triplane fracture is intra-articular. The joint surface is the single most important consideration when addressing this injury[64]; with this in mind, the approach is identical to that used for anatomic reduction of articular fractures in adults. Several authors have cited cases in which less than anatomic reduction has resulted in symptoms,[46,64,65] but there are no documented cases of end-stage arthritis due to an inadequately reduced articular component. Radiographic signs of arthrosis were reported in the studies of Beck and Engler[66] and Gerner-Smidt.[15]

Once the injury has been diagnosed, a single attempt should be made to reduce the displacement of the articular surface. This can be done in the operating room under a general anesthetic or under appropriate sedation in the emergency room. We prefer to use intravenous sedation if possible, especially in patients with minimally displaced fractures. General anesthesia is usually reserved for difficult patients or those in whom open reduction is probably required owing to marked displacement. The patient's knee is bent while forward traction is applied to the heel. The foot is simultaneously rotated internally (or externally, depending on the clinical presentation). The reduction is maintained temporarily with a short leg cast, and postreduction films are taken. If there is absolute anatomic reduction, the child is placed in a long leg cast with the foot in internal rotation. If there is any question as to the adequacy of reduction, a CT scan is obtained. If the displacement of the articular surface is more than 2 mm, open reduction is planned. Adequate closed reduction can be impeded by the periosteal sleeve, which often lodges in the fracture site. This is usually confirmed intraoperatively.

Variations of the above technique are acceptable. The closed reduction can be performed under image intensification, but with the realization that the fluoroscopic image may not be as representative of the reduction as a conventional radiograph. We prefer to try a single closed reduction under sedation and to rely on CT analysis of the reduction prior to planning more invasive treatment. If the plain films indicate that reduction is still unacceptable, immediate open reduction can take place without a CT scan. This is recommended only when the radiographic profile suggests a relatively simple fracture configuration and the surgeon is experienced in the operative management of this injury.

Postreduction management consists of a long leg cast with the foot internally rotated for 3 to 4 weeks, followed by a short leg weight-bearing cast for another 3 to 4 weeks. Careful inspection of interim radiographs is necessary as alterations in the treatment plan may become necessary if displacement occurs.

## Open Reduction

If open reduction is indicated, it should be performed as soon as possible after the injury. Thorough preoperative planning based on scrutiny of CT or conventional tomograms will allow treatment to progress smoothly. Anticipation of the fracture configurations will facilitate precise intraoperative technique. However, subtle separations of the epiphysis may be seen only during intraoperative inspection of the fragments.

A two-incision approach is often indicated in order to completely visualize the pathology. We recommend this approach in all cases unless there is absolutely no doubt that the surgeon is dealing with a "simple" two-part fracture, in which case a single anterolateral approach is sufficient. The first incision is made over the tibiofibular junction in longitudinal fashion. The anterior muscle group is retracted medially, along with the vital structures. Once the fracture line has been identified in the epiphysis, the foot is externally rotated to disimpact the fracture and allow for excavation of the gap. Often the periosteal sleeve will occupy this position, and it can be carefully removed. The extent of the anterolateral piece of epiphysis can also be identified. If the injury is clearly a two-part fracture, a manipulative reduction is performed and fixation is introduced in the same fashion as in the operative management of the Tillaux fracture. If the fracture is more complex, additional exposure is necessary. The second incision is made just medial to the medial gutter, also in longitudinal fashion. Occult separations of the medial epiphysis are sought.

Anatomic restoration of the distal tibial epiphysis is accomplished next. In the case of the three- or four-part fracture, reduction of the posterior metaphyseal flag is necessary for proper orientation. This is accomplished by anterior traction on the heel, with internal rotation of

the foot. A joker or elevator may be introduced through the sagittal fracture to aid in mobilization; this will usually allow for relocation of the free anterolateral fragment. If the fibula is fractured, it may be necessary to disengage the fibular fracture fragments in order to reduce the anterolateral piece and the posterior metaphyseal fragment. In rare instances interfragmentary screw or plate fixation of the fibula is indicated to aid in stabilizing the complex. We prefer the use of 3.5- or 4.0-mm cancellous cannulated screws across the epiphysis from medial to lateral into the free fragment. As will be discussed, growth disturbance in this injury is unusual, but protection of the physis and articular cartilage from iatrogenic injury is still prudent. With adequate visualization, noncannulated hardware can be used.

In the three- or four-part fracture there is only relative stability of the epiphyseal-metaphyseal junction. By virtue of transepiphyseal fixation and the presence of an intact fibula, the tendency for migration is lessened. However we recommend fixation of the reduced epiphyseal complex to the metaphysis. Some authors recommend screw fixation from anterior to posterior through the metaphyseal flag, but we prefer obliquely driven Kirschner wires that cross the physis. These are introduced from the medial side, usually through the medial malleolus (Fig. 22-22). Metaphyseal to epiphyseal fixation is definitely required if the fibula is fractured and is not fixed. Careful analysis of fracture geometry may dictate the use of additional fixation on an individual basis.

Postoperative management of this injury consists of a non-weight-bearing short leg cast for 3 to 4 weeks followed by a weight-bearing short leg cast for an additional 3 to 4 weeks. Hardware removal is usually indicated at 4 to 6 weeks for the transphyseal Kirschner wires and at 3 months for transepiphyseal hardware. We prefer to leave all hardware in place for 3 to 4 months and to remove it in one surgical session.

## Complications of Triplane Fractures

Complications from the triplane injury are uncommon. This is primarily due to the fact this is a transitional fracture, and aberrations of the usually vulnerable growth plate are negligible by virtue of the usual age of the patients.[39,48] It should be noted that occurrence of this fracture almost always precipitates complete closure of the growth plate, which in all likelihood is caused

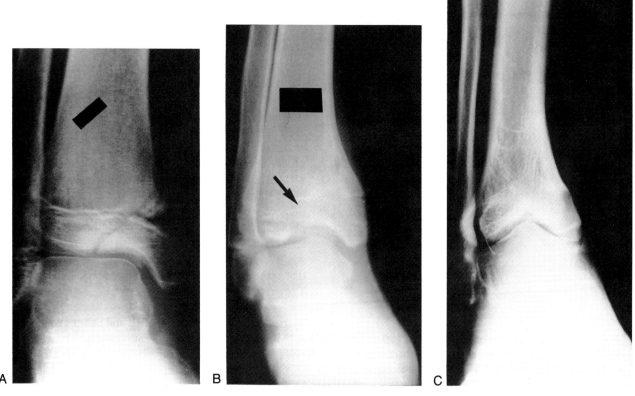

**Fig. 22-24.** (A) Salter IV injury of the medial tibial epiphysis, which was treated non operatively, in a 12-year-old boy. (B) Severe resultant varus angular deformity, which developed 14 months after injury. Note the transphyseal bridge (arrow) that developed in the area of physeal disruption. (C) Severe varus angulation deformity in a young man in his twenties who had suffered a medial physeal fracture as a child.

supply of the germinal cell layer of the physis, or occult damage to the epiphysis and metaphysis.[71] Bars that are relatively small initially may proliferate and manifest as problems only after subsequent enlargement. Transphyseal bars usually result in varus and valgus angular deformities. As already discussed, the greater the potential for growth, the greater the potential for an untoward result. Without follow-up treatment even the slightest incongruities will be progressive.

Salter V injuries to the foot and ankle are uncommon; there is even some question as to whether this type of injury exists at all.[72] However, there is at least some evidence that growth arrest does occur after some injuries without immediate radiographic evidence of physeal injury.[73] The most common manifestation is that of progressive limb length discrepancy. There may be a con-

comitant angular component to the deformity, which results from asymmetric loading of the physis. Other patterns of physeal injury, both within and outside the Salter-Harris classification, may occur simultaneously. The deformity may evolve in a totally unexpected direction, and therefore the solution to the problem may not become evident until sufficient time has passed. Treatment should not commence until the pattern of deformity is well established. However, one should not wait indefinitely and waste valuable growth potential for correction of the problem.

Complications following the uncommon type VI injury are actually quite frequent. They usually result either from burns or from open fractures in which the foot is abraded against the pavement; less common mechanisms include infection and iatrogenic causes. Once the able, immediate open reduction can take place without a CT scan. This is recommended only when the radiographic profile suggests a relatively simple fracture configuration and the surgeon is experienced in the operative management of this injury.

Postreduction management consists of a long leg cast with the foot internally rotated for 3 to 4 weeks, followed by a short leg weight-bearing cast for another 3 to 4 weeks. Careful inspection of interim radiographs is necessary as alterations in the treatment plan may become necessary if displacement occurs.

*Open Reduction*

If open reduction is indicated, it should be performed as soon as possible after the injury. Thorough preoperative planning based on scrutiny of CT or conventional tomograms will allow treatment to progress smoothly. Anticipation of the fracture configurations will facilitate precise intraoperative technique. However, subtle separations of the epiphysis may be seen only during intraoperative inspection of the fragments.

A two-incision approach is often indicated in order to completely visualize the pathology. We recommend this approach in all cases unless there is absolutely no doubt that the surgeon is dealing with a "simple" two-part fracture, in which case a single anterolateral approach is sufficient. The first incision is made over the tibiofibular junction in longitudinal fashion. The anterior muscle group is retracted medially, along with the vital structures. Once the fracture line has been identified in the epiphysis, the foot is externally rotated to disimpact the fracture and allow for excavation of the gap. Often the periosteal sleeve will occupy this position, and it can be carefully removed. The extent of the anterolateral piece of epiphysis can also be identified. If the injury is clearly a two-part fracture, a manipulative reduction is performed and fixation is introduced in the same fashion as in the operative management of the Tillaux fracture. If the fracture is more complex, additional exposure is necessary. The second incision is made just medial to the medial gutter, also in longitudinal fashion. Occult separations of the medial epiphysis are sought.

Anatomic restoration of the distal tibial epiphysis is accomplished next. In the case of the three- or four-part fracture, reduction of the posterior metaphyseal flag is necessary for proper orientation. This is accomplished by anterior traction on the heel, with internal rotation of the foot. A joker or elevator may be introduced through the sagittal fracture to aid in mobilization; this will usually allow for relocation of the free anterolateral fragment. If the fibula is fractured, it may be necessary to disengage the fibular fracture fragments in order to reduce the anterolateral piece and the posterior metaphyseal fragment. In rare instances interfragmentary screw or plate fixation of the fibula is indicated to aid in stabilizing the complex. We prefer the use of 3.5- or 4.0-mm cancellous cannulated screws across the epiphysis from medial to lateral into the free fragment. As will be discussed, growth disturbance in this injury is unusual, but protection of the physis and articular cartilage from iatrogenic injury is still prudent. With adequate visualization, noncannulated hardware can be used.

In the three- or four-part fracture there is only relative stability of the epiphyseal-metaphyseal junction. By virtue of transepiphyseal fixation and the presence of an intact fibula, the tendency for migration is lessened. However we recommend fixation of the reduced epiphyseal complex to the metaphysis. Some authors recommend screw fixation from anterior to posterior through the metaphyseal flag, but we prefer obliquely driven Kirschner wires that cross the physis. These are introduced from the medial side, usually through the medial malleolus (Fig. 22-22). Metaphyseal to epiphyseal fixation is definitely required if the fibula is fractured and is not fixed. Careful analysis of fracture geometry may dictate the use of additional fixation on an individual basis.

Postoperative management of this injury consists of a non-weight-bearing short leg cast for 3 to 4 weeks followed by a weight-bearing short leg cast for an additional 3 to 4 weeks. Hardware removal is usually indicated at 4 to 6 weeks for the transphyseal Kirschner wires and at 3 months for transepiphyseal hardware. We prefer to leave all hardware in place for 3 to 4 months and to remove it in one surgical session.

## Complications of Triplane Fractures

Complications from the triplane injury are uncommon. This is primarily due to the fact this is a transitional fracture, and aberrations of the usually vulnerable growth plate are negligible by virtue of the usual age of the patients.[39,48] It should be noted that occurrence of this fracture almost always precipitates complete closure of the growth plate, which in all likelihood is caused

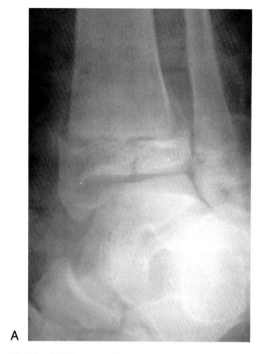
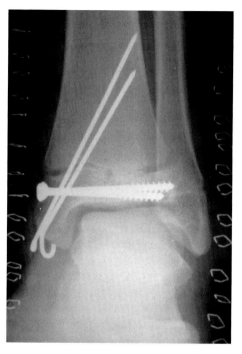

A

B

**Fig. 22-22. (A)** Preoperative anteroposterior radiograph showing a four-part triplane fracture, as evidenced by the separation of the medial epiphysis and metaphysis. Note the intra-articular displacement. **(B)** Postoperative anteroposterior radiograph showing the transepiphyseal screw fixation and transphyseal Kirschner wire fixation. The intra-articular displacement has been reduced.

by a combination of natural progression and post-traumatic influences. Very small and insignificant limb length discrepancies may result.

However, intra-articular defects are definitely areas of concern with regard to post-traumatic arthrosis. In many respects the attention to anatomic reduction in the pediatric patient should be no less than that afforded the adult patient. Most surgeons would not hesitate to operate on a displaced intra-articular fracture in adults under a certain arbitrary age. The vast majority of reported complications from this injury are the consequences of unrecognized or untreated intra-articular deficits.[27,46,60,64,65] These reports only vaguely describe the complication as arthrosis. Most of the children with complications experienced aching pain in the involved ankle. No specific mention of disabling degenerative arthritis is noted in the literature. Perhaps longer follow-up is needed to accurately assess the effects of malunited triplane fracture. The usual guideline of following growth plate injuries to skeletal maturity may be insufficient in this injury (Fig. 22-23).

## COMPLICATIONS OF PHYSEAL INJURIES

Complications resulting from injuries involving the growth plates about the ankle can have significant consequences. In general, the earlier the injury occurs in the patient's life, the more significant will be the complication. This is because disturbances of the growth plate have more time to manifest as deformities and subsequent functional deficits. On the other hand, the additional time may allow for potential remodeling of growth disturbances once treatment is initiated. Many of these complications can be avoided with strict adherence to the treatment principles for physeal fractures, but others may occur largely as a consequence of the injury regardless of treatment.

The distal tibia and fibula are particularly vulnerable to growth arrest resulting from high-energy trauma, which often occurs in lower extremity injuries. The complex geometry and mechanics of the ankle joint also contribute to the consequences of seemingly minor growth

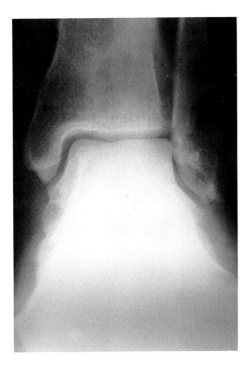

**Fig. 22-23.** Anteroposterior radiograph of patient in Fig. 22-21, 4 years after open reduction and internal fixation. Physeal closure occurred shortly after the original injury. There are no signs of early degenerative change.

aberrations. Most of the complications reported in the literature involve the medial side of the distal tibial epiphysis. This is in part due to the fact that if the medial aspect can be fractured, the tibial physis has not yet begun to close. In the second place, the common supinatory mechanism of ankle injury in children usually involves the medial structures. If only the lateral aspect is injured, the injury is usually a transitional fracture in an older child with some degree of antecedent physeal closure. When the fibular physis is involved, it is usually as a result of rotational or avulson-type injuries. Therefore transphyseal injuries to the fibula are rare. Usually very little axial load is imparted to the fibula, in contradistinction to tibial injuries.

Growth disturbances fall into four different categories, each with its own prognostic factors. The resultant deformity can be in the frontal plane (varus or valgus), the sagittal plane (equinus or calcaneus), or the transverse plane (rotational deformity), or can be a limb length discrepancy. Avascular necrosis of the distal tibial

epiphysis[67] and degenerative arthritis of the ankle are extremely rare sequelae of injury to the ankle.

It is generally accepted that the higher the Salter-Harris classification number, the higher the potential for complication. Salter I injuries rarely result in growth disturbance. Residual rotational deformities may result if the tibia or fibula is reduced in a nonanatomic position, but this is unlikely in the ankle unless there is concomitant fracture of the adjacent bone. Although both bones are frequently fractured, the residual rotation of the foot would be obvious in a malreduced position. Salter II injuries to the distal tibia are also expected to heal well without significant growth disturbancs. However Spiegel et al.[27] found that the actual occurrence of complications was related more to the amount of residual displacement than to the type of injury. These authors further indicated that the Salter II fractures in their study were all treated without open intervention and that some of the fractures were inadequately reduced. They concluded that anatomic reduction will decrease the incidence of angular growth deformities in Salter II injuries of the distal tibia. Salter III and Salter IV injuries entail significant risk of complication because these injuries are both intra-articular and transphyseal. This implies that there is a discontinuity of the physis, resulting in epiphyseal to metaphyseal bone contact. Without reduction the fracture gap can be expected to fill in with bone,[31] which will cause the metaphysis to become fused to the epiphysis. The larger the gap, the larger the bridge becomes. Although the physis of the displaced fragment will continue to grow,[68-70] the adjacent bridge serves as a hinge, and the growth will be asymmetric and angular (Fig. 22-24).

Spiegel and colleagues[27] suggest that the upper acceptable tolerance of displacement is 2 mm. However, others have suggested that only anatomic reduction is acceptable. The exact amount of displacement may show a spurious decrease on plain radiographs owing to projectional differences. One may inadvertently accept displacement that appears to be less than 2 mm but in actuality is more significant. The use of CT or plain tomography may clarify the exact amount of potential morbidity in questionable cases.

In spite of precise anatomic operative reduction some patients will develop growth disturbances. This suggests that there must be multiple types of physeal damage leading to formation of a bar. This may include unrecognized damage to the physeal cells, damage to the blood

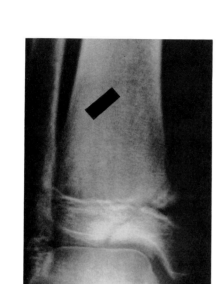
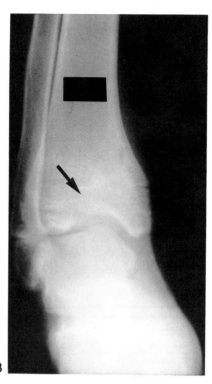
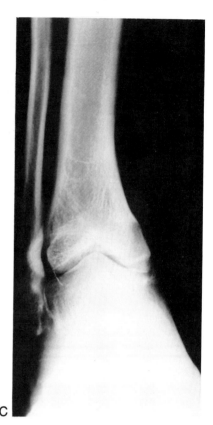

A                         B                          C

**Fig. 22-24.** **(A)** Salter IV injury of the medial tibial epiphysis, which was treated non operatively, in a 12-year-old boy. **(B)** Severe resultant varus angular deformity, which developed 14 months after injury. Note the transphyseal bridge (arrow) that developed in the area of physeal disruption. **(C)** Severe varus angulation deformity in a young man in his twenties who had suffered a medial physeal fracture as a child.

supply of the germinal cell layer of the physis, or occult damage to the epiphysis and metaphysis.[71] Bars that are relatively small initially may proliferate and manifest as problems only after subsequent enlargement. Transphyseal bars usually result in varus and valgus angular deformities. As already discussed, the greater the potential for growth, the greater the potential for an untoward result. Without follow-up treatment even the slightest incongruities will be progressive.

Salter V injuries to the foot and ankle are uncommon; there is even some question as to whether this type of injury exists at all.[72] However, there is at least some evidence that growth arrest does occur after some injuries without immediate radiographic evidence of physeal injury.[73] The most common manifestation is that of progressive limb length discrepancy. There may be a con-

comitant angular component to the deformity, which results from asymmetric loading of the physis. Other patterns of physeal injury, both within and outside the Salter-Harris classification, may occur simultaneously. The deformity may evolve in a totally unexpected direction, and therefore the solution to the problem may not become evident until sufficient time has passed. Treatment should not commence until the pattern of deformity is well established. However, one should not wait indefinitely and waste valuable growth potential for correction of the problem.

Complications following the uncommon type VI injury are actually quite frequent. They usually result either from burns or from open fractures in which the foot is abraded against the pavement; less common mechanisms include infection and iatrogenic causes. Once the

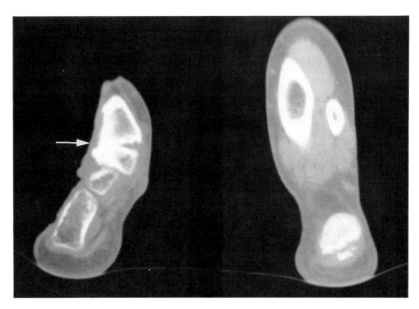

**Fig. 22-25.** CT scan through an ankle joint in a 6-year-old patient, the lateral aspect of whose foot was abraded in an automobile accident 9 months prior. The fibula was destroyed, and the lateral perichondrial ring was damaged. Note the resultant peripheral bridge of the lateral aspect of the tibia (arrow).

perichondrial ring is damaged, peripherally based physeal bars are quite common (Fig. 22-25). This usually results in marked angular deformity that are due to the geometry of the situation. There a very long lever arm emanating from the tethered point at the periphery of the physis, and therefore progressive angular deformities occur rapidly.

## Treatment

Treatment of the complications associated with physeal injuries requires a thorough understanding of the principles discussed in Chapters 20 and 22. Prompt recognition of the complication may enable the surgeon to take advantage of any remaining growth potential and actually correct the resultant deformity. In rarer instances it is better to wait until skeletal maturity has occurred before addressing the deformity. Careful analysis of the remaining amount of growth will dictate the best treatment scheme. Only experience and careful application of the physiologic process will permit optimal correction of these complications.

Often two or more techniques may need to be applied because the resultant deformities are multiplanar. Over-

all length insufficiency combined with angular deformity may require correction of both components, but simultaneous resolution of both is often impossible unless several techniques are utilized. The procedures may be carried out concurrently or in separate surgical sessions, depending on the individual case.

### Limb Length Inequalities

A limb length discrepancy may develop as an isolated event or may appear in conjunction with an angular or rotational deformity. Some physeal fractures result in premature closure of the plate, and a leg length inequality ensues without other sequelae.

In the child with isolated leg length inequality, contralateral epiphysiodesis is often the procedure of choice. Factors such as the child's expected height, bone age, and chronological age all play important roles in the selection of the proper procedure. Because more longitudinal growth proceeds from sites about the knee joint, larger discrepancies are often treated at that level. Smaller inequalities may be addressed at the level of the contralateral ankle. When only one bone of the ankle is involved in the injury, epiphysiodesis of the contralateral limb must be accompanied by arrest of the adjacent bone of the injured ankle in order to prevent subsequent development of a new angular deformity.

Lengthening procedures are technically more demanding and more prone to complications but may be offered to the child of predictably shorter stature or one who will not accept any further growth retardation. As experience is gained with the bone transport techniques of Ilizarov, these problems may be more amenable to lengthening procedures.

## Angular Deformities

In the child with an angular deformity following partial growth arrest, the question of whether treatment is indicated must first be addressed. Small deviations from each of the cardinal body planes are probably well tolerated.[21,24,33,36,39,74,75] In fact, we have observed several

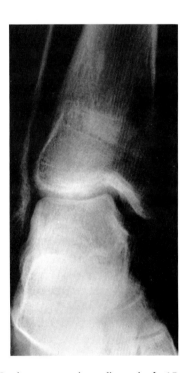

**Fig. 22-26.** Anteroposterior radiograph of a 15-year-old boy who had sustained a Salter-Harris IV fracture of the distal tibia with initial nonoperative treatment 3 years before (same patient as in Fig. 22-24A). Subsequent opening wedge grafting left a 20-degree varus deformity of the ankle. The patient functioned quite well in spite of the deformity and was able to play high school football.

patients with angular deformities due to fractures that occurred many years previously who had minimal locomotor difficulties (Fig. 22-26). Certainly some remodeling can take place, especially in the sagittal plane deviations. Karrholm et al.[75] have demonstrated changes in the migration of the distal aspect of the fibula in response to angular deformities, which were mediated through the distal tibial epiphysis. This intrinsic physiologic mechanism can often spontaneously correct an angular deformity. The process is believed to be controlled through differential growth of the proximal fibular epiphysis and a response to traction of the lateral ankle ligaments on the distal fibula. These processes however, are age-dependent. Currently, significant angular deformities are probably best treated by corrective procedures until further long-term studies of patients with such deformities are published.

The management of angular deformities can be quite complex, especially during the period of continued growth. Generally the treatment can be conservative, taking the form of orthoses and benign neglect, or surgical, by means of osteotomy, bridge resection, or selected epiphysiodesis of the same ankle or adjacent bone.

### Osteotomy

Osteotomy can be performed at any time after the complication is recognized. Although growth may be available at the physis and the deformity may subsequently worsen, realignment of the articular surface and redirection of weight-bearing forces may influence further development in the direction of correcting the deformity. Early surgery may serve to prevent premature arthrosis, but there is no conclusive long-term evidence to support this view. If substantial growth remains, osteotomy could be combined with physeal bridge resection. If growth potential is slight, correction should be aimed at maintenance of normal articular orientation to the supporting surface as well as establishment of normal tibiofibular relationships.

In most cases the osteotomy should be of the opening wedge type because of the need to restore length to the limb. Even if there is no excessive shortening, preservation of existing length is paramount. Preoperative assessment of leg length, including segmental radiographic measurements, are important in attaining the optimal result. We favor the use of corticocancellous bone grafts in these cases (Fig. 22-27). When large degrees of

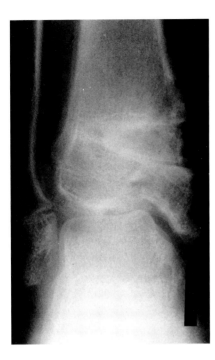

**Fig. 22-27.** Postoperative radiograph showing insertion of iliac crest corticocancellous graft after tibial osteotomy (cf. Fig. 22-24B). Note the improvement of the angular position of the distal tibial articular surface.

correction are necessary, allograft may be necessary because of the difficulty in obtaining large solitary portions of autograft. When small amounts of bone graft are required, we prefer to use autogenous bone from the iliac crest.

*Bridge Resection*

The excision of physeal bars with interposition of inert material is an intriguing concept. This technique has been fairly well studied in animal models and to a slightly lesser extent in human subjects. In the first clinical case, reported by Langenskiold[76,77] genu recurvatum was corrected by the use of an interposition fat graft. Several other interposition materials have been used with varying degrees of effectiveness; these include Silastic,[78] bone wax,[69] cranioplast,[79] cartilage,[80] and methyl methacrylate.[81,82] Each particular material has its own advantages and disadvantages, although not all have been used in a clinical setting.[79]

The indications for surgical resection of transphyseal

bars of the foot and ankle are fairly narrow. The general guidelines have been discussed above, but it should be stressed that the amount of expected deformity and morbidity without treatment should always be considered since nontreatment may be an acceptable alternative in some cases. The most important consideration is that of the skeletal age of the child. The earlier the attempt to reverse the aberrant physiologic process, the more time there is for the corrective procedure to eliminate the deformity. Once the growth process has been normalized by a surgical procedure, the usual mechanisms of physeal function can proceed. Contrarily, there is more potential for an unsuitable angular deformity to occur. Other considerations include the shape and contour of the physis, the shape of the bar, and the size of the bridge. It is generally accepted that bridges over 50 percent of the surface area of the physis cannot be treated by resection and are best treated by corrective osteotomy.

The principles of bridge resection must be followed in order to ensure optimal results from this difficult and challenging procedure. Complete resection of the bar is mandatory; however, preservation of as much of the normal physis, which is only possible with precise preoperative planning and imaging of the bar, is also desirable. Specific mapping of the extent of the bar and the location of the lesion in the epiphysis is essential prior to the operation. This can be done through a variety of imaging techniques. Although plain radiographs can provide essential information regarding the location of the bar, they usually cannot delineate the exact topography of the bar. Tomography has long been the standard in evaluating the extent of the bar. Although variations in technique may be utilized for the tomographic image,[77,79,83,84] it is generally accepted that plain tomography is inadequate for accurate mapping of the physeal bridge. More recently, CT has been shown to provide accurate representations of the extent of the bar[85] (Fig. 22-28). Assessment of leg length is also important in determining the need for additional procedures; preoperative scanograms are mandatory to assess discrepancies. Finally, bone age should be determined when there is any question of the remaining growth potential or when there is any gross disparity between physiologic age and chronological age.

The surgical approach is determined by analysis of the location of the bar and its configuration. Peripheral bridges are best directly resected from the side of the

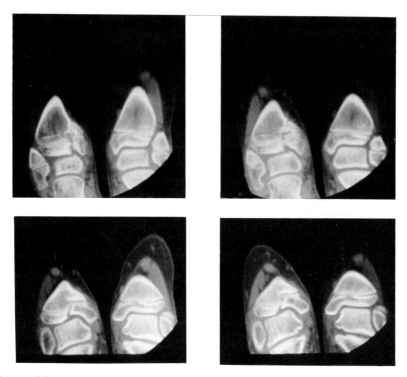

**Fig. 22-28.** CT scan of four representative sequential sections through the ankle joint showing the extent of the physeal bridge. The left upper quadrant is the posterior aspect of the ankle, and the right lower quadrant is the anterior aspect of the joint. The bridge, extending from the anterior aspect of the talus to the posterior aspect, is relatively narrow.

bone (Fig. 22-29). Visualization should be relatively good. A rotating burr can be used to resect the bar completely until normal physis is visualized. Magnification may be useful to improve the ability to distinguish normal from abnormal tissue. Copious irrigation is necessary during the process in order to improve visualization and avoid overzealous resection of the physis. This will also allow for heat dissipation, although no real harmful effect to the physis from heat has been demonstrated.

Centrally located bars are more difficult because of the problem of exposure. They are best approached from the metaphyseal side of the bar in order not to violate the articular surface or the perichondrial ring of Ranvier, although this approach is theoretically suboptimal because it is best to not leave any interposition material in the metaphyseal side if possible. A cortical window is made in the metaphysis in a location predetermined by the physeal map. Bone is removed from the metaphysis until the physis is reached, and additional bone is then

removed until the normal physis is seen circumferentially around the entire cavity. Visualization is aided by flexible fiberoptic surgical lights and in some cases by small dental mirrors. Once the proper amount of bone has been resected, the cavity is filled with the material of choice. Whatever substance is used should be confined to the epiphyseal side of the cavity in order to allow for the physeal cells to migrate over the inert substrate and produce additional metaphyseal bone (Fig. 22-30).

Peterson[79] contends that metal markers should be placed in the cancellous bone so that postoperative correction can be monitored. Correction of angular deformity can also be monitored with Kirschner wires placed in the respective sides of the bar. Either technique will allow early reoperation if the bar grows back and will also tell the surgeon whether or not there has been spontaneous compensation of the discrepancy by overgrowth of a more distant physis. Although some of the advantages of monitoring the early response may have limited value except in an academic setting, analysis of

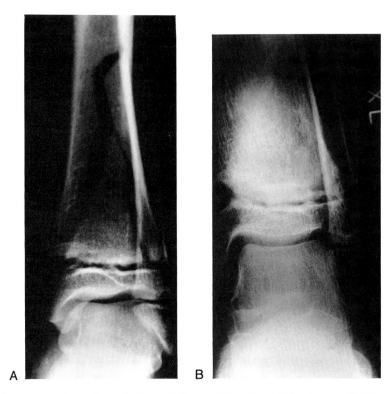

**Fig. 22-29.** (A) Anteroposterior radiograph of a grade II open Salter-Harris II fracture in which the perichondrial ring was damaged. At the time of initial debridement the injured portion of the physis was resected. (B) Follow-up radiograph 6 months after the injury showing adequate gap between the epiphysis and metaphysis. There is no evidence of growth disturbance.

large numbers of cases will permit optimal results for those surgeons performing only a few of these procedures.

Postoperative care for these patients depends on the amount of destabilization of the bone and an analysis of force vectors. Generally, structural integrity is not sufficiently weakened to preclude early weight-bearing, but in some cases significant stress risers may be created to preclude immediate weight-bearing. Cavities filled with methyl methacrylate are usually stronger than those filled with other materials. Long-term follow-up until physeal closure has occurred is mandatory, as these bars may re-form in the later stages of skeletal maturity.

### Partial Epiphysiodeses

There are relatively few indications for the isolated use of partial epiphysiodesis because most deformities that warrant correction result from injuries occurring well before skeletal maturity. The necessary maintenance of limb length cannot be accomplished with partial epiphysiodesis in the younger age group.

Partial epiphysiodesis to correct an angular deformity has a limited window of time in which it can be performed effectively. It is best utilized in the child who has a mild to moderate deformity and only a few years of growth left; this will minimize the limb-shortening effect of the procedure. However, this procedure can often be applied in conjunction with several growth arrest strategies to optimize the result in the growing child. The remaining growth of the involved physis can be arrested in the child who only has a few years of growth left and in whom the resultant limb length discrepancy will be minimal. This can be combined with complete growth arrest of the accompanying bone of the ankle. If these procedures are performed at an age at which significant growth potential remains, arrest of the contralateral physes should also be considered.

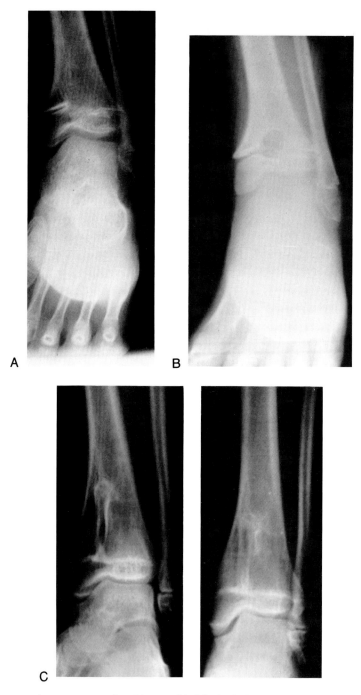

**Fig. 22-30.** (A) Preoperative tomogram of an 11-year-old girl who had sustained a Salter IV fracture of the medial tibial epiphysis 1 year previously. There is partial closure on the medial side. (B) Immediate postoperative radiograph demonstrating the cortical window made in the metaphyseal region. The bridge was resected, and the defect was filled with fat. (C) Radiograph at 18 months postsurgery, showing resolution of the deformity and absence of the bar. Note the apparent migration of the defect as the physis continues to grow normally.

The procedure itself is relatively benign, with a low incidence of complications. In the setting of angular deformity, timing of the procedure is more difficult than with complete growth arrest but on the other hand is less critical. Estimation of the final angular deformity and the exact age at skeletal maturity is critical for accurate results, but this is difficult even without a bony transphyseal bridge. The asymmetric growth within the same physis makes it clearly unpredictable in the traumatically induced setting. However, under- or overcorrection is seldom clinically significant and can be addressed with a secondary procedure.

# REFERENCES

1. Landin LA, Danielsson LG: Children's ankle fractures. Classification and epidemiology. Acta Orthop Scand 54:634, 1983
2. Carothers CO, Crenshaw AH: Clinical significance of a classification of epiphyseal injuries at the ankle. Am J Surg 89:879, 1955
3. Rogers LF: The radiography of epiphyseal injuries. Radiology 96:289, 1970
4. Boissevain ACH, Raymakers ELFB: Traumatic injury of the distal tibial epiphysis. An appraisal of forty cases. Reconstr Surg Traumatol 17:40, 1979
5. Peterson CA, Peterson HA: Analysis of the incidence of injuries to the epiphyseal growth plate. J Trauma 12:275, 1972
6. Bisgard JD, Martenson L: Fractures in children. Surg Gynecol Obstet 65:464, 1972
7. Lipschultz O: The end results of injuries to the epiphyses. Radiology 28:223, 1937
8. Compere EL: Growth arrest in long bones as a result of fractures that included the epiphysis. JAMA 105:2140, 1935
9. Ashhurst APC, Bromer RS: Classification and mechanism of fractures of the leg bones involving the ankle. Arch Surg 4:51, 1922
10. Bishop PA: Fractures and epiphyseal separation fractures of the ankle. A classification of three hundred and thirty two cases according to the mechanism of their production. AJR 28:49, 1932
11. Crenshaw AH: Injuries to the distal tibial epiphysis. Clin Orthop 41:98, 1965
12. Lauge-Hansen N: Fractures of the ankle. II: Combined experimental surgical and experimental roentgenologic investigations. Arch Surg 67:57, 1950
13. Danis R: Les Fractures Malléolaires. Théorie et Pratique de l'Ostéosynthese. Masson, Paris, 1949
14. Weber BG: Die Verletzungen des Sprunggelenkes. Aktuelle Probleme in der Chirugie. Hans-Huber, Bern, 1966
15. Gerner-Smidt M: Ankelbrud has Born. Thesis. Nyt Nordisk Forlag, Copenhagen, 1963
16. Dias LS, Tachdjian MO: Physeal injuries of the ankle in children. Clin Orthop 136:230, 1978
17. Gross RH: Ankle fractures in children. Bull N Y Acad Med 63:739, 1987
18. Dias LS: Fractures of the distal tibial and fibular physes. p. 1014. In Rockwood CA Jr, Wilkins KE, King RE (eds): Fractures in Children. JB Lippincott, Philadelphia, 1984
19. Lovell ES: An unusual rotatory injury of the ankle. J Bone Joint Surg [AM] 50:163, 1968
20. DeValentine SJ: Evaluation and treatment of ankle fractures. Clin Podiatr Med Surg 2:235, 1985
21. Karrholm J, Hansson LI, Laurin S: Supination adduction injuries of the ankle in children. Radiographic classification and treatment. Arch Orthop Trauma Surg 101:193, 1983
22. Salter RB: Injuries of the ankle in children. Orthop Clin North Am 5:1, 1974
23. Blount WP: Fractures in Children. Williams & Wilkins, Baltimore, 1958
24. Kärrholm J, Hansson LI, Selvik G: Roentgen stereophotogrammetric analysis of growth pattern after supination-adduction ankle injuries in children. J Pediatr Orthop 2:271, 1982
25. MacNealy GA, Rogers LF, Hernandez R et al: Injuries of the distal tibial epiphysis: systematic radiographic evaluation. AJR 138:683, 1982
26. Kling TF, Bright RW, Hensinger RN: Distal tibial physeal fractures that may require open reduction. J Bone Joint Surg [Am] 66:647, 1984
27. Spiegel PG, Cooperman DR, Laros GS: Epiphyseal fractures of the distal end of the tibia and fibula. A retrospective study of two hundrd and thirty seven cases in children. J Bone Joint Surg [Am] 60:1046, 1978
28. Johnson EW, Fahl JC: Fractures involving the distal epiphysis of the tibia and fibula in children. Am J Surg 93:778, 1957
29. Landin LA, Danielsson LG, Jonsson K et al: Late results in 65 physeal ankle fractures. Acta Orthop Scand 57:530, 1986
30. Bright RW: Physeal injuries. In Rockwood CA, Wilkins KE, King RE (eds): Fractures in Children. JB Lippincott, Philadelphia, 1984
31. Salter RB, Harris WR: Injuries involving the epiphyseal plate. J Bone Joint Surg [AM] 45:587, 1963
32. Bright RW, Burstein AH, Elmore SM: Epiphyseal plate cartilage. J Bone Joint Surg [AM] 56:588, 1974
33. Karrholm J, Hansson LI, Laurin S: Pronation injuries of the ankle in children. Retrospective study and radiological classification and treatment. Acta Orthop Scand 54:1, 1983

34. Cameron HU: A radiologic sign of lateral subluxation of the distal tibial epiphysis. J Trauma 15:1030, 1975
35. Weber BG, Sussenbach F: Malleolar fractures. p. 350. In Weber BG, Brunner CH, Freuler F (eds): Treatment of Fractures in Children and Adolescents. Springer-Verlag, Berlin, 1980
36. Karrholm J, Hansson LI, Laurin S: Supination-eversion injuries of the ankle in children: a restrospective study of radiographic classification and treatment. J Pediatr Orthop 2:147, 1982
37. Lauge-Hansen N: Ankelbrud. Munksgaard, Copenhagen, 1942
38. Thomasen E: Ankelbrud. Om der genetiske diagnose or reposition; Hansen N. Et kritisk referat. Nord Med 25:689, 1945
39. Karrholm J, Hansson LI, Selvik G: Roentgen stereophotogrammetric analysis of growth pattern after supination-eversion ankle injuries in children. J Pediatr Orthop 2:25, 1982
40. Broock GJ, Greer RB: Traumatic displacements of the distal tibial growth plate. J Bone Joint Surg [AM] 52:1666, 1970
41. Nevalos AB, Colton CL: Rotational displacement of the lower tibial epiphysis due to trauma. J Bone Joint Surg [AM] 59:331, 1977
42. Henke JA, Kiple DL: Rotational displacement of the distal tibial epiphysis without fibular fracture. J Trauma 19:64, 1979
43. Koval KJ, Lehman WB, Koval RP: Rotational injury of the distal tibial physis. Orthop Rev 9:987, 1989
44. Kleiger B, Mankin HJ: Fracture of the lateral portion of the distal tibial epiphysis. J Bone Joint Surg [AM] 46:25, 1964
45. Tillaux PJ: Traité d'Anatomie Topographique avec Applications à la Chirugie. Asselin et Hozeau, Paris,1892
46. Dias LS, Giegerich C: Fractures of the distal tibial epiphysis in adolescence. J Bone Joint Surg [Am] 65:438, 1983
47. Tachdjian MO: The Child's Foot. WB Saunders, Philadelphia, 1985
48. Von Laer L: Classification, diagnosis, and treatment of transitional fractures of the distal part of the tibia. J Bone Joint Surg [Am] 67:687, 1985
49. Molster A, Soreiide O, Solhaugh JH et al: Fractures of the lateral part of the distal tibial epiphysis (Tillaux or Kleiger fracture). Injury 8:260, 1977
50. Britton PD: Adolescent-type Tillaux fracture of the ankle: two case reports. Arch Emerg Med 5:180, 1988
51. Spinella AJ, Turco VJ: Avulsion fracture of the distal tibial epiphysis in skeletally immature athletes (juvenile Tillaux fracture). Orthop Rev 12:1245, 1988
52. Stefanich RJ, Lozman J: The juvenile fracture of Tillaux. Clin Orthop 210:219, 1986
53. DeValentine SJ: Foot and ankle fractures in children. p.

473. In Scurran BL (ed): Foot and Ankle Trauma. Churchill Livingstone, New York, 1989
54. Yao J, Huurman WW: Tomography in a juvenile Tillaux fracture. J Pediatr Orthop 6:349, 1986
55. Dingeman RD, Shaver GB: Operative treatment of displaced Salter Harris III distal tibial fractures. Clin Orthop 135:101, 1978
56. Lynn MD: The triplane distal epiphyseal fracture. Clin Orthop 86:187, 1972
57. Marmor L: An unusual fracture of the tibial epiphysis. Clin Orthop 73:132, 1970
58. Rang M: Children's Fractures. JB Lippincott, Philadelphia, 1974
59. Karrholm J, Hansson LI, Laurin S: Computed tomography of intraarticular supination-eversion fractures in adolescents. J Pediatr Orthop 1:181, 1981
60. Cooperman DR, Spiegel PG, Laros GS: Tibial fractures involving the ankle in children. The so-called triplane epiphyseal fracture. J Bone Joint Surg [Am] 60:1040, 1978
61. Izant TH, Davidson RS: The four part triplane fracture: a case report of a new patten. Foot Ankle 10:170, 1989
62. Seitz WH, LaPorte J: Medial triplane fracture delineated by computerized axial tomography. J Pediatr Orthop 8:65, 1988
63. Denton JR, Fischer SJ: The medial triplane fracture: report of an unusual injury. J Trauma 21:991, 1981
64. Spiegel PG, Mast JW, Cooperman DR, Laros GS: Triplane fractures of the distal tibial epiphysis. Clin Orthop 188:74, 1984
65. Ertl JP, Barack RL, Alexander AH et al: Triplane fracture of the distal tibial epiphysis. Long term follow-up. J Bone Joint Surg [Am] 70:967, 1988
66. Beck E, Engler I: Zur Prognose der Epiphysenverletzungen am distalen Schienbeinende. Arch Orthop Trauma Surg 65:47, 1969
67. Ogden JA: Injury to the growth mechanisms of the immature skeleton. Skeletal Radiol 6:237, 1981
68. Barash ES, Siffert RC: The potential for growth of experimentally produced hemiepiphysis. J Bone Joint Surg [AM] 48:1548, 1966
69. Friedenberg ZB: Reaction of the epiphysis to partial surgical resection. J Bone Joint Surg 39:332, 1956
70. Friedenberg ZB, Brashear R: Bone growth following partial resection of the epiphyseal cartilage. Am J Surg 91:362, 1956
71. Cass JR, Peterson H: Salter-Harris type IV injuries of the distal tibial epiphyseal growth plate, with emphasis on those involving the medial malleolus. J Bone Joint Surg [Am] 65:1059, 1983
72. Peterson HA, Burkhart SS: Compression injury of the epiphyseal growth plate: fact or fiction? J Pediatr Orthop 1:377, 1981

73. Pozarny E, Kanat IO: Epiphyseal plate fracture: Salter and Harris type V. J Foot Surg 26:204, 1987

74. Kärrholm J, Hansson LI, Svensson K: Prediction of growth after ankle fractures in children. J Pediatr Orthop 3:319, 1983

75. Kärrholm J, Hansson LI, Selvik G: Changes in tibiofibular relationships due to growth disturbances after ankle fractured in children. J Bone Joint Surg [Am] 66:1198, 1984

76. Langenskiold A: The possibilities of eliminating premature partial closure of an epiphyseal plate caused by trauma or disease. Acta Orthop Scand 38:267, 1967

77. Langenskiold A: An operation for partial closure of an epiphyseal plate and its experimental basis. J Bone Joint Surg [Br] 57:325, 1975

78. Bright RW: Operative correction of partial epiphyseal plate closure by osseous-bridge resection and silicone rubber implant. J Bone Joint Surg [Am] 56:655, 1974

79. Peterson HA: Partial growth plate arrest and its treatment. J Pediatr Orthop 4:246, 1984

80. Oesterman K: Operative elimination of partial premature epiphyseal closure: an experimental study. Acta Orthop Scand Suppl 147:1, 1972

81. Vickers DW: Premature incomplete fusion of the growth plate: causes and treatment by resection (physolysis) in fifteen cases. Aust NZ J Surg 50:393, 1980

82. Mallet J: Les épiphysiodèses partielles traumatiques de l'extremetée inferieure du tibia chez l'enfant: leur traîtement avec désépiphysiodèse. Rev Chir Orthop 61:5, 1975

83. Bright RW: Partial growth arrest: identification, classification, and results of treatment, abstract ed. Orthop Trans 6:65, 1982

84. Langenskiold A: Surgical treatment of partial closure of the growth plate. J Pediatr Orthop 1:3, 1981

85. Porot S, Nyska A, Fields S: Assessment of bony bridge by computed tomography: experimental model in the rabbit and clinical application. J Pediatr Orthop 7:155, 1987

# 23
# Soft Tissue Trauma in Children

*BARRY L. SCURRAN*
*LAURI McDANIEL*

Management of pediatric trauma, like that of adult trauma, consists of establishing tissue homeostasis and aiding in the rapid return to normal function, which is best achieved by appropriate assessment and therapeutic intervention when indicated. Wound management begins with the emergent care of the entire patient, as soft tissue trauma affects a system of closely integrated metabolic and physiologic components. Certainly life-threatening injuries are addressed initially. Once the patient is medically stable, evaluation of soft tissue and other associated trauma can ensue.

Trauma to the foot and ankle more often than not involves more than just the soft tissues; therefore each specific tissue system must be evaluated and assessed. The primary principles of treatment include maintenance of adequate blood supply, realignment of osseous structures, appropriate and thorough debridement, prevention of infection, and finally restoration of skin coverage. The clinician's goal should be to restore anatomic structure and, most importantly, function while attempting to achieve cosmetically acceptable results. Children present special problems relating in part to the effect of trauma on growing bone and the potential for further or progressive deformity.[1]

## INCIDENCE OF TRAUMA IN CHILDREN

Accidents are the leading cause of death in children less than 14 years of age. Izart and Hubey[2] found that in 49 percent of all emergency room visits the patients were children. The most common injuries included lacerations (32 percent), contusions and abrasions (22 percent), and fractures and dislocations (8.7 percent). Falls accounted for 45 percent of the injuries, of which 71 percent occurred in the home or yard, and 43 percent resulted from sports injuries, with football being the most frequently responsible. Peterson and Peterson[3] reviewed 330 growth plate injuries seen in the Mayo Clinic and found that boys were injured more than twice as often as girls. The foot-ankle complex is one of the most frequently injured areas. It has been estimated that 12 percent of all injuries are of the ankle,[4] with a higher incidence reported in violent sports, ballet,[5] and motor vehicle accidents.[6] With the growing emphasis on sports and physical activities, the incidence of injuries to the extremities is increasing, being greater in nonorganized than in planned activities.[7]

## CLINICAL EVALUATION
### History

A thorough history can be useful in determining the extent of the wound and possible underlying damage. The history should include a description of the injury, the nature and time of injury, the object causing injury, the environment in which the injury occurred, the amount of blood loss, and any initial treatment rendered. The approximate time at which the child last ate should also be obtained in the event that surgery under general anesthesia is contemplated. Previous injuries, drug allergies, significant past medical history, and tetanus immunization status should also be determined.

577

## Physical Examination

Initial examination of the injury should include a thorough evaluation of neurovascular status before any anesthetic is given. Neurologic examinations may be particularly difficult in young children. The patency of the dorsalis pedis and posterior tibial vessels should be noted. If pulses are nonpalpable, a Doppler ultrasound evaluation should be made to assess patency. During the examination direct pressure hemostasis or use of a proximal tourniquet should be attempted to allow better visualization, with care taken not to induce further ischemic damage. If fracture, dislocation, or foreign body is suspected, radiographs should be taken and reviewed prior to any manipulation that might be required for accurate examination. Comparison views should be taken when indicated. Appropriate anesthesia should be achieved to allow detailed assessment without excessive discomfort to the patient. Sedation may be helpful in treating young children. Increased local tissue pressures and vasoconstriction often occur with the use of local anesthetics but can be minimized by peripheral nerve blocks or proximal infiltration with use of smallest effective dose of anesthesia without epinephrine. A Papoose or other restraint may be useful if an adequate evaluation cannot be accomplished. It should, however, not be used until all proximal traumatic involvement has been ruled out.

Prior to deep exploration, the skin is gently cleansed with a mild antiseptic. The wound is then explored with use of aseptic technique. Deep wound cultures and Gram stains should be obtained. The laboratory evaluations should include a complete blood count (CBC) and urinalysis and electrolyte determinations, with other specific laboratory data obtained when indicated.

## CLASSIFICATION

Several wound classification systems have been proposed,[8-10] including that of Rank[11] and Thompson,[12] who proposed four categories for wound classification: tidy (clean), untidy (contaminated), wounds with soft tissue loss, and infected wounds (Table 23-1). Injuries are also described according to the specific tissue damage involved.

A clean wound has minimal soft tissue damage and minimal contamination. Extensive debridement is generally not necessary prior to closure, as these wounds are

**Table 23-1. Wound Classification**

Tidy wound
  Surgical incision
  Laceration
Untidy wound
  Crush
  Avulsion
  Abrasion
Wound with tissue loss
  Excision
  Burn
  Ulcer
  Avulsion
Infected wound
  Established (cellulitis, lymphangitis, abscess, burn, vasculitis)
  Incipient (burn, contaminated wound, abrasion)

(From Noe JM, Kalish S: Wound Care. Chesebrough-Pond, Inc., Greenwich, CT, 1975,, with permission.)

not likely to become infected. Included in this category are those wounds that can be converted to "clean" by appropriate debridement and copious lavage. Incisions and lacerations without undue contamination are but a few examples. Clean wounds may be closed primarily (Fig. 23-1).

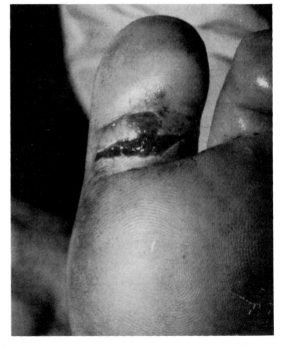

**Fig. 23-1.** Tidy, clean laceration. (From Scurran,[65] with permission.)

Contaminated wounds are associated with a higher degree of soft tissue damage and are more predisposed to infection (Fig. 23-2). A clean wound may become a contaminated wound if it is left exposed and untreated for longer than approximately 6 hours after the initial trauma owing to the amount of tissue desiccation and bacterial colonization potentially present. Factors that tend to increase the potential for wound infection include significant amounts of contamination or retained foreign or necrotic material, vascular compromise, extensive tissue loss, and excessive desiccation. Contaminated wounds should not be closed primarily unless they can be appropriately converted to clean wounds. Loose closure over a drain may be preferred, although removing a drain in a child may prove unpleasant to patient and physician alike.

Infected wounds are those that exhibit clinical signs of infection or gross contamination. Infected wounds are not closed until there is a clear transformation to a clean wound. This transformation involves the use of systemic antibiotics, debridement of all foreign bodies and necrotic tissue, and extensive local wound care until clinical signs of resolution, which may be supported by serial negative bacterial cultures. Skin grafting may be done, if indicated, once the infection has been resolved.

Wounds may also be described by their effect or action upon the skin and surrounding tissues (e.g., shearing, tearing), or they may be classified as open versus closed. They are considered closed when there has been no interruption of the skin; such wounds may be simple or complex and usually result from blunt trauma causing a contusion, compression, or crush injury. Variable amounts of ecchymosis and edema occur without external bleeding. Possible complications from closed injuries include hematoma and compartment syndrome.[13]

Open wounds include abrasions, lacerations, avulsions, degloving injuries, burns, gunshot wounds, and puncture wounds (Fig. 23-3). Abrasions are superficial wounds with only partial thickness loss, whereas a laceration is generally a full thickness injury. Avulsion and degloving injuries involve undermining through the subcutaneous plane tissue, with variable amounts of tissue loss.

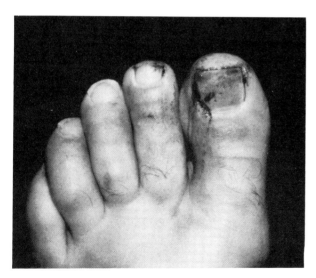

**Fig. 23-2.** Crush wound inflicted by 200-lb weight dropped on first and second digits. (From Scurran,[65] with permission.)

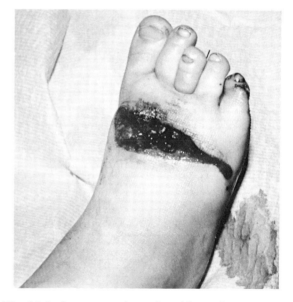

**Fig. 23-3.** Lawn mower laceration with associated tissue loss in a 22-month-old boy. Extensor tendons are repaired. (From Scurran,[65] with permission.)

## TREATMENT — GENERAL PRINCIPLES

Minor soft tissue trauma may be treated with ice, elevation, compression, and cleansing of superficial abrasions. Surgical debridement is performed to remove all devitalized tissue.[14] Only that tissue that is clearly nonviable, avascular, or necrotic is debrided. Hemostasis must be optimal. Bleeding vessels, once visualized and isolated, are cauterized or clamped and ligated. Atraumatic tissue handling is essential.[15] Skin edges should be retracted with sharp instruments rather than with blunt forceps or clamps, which may further damage devitalized tissues. Foreign debris and only very small, separate fragments of bone should be removed. Secondary debridement after demarcation of devitalized tissues may be necessary. Existing hematoma should be evacuated. The use of drains independent wound margins, wound packing to decrease dead space, and pressure dressings may be necessary to prevent further hematoma formation.

Thorough irrigation aids debridement, decreases wound flora, and is useful in preventing tissue desiccation. A topical irrigant will only remove surface flora, whereas jet lavage has been shown to decrease the number of bacteria in deeper tissues.[16] Strong antiseptics may be locally toxic to tissues, and their use is especially discouraged in children.[17] Most wounds remain to some degree contaminated after cleansing and irrigation, but not all become clinically infected. Children tend to become systemically ill quite rapidly, and the astute clinician continues treatment of all contaminated wounds until clinically resolved.

In summary, wound care principles necessary to decrease the likelihood of infection include the following: copious irrigation to decrease the bacterial count; adequate debridement to remove compromised, nonviable tissue and debris, and appropriate systemic antibiotics. Wounds suspected of contamination include those that are exposed for long periods of time and those with excessive soft tissue damage. Primary closure is generally not recommended in these instances. In children, sedation with treatment in an operative theater should be considered to decrease the psychological trauma of multiple interventions.

### Sequence of Treatment

The skin edges are thinly debrided, with care taken to preserve the subcutaneous layers unless they are already exposed. Muscle tissue is debrided until fresh bleeding occurs. The muscle may appear beefy red at first but turn dusky after 48 to 72 hours, necessitating serial debridement. An electrocautery device may also be utilized to assess tissue contractility. Tendons are identified and, if lacerated, either repaired primarily or tagged for delayed repair. Tendons may not need repair in some cases (e.g., lesser extensor digital tendons) as spontaneous repair with return of function is often noted (Fig. 23-3). Trauma to neurovascular structure should be clearly documented and immediately addressed when appropriate. Excessive debridement of small pieces of isolated bone is not necessary and may, in fact, hinder further osseous repair.

### Closure

Primary closure may be performed on clean wounds after gentle scrubbing with a mild antiseptic and water or other appropriate physiologic solution. Skin edges are reapproximated under minimal tension, the use of absorbable sutures being avoided when possible as they tend to lower local tissue resistance to infection. In children skin sutures should remain in the foot and leg for aproximately 14 days or up to 21 days on the plantar aspect of the foot or until clinically able to withstand the forces of weightbearing and gait. Of course, in the infant this becomes less of a factor.

Other types of closure include delayed primary closure, healing by secondary intention, coverage with skin grafts, and use of local or distant neurovascular flaps. Delayed primary closure is usually undertaken 4 to 6 days after the initial injury, when the viability of surrounding tissues has been established and the wound (when appropriately treated) can be considered clean. The technique is similar to that for primary closure. Contaminated or potentially contaminated wounds may be closed loosely over a dependent drain. Drains should be removed or changed every 24 to 48 hours until one is certain that wound healing has progressed satisfactorily without infection or complication. Again, sedation with or without restraint may be indicated in the tearful or uncooperative child.

## COMPARTMENT SYNDROME

Compartment syndrome is an increase in intracompartmental pressures resulting from excessive edema of the foot or leg. This can be secondary to a crush injury,

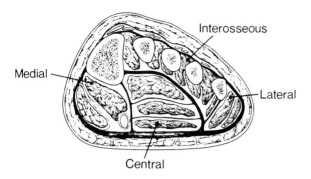

**Fig. 23-4.** Compartments of the foot, illustrated with their muscular contents through a coronary section at the level of the metatarsals base. (From Myerson,[66] with permission.)

contusion, burn, or infection. Muscle compartments (Fig. 23-4), which are bordered by bone and inelastic fascia, can become constricting forces with increasing volume from expanding tissues. Compartments then become tense, causing an increase in the intracompartmental pressures. Clinical signs of compartment syndrome include paresthesia, pallor and/or decreased or absent pulses, pain out of proportion to the underlying trauma, and rapidly advancing trophic changes. Compartment syndrome must be addressed immediately so that permanent sequelae from neurovascular compromise does not occur. Compartmental pressures can be measured to confirm a diagnosis. Treatment consists of early identification and compartmental fasciotomies when indicated.

## FOREIGN BODIES

Foreign bodies are common causes of injuries in children (Fig. 23-5). There may be no clear history of a penetrating injury, and radiographs may be negative, which challenges the physician to formulate an effective treatment plan (Fig. 23-6). Fortunately, a clear history of penetration is usually obtained. Localized erythema, edema, and tenderness should raise a degree of suspicion that a retained foreign body is the source.

Pins or needles are the most commonly encountered foreign bodies in the foot.[18] The object is usually superficial, but it may migrate into deeper tissues with weight-bearing.[19] Removal is often not necessary unless there is bone, joint, or neurovascular involvement. Other indications for removal include persistent discomfort with or without weight-bearing or the presence of a chronically draining or infected wound.[20] Initial identification and localization are done radiographically. Intraoperative localization can be difficult. Several methods have been devised to localize metallic foreign bodies, including use of electromagnetic metal detectors, triangulation with

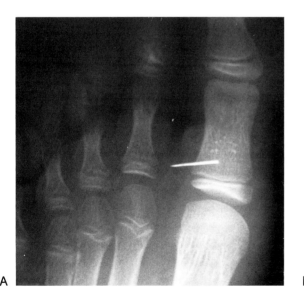
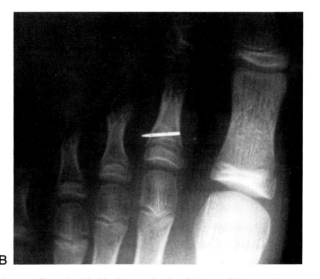

A   B

**Fig. 23-5.** **(A)** Initial radiograph of a child's foot with a sewing needle embedded in the proximal soft tissue of the great toe. **(B)** Demonstrates migration of the needle to the level of the proximal phalanx of the second toe, which was found to be penetrated at the time of surgery. (From Cooke,[19] with permission.)

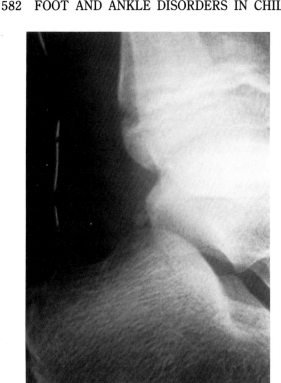

**Fig. 23-6.** Multiply fragmented needle extending through the substance of the Achilles tendon in a young child. No history of trauma. Possible child abuse must be considered. (From Cooke,[19] with permission.)

hypodermic needles, and C-arm or "mini" fluoroscopy.[21-25]

Frequently encountered nonmetallic foreign bodies include wood splinters, toothpicks, and thorns. Wood is often not detected on standard radiographs,[26]; thus these foreign bodies are the most difficult to diagnose and treat. Xerography is no more effective than standard radiography.[27] Computed tomography (CT) is the most reliable method of localizing retained wooden foreign bodies[19,28] (Fig. 23-7). Signs and symptoms include localized pain, erythema, edema, and puncture site. Superficial injuries often require only local debridement with removal of the foreign body. Deep wooden foreign bodies often become asymptomatic but may eventually become symptomatic. Reactions differ depending on the tissue involved. Synovitis can occur from intra-articular lesions.[29] If the bone has been penetrated, a periosteal reaction with cortical thickening as well as osteolysis may be demonstrated.[6-9] Foreign body granulomas are often found as a late result of a retained wooden foreign body and can be manifested as areas of joint destruction, osteolysis, and periostitis.[26,29-31] These changes can simulate Ewing's sarcoma, which should be included in the differential diagnosis. Foreign body granulomas commonly form chronically draining wounds, which are generally sterile but may become secondarily infected.

Glass foreign bodies are often the direct result of a plantar puncture wound, with the glass becoming embedded subcutaneously. Glass is frequently visible on standard radiographs, depending on size, location, and density. Pigmented or lead glass is easily visualized. Infection is uncommon when the penetrating or retained foreign body is glass; removal is not always indicated. Again, removal is indicated for those foreign bodies that are intra-articular, involve bone, threaten neurovascular structures, limit function, or remain symptomatic after conservative treatment. Wounds due to foreign bodies that were grossly contaminated before penetration should be debrided and observed closely for signs and symptoms of infection. Glass wounds frequently cause more extensive deep lacerations than the superficial location of the glass might suggest. Tendon and neurovascular function should be carefully evaluated in all glass laceration wounds.

## BITE WOUNDS

Mammal, insect, and reptile bites occur with high frequency. National estimates of animal bites range from 300 to 700 bites per 100,000 population each year.[32] Children 5 to 9 years old are overwhelmingly the primary victims of animal bites with more than 5 percent of that age group receiving at least one reported bite each year.[32] Children 9 to 14 years old are the next most frequent victims. Dogs are the most common offender in animal bite incidents, followed by cats, humans, and rats. In the majority of animal bite cases the offending animal belongs to the victim, a neighbor, or a friend.[33]

### Dog and Cat Bites

The incidence of dog bites increases in the early afternoon, especially during warm weather.[34] These injuries are rarely seen in an emergency room or physician's office because the majority inflict only minor damage, although the wounds are potentially serious. Bite wounds

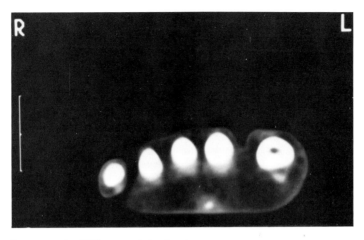

**Fig. 23-7.** Computed tomography (CT) scan of the forefoot demonstrating a wooden foreign body inferior to the second interspace. Standard radiographs were negative. (From Cooke,[19] with permission.)

include tears, avulsions, punctures, and scratches. Crush injury with swelling, ecchymosis, and devitalized tissue may also be present[34] (Fig. 23-8). The potential for infection varies. Although less than 5 percent of dog bites become infected, up to 50 percent of cat bites do.[32] The spectrum of pathogenic bacteria that cause bite infections is broader than is generally appreciated and includes both aerobic and anaerobic bacteria. *Pasteurella multocida* is found in only 20 to 25 percent of dog bite wounds.[34]

## Treatment

Animal bites should be evaluated in a manner consistent with that used for other forms of significant blunt trauma. After the patency of the patient's airway, breathing, and circulation has been ascertained, a careful search for associated fractures and other internal injuries is undertaken, especially if the animal was large.[35] Tetanus immunization should be ascertained and updated. Most children's animal bites can be treated on an outpatient basis. Meticulous wound cleansing, thorough debridement, and high-pressure irrigation should be performed when indicated. Careful debridement of all visible devitalized subcutaneous tissue and dermis is extremely important, especially in small puncture wounds. The wound should also be explored for injuries to tendons, nerves, joint capsule, cartilage, or bone, as previously described.

There is no evidence that prophylactic antibiotics are beneficial, except possibly in patients with significant hand wounds or wounds from cat bites.[35] Empiric antibiotic therapy should provide coverage for *P. multocida, Staphylococcus aureus,* streptococci, and possibly anaerobic bacteria.[30] Penicillin is the standard treatment for *P. multocida.* If *S. aureus* is present or suspected, however, an antistaphlococcal agent should be given in addition to penicillin.[32]

## Human Bites

Human bites most often occur in young males, the peak occurring in the spring and early summer and on weekends. They also occasionally occur in cases of child abuse. Most states have statutes requiring reporting of suspected child abuse to law enforcement authorities. They may also be self-inflicted. There are two types of human bites: occlusional and clenched fist injuries. Occlusional bites occur when the teeth are sunk into the skin. The infection rate for occlusional bites appears to be just slightly higher than the infection rates for more common lacerations. Clenched fist injuries are the most serious of human bite wounds. They occur when the closed fist of one person meets the teeth of another. A variety of infections can occur, including cellulitis, lymphangitis, and osteomyelitis. In 50 to 55 percent of human bite wounds anaerobic bacteria can be isolated.[32] The most commonly involved organisms are streptococci, staphy-

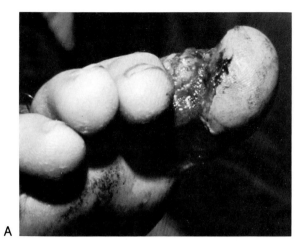

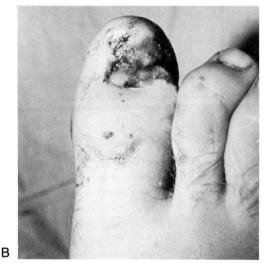

**Fig. 23-8. (A&B)** Dog bite to the hallux treated locally and granulated to heal without sequelae. The nail plate was removed to clean the wound adequately. (From Silvani,[33] with permission.)

lococci, and *Eikenella. Peptococcus* and *Bacteroides* are also often found.[35] The management of these wounds is similar to that of other bite wounds.

## Spider Bites

The very young are the most susceptible to death secondary to spider bites. Spiders that are able to penetrate the skin with bites are tarantulas, brown recluse spiders, and black widows.[36] Tarantulas have urticaria-producing hairs on the dorsal surface of the abdomen, which cause edema and pruritis. These may be treated with topical corticosteroids or oral antihistamines. If the reaction is severe, oral prednisone may be indicated.

Brown recluse spider bites cause severe necrotic tissue destruction called *necrotic arachnidism* (Fig. 23-9). Most commonly, bites to the foot occur while the patient is walking barefoot outdoors. Initial symptoms include stinging, pain, and pruritus. Necrotic arachnidism presents as a blue halo at the puncture site, which indicates local cyanosis; this usually progresses to a large ulceration, which may take several months to heal. As the lesion enlarges, systemic signs may appear, including restlessness, generalized urticaria, arthralgias, myalgias, hemolysis, disseminated intravascular coagulation, fever, diarrhea, proteinuria, hematuria, shock, and coma.[38] Patients with a necrotic bite greater than 1 cm in diameter should be tested for progressive hemolytic anemia or thrombocytopenia. If this has not occurred by 10 to 12 hours postbite, the likelihood of a severe systemic reaction appears low.[39]

### Treatment

Treatment remains controversial.[37-41] Common treatment methods include cleansing of the wounds, sterile nonadherent dressings, rest, and analgesics. Other recommended treatments include intralesional and oral corticosteroids and surgical debridement. Oral steroids may be indicated if the necrotic area appears greater than 3 to 4 cm or if coagulopathies or renal complications develop. Most ulcers epithelialize after several months in response to local wound care.

The venom of the black widow spider causes neurotoxic symptoms by depleting acetylcholine or catecholamines and thereby blocking neuromuscular transmission. Antivenin inhibits this reaction.[42] The bite presents initially as two fang puncture sites with slight surrounding erythema. Systemic symptoms may be most severe in the legs and abdomen and may mimic an acute abdomen. Symptoms peak several hours after the bite and may last several days. Anxiety, dizziness, weakness, fever, headaches, nausea, vomiting, chest tightness, respiratory distress, urinary retention, muscle fasciculation, and paresthesias may also be present. Limbs may be contracted, with flexor muscle spasms, and there may be burning paresthesias of plantar pedal surfaces. Renal damage, shock, cardiac and respiratory failure, cerebral

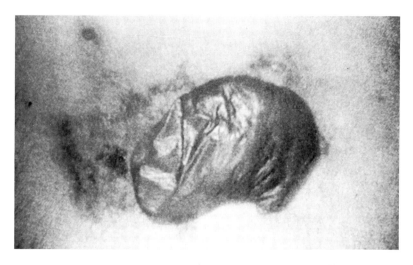

**Fig. 23-9.** A brown recluse spider bite (after 3 days). (From Silvani,[33] with permission.)

hemorrhage, and local bacterial infection may also occur. Envenomation, however, is usually self-limited, with symptoms peaking in severity within 3 to 4 hours, and usually only symptomatic treatment is required.

There is controversy about the use of horse serum antivenin. Hospitalization and the use of one ampule of *Latrodectus maetans* antivenin is recommended for patients with severe symptoms. Severe allergic reactions to the antivenin may occur despite a negative skin test for horse serum. Therefore, the antivenin should be administered with extreme caution and close observation. Serum sickness may also occur. Some authors have noted a higher incidence of severe reactions to the serum than to the envenomation.[43] Alternative medications include calcium gluconate, muscle relaxants, methocarbonate, and corticosteroids. Hospitalization and close observation are always indicated with pediatric patients until stability is ensured. Local wound care should be provided at the site of the bite wound.

## Snake Bites

The treatment of poisonous snake bites is controversial. Several deaths from snake bites are reported annually in the United States. Common complications include permanent deformities and amputation of the affected extremity (Fig. 23-10). The feet are frequently involved.

Poisonous snakes in the United States include the coral snake, rattlesnake, water moccasin, and copperhead. Most envenomation from rattlesnakes occurs in older adolescents and young adults.[44] Children may receive a higher dose of venom per kilogram and thus exhibit more intense symptomatology. Since snake venoms contain various amounts of neurotoxin, hemolysin, cardiotoxin, cholinesterase, phosphatase, nucleotidase, cytochrome oxidase inhibitor, hyaluronidase, and proteolytic enzymes, all body tissues are subject to attack. Toxic systemic effects and local cellular destruction at the puncture site are all caused by envenomation. The venom is activated by local body temperature and pH when it is first injected into the subcutaneous tissue. The immediate cellular destruction as well as destruction of local lymphatic and blood vessels occurs by hydrolysis. Swelling rapidly follows and is generally accompanied by severe local pain. Ecchymosis and bulla formation occur at or proximal to the site of the bite, which may progress to local gangrene of the skin and underlying structures as a result of profound local ischemia. Direct systemic effects may occur if venom is injected into intact vessels.

### Treatment

Initial treatment includes wound cleansing, tetanus prophylaxis, and sequential circumferential measurements of the involved area every 30 minutes to assess progression. Acetaminophen and opiate analgesics may be used when appropriate. One should avoid the use of aspirin

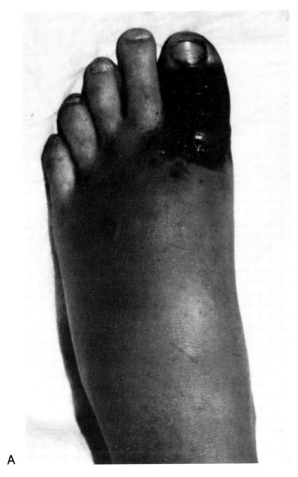

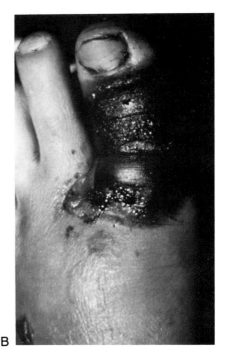

A                                                        B

**Fig. 23-10.** A rattlesnake envenomation of the left foot. **(A)** Left foot 3 days postbite showing marked edema (to the thigh), bleb formation, and necrosis surrounding the bite. The patient had received nine vials of Crotalidae antivenin initially. **(B)** Extreme gangrene (well demarcated) is present 9 days postbite. This extended deep, reaching the extensory tendons, joint capsule, and cortex or the phalanx. *(Figure continues.)*

because of its effect on platelets. All children should be observed for 24 hours even if the bite appears to be minor in nature, particularly with bites from the Mojave rattlesnake.[42]

In all envenomations, intravenous access should be established rapidly, as the patient may deteriorate acutely. Laboratory studies should include a CBC, prothrombin time, partial thromboplastin time, fibrinogen, fibrin degradation products, platelet count, serum creatinine, and creatinine kinase. These values should make possible an assessment of the effects on coagulopathies, muscle breakdown, and red blood cell count.

In patients with moderate to severe envenomation,

antivenin therapy should be strongly considered. The dose in children is 10mg/kg. Once the decision has been made to start antivenin therapy, one should consider skin testing for hypersensitivity. Since skin test material may sensitize patients to horse proteins, a skin test should not be applied for the mild or nonvenomous bites in order to avoid sensitization if the need for therapy should arise. Prior to initiation of therapy, volume expansion with normal saline should be undertaken to ensure that adequate intravascular volume is present. Debridement of the wound is reserved for patients who exhibit moderate to severe toxic systemic side effects and local tissue damage. Early fasciotomy remains controversial.

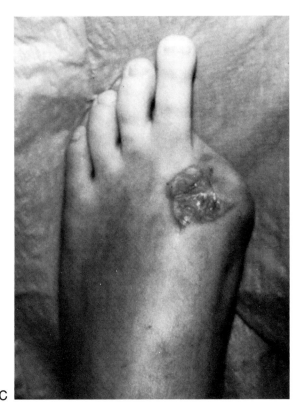

C

**Fig. 23-10** *(Continued).* **(C)** The hallux was amputated 20 days postbite (after three debridements), and wound closure was achieved by a plantar flap and split thickness skin graft. (From Silvani,[67] with permission.)

# THERMAL INJURIES

## Burns

The highest incidence of burn injury occurs in young children.[45] Burns to the skin can cause changes in all body systems and can cause severe metabolic and physiologic disorders, including fluid loss with subsequent hypovolemia and hypermetabolic state, which increases catabolism and weight loss.

The depth of a burn depends on the thickness of the skin at the site of the injury, the heat of the burning agent, and the length of time the agent was in contact with the skin. Burns are of either partial thickness (first or second degree) or full thickness (third degree). A first-degree burn is characterized by erythema without blister formation. Second-degree burns may be either superficial or deep[46]: superficial second degree burns are erythematous with blisters and are painful (Fig. 23-11); deep second degree burns may or may not have blisters, may be dry and anesthetic, and may appear mottled (Fig. 23-12). Third-degree burns involve destruction of the full thickness of the skin and its appendages. They are anesthetic, leathery, and whitish to dark in color and may have thrombosed vessels.

Types of burns include scalds, contact dry burns, burns from flames, cigarette burns, and radiant burns. Scalds are produced by hot water and cause the affected skin to peel off in sheets and become soggy. The depth of injury is varied and contoured. Contact dry burns are caused by hot objects, usually metallic or electrical. The injury is sharply demarcated, dry, and usually of uniform depth. Burns from flames are caused by fires and matches and may be identified by charring and singed hairs. Cigarette burns leave a circular mark. Electrical burns are small but deep, with exit and entry points. In friction burns, bony prominences may be affected and blisters are generally broken. In radiant burns, caused by radiant energy such as fire or the sun, injury varies from moderate to extensive, and the skin shows erythema and blistering,[47] dependent upon sensitivity, as previously discussed. Chemical burns from acids or bases may cause staining and scarring of the skin.

## Treatment

### Initial Measures

If a major burn has occurred, fluid resuscitation should begin as soon as possible to replenish intravascular volume and thus maintain tissue and organ perfusion. The amount of fluid necessary to maintain perfusion is proportionate to the patient's size and to the extent of the burn.

The circulation to the digits or to the entire foot may be compromised from circumferential burns, postburn edema, or burns with constricting eschar (Fig. 23-13). Therefore the circulatory status of the extremity must be assessed immediately and on a continual basis. When vascular compromise is present, an escharotomy must be performed. This is often done without anesthesia because eschar is frequently anesthetic. Prophylactic antibiotics, including penicillin or erythromycin, are given to children to prevent cellulitis from the streptococci that normally inhabit the skin.[48] Late gram-negative infections must also be considered in longer, deeper burns.

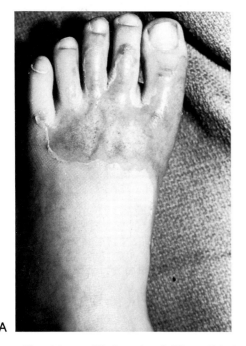
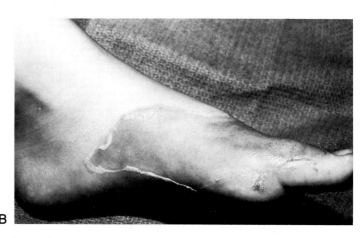

A                                                    B

**Fig. 23-11.** **(A)** Dorsal and **(B)** medial views of superficial second-degree burn. Blisters have broken, but the erythematous base is present. (From Tuerk,[45] with permission.)

During the initial evaluation burn wounds may be covered with sponges or gauze soaked in cool saline or water. The wounds are gently cleansed with a mild soap or detergent. Broken blisters are debrided, but intact blisters are generally left intact unless infection is present or likely.[49] Blisters are also debrided if their size and location interfere with joint motion and function. In deep burns optimal results are obtained if the broken blisters are covered with biologic dressings (e.g., porcine skin grafts or amniotic membranes). Unbroken blisters are also effective but not as effective as porcine skin in preventing tissue necrosis.[50]

*Dressings*

Feet are considered a critical area by the American Burn Association Severity Grading System.[51] Patients with circumferential burns or burns involving more than 5 percent of this critical area should be hospitalized. Infection of burn wounds is the most common cause of morbidity and mortality in burn patients; therefore control of contamination, which may be achieved by applying a topical antibiotic cream until wound covering is complete, is important in initial treatment. The most common topical antibiotic used is silver sulfadiazine; other topicals include mafenide, 0.5 percent silver nitrate solution, gentamicin cream, and povidone-iodine ointment. Systemic penicillin or erythromycin may also be indicated.

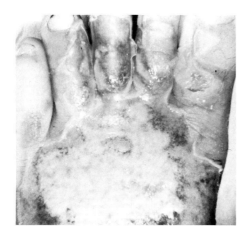

**Fig. 23-12.** Deeper second-degree burn with characteristically mottled appearance. (From Tuerk,[45] with permission.)

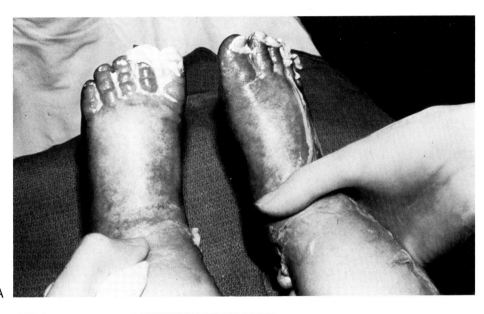

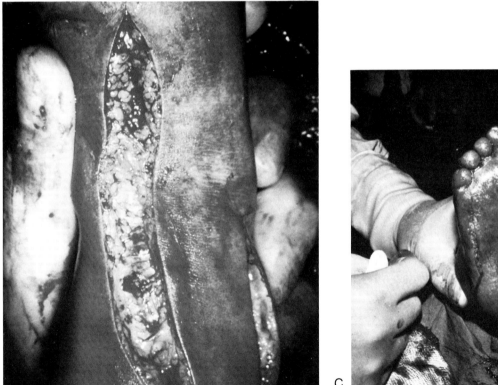

**Fig. 23-13.** **(A)** Child with second- and third-degree scald burns of both legs and feet following immersion in a bathtub. **(B)** Escharotomy on the right foot was required at 24 hours because of distal circulatory compromise secondary to edema. Escharotomy was also required on the left foot. **(C)** View of the plantar surface, showing the two escharotomy incisions needed to decompress the right foot. Adequacy of the escharotomy is judged by return of both the arterial pulse (by palpation or Doppler ultrasound) and the capillary circulation. *(Figure continues.)*

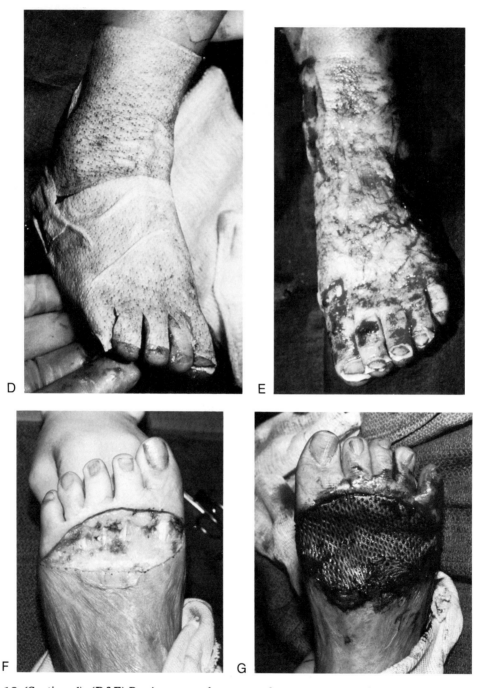

**Fig. 23-13** *(Continued)*. **(D&E)** Porcine xenografts were used to promote a vascular granular bed that would be acceptable for applications of a meshed split thickness skin graft. **(F)** Both feet were grafted prior to discharge. Over the next several years the child developed a contracture of the skin of the dorsum of the foot requiring secondary reconstruction. This view shows the amount of skin graft required following a simple incision of the dorsal burn scar contracture of the left foot. **(G)** A meshed split thickness skin graft has been placed on the right foot following release of the scar contracture. *(Figure continues.)*

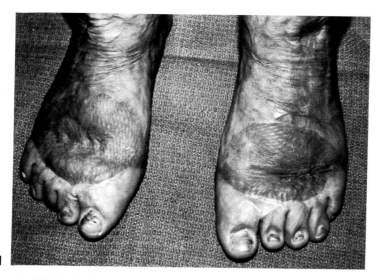

**Fig. 23-13** *(Continued).* **(H)** The healed grafts following scar release. In the future further scar releases and grafting may be required with growth of the child. If necessary, burn scar contractures of the dorsal web spaces can be corrected by double opposed Z-plasties. (From Tuerk,[45] with permission.)

The wounds are re-dressed once or twice daily, one dressing change being made during hydrotherapy once the patient has been stabilized. Hydrotherapy removes the old antibiotic creams as well as aiding in debridement of the wound. Second-degree burn wound dressings, which may be medicated gauze dressings such as Xeroform, with or without antibiotic cream, are changed every 1 to 2 days. The dressing change may also be facilitated by soaking in a tub.

*Care of Second- and Third-Degree Burns*

Second-degree burns generally heal within several weeks. Some authors believe that if healing takes longer than 2 weeks, skin grafts should be applied,[49] whereas others disagree and depend on exercise, splinting, and compression dressings.[52,53] Third-degree burns are best treated with skin grafting. Necrotic tissue must be debrided, infection must be controlled, and a well vascularized recipient bed must be established to support the graft. Grafts can be placed directly on paratenon, perineurium, or periosteum but not bare tendon, nerve, or bone. Grafts are harvested with an air-driven or electrical dermatome. Donor sites are covered with Op-Site, which is generally left intact for 7 to 10 days. Partial thickness grafts can be used as a sheet or meshed. A light compressive dressing is applied over an Interface dressing and left in place for 1 to 2 days before daily inspection is begun. The limb is left elevated for 3 to 4 days postoperatively. Loose compression is important once the limb is allowed to become dependent. For brief periods, pressure is applied to the wound by means of an Ace bandage or Tubi-Grip; this treatment is continued for up to 1 year to prevent hypertrophic scarring.

Complications

Hypertrophic scarring and contractures are common postburn complications in children. Delayed reconstruction may be necessary; children should be assessed periodically. Scar contracture can worsen with time, not only because of contracture of the scar but also because of normal growth of the surrounding tissues as the child develops.[54] This condition, if untreated, can result eventually in growth alterations of the underlying bone. Hypertrophic scars that interfere with the wearing of shoes, become irritated by mechanical friction, or cause significant deformity may require serial intralesional steroid injections or excision and replacement with skin grafts. Linear contractures that interfere with joint range of motion may require Z-plasties or the addition of skin by further grafting. It has been recommended that for best

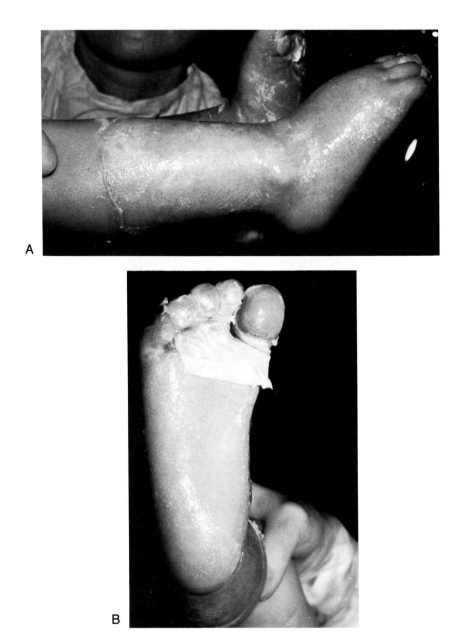

**Fig. 23-14. (A)** Child with second-degree scald burns of both legs and feet following immersion in a bathtub. The blisters have broken and have been debrided in the whirlpool. Notice the edema of the dorsum of the foot, requiring continuing assessment of the distal circulation. **(B)** View of the plantar surface of the feet of the same child. Because the plantar skin is thicker than the skin of the instep, injuries that cause third-degree burns of the instep may result in only second-degree burns of the sole. *(Figure continues.)*

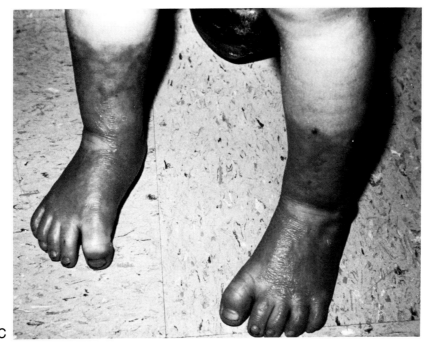

C

**Fig. 23-14** *(Continued).* **(C)** Two months following the injury, the second-degree burns have healed with the use of daily whirlpool and silver sulfadiazene cream dressings. After healing, the child is measured for individually fitted pressure garments, which are worn continuously to prevent burn scar hypertrophy. (From Tuerk,[45] with permission.)

results all skin releases in the foot be immobilized with either Kirschner or dynamic splints for a minimum of 2 weeks postoperatively.[54]

## Prevention

Children are at risk of burns in both the kitchen and the bathroom caused by hot water (Fig. 23-14). Preventive measures include turning hot water heaters down below 137°F (57°C) and adequate supervision in the bathtub and around the stove.[55] The possibility of child abuse should also be considered, especially in immersion scald burns.

## Cold Injuries

The mildest form of cold injury is frostnip, which tends to occur in apical structures (nose, ears, hands, feet), where blood flow is most variable because of the richly innervated arteriovenous anastomoses. This is most often seen in skiers exposed to fast-moving cold air.[56] Children are especially prone as they may often remove restric-tive yet protective clothing. Simple warming by the pressure of a warm hand is sufficient treatment. More consequential cold injuries may be divided into freezing (frostbite) and nonfreezing (immersion foot) injuries. The diagnosis of freezing versus nonfreezing injuries generally can be made on the basis of history and clinical manifestations.

Immersion foot, or trench foot, is a disease of the sympathetic nerves and blood vessels in the foot. It is seen when the feet remain wet, at ambient temperatures near or slightly above freezing, for long periods. It is usually associated with dependency and immobilization of the lower extremities; constriction of the limb by shoes and clothing may be contributing factors. Immediate symptoms include numbness and tingling, with itching and pain, progressing to leg cramps and complete numbness. The skin is initially red, later becoming progressively pale and mottled and still later gray and blue. The injury often produces a superficial, moist, liquification gangrene. Management entails careful washing and drying of the feet, gentle rewarming, and slight elevation of the extremity. Early physical therapy is essential.[56] The injury is uncommon in children.

## Frostbite

Several days after the injury, frostbite can be classified into four degrees of severity. In first-degree frostbite, hyperemia and edema are evident. Second-degree frostbite is characterized by hyperemia, edema, and large, clean blisters. Third-degree frostbite is characterized by hyperemia, edema, and vesicles filled with hemorrhagic fluid, which are usually smaller than the blisters occurring in second-degree frostbite. Fourth-degree frostbite involves complete necrosis with gangrene, with potential loss of the affected part.[53] Freezing causes a profound redirection of blood flow to the extremity, resulting in rupture of small blood vessels and edema. When the tissues thaw, intense vasoconstriction occurs at both involved and uninvolved areas.[1]

## Treatment

The patient must be removed from the cold environment; treatment should not be attempted in the field. Normal core body temperature should be restored before treating the local injury. The preferred initial therapy for frostbite is rapid rewarming in a water bath at a temperature of 39 to 42°C. Strict aseptic technique should be employed during the warming process and during subsequent wound treatments. Rewarming is continued until the frostbitten tissue has a flushed appearance, demonstrating that the circulation has been re-established. This process usually lasts 30 to 45 minutes. Narcotics and analgesics may be required to relieve ischemic pain during the rewarming process. After rewarming, the skin is washed gently. The limb should be elevated to minimize edema, and weight-bearing and friction should be avoided. Necrotic tissue should be allowed to demarcate and mummify before surgical debridement is performed unless severe infection with sepsis develops. Amputation may be electively performed on mummified tissue once it has clearly demarcated.

Late sequelae of significant cold injury include premature closure of epiphyses, decreased resistance to recurrent or future cold injury, chronic pain syndrome, hyperhidrosis, and late development of squamous cell carcinoma.[57,58] Articular surface irregularities and subchondral cysts may occasionally develop in both children and adults. Actual joint space narrowing is uncommon following frostbite.[58] Care should be taken to prevent prolonged exposure of acral body parts in children, who are often prone to remove protective clothing.

# TENDON INJURIES

Tendon injuries to the foot in children are relatively uncommon. They may, however, result in instability and joint destruction if they are not properly diagnosed and adequately treated.

## Healing

Primary healing occurs when sutures are used to repair the laceration or rupture, whereas secondary healing occurs when the tendon ends are left to heal in loose connective tissue. In primary healing if the tendon repair is successful, the collagen between the ends of the repaired tendon will reorganize into parallel bundles, which lends great tensile strength. The collagen between the tendon and surrounding tissue remains randomly oriented and highly elastic or mobile.[59] In secondary healing the gap between the tendon ends is bridged first with gelatinous and later with dense fibrous scar tissue.[60] Remodeling of the scar then occurs. The scar tissue is both quantitively and qualitatively different from normal tendon. There is poor continuity between the scar tissue and the tendon ends, which decreases the gliding function of the tendon.

Tendon rupture occurs when a tendon is extended beyond its point of elasticity, which is approximately an 8 percent extension of its total length.[61] The most common mechanism of rupture is sudden application of a stretching force to a muscle that is strongly contracting. Rupture may occur at the insertion to bone, at the musculotendinous junction, or through the muscle belly or muscle origin. In children, the physeal plate may fracture before tendon rupture occurs.

In our experience, tendon laceration occurs much more frequently in children than does tendon rupture (Fig. 23-15). When a tendon is lacerated, the time, the type, and the location of the wound are important factors in considering primary versus secondary repair. The ideal time for treating tendon lacerations is within 4 to 6 hours of the injury. If optimum primary healing of the

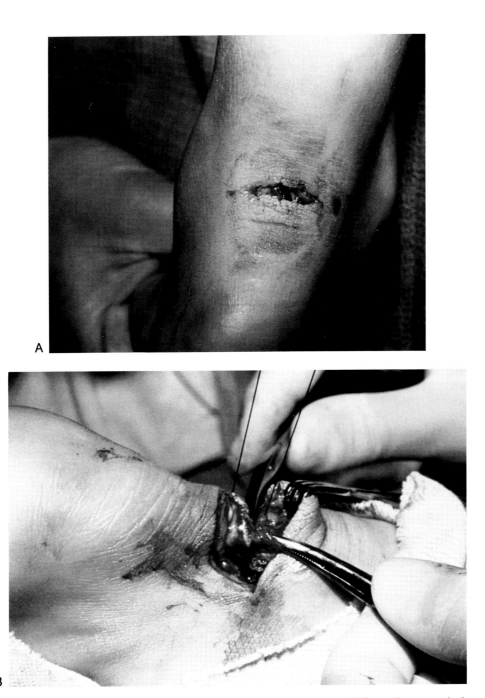

**Fig. 23-15.** (A) Lacerated Achilles tendon following a kick to a glass shower door. (B) Bunnell-type repair shown here was reinforced with circumferential simple interrupted sutures. (From Sheinberg and Bayne,[68] with permission.)

skin is expected to take place, the tendon should be sutured at the same time as the skin. A lacerated crush wound with skin avulsion or skin loss should not be closed if a large amount of tissue damage is present, as these wounds have a greater propensity for inflammation and infection. If initial cultures are negative and no clinical sign of infection is noted, secondary closure may be done in 4 to 6 days. Skin coverage over a tendon repair is essential to ensure gliding function.

As with all soft tissue injuries, a history of tetanus immunization should be obtained. Gram stain and wound culture and sensitivity should be obtained on initial examination before prophylactic or therapeutic antibiotics are administered. The type of wound and host determine the use of appropriate antibiotics. Children must be closely monitored, and immediacy is required if infection is suspected. Surgical debridement should be performed to remove gross contamination and nonvital tissue and permit identification of the damage to the tendon and surrounding tissue. Pulsatile irrigation should be performed to remove clotted blood, necrotic tissue, foreign bodies, dirt, and other debris.

If the ends of the tendon have retracted, they may be retrieved with a hemostat placed inside the tendon sheath. If this is not possible, a small incision should be made where the stump of the tendon is most likely to be found. The tendon ends are then debrided of irregular or devitalized ends and reapproximated. Buried sutures should be kept to a minimum. A compressive dressing and elevation are used to prevent swelling. The tendon repair is then protected with appropriate immobilization for 3 to 6 weeks. The ideal suture material should be nonreactive, small caliber, strong, and easy to handle and should hold a good knot.[62] Synthetic nonabsorbable suture material such as nylon, polypropylene, or polyester may be used. Monofilament stainless steel may also be used as a pull-out suture; however this is often uncomfortable, especially in children, and in our opinion should be avoided in younger patients.

Maintenance of the tendon repair depends on the suture material, suturing technique, and postoperative management. The repair is strongest when sutures are perpendicular to both the collagen bundles of the tendon and the stress applied to the repair.

## BICYCLE SPOKE INJURIES

Bicycle spoke injuries occur when the child's foot, ankle, or heel becomes trapped in and is dragged by the spokes of the wheel, resulting in the typical pattern known as

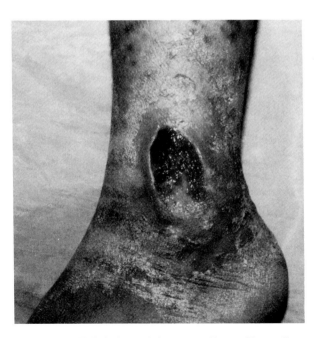

**Fig. 23-16.** Full thickness defect created by catching malleolus in a bicycle spoke. (From Scurran,[65] with permission.)

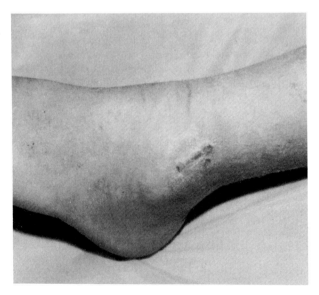

**Fig. 23-17.** Appearance of same wound as in (23-16) 2½ weeks after conservative treatment with Unna boots, changed at 5-to-7 day intervals. (From Scurran,[65] with permission.)

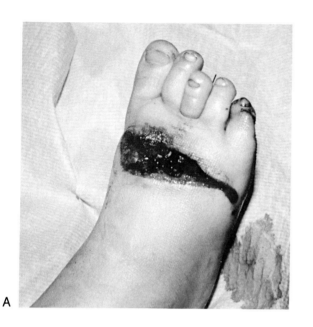

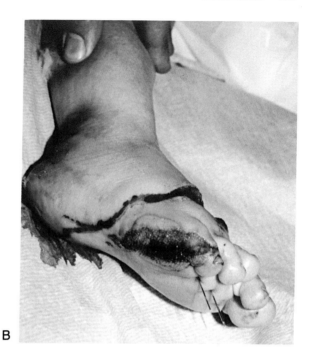

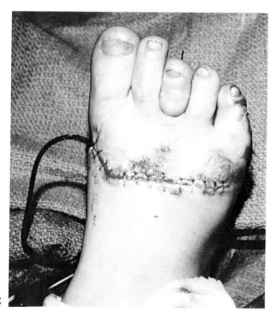

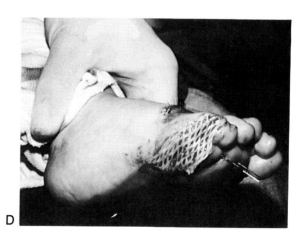

**Fig. 23-18.** **(A&B)** Dorsal and lateral views of 19-month-old male, run over by a riding-type power mower. Injuries appear to be dorsal, full thickness, multi-tissue loss, and lateral partial thickness skin loss. Initial treatment consisted of irrigation, identification of traumatized structures, debridement, and stabilization of fractures. No primary closure attempted. **(C&D)** 6 days later the skin was primarily closed over a drain (indicating original suspicion of full thickness loss was in error). Lateral wound was deeper than originally suspected and split thickness skin grafting was required. *(Figure continues.)*

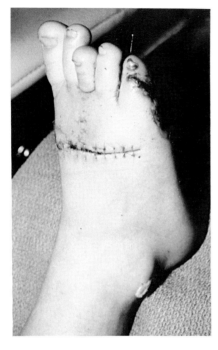
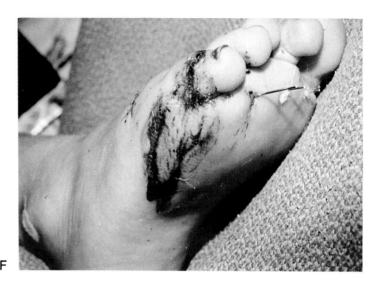

**Fig. 23-18** *(Continued).* **(E&F)** 10 days postoperation. Both wounds healing uneventfully. Patient began weight bearing at 5 weeks due to bone loss at 3rd metatarsal fracture site.

spoke wheel injuries (Figs. 23-16 and 23-17). These injuries initially appear minor and may not be given much attention by parents and physicians. Thus, significant consequences such as skin necrosis, sepsis, fractures, physeal injury, and even tetanus may often result.[63]

This injury usually occurs when two children or an adult and child are riding on one bicycle, particularly when the child is riding on the rear carrier.[63] Usually these injuries result from entrapment of the heel or foot between the spokes and the rigid fork of the moving bicycle. With a sudden deceleration of the moving vehicle, the kinetic energy of the bicycle is transferred to the entrapped limb with a crushing impact. This results in lacerations or a shearing injury from the spoke or to a crush injury due to impingement of the foot between the wheel and the frame of the bicycle. Laceration usually occurs at the malleoli, Achilles tendon or dorsum of the foot.[1]

Compression necrosis secondary to injured blood vessels that have thrombosed and soft tissue that has been sheared from underlying fixed points may not become apparent for 3 to 4 days following the injury.[71] Definitive treatment such as skin grafts must be delayed until after clear delineation and debridement of necrosis.

Abrasions and tissue loss areas are treated with appropriate dressings, mild compression, elevation, and splint immobilization. The vasculature should be continually assessed, and further debridement is done as indicated at frequent dressing changes. Early skin grafts to the dorsum of the foot and malleoli may be performed. Lacerations may be primarily closed after careful debridement. Unna boot immobilization with appropriate interval debridement has proved successful in our experience if wounds are less than 2 to 3 cm in diameter.

Many of these injuries could be prevented if spoke shields were installed over the front and back wheels, if no more than one person were permitted to ride on the bicycle, and if any injury, no matter how benign in appearance, were appropriately evaluated.[63]

## LAWN MOWER INJURIES

Power mowers can produce devastating damage, (Fig. 23-18), including partial to complete amputation of the foot or leg, major lacerations, and fractures. Missile injuries from flying objects on the ground thrown by the lawn mower at high speeds may also occur. The initial injury may appear small, but an underlying deep injury or foreign body may result in infection.[1]

These injuries usually occur when children are allowed too close to a mower being operated by their parents or siblings, when children are carried as passengers on a "ride-on" mower, and when children, not yet in their teens, are allowed to use the mower.[61] Ride-on lawn mowers cause the most severe trauma, often resulting in prolonged hospitalization and major residual deformity, with the foot being commonly involved.[64]

Power mower injuries must be assumed to be contaminated with both aerobic and anaerobic bacteria and thus should not be closed primarily. Tetanus immunization should also be assessed and updated as required. These wounds should be treated initially with broad-spectrum antibiotics. Thorough debridement with exploration under anesthesia is necessary, as the depth of the wound is often deceptive. (Management of contaminated wounds has been described elsewhere in this chapter.) Most of these injuries can be prevented if young children are not permitted to use power mowers, particularly the ride-on variety, and if all children are kept well away from the area where the mower is being used.[64]

# REFERENCES

1. Siffert RS, Feldman DJ: Trauma to the child's foot and ankle, including growth plate and epiphyseal injuries. p. 1660. In Jahss MH (ed): Disorders of the Foot. Vol. 2.
2. Izart RJ Jr, Hubay CA: The annual injury of 15,000,000 children: a limited study of childhood accidental injury and death. J Trauma 6:65, 1966
3. Peterson CA, Peterson HA: Analysis of the incidence of injuries to the epiphyseal growth plate. J Trauma 12:275, 1972
4. Blais MM, Green WT, Anderson M: Lengths of the growing foot. J Bone Joint Surg [AM] 38:998, 1956
5. Siffert RS, Levy RN: Athletic injuries in children. Pediatr Clin North Am 12:1027, 1965
6. Huelke DF: Extremity injuries produced in motor vehicle collision. J Trauma 10:189, 1970
7. Keddy JA: Accidents in childhood: a report on 17,141 accidents. Can Med Assoc J 91:675, 1964
8. Grossman JA: The repair of surface trauma. Emerg Med Clin North Am 12:220, 1982
9. Hirata I: Soft Tissue Injuries. College Health 23:215, 1975
10. Mills J et al: Current Emergency Diagnosis and Treatment. Lange Medical Publications, Los Altos, CA, 1985
11. Rank BK: Surgery of Repair as Applied to Hand Injuries. 3rd Ed. Williams & Wilkins, Baltimore, 1968, p. 88
12. Thompson RVS: Primary Repair of Soft Tissue Injuries. Melbourne University Press, Melbourne, 1969
13. Daly N, Vascular trauma. In Scurran BL (ed): Foot and Ankle Trauma. Churchill Livingstone, New York, 1989
14. American College of Surgeons, Committee on Trauma: A Guide to Initial Therapy of Soft Tissue Wounds. Am College of Surgeons, ?, June 1974
15. Converse JM: Plastic and Reconstructive Surgery, Vol. 1. WB Saunders, Philadelphia, 1964
16. Krizek TJ: Local factors influencing incidence of wound sepsis. Contemp Surg 10(4):45, 1977
17. Hoover NW, Ivins JC: Wound debridement. Arch Surg 79:701, 1959
18. Mann R: Surgery of the Foot. 5th Ed. CV Mosby, St. Louis, 1986
19. Cooke R: Foreign bodies. p. 119. In Scurran BL (ed): Foot and Ankle Trauma. Churchill Livingstone, New York, 1989
20. Jahss MA: Pseudotumors of the foot. Orthop Clin North Am 5:67, 1974
21. Jeffery JI: Surgical excision of foreign bodies. J Am Podiatr Med Assoc 74:229, 1984
22. Rickoff SE, Bauder T, Kerman BL: Foreign body localization and retrieval in the foot. J Foot Surg 71:84, 1975
23. Hunt GB: Triangulation for removal of foreign bodies: two illustrative cases. Tex Med 71:84, 1975
24. Puhl RW, Altman MI, Seta JE, Nelson GA: The use of fluoroscopy in the detection and excision of foreign bodies in the foot. J Am Podiatr Med Assoc 73:514, 1983
25. Wilner JM, Lepon GM: The use of C-arm fluoroscopy and its application to podiatric surgery. J Foot Surg 22:283, 1985
26. Charney DB, Manzi JA, Turlik M, Young M: Non-metallic foreign bodies in the foot: radiography vs. xerography. J Foot Surg 25:44, 1986
27. Kuhns LR, Borlaza GS, Seigel RS, et al: Technical Notes: an in vitro comparison of computed tomography, xeroradiography and radiography in detection of soft tissue foreign bodies. Radiology 132:218, 1979
28. Bernardino MD, Jing BS, Thomas J, et al: The extremity soft tissue lesion: a comparative study of ultrasound, computed tomography, and xerography. Radiology 139:53, 1981
29. Cracchiolo A: Wooden foreign bodies in the foot. Am J Surg 140:585, 1980
30. Swischuk LE, Jorgensen F, Jorgensen A, Capen D: Wooden splinter induced "pseudotumor" and osteomyelitis-like lesions of bone and soft tissue. AJR 122:176, 1974
31. Simmons BP, Southmayd WW, Schwartz HS, Hall JE: Wood: an organic foreign body of bone. Clin Orthop 106:276, 1975

32. Wishon PM, Huang A: The trouble with children's best friends. Children Today, May-June 1979
33. Silvani S: Animal Bites. p. 131. In Scurran BL (ed): Foot and Ankle Trauma. Churchill Livingstone, New York, 1989
34. Goldstein EJ: Management of human and animal bite wounds. J Am Acad Dermatol 21:6, 1989
35. Callahan ML: When an animal bites. Emerg Med Clin North Am 119, June 1988
36. Hunt GR: bites and stings of uncommon arthropods. I: Spiders. Postgrad Med J 70:91, 1981
37. King CE, Rees RS: Management of brown recluse spider bites. JAMA 251:889, 1984
38. Pitts NC: Necrotic arachnidism. N Engl J Med 267:400, 1962
39. Dillaha CS, Jansen GT, Honeycutt WM: North American laxoscelism. JAMA 188:33, 1964
40. Russell FE, Gertsch WJ: Letter to the editor. Toxicology 21:337, 1983
41. Berger RS: A critical look at therapy for the brown recluse spider bite. Arch Dermatol 107:298, 1973
42. Bettini S: On the mode of action of Lactrodectus species venom. Ann First Super Sanita 7:1, 1971
43. Moss HS, Binder LS: A retrospective review of black widow spider envenomation. Ann Emerg Med 16:188, 1987
44. Banner W: Bites and stings in the pediatric patient. Curr Probl Pediatr 18(1), 1988
45. Tuerck D: Burns and Frostbite. p. 153. In Scurran BL (ed): Foot and Ankle Trauma. Churchill Livingstone, New York, NY, 1989
46. Warden GD: Outpatient care of thermal injuries. I. Surg Clin North Am 67:147, 1987
47. Hobbs CJ: Burns and Scalds. Br Med J 298:1302, 1989
48. Zachery LS, Heggers JP, Robson MC et al: Burns of the feet. J Burn Care Rehabil 8:192, 1987
49. Warden GD: Outpatient care of thermal injuries. II. Surg Clin North Am 67:151, 1987
50. Zawacki BE: Reversal of capillary stasis and prevention of necrosis in burns. Ann Surg 180:98, 1974
51. Hunt JL, Purdue G: Acute burns. Selected Readings Plast Surg 4:2, 1987
52. Schuck JM: Preparing and closing the burn wound. Plast Surg Clin North Am 1:584, 1974
53. Habal MB: The burned hand: a planned treatment program. J Trauma 18:589, 1978
54. Waymack JP, Fidler J, Warden GD: Surgical correction of burn scar contractures of the foot in children. Burns Incl Therm Inj 14(2):156, 1988
55. Maley MP, Achauer BM: Prevention of tap water scald burns. J Burn Care Rehabil 8:62, 1987
56. Edlich RF, Chang DE, Birk KA et al: Cold injuries. Compr Ther 15(9):13, 1989
57. Purdue GF, Hunt JL: Cold injury: A collective review. J Burn Care Rehabil 7:331, 1986
58. House JH, Fidler MO: Frostbite of the hand. p. 1553. In Green, DP (ed): Operative Hand Surgery. Churchill Livingstone, New York, 1982
59. Beasley RW: Tendon injuries. In Beasley RW (ed): Hand Injuries. WB Saunders, Philadelphia, 1981
60. Peacock EE: Research in tendon healing. In Tubiana R (ed): The Hand. WB Saunders, Philadelphia, 1981
61. Williams IF: Cellular and biochemical composition of healing tendon. In Jenkins HR (ed): Ligament Injuries and Their Treatment. Aspen, Rockville MD, 1985
62. Leddy JP: Flexor tendons: acute injuries. In Green DP (ed): Operative Hand Surgery. Churchill Livingstone, New York, 1982
63. Sankhala SS, Gupta SP: Spoke-wheel injuries. Indian J Pediatr 54:251, 1987
64. Johnstone BR, Bennett CS: Lawn mower injuries in children. Aust N Z J Surg 59:713, 1989
65. Scurran BL: Soft Tissue Injuries. p. 978. In McGlamry ED (ed): Comprehensive Textbook of Foot Surgery. Williams & Wilkins, Baltimore, 1987
66. Myerson MS: Experimental decompression of the fascial compartments of the foot — the basis for fasciotomy in acute compartment syndromes. Foot Ankle 8:308, 1988
67. Silvani SH, Karlin JM, DeValentine SJ, Scurran BL: Poisonous snake bites of the extremities. J Am Podiatr Med Assoc 70:122, 1980
68. Sheinberg R, Bayne O: Concepts in the management of tendon trauma to the foot and ankle. p. 167. In Scurran BL (ed): Foot and Ankle Trauma. Churchill Livingstone, New York, 1989

# SUGGESTED READINGS

Gore D, Desai M, Herndon DN et al: Comparison of complications during rehabilitation between conservative and early surgical management in thermal burns involving the feet of children and adolescents. J Burn Care Rehabil 9:92, 1988

Griffiths DM, MacKelly A: Bicycle-spoke and "doubling" injuries. Med J Aus 149:618, 1988

Osgood PF, Szyfelbein SK: Management of burn pain in children. Pediatr Clin North Am 36:1001, 1989

Rivlin E: The psychological trauma and management of severe burns in children and adolescents. Br J Hosp Med 40:210, 1988

Subrahmanyam M, Date VN, Samant NA et al: Bicycles and injuries in children. J Indian Med Assoc 75:205, 1980

Thurston AJ: Foot injuries caused by power lawn mowers. N Z Med J : 131 Feb. 1980

# 24

# Infections of Bones, Joints, and Soft Tissues

ANVAR M. VELJI
STEVEN J. DeVALENTINE
CLINT M. THORNTON

Major advances have occurred over the last several years in the various aspects of diagnosis and therapy of bone, joint, cartilage, and soft tissue infections. Nevertheless, sepsis continues to be a major problem, and a high index of suspicion is a requisite for a better outcome. Isolation of the causative organism (s) is crucial. Surgical drainage and evacuation of pus are of paramount importance in order to achieve diagnostic and therapeutic goals. Appropriate choice of antimicrobials, duration of therapy, and mode of delivery have also acquired increased significance in this cost containment era. Increased study of host defense mechanisms and inherent patient and surgical risk factors are new directions of research that seek to improve the overall quality of treatment.

## HOST FACTORS

Normal host resistance factors are extremely complex, and there is a continuous and dramatic addition to our knowledge base with the advent of monoclonal and DNA technology. Nonspecific factors in host defenses have classically included mechanical barriers; nutrition; age; heredity; local indigenous microflora; fever response; hormonal factors; inflammatory mediators, including leukotrienes and prostaglandins; acute phase reactants such as opsonins, interferons, and complement; chemotactic factors; and phagocytosis.

The most significant gains in the field of infectious diseases have occurred in the area of the *specific immune system*. Cell-mediated immunity (CMI), generally tested by the delayed cutaneous hypersensitivity reactions to antigens, includes various factors aside from the T lymphocyte. For example, interaction occurs between T and B lymphocytes. Macrophage regulation may occur as the result of cell activation and by interaction with T-suppressor cells. Various subsets of T cells, including T-helper, T-suppressor, T-amplifier, and T-effector cells, have also been shown to perform complex and specific cell-mediated immune function.

Mechanical factors such as increased tissue pressure and physical factors such as reduced pH and $PO_2$ which result from abscess formation, may limit host defenses or may be injurious to host tissue; multiple microbial enzymes and toxins and tissue oxidation may cause rapid irreversible tissue necrosis. Hence, it is crucial that a "shotgun" approach not be used to treat these infections, as chronicity and or limb loss may result.

In the following review emphasis will be placed on selected classical infections, with a brief review of pathogenesis, clinical presentation, diagnosis, and therapy. Relatively newer entities such as Lyme disease will also be discussed. A detailed review of important newer anti-

601

microbials and advances in surgical techniques will be undertaken.

# OSTEOMYELITIS

Osteomyelitis is an infection of bone, which may be caused by multiple pathogens, including pyogenic bacteria, mycobacteria, fungi, and, rarely, viruses. Bone infections were described by Hippocrates and have been identified in ancient Egyptian mummies as well. Osteomyelitis in children is most commonly a hematogenous infection but may occasionally occur by direct extension from an adjacent focal area of infection. It is generally classified into the following types: (1) hematogenous osteomyelitis; (2) osteomyelitis secondary to a contiguous focus of infection; and (3) osteomyelitis secondary to peripheral vascular disease. In children the first two types predominate.

## Hematogenous Osteomyelitis

The peak incidence of hematogenous osteomyelitis occurs in two different age groups: children and adults over 50 years old. Males are generally affected more often than females.

### Pathogenesis

The most common sites of hematogenous bone infection are the metaphyseal areas of long bones such as the humerus, femur, and tibia. Branches of the nutrient arteries to long bones form communicating loops with large metaphyseal venous sinusoids near the metaphyseal border of the physis (Fig. 24-1). These vessels do not cross the physis in skeletally immature children older than 8 to 12 months. When bacteremia occurs, the bacteria enter the bone through the nutrient artery and congregate in these venous metaphyseal sinusoids, where blood flow is sluggish. Koch showed that bacteria injected intravenously into skeletally immature animals tend to localize in these metaphyseal sinusoids within 2 hours of infection.[1] The infection usually begins in the metaphysis near the physis in children who develop hematogenous osteomyelitis, and it usually does not cross the physis into the epiphysis or enter the joint space (except in the case of intra-articular epiphyses, such as the femoral head). Inflammation, vascular engorgement, and abscess formation result in thrombosis of nutrient metaphyseal vessels, which causes bone necrosis. Infection generally spreads to the medullary canal away from the physis and to the easily dissected subperiosteal space through the haversian canal system.

Chronic infection results in the formation of islands of

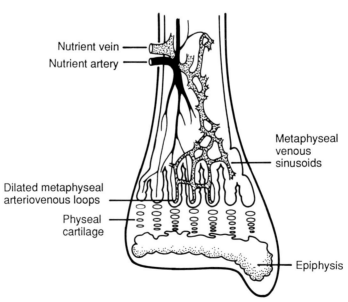

**Fig. 24-1.** Blood flow through the large venous metaphyseal sinusoids and dilated arteriovenous loops is sluggish, which results in a higher probability of bacterial localization in the metaphyseal area of children's long bones.

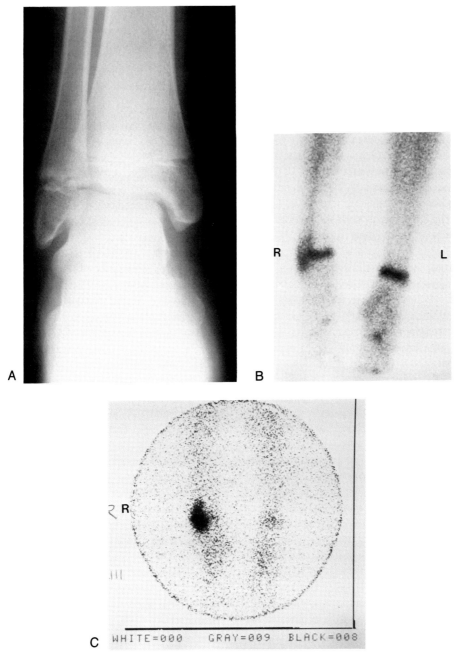

**Fig. 24-2.** (A) Normal plain radiograph of a 13-year-old boy presenting with right lateral malleolar pain, swelling, and fever 2 days after a direct blow to the ankle during a basketball game. (B) Technetium 99 bone scan shows slightly increased tracer uptake of the right lateral malleolus (an asymmetric but equivocal response), which could be characteristic of early osteomyelitis. (C) Intense asymmetric uptake of indium 111 is more conclusive of acute hematogenous osteomyelitis. Bone aspiration yielded *Staphylococcus aureus*. The patient was treated with 10 days of intravenous nafcillin followed by 4 weeks of oral antibiotic.

necrotic cortical bone *(sequestrum)*. New periosteal bone *(involucrum)* forms around the area of sequestrum and intramedullary granulation tissue. The subcortical cavities that are formed often become filled with pus and may spontaneously drain, emitting fragments of sequestrum through cutaneous sinus tracts. Once the child achieves skeletal maturity, vascular channels invade and cross the physis, thus hematogenous osteomyelitis in the mature individual is equally likely to affect the epiphysis as in the child and is more likely to penetrate the joint space.[2] Trueta demonstrated that the metaphyseal vessels of the infant (less than 8 to 12 months of age) also penetrate the physis.[3,4] Thus, osteomyelitis in an infant long bone, as in an adult long bone, is more likely to involve the epiphysis as well as the metaphyseal area and therefore is more likely to invade the joint space.[2,5,6]

At least one-third of patients presenting with hematogenous osteomyelitis have a history of blunt trauma to an area subsequently involved (Fig. 24-2). A number of predisposing conditions have been identified in children who develop hematogenous osteomyelitis. Skin, urinary, pelvic, dental, gastrointestinal, and respiratory infections and bacterial endocarditis may result in hematogenous bacteremia that is likely to localize to bone. Burns, narcotic addiction, hemodialysis, immunosuppressive therapy, sickle cell anemia, and leukocyte dysfunction (granulomatous disease of childhood) have also been identified as predisposing conditions.

The foot has traditionally been considered an unusual location for osteomyelitis in children. Jacobs, however, reported that 10 percent of children with osteomyelitis in his review presented with foot involvement.[7] These cases included both hematogenous osteomyelitis and that due to contiguous foci of infection (mostly puncture wounds). The calcaneus is the most frequent site of involvement, followed by the metatarsal and other tarsal bones.

*Staphylococus aureus* is isolated in at least 60 to 90 percent of cases,[7-9] and gram-negative organisms are isolated in about 7 to 10 percent, with streptococci, *Staphylococus epidermidis,* and *Hemophilus influenzae* found in most of the remaining cases. Other organisms may be responsible for hematogenous osteomyelitis in patients with modified host factors. Salmonellae are prevalent in patients with sickle cell anemia and other hemoglobinopathies, and *Pseudomonas aeruginosa* is an important isolate in "older" narcotic addicts. Mycotic osteomyelitis occurs in immunocompromised hosts and has a propensity to involve the bones of the hands and feet and the vertebrae.

## Clinical Features

Systemic signs and symptoms of acute hematogenous osteomyelitis may include a history of fever, chills or sweats, nausea, vomiting, evidence of dehydration, or sepsis. Lack of systemic response is possible. Irritability or lack of hunger may be the only systemic signs of infection is some cases, especially in neonates. Marked pain with direct palpation of the affected bone is one of the most consistent local findings in acute cases. Other important local signs may include decreased range of motion of the affected limb or joint, inability to bear weight or to ambulate on the affected lower extremity, and redness, edema, and increased temperature at the infection site. Pseudoparalysis is common in the very young child, but the protective muscle spasm that occurs with attempted movement of the affected limb will help to rule out other neuromuscular etiologies.

Subacute hematogenous osteomyelitis is an entity that has been described by numerous authors.[10-13] Typical signs of systemic infections are usually absent, and the child may not present for evaluation for months or even years after the initial infecting event.[14] The only clinical findings may be local tenderness and swelling. The leukocyte count is usually normal, but the erythrocyte sedimentation rate (ESR) may be elevated. The radiographic appearance has been classified by King and Mayo,[13] and is usually that of a low-grade inflammatory lesion, and the differential diagnosis will usually include benign bone tumors. The radiographic appearance is often that of a localized lytic lesion surrounded by a reactive sclerotic margin (Brodie's abscess)[15] (Fig. 24-3A). The clinical phenomenon of subacute hematogenous osteomyelitis or Brodie's abscess is probably primarily a manifestation of decreased bacterial virulence or vigorous host immune response resulting in a containment of infection resembling a foreign body inclusion cyst. Treatment requires surgical drainage and curettage of the cyst contents and any necrotic tissue or bone. Wounds are closed over a drain. Parenteral or sequential parenteral-oral antimicrobial therapy should be continued for at least 6 weeks.

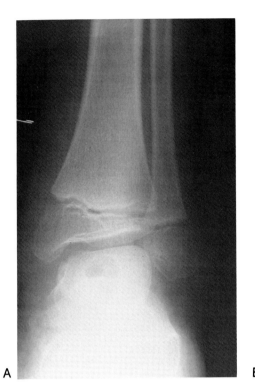

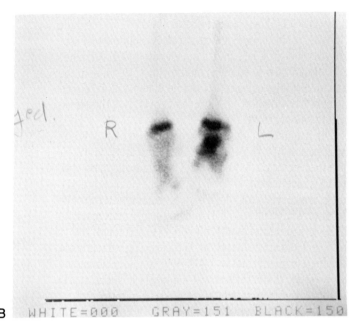

A

B

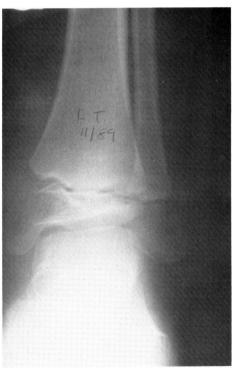

C

**Fig. 24-3.** An 8-year-old boy with subacute onset pain and swelling of left ankle area. History was remarkable for clubfoot release with talonavicular pinning as an infant. (**A**) Plain radiograph shows a well defined Brodie's abscess of the talar body. (**B**) Technetium 99 bone scan shows markedly increased uptake of the left talar body. (**C**) Appearance on radiograph 8 months after incision, drainage, and curettage of Brodie's abscess.

## Laboratory and Radiographic Findings

Laboratory findings of acute bone infection may include elevated white count, elevated polymorphonuclear leukocytes (possible left shift), and elevated ESR. Changes in ESR may also be useful in monitoring the course of the infection. Blood cultures should be drawn before an anticipated fever spike, as bacteremia precedes the elevation of temperature.

The diagnosis of acute hematogenous osteomyelitis is best established or refuted by obtaining an aspirate for culture from the affected area. This is usually done with an 18 gauge needle or lumbar puncture needle directed at the suspected area of bone involvement with the child sedated. Image intensification fluoroscopy may be useful if the affected area is difficult to locate (although this is not usually the case in the foot and lower leg). If pus is not obtained from soft tissue aspiration, the bone should be penetrated. If the differential diagnosis includes septic arthritis, the joint should be aspirated separately.

Radiographs taken during the first 1 to 2 weeks of infection may be completely unremarkable or may show only soft tissue manifestations of inflammation. The first soft tissue abnormality on plain films is often obliteration by edema of deep, radiographically lucent intramuscular tissue planes. Later, more superficial intramuscular tissue planes may be obliterated and subcutaneous edema may be present. Comparison views of the unaffected extremity may be helpful. Variable cancellous bone density and metaphyseal rarefaction due to hyperemic bone resorption and bone destruction are usually present between 1 and 3 weeks following onset of untreated infection in children. Periosteal elevation may occur if subperiosteal abscess develops, and new periosteal bone formation (involucrum) also may occur between 2 and 3 weeks. Late radiographic signs consistent with severe bone destruction (usually occurring more than 2 to 3 weeks after onset of infection) include patchy, irregular areas of lytic and sclerotic bone. Areas of sclerotic and necrotic bone (sequestrum), which lose their blood supply and cannot undergo demineralization, appear relatively radiodense as compared with surrounding areas of "excessively" vascularized bone that have undergone considerable resorption.

Radionuclide scans may also be helpful. Three-phase technetium 99 bone scans are highly sensitive but relatively nonspecific. Bone scans may occasionally show no uptake in very early hematogenous osteomyelitis if con- siderable vascular thrombosis has occurred. Use of a technetium 99 bone scan in combination with either a gallium 67 citrate or an indium 111 radionuclide scan provides considerably more specificity in detecting acute bone infection and is discussed in greater detail in Chapter 4.

A differential diagnosis in a child who presents with acute or subacute onset bone pain and swelling should include trauma, fracture, acute rheumatic fever or arthritis, septic arthritis, malignant bone tumor (e.g., Ewing's or osteogenic sarcoma), acute leukemia, and infantile cortical hyperostosis.

## Treatment

### Medical Management

Acute hematogenous osteomyelitis in children is primarily a medically treated disease, which can usually be managed with specific intravenous antimicrobial therapy alone without need for surgical debridement. Antibiotic therapy is specifically adjusted to eradicate expected organisms of the child's age group on the basis of positive blood culture or biopsy results (Fig. 24-4). Surgical intervention is necessary for those children who do not respond adequately within 48 hours to specific antimicrobial therapy or those with evidence of joint sepsis or abscess.

Initial empiric parenteral antibiotic therapy based on the most likely organism is the initial course of treatment. The bacteriology of pediatric hematogenous osteomyelitis changes with the age and developing immune system of the child. The most common organism found in children over 3 years of age and in adults with uncomplicated hematogenous osteomyelitis, is *S. aureus,* with streptococci occasionally present.[7-9] A β-lactamase (penicillinase)-resistant penicillin (e.g., nafcillin) or alternatively a first-generation cephalosporin usually provides adequate coverage as initial empiric antimicrobial therapy in this age group. *S. aureus* osteomyelitis is also quite common in younger children. Neonates, however, also are more likely to develop osteomyelitis secondary to group B streptococci or gram-negative Enterobacteriaceae and therefore require gram-negative coverage (e.g., by an aminoglycoside or a second-or third-generation cephalosporin) in addition to a β-lactamase-resistant penicillin. *H. influenzae* osteomyelitis is common in children between the neonatal period and 3 years of

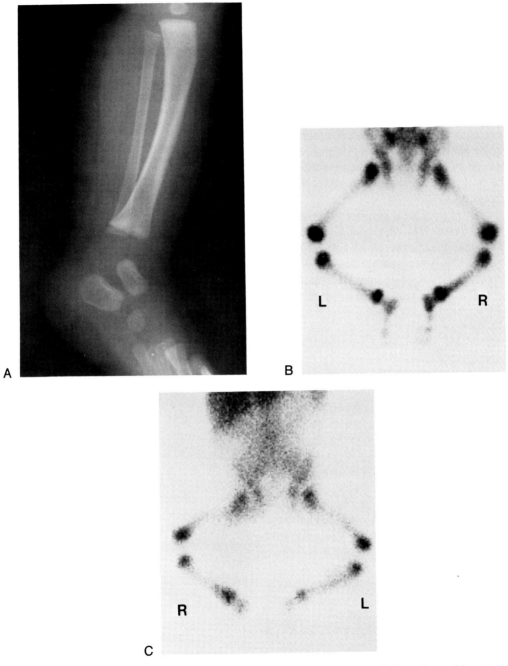

**Fig. 24-4.** A 3-month-old boy admitted with a tender, warm swelling of the distal right lower leg and fever to 104°F without a history of trauma. He did have a history of otitis media, which was treated 1 week prior to admission. Blood cultures yielded *S. aureus*. **(A)** Plain radiographs are unremarkable. **(B)** Technetium 99 bone scan reveals asymmetric tracer uptake in the right distal tibial metaphysis **(C)** Gallium 67 citrate scan also shows increased uptake. The patient was treated with intravenous nafcillin for 10 days followed by oral antibiotics for 1 month.

age.[7,9] *H. influenzae* meningitis has also been associated in some cases with osteomyelitis in this age group. Appropriate antimicrobial coverage for staphylococci, streptococci, and *H. influenzae* with adequate blood-brain barrier penetration should be selected as initial empirical therapy in this age group.

Subsequent choice of antimicrobials is based on identification of the causative organism as well as the minimum inhibitory concentration (MIC) and minimum bactericidal concentration (MBC) of the selected antimicrobial drug. Adequate MICs and MBCs ensure a good or excellent therapeutic to toxic ratio and an adequate serum levels of the antimicrobial and help prevent the phenomenon of tolerance.

Sequential use of parenteral antimicrobial treatment followed by oral antimicrobial regimens for suppurative skeletal infections has a number of advantages and has been fairly successful. The advantages include obviating the technical difficulties of maintaining intravenous lines for several weeks and decreasing the inherent risks of nosocomially acquired infection, the cost of hospitalization, and the cost of parenteral preparations. Certain caveats exist for safe, successful management. Initially, between 5 and 10 days of parenteral inpatient therapy is required, after which the patient is converted to an appropriate oral antimicrobial. Patients are seen frequently to ensure compliance. Serum antimicrobial concentrations are obtained to ensure adequate serum bactericidal activity (at least 1:8 to 1:16). Successful use of oral antimicrobial therapy requires that the patient remain free of major side effects, including pseudomembranous colitis. Appropriate blood tests, including white blood cell (WBC) count and ESR, are made at regular intervals. There is ample evidence now to conclude that adequate concentrations of antimicrobials can be attained in synovial fluid to treat acute pyogenic arthritis and acute osteomyelitis by this method.[16-21] The length of treatment is variable, depending upon the site and severity of infection, the extent of surgical decompression if any, and other host factors. Most uncomplicated cases of hematogenous osteomyelitis in children are treated with a minimum of 4 to 6 weeks of antimicrobial therapy.

A special situation exists in patients with sickle cell disease. Bone infarction and infection, both of which occur in the diaphysis of long bones, are difficult to differentiate clinically. Fever, ESR, and WBC counts are, however, usually higher in acute osteomyelitis. Bone

scan may be helpful to differentiate bone infarction from bone infection. Salmonella is the predominant organism found in sickle cell anemia-related osteomyelitis, which is thought to result from bacteremia following ingress of organisms through microinfarcts in the wall of the gastrointestinal tract. *S. aureus* is also commonly isolated.

### Surgical Management

Surgical intervention may include: (1) open biopsy to establish a diagnosis or identify a causative organism when needle aspiration or other more conservative techniques are not conclusive; or (2) surgical drainage of abscess or debridement of necrotic bone and infected granulation tissue. Surgical evacuation is generally indicated if an adequate response to parenteral therapy has not occurred within 48 hours or if abscess is present. An adequate response to parenteral therapy should include lessening signs of sepsis and local tenderness. The presence of abscess or sequestered or necrotic bone is always an indication for surgical drainage.

Surgical decompression and drainage are performed through a cortical window of about $1 \times 2$ cm size depending upon location. Fluoroscopic control may be helpful in localizing the area of involvement without physeal damage. Care should be taken to avoid excessive periosteal stripping, dissection about the perichondrial ring and physis, and excessive structural weakening of bone. Aerobic, anaerobic, acid-fast bacillus (AFB), and fungal cultures should always be obtained. The wound should be irrigated copiously, preferably with a pulsing power lavage. Deep soft tissue coverage of bone over a perforated closed suction Silastic drain is preferred to leaving a completely open wound. The remainder of the wound can be packed open or closed depending upon the extent of abscess. The drain is removed once drainage stops and systemic and local signs of infection show improvement, usually within 3 to 5 days.

## Osteomyelitis Secondary to a Contiguous Focus of Infection

Osteomyelitis that occurs as a result of spread from an adjacent infection site may have multiple and diverse etiologies. The spectrum runs from infections following puncture wounds, cat bites, and thermal burns to those following surgical fracture correction and reconstruction. These traumatic or surgical insults result in the implantation of the organism directly into bone or into the adjacent soft tissue. Direct implantation of the organism subepidermally into bone via trauma may delay diagnosis or suspicion of osteomyelitis, especially when multiple trauma is involved.

Early deep wound infections due to ordinarily noninvasive bacteria such as *S. epidermidis* or diphtheroids are usually low-grade and insidious. The only sign of infection may be persistent brawny edema and mildly increased local temperature. An elevated ESR along with drainage of seropurulent material from the wound may clarify the diagnosis. Bone involvement is often present. Systemic signs are usually absent in early phases of the infection but may appear as infection progresses. Specimens for bacteriologic study may be obtained from the wound (although these are not definitive), sinus tract, deep tissue, or a bone biopsy.

## Puncture Wounds

Osteomyelitis associated with puncture wound injuries commonly involve the foot or the patella and have, inappropriately, been broadly termed *inoculation osteomyelitis* in the earlier literature. The latter terminology may be used if there is documented osteomyelitis following inoculation. In children, osteochondritis (inflammation of bone and cartilage) tends to result more often than true osteomyelitis. Nail puncture wounds account for the vast majority (90 percent or more) of puncture wounds to the feet of children in most studies.[22] In general, puncture wounds to the foot account for almost 1 percent of all

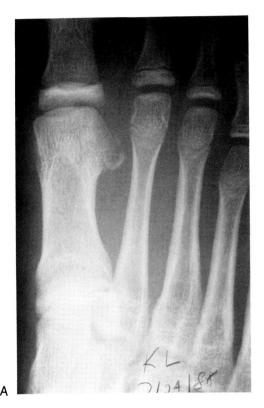
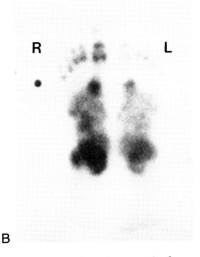

**Fig. 24-5.** A 13-year-old boy who stepped on a nail, which penetrated his tennis shoe plantar to the first metatarsophalangeal joint, 10 days prior. Erythema and first metatarsophalangeal joint effusion were present. **(A)** Oblique radiograph shows destructive changes of the fibular sesamoid bone. **(B)** Technetium 99 bone scan shows intense asymmetric uptake about joint. Joint aspiration yielded *P. aeruginosa*. Treatment consisted of incision, drainage, and excision of the fibular sesamoid bone through a plantar approach as well as intravenous tobramycin for 6 weeks.

visits to emergency rooms for children age 15 and under.[23] Acute or subacute onset soft tissue infection probably occurs in about 10 percent of these cases, and osteomyelitis occurs in about 1.5 percent of all cases.[24-26]

*P. aeruginosa* is the predominant organism responsible for more than 90 to 95 percent of cases of post-puncture wound osteomyelitis of the foot[27-31] (Fig. 24-5). It is frequently recovered from the inner foam layer of the sole of sneakers,[32,33] which acts as a reservoir for the eventual inoculum when a penetrating injury occurs. The perfect milieu for the proliferation of *Pseudomonas* is created by the persistently damp sneaker environment that occurs secondary to perspiration, lack of adequate aeration, and increased water permeability with shoe wear. Occasionally, *S. aureus,* streptococci, or other species of *Pseudomonas* may be responsible for puncture wound-associated infections. However, *P. aeruginosa* organisms have a high predilection for infecting the cartilage.[34] The practice of using $\beta$-lactam-based antimicrobials orally or as topical agents tends to encourage the growth of the *Pseudomonas* superinfection.

Puncture wounds of the patella are generally accidental and are incurred during play when pine needles, cactus thorns, or wooden splinters are embedded. The most common age group is between 5 and 15 years, when the patella is still in its "vascular phase." In adulthood the patella becomes almost totally avascular. A typical history of inoculation is generally present, and signs of osteomyelitis usually appear about 7 to 10 days following the event. *S. aureus* is the most common organism isolated in osteomyelitis of the patella secondary to puncture wounds. Sporotrichosis or trichosporon is more commonly associated with puncture wounds secondary to thorn injuries.

### Clinical Features

Examination of the wound site is necessary to exclude the presence of any residual foreign body. Riegler and Routson reported the presence of foreign material in as many as 50 percent of cases when infection occurred following puncture wounds even though previous emergency room treatment had been rendered.[35] A hyperkeratotic layer of tissue, which must be debrided, may be present at the puncture entry site before proper wound exploration can be performed.

The initial pain and swelling associated with puncture wounds of the foot may be poorly localized. Point tenderness with localized swelling and erythema usually occurs by the third or fourth postinjury day. Generally, no fever or leukocytosis is present, and the ESR is not helpful in evaluating disease activity.

In patellar involvement no constitutional signs are noted, but significant patellar pain results upon extension of the leg. The diagnosis may be confirmed when changes are visible radiographically 2 to 3 weeks later. Computed tomographic (CT) views of the patella may be helpful and may indicate rarefaction or sclerosis. The treatment is directed toward the appropriate organism (s), and debridement may also be required. In resistant cases a search should be made for fungal elements.

### Treatment

Most children (i.e., more than 90 percent) who suffer puncture wounds to the foot do not develop infection, and very few develop osteomyelitis (fewer than 1 to 2 percent). It is difficult to predict those children who will develop late onset indolent gram-negative osteomyelitis on the basis of initial presentation. In addition no useful oral prophylactic agents are available. It is unreasonable to subject every child who presents with a puncture wound to surgical wound exploration or hospitalization and parenteral antimicrobial administration. Until recently no useful predictor was available to identify high-risk patients. In 1989 Patzakis et al. classified the sole of the foot into three anatomic zones according to risk of infection or late osteomyelitis with puncture wounds on the basis of a retrospective review of 81 cases[36] (Fig. 24-6). Of those infections requiring hospitalization 50 percent occurred in zone 1, 33 percent in zone 3, and 17 percent in zone 2. The vulnerable subcutaneous location of the metatarsophalangeal joint (zone 1) and the high impact weigh-bearing of the heel (zone 3) make these areas particularly susceptible to deep penetrating injury and bone and joint inoculation. Wounds in zone 2 or very superficial wounds without local or systemic signs of infection or gross contamination can usually be managed with warm soaks, tetanus prophylaxis, and observation. Deep penetrating wounds of zones 1 and 3 can usually be managed on an outpatient basis by close observation and local wound care if no signs of systemic or local infection or foreign body are present. Patients should be followed at weekly intervals for up to 3 weeks. Wound exploration

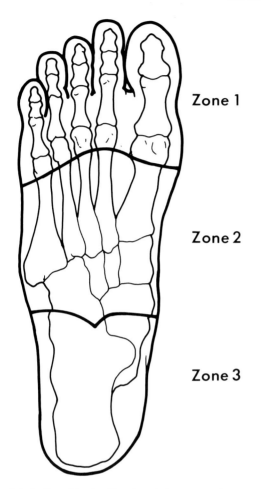

Zone 1

Zone 2

Zone 3

**Fig. 24-6.** Patzakis classification of plantar puncture wounds of the foot. Puncture wounds are classified as involving high risk (zone 1), moderate risk (zone 3) and relatively low risk (zone 2) of osteomyelitis or deep infection. (From Patzakis et al.,[36] with permission.)

and debridement are considered in the basis of degree of local edema, erythema, and degree of contamination. We recommend the use of an oral quinolone plus a $\beta$-lactam-based antimicrobial (e.g., cephalexin) in high-risk patients over the age of 16 years; however, with high-risk children under 16 years of age with signs of infection requiring hospitalization, parenteral nonquinolone antipseudomonal therapy [e.g. ceftazidime alone or cefoperazone, a monobactam (aztreonam), or a ureidopenicillin, in combination with an aminoglycoside] is preferable.

The "ideal" duration of therapy for documented os-

teomyelitis is considered to be a minimum of 4 weeks. We, along with others, have noted that when parenteral therapy is combined with thorough surgical drainage and debridement, local signs and symptoms often resolve within 4 to 5 days. We prefer to continue parenteral antimicrobial therapy for about 10 to 12 days after the first thorough debridement. A recent prospective study evaluated a treatment regimen with a shorter (7-day) duration of intravenous antimicrobials following effective surgical drainage and debridement. A clinical course without relapse was produced in 75 of 77 patients.[7]

## Chronic Osteomyelitis

Osteomyelitis that is hematogenous, secondary to a contiguous focus of infection, or secondary to a vascular insufficiency may present as either an acute or chronic process. The criteria for chronicity are still not agreed upon. Chronic osteomyelitis has been defined in various ways, including osteomyelitis present for more than 3 weeks prior to initiation of treatment; persistence of a draining sinus for at least 5 to 8 weeks; osteomyelitis with recurrent admissions; and pain with or without a draining sinus for 8 weeks.[37]

The therapy of acute osteomyelitis is relatively well defined, but that of chronic osteomyelitis has not been well established. Selection of optimal antimicrobials, duration of therapy, and potential recurrence after many years of quiescence are major considerations in the management of chronic osteomyelitis. Incision and drainage of any abscess, surgical debridement of any necrotic bone and sequestrum, and adequate soft tissue bone coverage, which may require muscle or skin flap replacement, are important mainstays of therapy (Fig. 24-7). Debridement should include complete excision of all devitalized bone, scars, and chronic granulation tissue. Bone should be curetted to healthy-appearing bleeding bone; however, the structural integrity of important bones must be maintained. The wound is usually packed open if abscess is present or extensive drainage is required. Delayed partial wound closure can usually be performed in 2 to 5 days. Alternatively, the wound can be closed over perforated closed suction Silastic drains. It is important to provide deep soft tissue coverage of exposed bone as soon as possible to prevent desiccation and further necrosis. The superficial portion of the wound is often left open to heal secondarily. The Mayo Clinic has

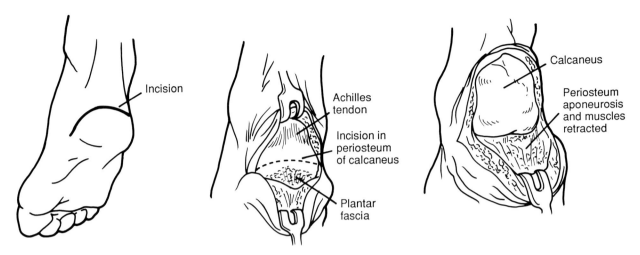

**Fig. 24-7.** Surgical exposure of the calcaneus. (Modified from Tachdjian,[37] with permission.)

reported 76 percent short-term and 66 percent one-year success rates with aggressive combination surgical and antimicrobial therapy in the management of chronic bone infection.[38]

Selection of an appropriate antimicrobial should be based upon bone cultures taken at the time of debridement. It is often difficult, however, to culture the offending organism from areas of chronic bone infection, and blood cultures are usually not helpful. This may be due in part to chronic and frequent antimicrobial therapy received by many of these patients. In cases in which no organism can be recovered, treatment should be based upon previous cultures, if available, or the most likely organism (usually *S. aureus*) should be assumed to be the offending agent. The duration of therapy for *S. aureus* infection is 4 to 6 weeks of parenteral antibiotics followed by oral therapy of up to 3 to 6 months. If *P. aeruginosa* is involved or a mixed infection is present, therapy may need to be much longer, and repeated surgical intervention is often necessary. The availability of home-based therapy using Hickman, Groshong, or other similar central venous line catheters has helped to decrease lengthy hospitalization. ESR, WBC count activity, and newer types of diagnostic imaging techniques are helpful but not totally reliable in determining the activity of infection. Implantation of gentamicin- or tobramycin-containing beads made of methyl methacrylate bone cement has also been used in the management of chronic bone infection for both gram-negative and gram-positive bacterial infections. This technique provides very high prolonged local tissue levels of antimicrobial at the site of chronic infection, where vascular supply and thus systemic antimicrobial penetration is usually poor while avoiding much of the potential toxicity of prolonged systemic treatment.

## Septic Arthritis

### Pathogenesis

Acute septic arthritis (also known as septic joint, pyarthrosis, and suppurative arthritis) is a relatively uncommon disease. Septic arthritis results from bacterial invasion of the joint secondary to hematogenous seeding, from a contiguous focus of osteomyelitis, or from a long-standing soft tissue infection. Common organisms include *S. aureus,* group B streptoccocci, *H. influenzae,* and gram-negative organisms. *Pseudomonas* is a common isolate when infection is associated with puncture wounds. In the child 1 to 11 years of age the hematogenous route is most common owing to the vascular anatomy of the physis and epiphysis. Joint infection may occur secondary to hematogenous seeding from systemic ailments such as pneumonia, endocarditis, or sexually transmitted diseases. In the age group between 6 months and 5 years, *H. influenzae* type B is common and may even be the predominant organism. *Neisseria gonorrhoeae* should be kept in mind in the adolescent presenting with polyarthritis.

## Clinical Features

A septic joint is painful and warm and often demonstrates marked effusion. Muscle splinting and pseudoparalysis may be evident at the jolint level and may be the presenting picture in the neonate or toddler. Extremity muscle splinting, irritability, and refusal to ambulate are common presenting signs in the older child. Systemic signs of infection (e.g., fever, malaise, tachycardia) may be present. The diagnosis is obtained by aspiration of the affected joint after a local field block. Care is taken not to penetrate adjacent cartilage or bone during the procedure. After arthrocentesis, the specimen is sent for Gram stain, culture, and joint fluid analysis (Table 24-1). A complete blood count (CBC) with differential and an ESR should be obtained to monitor the course of the infection. Joint aspiration in septic arthritis yields fluid that varies in color from cloudy yellow to creamy white. The WBC count in the aspirate is generally in the range of 50,000 to 100,000, but in gonococcal arthritis it may be lower than 50,000 cells per cubic millimeter. However, in all bacterial effusions (except those due to mycobacteria and brucellosis) there is a predominance of polymorphonuclear leukocytes (90 to 95 percent). Gram smear often reveals the etiologic organism. Glucose determination along with concomitant blood glucose may also aid in the diagnosis. In situations in which antimicrobials have been used, latex agglutination or counterimmunoelectrophoresis techniques are often helpful. Blood cultures should be obtained in all situations.

## Treatment

Joint sepsis should be considered an intra-articular abscess; hence surgical drainage is necessary. Repeated aspiration or arthroscopic drainage and irrigation may be adequate in larger joints (ankle or knee). Repeated accumulation of fluid in larger joints and sepsis of the small joints of the foot usually require open drainage and irrigation. When osteomyelitis is present, debridement of infected bone must also be performed. Bacteremia, if present, should also be evaluated with blood cultures and managed with appropriate systemic antimicrobial therapy.

Antimicrobials are always started early and are given parenterally as soon as the relevant cultures are obtained. An antistaphylococcal antimicrobial is always included. In neonates and in the age group in which *H. influenzae* is likely to be present gram-negative antimicrobial coverage must be included. We prefer either cefotaxime or cefuroxime as our initial empirical antimicrobial, as these also provide an excellent penetration of

Table 24-1. **Joint Fluid Analysis**

| Disease | Appearance | WBC[a] Count (cells per cubic millimeter) | Differential | Viscosity | Sugar | Protein | Bacteria | Crystals |
|---|---|---|---|---|---|---|---|---|
| Osteoarthritis | Yellow, clear | 200–10,000 | Lymphs[a] | Good | High | Low | None | None |
| Rheumatoid arthritis | Yellow, cloudy | 10,000–50,000 | Polys[a] | Poor | Middle | High | None | None |
| Lupus erythematosus | Yellow, cloudy | 5,000–25,000 | Polys and lymphs | Fair | Middle | High | None | None |
| Reiter's disease | Yellow, cloudy | 25,000–100,000 | Polys | Poor | Middle | High | None | None |
| Gout | Yellow, cloudy | 15,000–50,000 | Polys | Fair | High | High | None | Urate |
| Pseudogout | Yellow, cloudy | 15,000–50,000 | Polys | Fair | High | High | None | Pyrophosphate |
| Infection: viral | Yellow, clouds | 5,000–25,000 | Lymphs | Good | High | Middle | None | None |
| Infection: bacterial | Yellow, cloudy to purulent | 15,000–100,000 | Polys | Poor | Low | High | Present | None |
| Infection: mycobacterial | Yellow, cloudy | 15,000–100,000 | Lymphs and polys | Poor | Low | High | Biopsy positive | None |
| Infection: fungal | Yellow, cloudy | 15,000–100,000 | Polys | Poor | Low | High | May need special media | None |

[a] WBC = white blood cell; lymphs, lymphocytes; polys, polymorphonuclear leukocytes.

the blood-brain barrier, thereby ensuring adequate empirical concomitant coverage of potential *H. influenzae* meningitis or other gram-negative Enterobacteriaceae infections. These third-generation cephalosporins also provide adequate protection against *S. aureus*. If *S. aureus* alone is isolated on final cultures, a pure antistaphylococcal agent such as nafcillin or cefazolin is preferred. The duration of parenteral therapy is between 5 and 14 days. Longer therapy is necessary for concomitant osteomyelitis, as previously discussed. Following parenteral therapy, the child is given an oral antimicrobial such as dicloxacillin, cephalexin, or cefuroxime, depending upon the identity and sensitivity of the organism isolated, to complete a total antimicrobial course of 4 weeks for larger joints. Surgical drainage of gonococcal ankle joint sepsis is not required. Penicillin is the drug of choice, except in rare instances in which a resistant organism that produces β-lactamase is present, in which case alternate agents such as ceftriaxone may be used very effectively.

Local measures include extremity immobilization and wound care. Closed suction irrigation systems may be used for daily joint lavage. Joint motion should be maintained. Inadequately treated joint sepsis may lead to early arthritis or even ankylosis.

# SOFT TISSUE INFECTIONS

The dorsal and plantar aspects of the foot are especially vulnerable to numerous insults, including puncture wounds, blister formation, maceration of toe web spaces, animal bites, and direct and indirect injuries related to athletic activities. Some common types of soft tissue infections are reviewed below.

## Toe Web Space Infections

In toe web spacing infections the most frequently isolated organism is *P. aeruginosa,* with *Proteus mirabilis* the next most common cause.[39] Other bacteria, such as *S. aureus* and *Corynebacterium minutissum* may also cause toe web space infections. The tissue is generally damp, boggy, and macerated, and a purlent discharge may be noted. The third and fourth web spaces are the most common sites of involvement. Sinus tract formation is not uncommon and must be explored if present. Generally there is a preceding history of tinea pedis or of prolonged immersion or exposure to excessive perspiration. Treatment consists of debridement of any macer-

ated tissue combined with soaks, with or without broad-spectrum oral antimicrobial treatment, for mild infection. Treatment of more severe infections may require parenteral antimicrobials or oral quinolones in patients over 16 years of age.

## Tinea Pedis

The warm, moist, dark environment found in shoes provides an ideal habitat for the fungi that cause tinea pedis. Dermatophyte organisms can be found in a variety of places, including soil, shoes, and showers. The infection may be acute or chronic. Acute tinea pedis is characterized by vesicular eruptions, pruritus, erythema, and tenderness. Secondary bacterial infections with pustules are common findings. *Trichophyton mentagrophytes* is the responsible organism in the majority of acute cases. Chronic tinea pedis is characterized by scaling and peeling of the epidermis in a moccasin distribution. Re-exacerbation of infection is common, especially in summer months. The organism responsible for chronic tinea pedis in over 50 percent of cases is *Trichophyton rubrum.* Diagnosis is confirmed by the presence of fungal hyphae on microscopic examination of potassium hydroxide wet-mounted slides containing epidermal scrapings or by positive identification of dermatophytes on dermatophyte test medium (DTM) culture medium.

Treatment may include soaks with drying medication (e.g., Burow's solution) and topical antifungals (e.g., creams, powders, or sprays). The patient should be advised to wear sandals or other open-type shoes. Oral griseofulvin or ketoconazole may be used in severe acute or recalcitrant cases combined with topical antifungal medication.

## Paronychia

Paronychia can be defined as a periungual, subcuticular abscess. The offending nail border acts as a foreign body irritant; it should be debrided or resected to decompress any periungual abscess and eliminate mechanical irritation of surrounding soft tissues. The most common offending organism is *S. aureus*. Oral penicillinase-resistant penicillin or cephalosporins (e.g., dicloxacillin, cephalexin) are used to treat early paronychia without abscess or to hasten recovery in severe cases. Often saline soaks will suffice once the offending nail edge has been removed. Osteomyelitis secondary to paronychia in an uncompromised host is extremely rare. A *felon,* or digital terminal pulp abscess, can, however, result in osteomyelitis of the distal phalanx. Incision and drainage are necessary, along with appropriate oral antimicrobial management. The reader is referred to Chapter 16 for further discussion of the management of ingrown toenails.

## Animal Bites

Animal bites or scratches may inoculate local soft tissues, which may later infect bones and joints. The deeper bites may inoculate organisms directly into synovial sheaths and osseous or articular structures. Cat and dog bites make up the majority of animal bites. *Pasteurella multocida* is the predominant organism, along with *S. aureus* and streptococci. *P. multocida* is a nonmotile, non-spore-forming, gram-negative coccobacillus, which thrives in aerobic as well as anaerobic environments. A number of anaerobes may also be part of the flora inoculated. Since all animal bites should be considered tetanus prone, a history including the tetanus status of the patient and the immunization status of the animal is important. In addition to the superficial wound, localized cellulitis is a common finding. The causative organisms generally respond to penicillin unless they produce $\beta$-lactamase. It is important to ensure that the deeper structures have not been damaged, since otherwise, a chronic course ensues with involvement along fascial planes or in synovial sheaths or bone, which may require extensive surgery and result in permanent damage. Radiographic studies are necessary to rule out osseous involvement. Irrigation and cleansing of the wound, aggressive debridement of any devitalized tissue, and drainage of any suspected abscess should be performed. Lower extremity animal bite wounds should not be closed primarily.

## Marine Infections

Cellulitis, myositis, lymphangitis, and septicemia occur commonly when wounds in general have been exposed to marine or brackish water, shellfish, or other sea creatures.

*Vibrio vulnificus* infections may occur from ingesting raw shellfish or from direct contamination of open wounds exposed to contaminated seawater. Skin lesions are characterized by an intense, rapidly progressive subcutaneous cellulitis with extension into the dermis and muscle.[40] An overlying hemorrhagic bulla may be present. Within hours these areas may infarct, causing large areas of devitalized tissue. Morbidity and mortality are fairly high reaching approximately 15 to 25 percent in patients who are immunocompromised. The disease is less dramatic in the nonimmunocompromised host. Diagnosis is made by history of exposure to salt water and demonstration of curved gram-negative bacilli on Gram stain or culture. Treatment of wound and metastatic lesions consists of aggressive surgical debridement along with parenteral antimicrobials, preferably doxycycline in combination with cefotaxime, although an ideal regimen has not yet been established.[41] Carbenicillin, erythromycin, and gentamicin are generally not efficient.[42] Supportive care, intravenous fluids, and monitoring in an intensive care setting are necessary in severe cases.

If *Vibrio alginolyticus* is isolated from a wound infection, most superficial wounds will only require local care. Trimethoprim-sulfamethoxazole or doxycycline should be used in immunocompromised patients. Although doxycycline is generally contraindicated in children under 8 years of age, when life-threatening situations occur and no other choices are available, it may be used with care.

*Mycobacterium fortuitum* and *Mycobacterium chelonei* are found in soil and water and are inoculated in the wound following a cutting, scraping, or penetrating injury. *Mycobacterium marinum* is acquired during swimming accidents. These mycobacteria are resistant to antituberculous agents but are susceptible to amikacin, cefoxitin, sulfonamides, doxycycline, erythromycin, and the quinolones.[43]

## Cellulitis

Cellulitis results from infection of the subcutaneous tissue and rarely may lead to infection of deeper structures. Physical examination findings may include pain, swelling, erythema, and increased heat within the inflamed tissue. Red streaks may indicate lymphangitis. Systemic signs of infection are often present. Diagnosis is usually made by physical examination and confirmed with laboratory results. *S. aureus* and streptococci are usually implicated, but diverse organisms have been isolated, including *H. influenzae* and mycobacteria. Prognosis for recovery is normally good; however, in long-standing cases or in immunocompromised hosts, necrotizing infections may occur.

Parenteral therapy is indicated and blood cultures should be obtained when septicemia is present. A sterile nonbacteriostatic saline aspiration culture of infected areas can be used but usually is unnecessary. Empirical antimicrobial therapy with an antistaphylococcal antmicrobial (e.g., nafcillin, cephazolin) is usually adequate. Localization of infection in the form of focal abscess formation may occur after onset of treatment, requiring surgical drainage. Local measures include intravenous fluids, rest, leg elevation, and warm, moist dressings.

## Crepitant Cellulitis, Fasciitis, and Myositis

*Clostridial cellulitis* is characterized by a crepitant septic process involving the epifascial and subcutaneous tissue, usually in a traumatized lower extremity. Local pain and swelling are present. Gas formation may be extensive, but the wound often appears benign. The incidence of classical gas gangrene has decreased considerably as a result of debridement and the extensive use of prophylactic antimicrobials in treating traumatic wounds. The incubation period is shorter in clostridial myonecrosis (gas gangrene) than it is in clostridial cellulitis, and the disease is more aggressive, with a higher morbidity and mortality. In both situations *Clostridium perfringens* is the primary causative organism, and the damage is due to its various toxins. Therapy is surgical and is aggressive in both situations. Any sutured wound should be widely opened and debrided, and antimicrobials should be rapidly delivered. Gram-stained smears of wound exudate will show the characteristic predominant gram-positive bacilli, possibly along with gram-negative bacilli. Penicillin G is the antibiotic of choice, but Chloramphenicol, clindamycin, or cefoxitin may be added or may be substituted in cases of penicillin allergy. Guillotine amputation may be necessary if wide extensive debridement is not effective in controlling infection. Hyperbaric oxygen is a valuable adjunctive therapy if readily available.[44] Antisera have not been found effective.

In *necrotizing fasciitis* there is widespread fascial necrosis with relative sparing of skin and underlying muscle. Severe systemic toxicity is present.[45] Necrotizing fasciitis may be rapidly fatal unless prompt therapy is instituted. The most frequent sites of infection are the extremities, and infection usually develops following minor trauma. Skin abscesses, frostbite, insect bites, open fractures, and surgical wounds are common initiating factors. Initially a cellulitic, red, hot, swollen and tender area is noted. Later the erythema spreads, and the skin becomes shiny, smooth, and tense, after which it changes color to a dark dusky blue, with formation of

blisters and bullae. The bullae later become hemorrhagic. A foul-smelling dishwater like purulent drainage follows. Ecchymotic areas, with subsequent thrombosis of subcutaneous veins and nutrient arteries may follow, resulting in focal areas of necrosis. Gangrene of the skin follows the resulting ischemia, and the skin also develops anesthesia or hypoesthesia due do destruction of the subcutaneous nerves. Cutaneous anesthesia may precede the appearance of skin necrosis. Septic shock results and may be fatal if the patient remains untreated.

Facultative anaerobes such as streptococci (other than group A) are usually isolated in combination with obligate anaerobes such as *Bacteroides* and *Peptostreptococcus*. Members of the Enterobacteriaceae group may also be present. Obligate aerobes are usually not isolated. Initial culture material for Gram stain is best obtained from areas of necrotic cellulitis when the leading edge is aspirated. It should be noted that cultures should always be sent for aerobic and anaerobic isolation. Radiography detects gas in soft tissue readily when present and tends to point to the presence of anaerobes. Wide surgical drainage through extensive fasciotomy together with debridement of all necrotic tissue is of paramount importance. Frequent repeat debridement is often necessary. Adjunctive therapy with triple antimicrobials (e.g., penicillin, gentamicin and clindamycin or penicillin, gentamicin, and metronidazole), together with appropriate acid-base, electrolyte, and fluid correction, is instituted. Hyperbaric oxygen therapy, if readily available, may aid in halting the progression of the anaerobic process.

*Myositis* may have multiple etiologies, including spread from a contiguous source of infection to injured muscle; hematogenous seeding in muscle previously injured through trauma; and direct inoculation of organisms into the muscle itself (e.g., by injection with a dirty needle). This infection, rarely seen in the foot or ankle, produces cramping, splinting, pain, and swelling, with an increase in temperature present over the affected muscle. Induration may indicate abscess formation. In longstanding cases, severe damage to the muscle may occur with resultant loss of function. Acute presentation with systemic toxicity is not uncommon. Clinical entities that may be associated with myositis include clostridial myonecrosis, acute bacterial myositis, including staphylococcal and streptococcal necrotizing myositis, and following influenza.[46] Disseminated fungal myositis may result from *Candida* infection. Parasitic myositis has been described as a result of trichinosis, toxoplasmosis, and cysticercosis. Surgical debridement, if indicated, bed rest, elevation, and appropriate antibiotics are mainstays of therapy.

*Pyomyositis* is a disease of adolescents and young adults, although cases do occur in infants. Pyogenic intramuscular abscesses are more often seen in the tropics. These abscesses are usually associated with trauma, diabetes, intravenous drug use, poor hygiene, and poor nutrition. Solitary or multiple lesions may be present and may involve the thigh, calf, buttock, arm, scapula, and chest wall. The lesions appear "woody" to palpation and are tender and generally without fluctuance, erythema, or warmth. Diagnosis can be confirmed with ultrasound. Gallium 67 citrate scanning is the most sensitive diagnostic procedure for detecting small muscle abscesses.

## LYME DISEASE

Lyme disease is a complex, multisystem disorder, which begins with a bite by *Ixodes dammini* or related ixodid ticks. *Borrelia burgdorferi,* a spirochete, is transmitted to the host by the insect bite. The illness, like syphilis, has been divided into three clinical stages, based upon differences in appearance and organ system involvement, which often occur over a period of many months to years. Lyme disease primarily affects the skin, nervous system, heart, and musculoskeletal system. In stage I a unique lesion, erythema chronicum migrans, is noted in approximately 80 percent of individuals. Other skin manifestations also occur, and a flu-like illness, which includes arthralgias and bone pain, may be present. In stage II the nervous system, heart, and eyes are involved. In stage III the predominant manifestation is arthritis, which involves one or two joints at a time, is migratory, and involves large joints more commonly. Late neurologic complications may occur. An excellent review of the diagnosis and management of Lyme disease has been provided by Duffy.[47]

## ANTIMICROBIAL REVIEW

Antimicrobials play a pivotal role as adjunct therapy of lower extremity musculoskeletal infections. Newer penicillins, second-, third-, and fourth-generation cephalosporins, second- and third-generation quinolones, semisynthetic monobactams, thienamycins (penems), and combinations of antimicrobials with $\beta$-lactamase inhibitors have been developed since about 1975 by modification of the basic structure of the $\beta$-lactam ring or by addition of side chains, thus conferring greater stability and improving the spectrum of activity.

## The Penicillins

All penicillins have in common a $\beta$-lactam ring structure and the ability to inhibit bacterial cell wall synthesis (bacteriocidal activity) (Fig. 24-8). The specific antibacterial activity of the different penicillins is determined primarily by side chain substitutions. For purposes of discussion, the penicillins will be divided into the following six groups based upon their spectrum of antibacterial activity and chemical structure: (1) basic penicillins; (2) penicillinase-resistant penicillins; (3) aminopenicillins; (4) carboxypenicillins; (5) acylureidopenicillins; and (6) penicillins combined with $\beta$-lactamase inhibitors.

### The Basic Penicillins

The basic penicillins include antimicrobials such as penicillin V, penicillin G, procaine penicillin G, and benzathine penicillin G (Fig. 24-8). The basic penicillin spectrum of activity includes most streptococci, some anaerobes and gram-negative cocci, and non-penicillinase-producing staphylococci. Penicillinase, an enzyme produced by some bacteria, is capable of inactivating the $\beta$-lactam ring structure of the penicillins, which makes these antimicrobials ineffective against any penicillinase-producing organisms. The basic penicillins have limited usefulness in the management of lower extremity infections except when combined with other antimicrobial regimens, as the predominant organisms in most lower extremity musculoskeletal infections are penicillinase-producing organisms.

### Penicillinase-Resistant Penicillins

Minor modification of the $\beta$-lactam ring structure of the basic penicillin antibiotics has resulted in the development of antibiotics that are resistant to $\beta$-lactamase destruction (Fig. 24-9). The spectrum of these penicillinase-resistant penicillins is similar to that of the basic penicillins with the addition of $\beta$-lactamase-producing

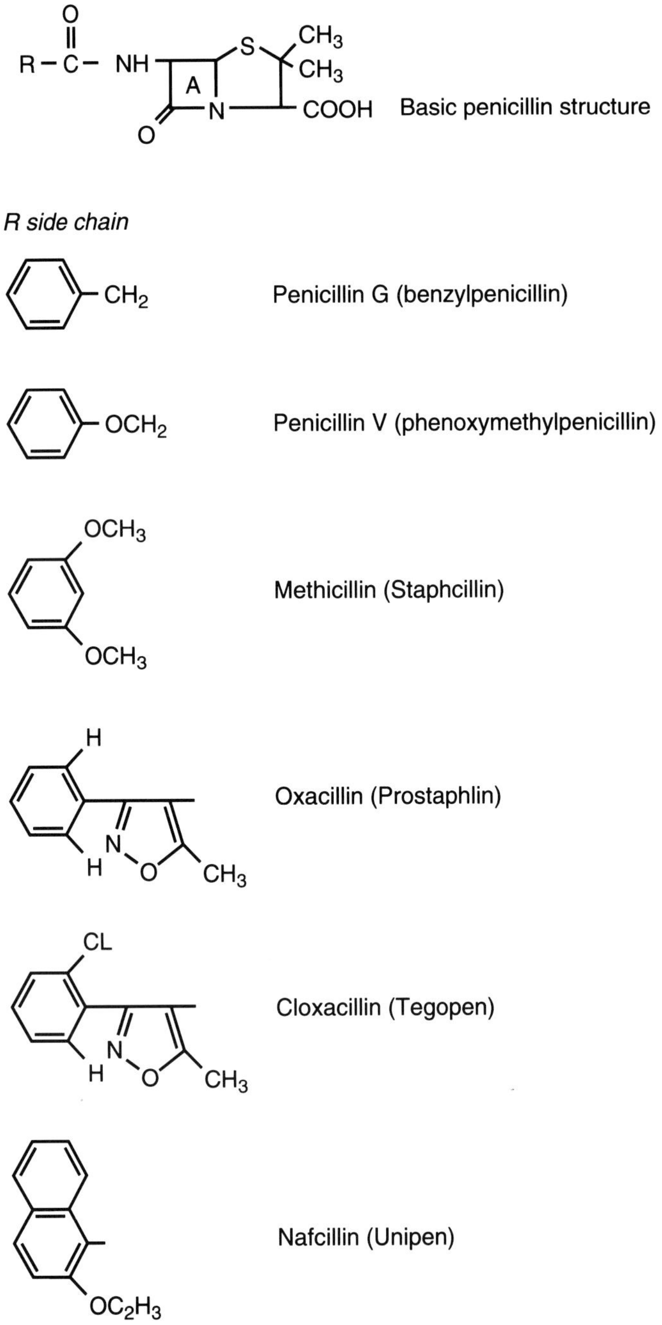

**Fig. 24-8.** Structural formulas of the basic penicillins.

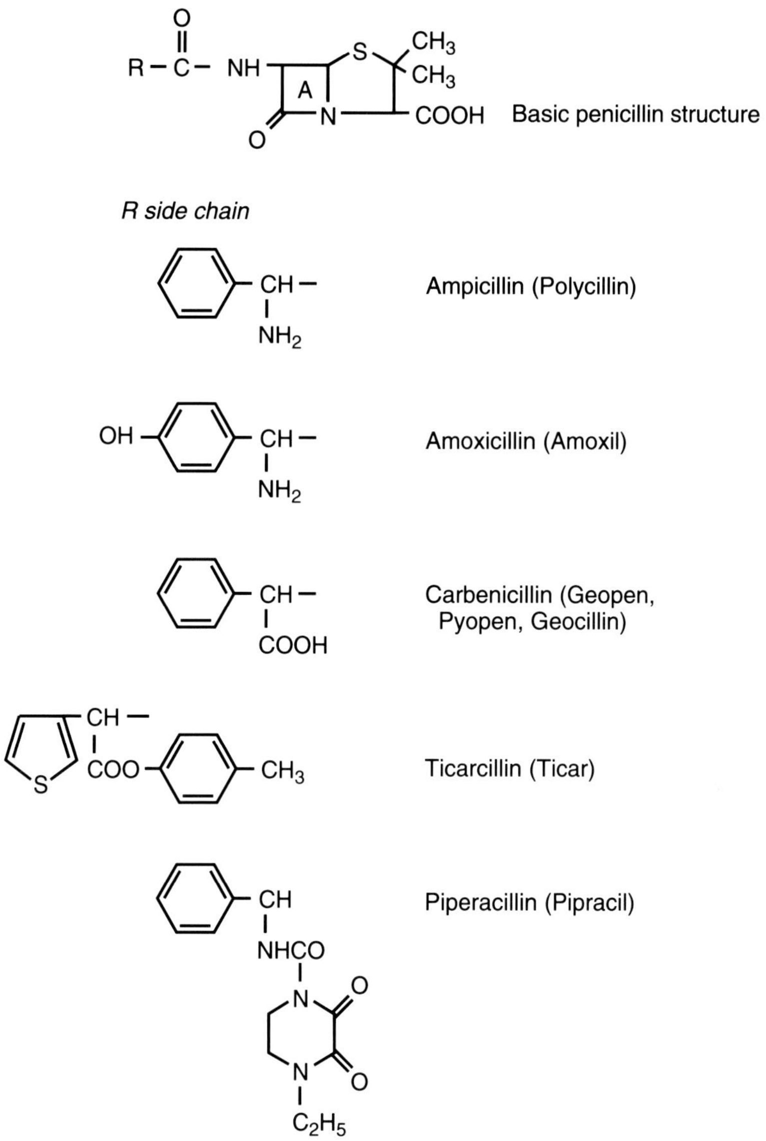

Fig. 24-9. Structural formulas of the newer penicillins.

staphylococci, which now cause the majority of lower extremity infections in both children and adults. Although serum concentrations of penicillinase-resistant penicillins are usually adequate to eradicate most streptococcal infections, these infections are generally more susceptible to and more appropriately treated with the basic penicillins. Available penicillinase-resistant penicillins include the oral forms of dicloxicillin and cloxicillin and parenteral forms of methicillin, nafcillin, and oxacillin.

### Aminopenicillins

The aminopenicillins include ampicillin and amoxicillin (Fig. 24-9). Their spectrum is similar to that of penicillin G, although their activity is weakened against organisms known to be sensitive to penicillin G. Their activity against gram-negative bacilli, including the enteric organisms and enterococci, however, is enhanced as compared with that of the basic penicillins.

### Carboxypenicillins

The carboxypenicillins were the first generation of penicillins to be developed with activity against *P. aeruginosa* (Fig. 24-9). They include the parenteral preparations of carbenicillin and ticarcillin. They may also be useful in the treatment of infections involving *Enterobacter* and *Proteus;* however their activity is limited, and when used in the management of serious infections, they should be combined with an aminoglycoside for synergy.

### Acylureidopenicillins

The acylureidopenicillins, which might be considered second-generation carboxypenicillins, were developed by substituting a ureido group (NH-CO-NR2) for the carboxy group, thereby maintaining ampicillin's valuable activity against *Streptococcus faecalis* while enhancing activity against gram-negative bacilli, including *P. aeruginosa, Proteus, Klebsiella,* and some anaerobes (Fig. 24-9). These antibiotics, which are only available in parenteral preparations, include piperacillin, mezlocillin, and azlocillin.

### Penicillins Combined with β-Lactamase Inhibitors

Clavulinic acid and sulbactam are two semisynthetic β-lactamase inhibitors with a broad range of activity against β-lactamase enzymes produced by various organisms, including *Bacteroides, Hemophilus, Klebsiella, Escherichia coli,* and *N. gonorrhoeae.* These inhibiting agents have been combined with various aminopencillins or ticarcillin, resulting in an enhanced activity and a spectrum that includes the above-mentioned β-lactamase-producing organisms. Amoxicillin combined with clavulinic acid is available in oral form (Augmentin), which is effective against minor staphylococcal and mixed gram-positive and gram-negative infections, including *Bacteroides.* It is useful in the treatment of human and animal bite wounds. Ampicillin combined with sulbactam (Unasyn) and ticarcillin combined with clavulinic acid (Timentin) are available in parenteral forms and are useful in the management of more severe infections of soft tissues, bones, and joints.

### Adverse Reactions

Up to 10 percent of the population may show some degree of hypersensitivity to the penicillins, which may manifest as fever, skin rash, urticaria, or bronchospasm. Anaphylaxis may occur, as may gastrointestinal intolerance especially with the ureidopenicillins. High doses of the penicillins are normally well tolerated by the majority of the population; the penicillins are excreted by the kidneys, however, and dosages may need to be adjusted when renal disease is present. Other potential problems include central nervous system dysfunction, hematologic reactions, electrolyte distrubance, and pseudomembranous colitis.

## The Cephalosporins

The cephalosporins contain the basic β-lactam ring structure common to the penicillins and have a somewhat similar spectrum of activity, with slightly greater effectiveness against β-lactamase-producing organisms and a somewhat broader antibacterial spectrum (Fig. 24-10). They have been divided into three groups based upon their chronologic development and variation in antibacterial spectrum: first-generation, second-generation, and third-generation cephalosporins.

### First-Generation Cephalosporins

The first-generation cephalosporins include oral forms such as cephalexin (Keflex) and cephradine (Velosef). Parenteral forms include cefazolin (Kefzol) and cephalothin (Keflin). These antimicrobials are most effective against gram-positive cocci and some anaerobes and show excellent activity against staphylococci (except those that are methicillin-resistant) and nonenterococcal streptococci (except penicillinase-producing pneumococci). First-generation cephalosporins also have moderate activity against gram-negative organisms, including *E. coli, Klebsiella pneumoniae,* and indole-negative *Proteus (P. mirabilis).*

### Second-Generation Cephalosporins

Second-generation cephalosporins include the oral form cefuroxime (Ceftin) and the parenteral forms cefoxitin (Mefoxin), cefamandole (Mandol), cefonicid (Monocid), cefuroxime (Zinacef), and cefotetan (Cefotan). Second-generation cephalosporins tend to be less active against gram-positive cocci than first-generation cephalospo-

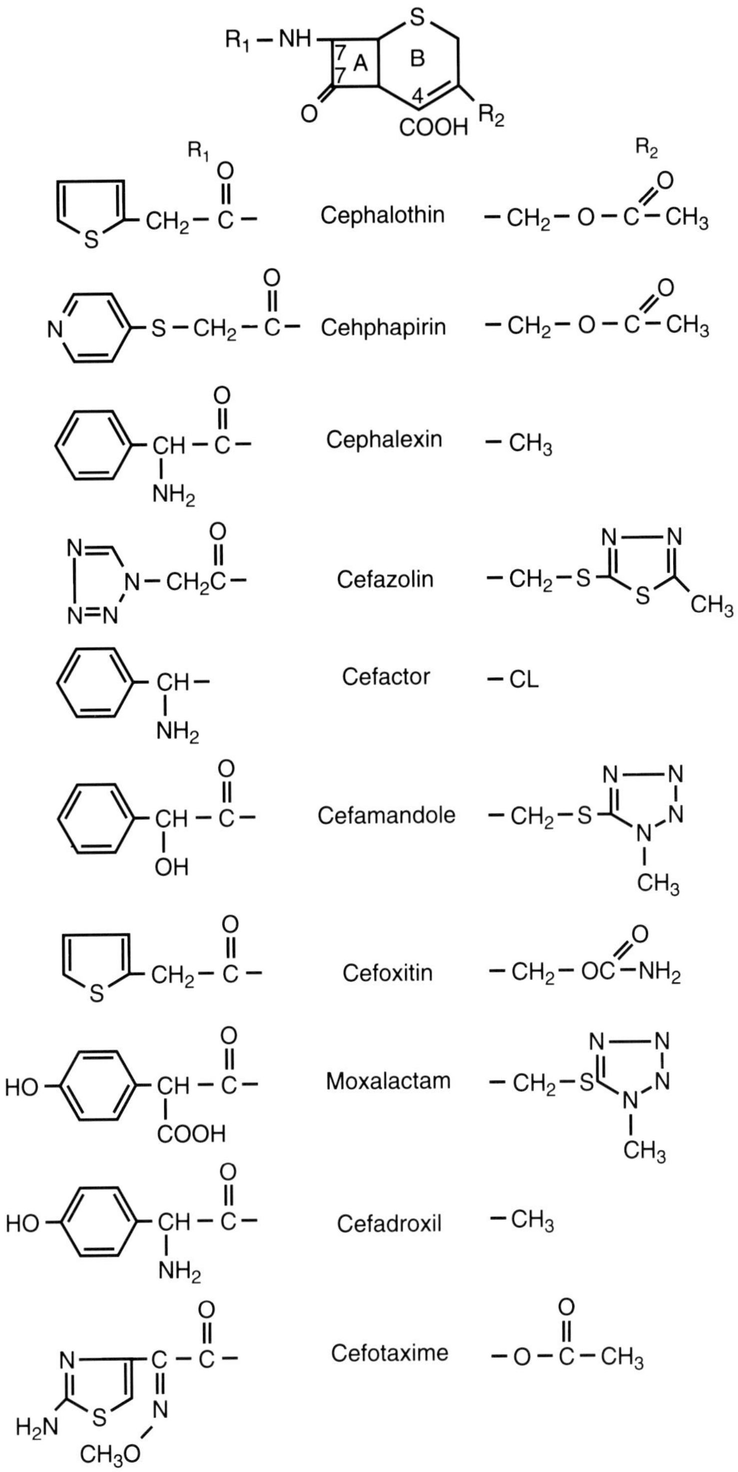

**Fig. 24-10.** Structural formulas of selected recently developed cephalosporins.

rins; however, they have enhanced activity against many gram-negative rods, including *H. influenzae, N. gonorrhoeae, Neisseria meningitidis,* some anaerobes, and many organisms in the Enterobacteriaceae group.

## Third-Generation Cephalosporins

Third-generation cephalosporins are even less active against gram-positive cocci than second-generation cephalosporins; however, they do exhibit enhanced activity against many gram-negative bacteria, particularly the Enterobacteriaceae. They are commonly divided into two groups based upon their activity against *P. aeruginosa.* The first group, which is most active against *P. aeruginosa,* includes ceftazidime (Fortaz, Tazidime, and Tazicef) and cefoperazone (Cefobid). The second group, which is less active against *P. aeruginosa,* includes cefotaxime (Claforan), ceftizoxime (Cefizox), and ceftriaxone (Rocephin). Cefotaxime is used most extensively worldwide and will be used as an index agent in this discussion. Cefotaxime inhibits more than 90 percent of strains of Enterobacteriaceae, including those producing β-lactamase and those resistant to aminoglycosides. Variable susceptibility of strains of *Acinetobacter, Enterobacter cloacae,* and *Serratia marcescens* occurs. Most strains of *P. aeruginosa* are resistant to cefotaxime. Cefotaxime has moderate activity against anaerobes, whereas second-generation antimicrobials such as cefoxitin and cefotetan offer markedly superior activity in this regard.

Ceftazidime is preferred over cefoperazone for treatment of *Pseudomonas* infections since it currently exhibits antibacterial activity against approximately 90 percent of strains. Ceftazidime, however, is relatively ineffective against anaerobes and is not as active against gram-positive cocci as cefotaxime. It is about equipotent to cefotaxime against Enterobacteriaceae. Ceftriaxone is useful because of its long half-life and once-a-day parenteral dosage, which may allow outpatient therapy.

## Adverse Reactions

Allergic reactions to cephalosporins occur in 5 to 10 percent of those patients who exhibit allergic reactions to the penicillins. The most common reactions include rash, which may be maculopapular or urticarial. The use of cephalosporins is absolutely contraindicated in patients who have exhibited urticarial or anaphylactic reactions to penicillins. Gastrointestinal distress, including diarrhea, may occur, and hematologic reactions, including thrombocytopenia, neutropenia, and bleeding disorders, have been described.

# Other β-Lactam Compounds

## Imipenem

Imipenem is a bicyclic β-lactam compound, which is administered with cilastatin in order to prevent its breakdown in the renal tubules. It has the broadest spectrum of the β-lactam antibiotics and has been shown to be as efficacious as third-generation cephalosporins in mixed polymicrobial soft tissue infections, particularly diabetes-related infections and osteomyelitis. It has no activity against methicillin-resistant staphylococci and certain enterococci. An organism resistance may develop during therapy in as many as 60 percent of cases, primarily in infections due to *P. aeruginosa* or other *Pseudomonas* species. Because of its expense and the potential risk of seizure, however, its use should be reserved for situations in which monotherapy is desirable in the seriously ill patient with multiple bacterial pathogens who needs an aminoglycoside-sparing regimen and is at high risk for ototoxicity and nephrotoxicity. This is generally not the case in infants and children.

## Aztreonam

Aztreonam is a synthetic monobactam with an antibacterial spectrum generally limited to gram-negative rods, which is bactericidal and highly resistant to β-lactamase destruction. It has minimal activity against anaerobes but is very effective against most Enterobacteriaceae. It inhibits 90 percent of *P. aeruginosa* at minimum inhibitory concentration (MIC) of 12.5 mg/ml, making it slightly less active against *Pseudomonas* than ceftazidime. Aztreonam is clinically indicated in limited situations involving patients with gram-negative infections who are allergic to penicillin and in whom the nephrotoxicity or ototoxicity of an aminoglycoside may be a problem. Such situations are unusual in infants or children. Aztreonam should not be used as a single agent for empirical management of infection or in any situation in which a gram-positive infection is a possibility.

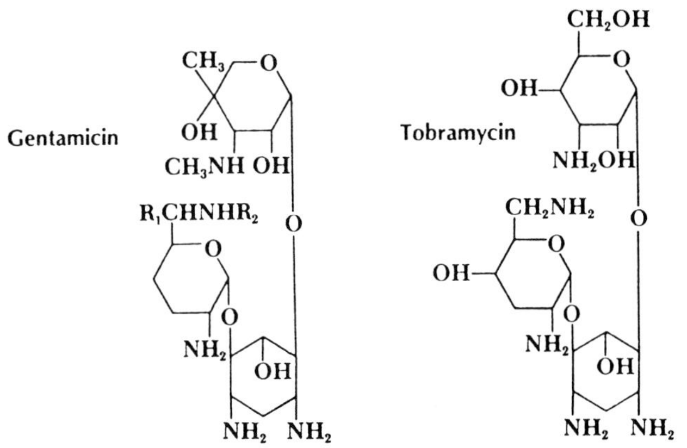

**Fig. 24-11.** Structural formulas of gentamicin and tobramycin (aminoglycosides).

## Aminoglycosides

The aminoglycoside antimicrobials have a broad spectrum of activity against both gram-positive and gram-negative organisms. Historically, they have been reserved primarily for serious gram-negative infections. The family of the aminoglycoside antimicrobials is defined by the presence of two amino sugars linked by glycosidic bonds to an aminocyclitol ring (Fig. 24-11). This group includes antimicrobials such as neomycin, kanamycin, gentamicin, tobramycin, and amikacin. Spectinomycin is often included as a member of this group; however, since it does not contain an amino sugar or glycosidic bond, it is technically not an aminoglycoside antimicrobial. The precise biochemical mechanism of the action of aminoglycosides remains an enigma. Aminoglycosides clearly inhibit bacterial protein synthesis, which appears to be contributory to their lethal effect; however, this activity alone does not provide a sufficient explanation for their lethality. The in vitro bacterial spectrum of the aminoglycosides includes primarily aerobic and facultative gram-negative bacilli and *S. aureus*. Although effective against *S. aureus* in vitro, aminoglycosides are generally not used for known staphylococcal infections since a number of antimicrobials with potentially lower toxicity and proven effectiveness are available. Aminoglycosides are considered an excellent choice for serious infections caused by aerobic or facultative gram-negative bacilli, including those caused by *P. aeruginosa*.

Dose-related toxicity has been a major consideration with the aminoglycosides. They are not metabolized by humans but are eliminated via the kidneys. Their principal toxicities include nephrotoxicity, ototoxicity, and neuromuscular paralysis. The pharmacokinetics of aminoglycosides differ significantly with age, primarily because of the significant differences in glomerular function that occur in newborn children, young adults, and the elderly. The volume of distribution is considerably larger as a percentage of body weight and the half-life of the drug is significantly prolonged in the newborn. After the newborn period, infants and children have volumes of distribution that are close to those of young adults, but the half-life of the drug is shorter than in young adults, presumably owing to more efficient glomerular function, which decreases with age. Serum concentration of aminoglycosides must be monitored during the course of therapy in order to ensure adequate serum concentration and prevent toxicity. Serum peak and trough levels should be drawn at the fourth dose and repeated periodically, with adjustment of dose as necessary. The patient should be watched for potential signs of toxicity, which should include laboratory monitoring of serum creatinine on a regular basis. Dosages also need to be decreased when decreased renal function is present.

## The Quinolones

The fluorinated quinolones are a new class of antimicrobials with a broad spectrum of activity against both aerobic gram-positive and aerobic gram-negative species, in-

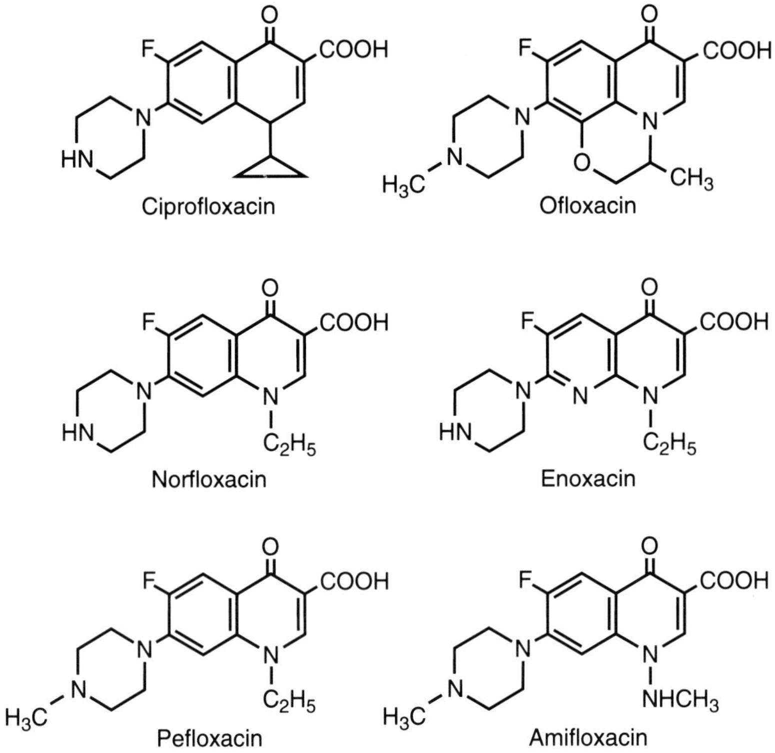

**Fig. 24-12.** Structural formulas of the fluorinated quinolones.

cluding *Pseudomonas* (Fig. 24-12). They are available and efficacious in oral form, providing a significant benefit over the aminoglycosides; however, they are currently not authorized for use in pregnant women or children and are not recommended prior to skeletal maturity. The quinolones interfere with bacterial DNA replication by targeting DNA gyrase. The quinolones have proved to be clinically efficacious in the management of aerobic gram-negative rod infections, particularly those caused by the Enterobacteriaceae. Their activity is limited against gram-positive cocci and poor against anaerobes, and they should not be used as sole agents in either of these infections. Adverse reactions that have been described include central nervous system effects, such as mild headache, dizziness, sleep disturbance, and, rarely, seizure disorder. Photosensitivity, diarrhea, and nausea may occur more frequently. Although this class of antimicrobials cannot be used in children, we have found it to be a useful oral agent in the management of gram-nega-

tive rod infections of the foot in skeletally mature adolescents, particularly those with *Pseudomonas* puncture wound infections.

## REFERENCES

### Osteomyelitis

1. Koch J: Untersuchungen über die Lokalisation der Bakterien, das Verhalten des Knochenmarkes und die Veränderungen der Knochen, insbesonder der Epiphysen, bei Infektionsskrank-heiten. Z Hyg Infektionsk 69:436, 1911
2. Ogden JA, Lister G: The pathology of neonatal osteomyelitis. Pediatrics 55:474, 1975
3. Trueta J: The normal vascular anatomy of the human femoral head during growth. J Bone Joint Surg [Br] 39:358, 1957
4. Trueta J: The three types of acute hematogenous osteomyelitis: a clinical and vascular study J Bone Joint Surg [Br] 41:671, 1959

5. Trueta J: Acute hematogenous osteomyelitis: its pathology and treatment. Bull N Y Acad Med 35:25, 1959
6. Trueta J: Acute hematogenous osteomyelitis: its pathology and treatment. Bull Hosp Jt Dis Orthop Inst 14:5, 1953
7. Jacobs JC: Acute osteomyelitis. NY State J Med 5:90, 1978
8. Dich VQ, Nelson JD, Haltalin KC: Osteomyelitis in infants and children. A review of 163 cases. Am J Dis Child 129:1278, 1975
9. Jackson MA, Nelson JD: Etiology and medical management of acute suppurative bone and joint infections in pediatric patients. J Pediatr Orthop 2:213, 1982
10. Bledhill RB: Subacute osteomyelitis in children. Clin Orthop 96:57, 1973
11. Roberts JM, Drummond DS, Breed AL, Chesney J: Subacute hematogenous osteomyelitis in children: a retrospective Study. J Orthop Pediatr 2:249, 1982
12. Green NF, Beauchamp RD, Griffin PP: Primary subacute epiphyseal osteomyelitis. J Bone Joint Surg [Am] 63:107, 1981
13. King DM, Mayo KM: Subacute hematogenous osteomyelitis. J Bone Joint Surg 51:458, 1969
14. Stephens MM, MacAuley P: Brodie's abcess. A long-term review. Clin Orthop 234:211, 1988
15. King DM, Mayo KM: Subacute hematogenous osteomyelitis. J Bone Joint Surg [Br] 51:458, 1969
16. Prober CG, Yeager AS: Use of the serum bactericidal titer to assess the adequacy of oral antibiotic therapy in the treatment of acute hematogenous osteomyelitis. J Pediatr 95:131, 1979
17. Nelson JD, Bucholz RW, Kusmiesz H, Shelton S: Benefits and risks of sequential parenteral oral cephalosporin therapy for suppurative bone and joint infections. J Pediatr Orthop 2:255, 1982
18. Tetzlaff TR, McCracken GH, Nelson JD: Oral antibiotic therapy for skeletal infections of children. J Pediatr 92:485, 1978
19. Tetzlaff TR, Howard JB, McCracken GH et al: Antibiotic concentrations in pus and bone of children with osteomyelitis. J Pediatr Orthop 92:135, 1978
20. Nelson JD, Howard JB, Shelton S: Oral antibiotic therapy for skeletal infection in children. J Pediatr Orthop 92:131, 1978
21. Bryson YJ, Connor JD, Leurs M, Giammona ST: High dose dicloxicillin treatment of acute staphylococcal osteomyelitis in children. J Pediatr 94:673, 1979
22. Verdile VP, Foreed MA, Gerard J: Puncture wounds to the foot. Emerg Med Rev 7:193, 1989
23. Edlich RF, Rodeheaver GT, Horowitz JH, Morgan RF: Emergency department management of puncture wounds and needlestick exposure. Emerg Med Clin North Am 4:581, 1986
24. Fitzgerald RH, Covan DE: Puncture wounds of the foot. Orthop Clin North Am 6:971, 1975
25. Fitzgerald RH, Landelle DG, Corvair DE: Osteomyelitis in children: Comparison of hematogenous and secondary osteomyelitis. Can Med Assoc J 1R:166, 1975
26. Crosby LA, Powell DA: The potential value of the sedimentation rate in monitoring treatment outcome in puncture woundrelated Pseudomonas osteomyelitis.
27. Brand RA, Black H: Pseudomonas osteomyelitis following puncture wounds in children. J Bone Joint Surg 56:1637, 1974
28. Lang AG, Peterson MA: Osteomyelitis following puncture wounds of the foot in children. J Trauma 16:993, 1976
29. Mahan KT, Kalish SR: Complications following puncture wounds of the foot. J Am Podiatr Med Assoc 72:497, 1982
30. Collins BS, Karlin JM, Silvoni SH, Scarren BL: Pseudomonas pyarthrosis and osteomyelitis from a puncture wound of the foot. J Am Podiatr Med Assoc 75:316, 1985
31. Miller EH, Semian DW: Gram-negative osteomyelitis following puncture wound of the foot J Bone Joint Surg 57:535, 1975
32. Fritz RH, Brosson FJ: Concerning the source of pseudomonas osteomyelitis of the foot. Unpublished material. Div. of Infectious Disease, Dept. of Pediatrics, The Johns Hopkins Hospital, Baltimore
33. Fisher MC, Goldsmith JF, Gilligan PH: Sneakers as a source of Pseudomonas aeruginosa in children with osteomyelitis following puncture wounds. J Pediatr 106:607, 1985
34. Johnson PH: Pseudomonas infection of the foot following puncture wounds. JAMA 204:170, 1968
35. Riegler HF, Routson GW: Complications of deep puncture wounds of the foot. J Trauma 19:18, 1979
36. Patzakis MJ, Wilkins J, Brien WW, Carter VS: Wound site as a predictor of complications following deep nail puncture to the foot. West J Med 150:545, 1989
37. Tachdjian MD: Pediatric Orthopedics. Vol. 2. WB Saunders, Philadelphia, 1990
38. Irons GB, Wood MB: Soft tissue coverage for the treatment of osteomyelitis of the lower part of the leg. Mayo Clin Proc 61:382, 1986

## Soft Tissue Infections

39. Gregory D, Schaffner W: Pseudomonas infections associated with hot tubs and other environments Infect Dis Clin North Am 1:635, 1989
40. Wickbolt LG, Sanders CV: Vibrio vulnificus infection. A

case report and update since 1970. J Am. Acad Dermatol 9:243, 1983

41. Hill MK, Sanders CV: Localized and systemic infection due to Vibrio species. Inf Dis Clin North Am 1:687, 1987

42. Bowden JH, Hull JH, Cocchetto M: Antibiotic efficacy aganist Vibrio vulnificus in the mouse: superiority of tetracycline. J Pharmacol Esp Ther 225:595, 1983

43. Wallace: Non tuberculous mycobacteria and water: a love affair with increasing clinical importance. Infect Dis Clin North Am 1:677, 1987

44. Moehring HD: Post operative clostridial infection. A case report. Clin Orthop 228:265, 1988

45. Wilkerson MR, Paull W, Coville FV: Necrotizing fasciitis review of the literature and case report. Clin Orthop 216:187, 1987

46. Nather A, Wong FY, Balasubramanian PB, Pang M: Streptococcal necrotizing myositis: A rare entity. A report of 2 cases. Clin Orthop 215:206, 1987

47. Duffy J: Lyme disease. Infect Dis Clin North Am 1:511, 1987

## SUGGESTED READINGS

### Antimicrobial Review

Allan JD, Eliopoulos GM, Moellering RC Jr: Expanding spectrum of beta-lactam antibiotics. Adv Intern Med 31:119, 1986

Goth A: Medical Pharmacology. 11th Ed. CV Mosby, St. Louis, 1984

Green SA: Antibiotic update. Adv Orthop Surg 7:48, 1983

Handbook of Antimicrobial Therapy. Rev. Ed. The Medical Letter Inc., New Rochelle, NY, 1984

Hugar DW: Management of infection. p. 494. In Marcus SA, Block BIT (eds): American College of Foot Surgeons: Complications in Foot Surgery—Preventions and management. 2nd Ed. Williams & Wilkins, Baltimore, 1984

Klempner MS, Styst B: Prevention of recurrent staphylococcal skin infections with low-dose oral clindamycin therapy. JAMA 260:2682, 1988

Laden SK, Hamilton LW, Roankiewicz JA: Review of antipseudomonal antibiotics. p. 7. In Kowalsky SF, Echols RM (eds): Antipseudomonal Therapy: Consideration for Drug Selection. New Jersey Scientific Therapeutics Information, 1986

Mandell GL: Cephalosporin. In Mandell GL (ed): Anti-Infective Therapy. Churchill Livingstone, New York, 1985

Mandell GL, Douglas RG Jr, Bennett JE: Principles and Practice of Infectious Diseases. Churchill Livingstone, New York, 1990

Neu HC: Ciprofloxacin: an overview and prospective appraisal. Am J Med 82, suppl. 4A:395, 1987

Ristuccia AM: Aminoglycosides. p. 305. In Ristuccia AM (ed): Antimicrobial therapy. Raven Press, New York, 1984

Siekert RG (ed): Symposium on Anti-microbial Agents. Mayo Clin Proc 58(1):3, (2):79, (3):147, (4):217, 1983

The choice of antimicrobial drugs. Med Lett Drugs Ther 26:19, 1984

Thornsberry C: Review of in vitro activity of 3rd generation cephalosporin and other newer beta-lactam antibiotics against clinically important bacteria. Am J Med 79, suppl 2A: 14, 1985

Till K, Solomon MG, Ketman BL: Indications and uses of prophylactic antibiotics in podiatric surgery. J Foot Surg 23:166, 1984

Wexler HM, Harris B, Carter et al: In vitro efficacy of sulbactam combined with ampicillin against anaerobic bacteria, antimicrobial agents and chemotherapy. 27:876, 1985

# 25

# Bone Tumors and Tumor-like Malformations of the Lower Extremity

*KENT K. WU*

With a few exceptions, both benign and malignant bone tumors only occasionally affect children and young adults. Although bone tumors are truly rare, it is imperative that all clinicians who see children have a basic understanding of the evaluation and diagnostic workup of the patient with suspected or possible tumor. An early diagnosis will not be made without a basic knowledge of bone tumor types combined with a high index of suspicion, and although the overall incidence of tumor is very small, the potentially serious nature of these lesions requires that the clinician consider tumors in the differential of any adolescent or young adult patient with unexplained pain, edema, mass, fever, or other symptoms.

Diagnostic evaluation and management of most tumors requires a team approach involving a surgeon, a diagnostic radiologist familiar with bone lesions, a pathologist, and in many cases an oncologist and a radiotherapist. Communication among specialists is essential. The bone radiologist who is supplied with as much clinical information as possible will be able to make a more useful interpretation. The pathologist should usually be consulted in advance of biopsy in order to determine what type of specimen will be most useful. Above all, potentially malignant tumors should usually be referred to or managed in conjunction with an experienced tumor surgeon prior to biopsy.

The main purpose of this chapter is to provide a brief but comprehensive review of the various bone tumors, as well as an introduction to their evaluation and manage-

ment. Time and space limitations permit discussion only of those tumors that have a predilection for young people, although some tumors that chiefly affect middle-aged or older adults will be reviewed briefly.

## DIAGNOSTIC STUDIES
### General Considerations

A thorough history and physical examination of any patient with a suspected tumor or with unexplained symptoms is essential to accurate diagnosis. Severe clinical symptoms or constitutional symptoms such as weight loss, malaise, anorexia, fever, night sweats, or generalized weakness may be indicators of the potentially malignant nature of a bone tumor. A history of rapid tumor growth, large tumor size, pathologic fracture, chronic exposure to oncogenic agents, or past cancer surgery also may indicate a potentially malignant lesion.

Age, sex, and location are often important diagnostic considerations. Almost all bone tumors affect males more frequently than females. Chondrosarcoma has a predilection for older adults; osteogenic sarcoma for teenagers; Ewing's sarcoma for older children; and neuroblastoma metastatic to bone for infants. Certain bone tumors have a predilection for certain sites of involvement. For example, enchondroma most commonly affects the phalanges and metacarpals of the hand; chordoma the spheno-occipital and sacrococcygeal regions;

osteoblastoma the neural arches of the spine; giant cell tumor the ends of long tubular bones; and chondroblastoma the epiphyses of long tubular bones.

A careful physical examination should be made, including a specific, detailed examination of the involved extremity. A palpable extraosseous tumor mass, tumor-induced skin ulceration, increased cutaneous vascularity (redness, warmth, distended superficial veins, etc.), hepatosplenomegaly in the absence of other systemic diseases, and enlarged regional lymph nodes are among the conditions that are highly suggestive of the malignant nature of a bone tumor.

## Laboratory Studies

Laboratory studies that should be performed routinely in cases of suspected bone tumor include a blood count, urinalysis, and determinations of erythrocyte sedimentation rate, serum calcium, phosphorus, alkaline phosphatase, and protein. Additional studies that may be useful in select cases might include serum acid phosphatase, creatinine phosphokinase, and serum and urine electrophoresis. Secondary anemia, leukocytosis, and elevated erythrocyte sedimentation rate are general indicators of the fulminating nature of the bone tumor under study. In addition, elevated serum alkaline phosphatase is often associated with osteogenic sarcoma and pagetoid sarcoma, and elevated serum acid phosphatase often occurs with metastatic prostatic carcinoma. A typical electrophoretic curve and urinary Bence Jones protein are associated with multiple myloma, and increased urinary excretion of catecholamines and their metabolites is associated with metastatic neuroblastoma and pheochromocytoma. Large numbers of abnormal leukocytes in the peripheral blood are found in leukemia.

## Diagnostic Imaging

Routine radiographs (anteroposterior, lateral, and oblique views) of the tumor-bearing bone are invariably required. Cortical perforation and extraosseous tumor extension, poor tumor margins, permeative bone destruction, irregular or spiculated periosteal new bone formation, and tumorous new bone formation are radiologic signs that are highly suggestive of the malignant nature of the bone tumor. In the case of some typically benign bone lesions, the radiographic appearance may be so diagnostic that biopsy may not be necessary. More often, however, the radiologic diagnosis may be equivocal and histologic confirmation may be required. A thorough discussion of the radiographic characteristics of all bone tumor is beyond the scope of this chapter. However, some typical radiographic characteristics of the various bone tumors will be mentioned in the discussion of individual tumors.

*Technetium 99 bone scans* are extremely useful in detecting bone metastases as well as in determining the level of bone resection, because tumor tissue usually does not extend beyond the area of increased technetium uptake.

*Computed tomography (CT)* is very effective in demonstrating the extent of tumor involvement and the relationship of the tumor to nearby major vascular structures.

*Arteriograms* clearly show the relationship between the bone tumor and its nearby vascular structures and the exact location of the feeding and draining blood vessels. This information can be used to embolize the tumor, which may facilitate subsequent limb-salvaging operations.

*Magnetic resonance imaging* (MRI) is probably the most useful modality in demonstrating the size, shape, and extent of bone tumor involvement. In a metastatic lesion MRI is often capable of detecting the presence of metastasis to the bone even before bone destruction has taken place.

## Diagnostic Evaluation

### Biopsy

Biopsy is the ultimate diagnostic tool in the evaluation of bone tumors, and is necessary when the diagnosis cannot be satisfactorily determined by noninvasive diagnostic studies or when the diagnosis of a potentially malignant tumor is entertained. Biopsy may be accomplished by needle aspiration or by open techniques. Open biopsy may be performed in either of the following manners: (1) incisional biopsy which involves removing only a small portion of the tumor without disturbing the bulk of tumor mass; and (2) excisional biopsy which involves removal of the entire tumor mass, usually without a margin of surrounding normal tissue. Needle biopsy, or incisional biopsy is generally preferred for potentially malignant tumors. Careful technique is important so that minimal tissue contamination of tumor cells occurs.

## Open Biopsy

Open biopsy is the most commonly used method of biopsy for bone tumors. When the preoperative radiologic studies indicate the possibility of a malignant bone tumor, the biopsy should be performed by the same surgeon who intends to perform the subsequent definitive surgery (which can be either a limb-salvaging operation or an amputation). Since the definitive bone tumor surgery should remove the entire biopsy tract, any unwisely placed biopsy site may severely limit the feasibility of a limb-salvaging operation or an amputation at the proper level. In an open biopsy if the bone tumor has an extraosseous component, the biopsy specimen can be taken directly from the extraosseous portion of the tumor, which tends to be the most aggressive and fastest-growing portion of the tumor. If the bone tumor is still intraosseous (intracompartmental), all the overlying soft tissues should be widely retracted away from the bone biopsy site, where a round hole can be drilled through the cortex and the tumor tissue can be obtained with curettes of different sizes. Intraoperative frozen sections should be obtained to provide a tissue diagnosis and to make sure that adequate amounts of representative tumor tissue have been obtained. To prevent the spread of intraosseous tumor into the extraosseous tissue space, the bone biopsy window should be carefully and tightly sealed off with bone cement (methyl methacrylate). The biopsy site should then be thoroughly irrigated with copious amounts of normal saline to wash out all the loose tumor cells, which may be inadvertently splattered into the surrounding soft tissues. New drapes, gloves, gowns, sutures, and surgical instruments should be used to close the wound.

## Needle Biopsy

The obvious advantages of a needle biopsy include its simplicity and the minimal likelihood of morbidity and mortality. Its biggest drawback is the meager amount of tissue available for pathologic diagnosis. Amounts and quality of tissue obtained may not be sufficient for the pathologist to make a definitive diagnosis, or in some cases the needle biopsy may even contribute to an incorrect diagnosis. Needle biopsy is probably most useful for vertebral tumors and is rarely indicated in the foot and lower extremity since most tumors in these locations are easily accessible by open biopsy techniques with minimal morbidity.

## Histologic Features of Malignant Bone Tumors

Common histologic features of malignant bone tumors may include a marked increase in cellularity as well as cellular pleomorphism (significant variation in size and shape of tumor cells). Frequent mitotic figures, hyperchromatism, and the presence of sarcomatous giant cells, poorly differentiated and immature cell types, and cells of extraskeletal origins (carcinoma cells) may also indicate malignancy. Aggressive tumor behavior such as cortical perforation and invasion of adjacent soft tissues may also be present.

## Staging of Malignant Bone Tumors

Staging of malignant neoplasms is a useful method of allowing more careful comparisons of tumor behavior and response to treatment. Enneking et al. have shown that tumor staging most accurately predicts the type of surgical procedure that will be necessary to achieve local control of the tumor. Tumor staging is determined by data collected from history and physical examination, diagnostic imaging studies, and biopsy. The following system proposed by Enneking is most commonly used.

*Stage IA:* A low-grade intracompartmental bone tumor (lesion confined to a single anatomic compartment)

*Stage IB:* A low-grade extracompartmental bone tumor (lesion extends beyond a single anatomic compartment)

*Stage IIA:* A high-grade intracompartmental bone tumor

*Stage IIB:* A high-grade extracompartmental bone tumor

*Stage III:* Any bone tumor with regional or distant metastases

# CLASSIFICATION

Categorization of bone tumors is the first and most important step in the determination of prognosis and treatment. A useful classification system allows one to subdivide a general category of problems, to identify individual variations, and the through observation and adequate follow-up to determine more individually appropriate types of treatment and prognosis. Bone tumors are gen-

Table 25-1. **A Simplified Classification of Bone Tumors**

Osteogenic Tumors
    Osteogenic sarcoma (osteosarcoma)
    Parosteal (juxtacortical) osteogenic sarcoma
    Osteoid osteoma
    Osteoblastoma
Chondrogenic Tumors
    Chondrosarcoma
    Chondromyxoid fibroma
    Chondroblastoma
    Chondroma (enchondroma), Ollier's disease, and Maffucci's syndrome
    Osteochondroma (osteocartilaginous exostosis) and hereditary multiple exostoses
Fibrogenic Tumors
    Fibrosarcoma
    Desmoplastic fibroma
    Aneurysmal bone cyst
    Unicameral (solitary) bone cyst
    Fibrous (fibro-osseous) dysplasia
    Fibrous cortical (metaphyseal fibrous) defect and nonossifying (nonosteogenic) fibroma
Fibrohistiocytic Tumors
    Malignant fibrous histiocytoma
    Giant cell tumor
Vasogenic Tumors
    Hemangioendothelioma
    Hemangiopericytoma
    Hemangioma
Neurogenic Tumors
    Neurogenic sarcoma
    Neurilemmoma
    Neurofibroma and neurofibromatosis (von Recklinghausen's disease)
Lipogenic Tumors
    Liposarcoma
    Lipoma
Ewing's Sarcoma
Malignant Lymphoma
Multiple Myeloma
Leukemia
Metastasis
Mesenchymoma
Chordoma

erally classified on the basis of the originating tumor cell type. The simplified classification scheme outlined in Table 25-1 will be used in this discussion.

# Osteogenic Tumors

All osteogenic tumors have a large number of osteoblastic cells in different stages of differentiation and maturation in intimate association with new bone formation.

*Osteogenic sarcoma* and *parosteal osteogenic sarcoma* not only are locally infiltrative and destructive but also can produce fatal distant metastases. In contrast, osteoblastoma and osteoid osteoma are well localized benign bone tumors, which can be eradicated by local resection.

## Osteogenic Sarcoma

Osteogenic sarcoma (osteosarcoma) is one of the most malignant tumors and is also the second most common malignant primary bone tumor. Only multiple myeloma exceeds it in its frequency of occurrence. Osteogenic sarcoma has a predilection for the distal femur, proximal tibia, and humerus of male patients in the second decade of life. Anatomically, osteogenic sarcoma can be subdivided into intramedullary, parosteal (juxtacortical), and extraosseous, intracortical, and periosteal types. On an etiologic basis, osteosarcoma can be classified into primary osteosarcoma, which originates de novo, and secondary osteosarcoma, which arises from bones or soft tissues with pre-existing lesions or with a history of exposure to oncogenic chemical, physical, or biologic agents.

Common clinical signs include pain, swelling, palpable tumor mass, localized signs of hyperemia, muscle atrophy, and tenderness. Radiologically, intramedullary bone destruction and tumor bone formation, cortical perforation, periosteal new bone formation, and an extraosseous tumor extension are frequently present (Fig. 25-1). Microscopically, osteogenic sarcoma typically shows the presence of many malignant osteoblastic cells, which are actively producing tumor osteoid (Fig. 25-2).

## Parosteal (Juxtacortical) Osteogenic Sarcoma

Parosteal osteogenic sarcoma is a relatively uncommon but distinctive type of osteogenic sarcoma, which develops in close relationship to the surface of a bone and has a prognosis significantly better than that of a comparable intramedullary osteogenic sarcoma. Parosteal osteogenic sarcoma accounts for approximately 5 percent of all osteogenic sarcomas and under 2 percent of all primary malignant bone tumors. It preferentially attacks the long tubular bones (femur, tibia, humerus, and ulna), especially the posterior surface of the distal femur, of young adults with no apparent sex preference.

Clinically, a parosteal osteogenic sarcoma may be

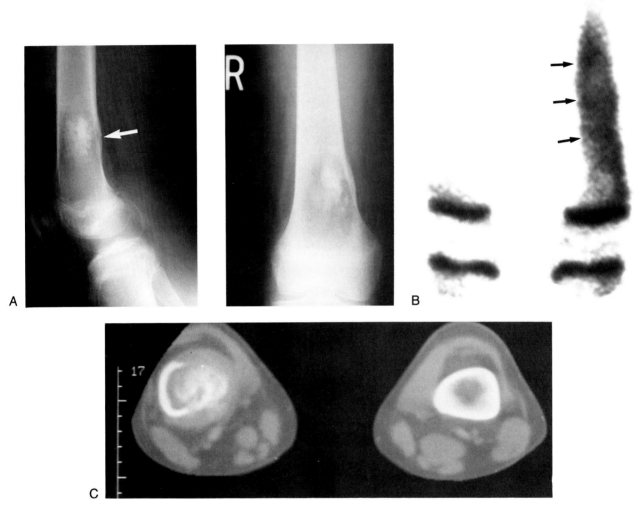

**Fig. 25-1.** (**A**) Anteroposterior and lateral distal femoral radiographs of a 14-year-old white boy show both host bone destruction and tumor bone formation in the medullary canal of the right distal femur. (**B**) Bone scan of the same distal femoral region shows a marked increase in the radionuclide uptake in this region. (**C**) CT scan of the same distal femur shows cortical perforation with extraosseous tumor extension into the posteromedial aspect of the distal thigh.

completely asymptomatic or may produce mild symptoms such as a painless swelling, mild aches, or some limitation of joint motion for months or years. Radiologically, this sarcoma is a large, lobulated, densely radiopaque tumor with a tendency to encircle the adjacent host bone. The broad tumor base tends to have the greatest degree of radiopacity. The peripheral portion of the tumor is somewhat irregular and often contains irregular radiolucent defects produced by foci of fibrous or cartilaginous tissues. Tumor-induced periosteal new bone formation is rarely seen, and occasionally cortical erosion and intramedullary tumor extension may also be visible on plain radiographs (Fig. 25-3). Microscopically, parosteal osteogenic sarcoma is characterized by the presence of intertwining bundles of proliferating fibrosarcomatous spindle cells with plump and somewhat pleomorphic nuclei in intimate association with tumor bone formation (Fig. 25-4).

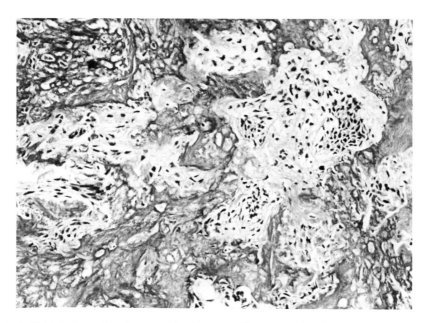

**Fig. 25-2.** A typical histologic section of an osteoblastic osteogenic sarcoma showing many hyperchromatic malignant osteoblastic cells actively producing tumor osteoid. (H&E, × 160.) (From Wu KK: Diagnosis and Treatment of Benign and Malignant Monostotic Tumors of the Spine. National Reproductions Corp., Detroit, 1985, with permission.)

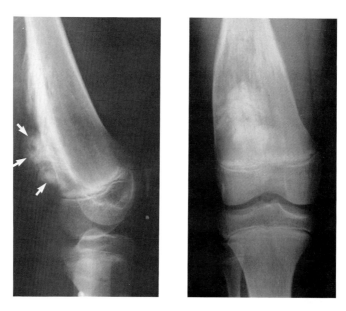

**Fig. 25-3.** Anteroposterior and lateral distal femoral radiographs of a 14-year-old boy show a lobulated parosteal osteogenic sarcoma on the posterior surface of the distal femur, with foci of radiolucent defects in these lobules caused by the presence of fibrous and cartilaginous tissues.

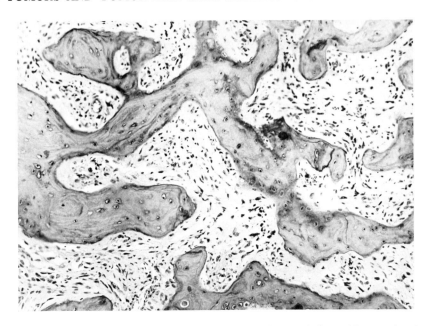

**Fig. 25-4.** Photomicrograph of a parosteal osteogenic sarcoma showing newly formed bony trabeculae produced by sheets of proliferating fibrosarcomatous spindle cells. (H&E, × 100.) (From Wu KK: Diagnosis and Treatment of Benign and Malignant Monostotic Tumors of the Spine. National Reproductions Corp., Detroit, 1985, with permission.)

## Osteoid Osteoma

Osteoid osteoma is a relatively uncommon bone tumor that accounts for less than 3 percent of all excised bone tumors. It preferentially attacks the diaphyseal and metaphyseal regions of long tubular bones, especially the femur and tibia, which account for approximately 50 percent of the reported cases. This tumor predominantly affects children and young adults in the 10- to 25-year age range, with a male to female ratio of more than 2 : 1.

Clinically, osteoid osteoma typically produces a localized pain, which tends to be worse at night and is frequently relieved by aspirin. The pain initially tends to be vague and intermittent but gradually becomes more severe and constant, to the point that the patient is compelled to seek medical attention. Radiologically, an osteoid osteoma typically has a radiolucent central nidus measuring less than 1 cm in diameter and is surrounded by a narrow zone of radiolucency which is in turn surrounded by a perinidal sclerosis of host bone (Fig. 25-5). Microscopically, the nidus of an osteoid osteoma usually consists of a network of osteoid trabeculae with varying degrees of mineralization in a fairly vascular fibrous connective tissue that also contains a variable number of benign giant cells and well differentiated osteoblasts. The perinidal osteosclerotic zone usually consists of well mineralized bone with dense cortical bone in intracortical osteoid osteoma, thickened trabecular bone in spongious osteoid osteoma, and abundant localized periosteal new bone formation in periosteal osteoid osteoma (Fig. 25-6).

## Osteoblastoma

Osteoblastoma is an uncommon bone tumor, accounting for 1 percent of all primary bone tumors. It preferentially attacks the spinal column and long tubular bones, especially the femur and tibia of patients in their second decade of life with a male to female ratio of approximately 2 : 1. Clinically, pain is the most common symptom; spinal osteoblastomas can also produce neurologic symptoms and signs. Radiologically an osteoblastoma usually appears as a well circumscribed, expansile and osteolytic lesion in which varying degrees of patchy or granular radiopacity can be found (Fig. 25-7A). Angiography often reveals increased vascularity of this lesion (Fig. 25-7B). The shape, size, and intraosseous and extraosseous involvement of the tumor are best demon-

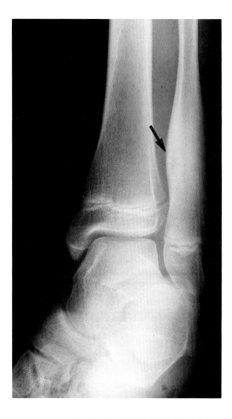

**Fig. 25-5.** An osteoid osteoma of the distal fibula in this 10-year-old boy shows a small radiolucent central nidus surrounded by a zone of perinidal cortical sclerosis of the host bone. (From Wu KK: Surgery of the Foot. Lea & Febiger, Philadelphia, 1986, with permission.)

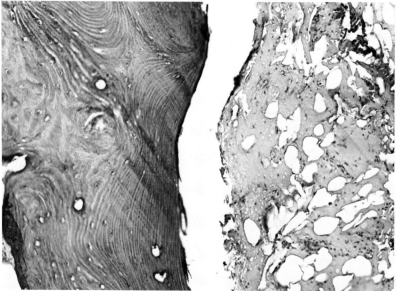

**Fig. 25-6.** Low-power photomicrograph of an intracortical osteoid osteoma showing dense cortical bone on the left and highly vascular benign osteogenic connective tissue on the right. (H&E, × 100.) (From Wu KK: Diagnosis and Treatment of Benign and Malignant Monostotic Tumors of the Spine. National Reproductions Corp., Detroit, 1985, with permission.)

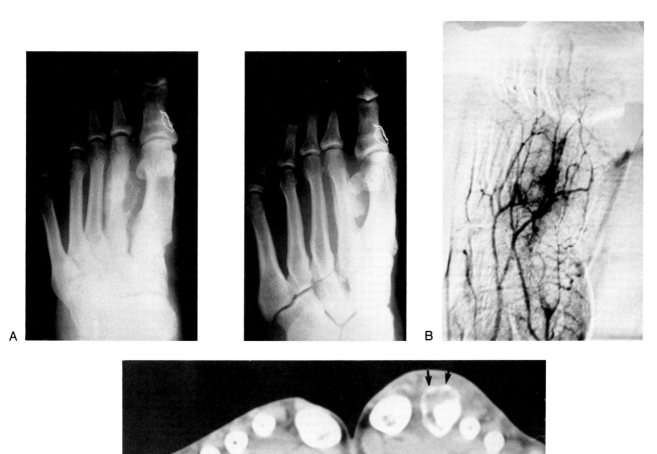

**Fig. 25-7.** **(A)** Anteroposterior and oblique foot radiographs of a 21-year-old man with an osteoblastoma in the left second metatarsal showing diaphyseal cortical destruction and expansion of the second metatarsal. **(B)** Digital subtraction angiography of the same foot showing increased vascularity of the second metatarsal. *(Figure continues).*

strated by means of CT scan and MRI (Fig. 25C–F). Microscopically osteoblastoma is characterized by an abundant amount of osseous tissue with varying degrees of mineralization and by osteoblastic cells in different stages of differentiation and maturation, accompanied by a very vascular connective tissue stroma in which a various number of benign-looking multinucleated giant cells can be seen (Fig. 25-8).

## Chondrogenic Tumors

Chondrogenic tumors belong to a family of cartilaginous tumors, the main histologic features of which are cartilage cells in different stages of maturation and differentiation and chondroid intercellular matrix produced by these cells. *Chondrosarcoma* is a malignant bone tumor with a propensity for local recurrence and late metas-

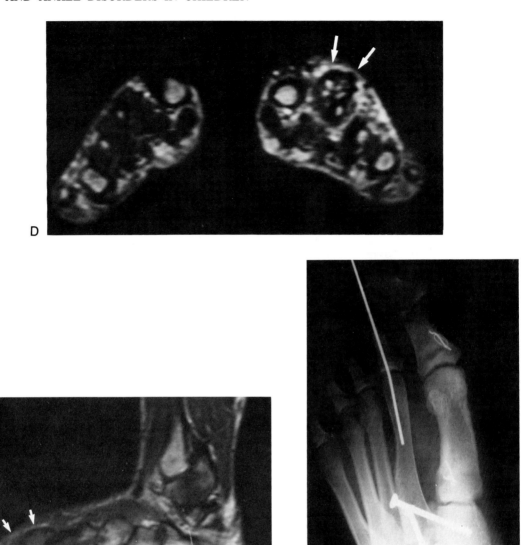

**Fig. 25-7** *(Continued).* (**C**) CT scan of the same foot showing marked cortical expansion of the left second metatarsal. (**D&E**) MRI images again showing marked cortical expansion in both the longitudinal and transverse planes. (**F**) The osteoblastoma was eradicated by a complete removal of the second metatarsal and insertion of a carefully sculptured bicortical iliac graft, whose proximal end was fused to the three cuneiforms. The fusion was successful, and the left foot had an excellent cosmetic and functional long-term result. (From Wu KK: Osteoblastoma of the foot. J Foot Surg 27:92, 1988, with permission.)

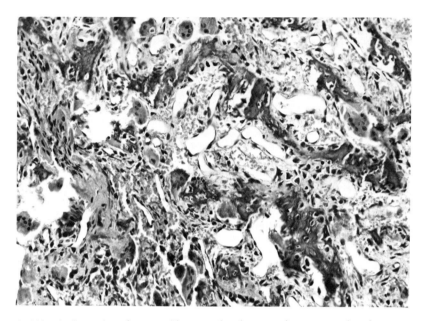

**Fig. 25-8.** A typical histologic section of an osteoblastoma showing many immature trabeculae accompanied by many osteoblastic cells in a highly vascular stroma in which quite a few benign-looking multinucleated giant cells are present. (H&E, × 157.) (From Wu KK: Diagnosis and Treatment of Benign and Malignant Monostotic Tumors of the Spine. National Reproductions Corp., Detroit, 1985, with permission.)

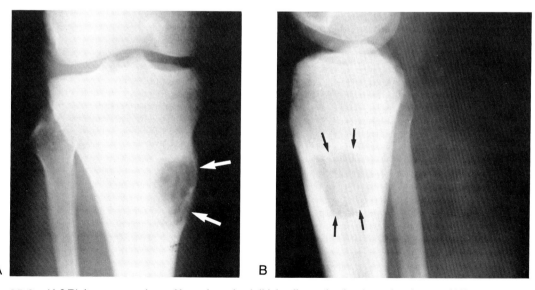

A    B

**Fig. 25-9.** **(A&B)** Anteroposterior and lateral proximal tibial radiographs showing a chondromyxoid fibroma, which is metaphyseally and eccentrically located, well circumscribed, oval, and radiolucent, with some cortical expansion and an osteosclerotic tumor border.

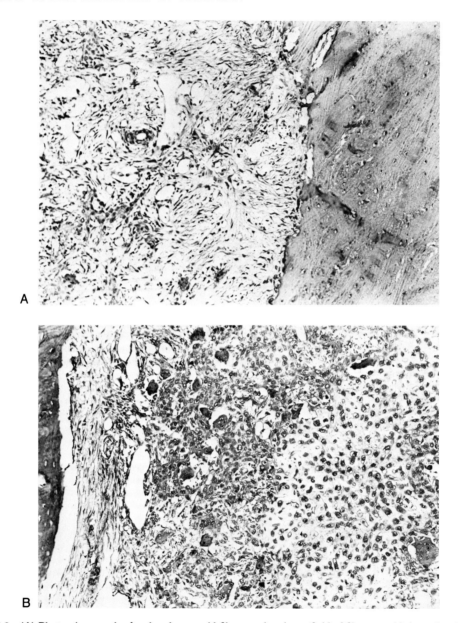

**Fig. 25-10.** (A) Photomicrograph of a chondromyxoid fibroma showing a field of fibromyxoid tissue in which many dilated vascular channels are present. (H&E, × 100.) (B) A different field of the same chondromyxoid fibroma showing a distinctive cartilaginous lobule with many chondroblasts and chondrocytes on the left and a fibrohistiocytic tissue with quite a few benign-looking giant cells on the right. (H&E, × 100.) (From Wu KK: Diagnosis and Treatment of Benign and Malignant Monostotic Tumors of the Spine. National Reproductions Corp., Detroit, 1985, with permission.)

tasis, whereas *chondromyxoid fibroma, chondroblastoma, chondroma,* and *osteochondroma* are benign cartilaginous tumors that respond to local surgical treatment with good to excellent results in the majority of the cases.

## Chondrosarcoma

Chondrosarcoma is a relatively common malignant bone tumor that accounts for about 10 percent of all malignant bone tumors. Its frequency of occurrence is surpassed only by that of multiple myeloma and osteogenic sarcoma. Chondrosarcoma preferentially attacks the long tubular bones (femur, tibia, humerus, etc.), and large flat bones (scapula and ilium) of adult patients, with a slight male preference. Primary chondrosarcoma arises de novo, whereas secondary chondrosarcoma originates in a pre-existing lesion or arises from bone previously exposed to oncogenic agents. Anatomically, chondrosarcoma can be divided into the following types: (1) central chondrosarcoma, which arises from the medullary portion of a bone; (2) peripheral chondrosarcoma, which arises from the cortical surface of a bone; (3) juxtacortical (periosteal) chondrosarcoma, which originates in the periosteal or juxtacortical soft tissues; (4) extraosseous

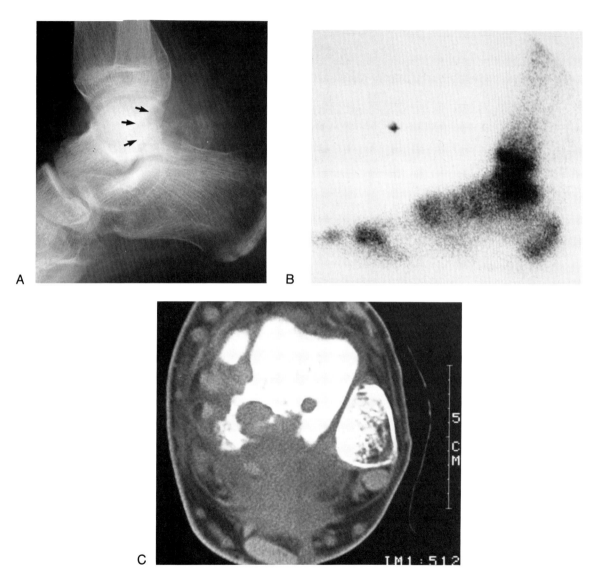

**Fig. 25-11. (A)** Lateral ankle radiograph of a teenage boy with a talar chondroblastoma showing destruction of the posterior aspect of the right talus, with extension of tumor tissue into the posterior aspect of the ankle region and a slightly sclerotic anterior tumor border. **(B)** Bone scan of the same ankle reveals that the entire posterior half of the talus is "hot." **(C)** CT scan of the same ankle shows extensive destruction of the posterior aspect of the right talus. (From Wu KK: Chondroblastoma of the foot. J Foot Surg 28:72, 1989, with permission.)

chondrosarcoma, which develops in the extraskeletal soft somatic tissues; (5) synovial chondrosarcoma, which arises from an intra-articular location; and (6) tenosynovial chondrosarcoma, which originates in the tendon sheath.

### Chondromyxoid Fibroma

Chondromyxoid fibroma is a fairly rare bone tumor, which accounts for less than 0.5 percent of primary bone tumors. It shows a predilection for long tubular bones of the lower extremity (femur and tibia) of adolescents and young adults, with a slight male preference. Clinically, its symptoms and signs may include mild pain for months or even 1 or 2 years, mild to moderate tenderness, slight swelling, a firm and palpable cortical mass, night pain, and pain aggravated by excessive use of the involved extremity. Radiologically, a chondromyxoid fibroma usually presents as an eccentric, well circumscribed, oval or roundish, and radiolucent metaphyseal lesion. Cortical bulging, a scalloped and sclerotic medullary border, coarse bony trabeculation, and the absence of periosteal new bone formation and intralesional calcification are the other frequent radiologic findings (Fig. 25-9). Microscopically, this tumor is characterized by the presence of

a mixture of benign-looking chondroid, myxoid, and fibrous tissues (Fig. 25-10).

### Chondroblastoma

Chondroblastoma is a relatively uncommon benign cartilaginous tumor that accounts for approximately 1 percent of all bone tumors. It shows a strong predilection for the epiphyseal ends of long tubular bones, especially the lower femur and upper tibia and humerus of patients in their second decade of life, with a male to female ratio of 2:1. Clinically, owing to its epiphyseal location this tumor frequently produces joint symptoms and signs, such as joint pain, synovial effusion, loss of normal joint motion, muscle atrophy, joint tenderness, flexion contracture, and limping.

Radiologically, a chondroblastoma usually appears as an oval or round, eccentric lesion, which often occupies less than half of the entire epiphysis, with a thin osteosclerotic tumor margin and a fuzzy, rarefied, and mottled appearance (Fig. 25-11A). Radionuclide bone scanning, CT scanning, and MRI are very helpful in delineating the intraosseous and extraosseous borders of the tumor (Figs. 25-11B and C and 25-12). Microscopically, the great majority of tumor cells in chondroblastoma are

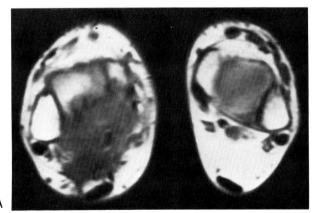
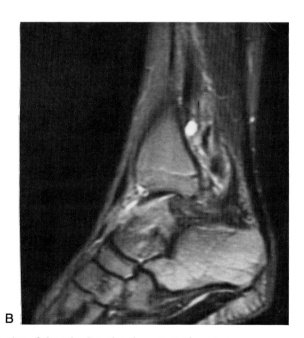

A        B

**Fig. 25-12.** (A&B) MRI shows not only the extent of destruction of the talus but also the extent of extraosseous tumor extension. (From Wu KK: Chondroblastoma of the foot. J Foot Surg 28:72, 1989, with permission.)

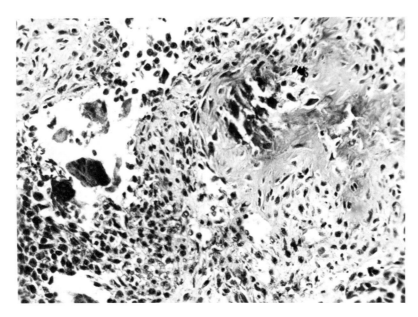

**Fig. 25-13.** Photomicrograph demonstrating all the important features of a chondroblastoma. These include many chondroblasts with distinct cytoplasmic borders, islands of cartilaginous tissue with chondrocytes in lacunae, osteoclast-like giant cells, and small foci of intralesional calcification. (H&E, × 250.) (From Wu KK: Diagnosis and Treatment of Benign and Malignant Monostotic Tumors of the Spine. National Reproductions Corp., Detroit, 1985, with permission.)

polygonal or round chondroblasts, which display round, oval, and slightly indented or lobulated nuclei; even chromatin and inconspicuous nucleoli; granular cytoplasm enclosed by a distinct cytoplasmic border; varying amounts of intracytoplasmic glycogen granules; and a variable number of mitotic figures. Islands of chondroid tissue, benign multinucleated giant cells, chicken-wire-like calcification, small foci of metaplastic new bone formation, and other features can also be seen (Fig. 25-13).

## Chondroma, Ollier's Disease, and Maffucci's Syndrome

Chondroma, also known as *enchondroma,* is a fairly common benign cartilaginous tumor, which is the most common bone tumor of the hands and feet. It can affect patients in a wide age range with no sex predilection. Clinically, it is usually asymptomatic and is often discovered accidentally following trauma or after a pathologic fracture has occurred. Radiologically, chondroma is a centrally located osteolytic lesion with a well circum-scribed margin and varying degrees of stippled or mottled calcification. Chondroma of short tubular bones can involve large portions of these bones, causing thinning and bulging of their cortices, and can even produce pathologic fractures (Fig. 25-14). Microscopically, chondroma is composed of benign-looking cartilaginous tissue in which the cartilage cells are often small and rarely share their individual lacunae. Giant cartilage cells, mitoses, increased cellularity, and other features of cellular pleomorphism are absent (Fig. 25-15).

Ollier's disease, also known as *enchondromatosis,* shows a strong predilection for phalanges and metacarpals of the hand and a lesser predilection for the femur, tibia, and ilium. It often shows an asymmetric involvement, tending to affect one side of the body more than the other, and has a propensity for chondrosarcomatous transformation (Fig. 25-16).

Maffucci's syndrome is a very rare form of enchondromatosis associated with multiple soft tissue hemangiomas. This tumor has a strong predilection for the hands and feet, and has a greater tendency toward malignant transformation than Ollier's disease.

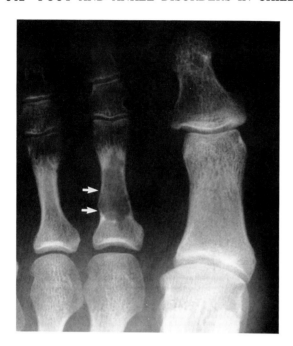

**Fig. 25-14.** Anteroposterior radiograph of the toes showing an enchondroma in the second proximal phalanx, which has slightly bulged the cortex and produced a pathologic fracture.

## Osteochondroma and Hereditary Multiple Exostoses

Osteochondroma (osteocartilaginous exostosis) is the most common benign bone tumor, accounting for about 50 percent of all benign bone tumors. Osteochondroma has a predilection for the long tubular bones of adolescents and young adults, its peak incidence occurring during the second decade of life, with a male to female ratio of approximately 2:1. Clinically, osteochondromas of the extremities are usually asymptomatic or minimally symptomatic. However, pain and other symptoms can be caused by irritation of surrounding muscles or tendons, bursa formation, fracture through the stalk of an osteochondroma, joint impingement, nerve compression, vascular disturbances, or other effects of the tumor. Radiologically, in a stalked (narrow-based) or sessile (wide-based) osteochondroma the cortical and trabecular bone is usually continuous with that of host bone. A young osteochondroma is generally covered by a smooth cartilaginous cap with varying degrees of radiopaque calcification. However, senescent osteochondromas may lose their round and smooth surfaces owing to replacement of the hyaline cartilage by bone through endochon-

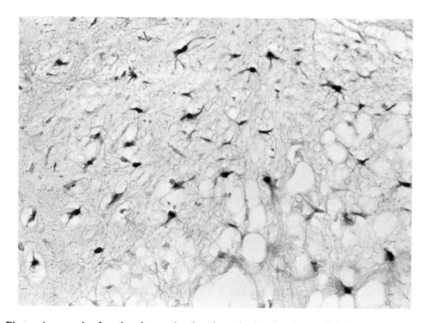

**Fig. 25-15.** Photomicrograph of a chondroma (enchondroma) showing low cellularity, small cartilage cells, and abundant amount of intercellular matrix. (H&E, × 250.) (From Wu KK: Diagnosis and Treatment of Benign and Malignant Monostotic Tumors of the Spine. National Reproductions Corp., Detroit, 1985, with permission.)

## Fibrogenic Tumors

Fibrogenic tumors share the common histologic features of having fibroblastic cells and associated collagenous intercellular matrix as the important components of their tumor tissues. *Fibrosarcoma* is a malignant tumor that is locally aggressive in producing local tumor recurrence following suboptimal resection and can also produce fatal distant metastases. The remainder of the fibrogenic tumors can all be considered to be benign bone tumors owing to their benign clinical course.

### Fibrosarcoma and Desmoplastic Fibroma

Fibrosarcoma is an uncommon bone tumor with a predilection for the metaphyses of long tubular bones of patients in a wide age range but without any apparent sex preference. Fibrosarcomas can be classified into central fibrosarcoma, which originates in the medullary portion of a bone, periosteal ( juxtacortical) fibrosarcoma, which arises from the cortical surface of a bone, and extraosseous fibrosarcoma, which can affect almost every organ in the body.

Desmoplastic fibroma is a very rare bone tumor, which affects the jaw bones, long tubular bones (femur, tibia, and humerus), and large flat bones (ilium and scapula) of patients in a wide age range without any special sex predilection.

### Aneurysmal Bone Cyst

Aneurysmal bone cyst is an uncommon bone tumor, which accounts for about 1 percent of biopsied primary bone tumors. It preferentially attacks long tubular bones of older children, adolescents, and young adults, about three-fourths of the reported cases occurring in patients under 20 years of age, with no apparent sex predilection. Clinically, pain, swelling, and tenderness of several months to a few years duration are the most common symptoms and signs. Loss of joint motion, muscle atrophy, and pathologic fracture can also occur. Radiologically, aneurysmal bone cyst is an oval or round, eccentrically located, metaphyseal or diaphyseal, osteolytic lesion with varying degrees of intralesional trabeculation and cortical thinning and expansion. The eggshell-thin and balloon-like radiographic appearance is the distinctive hallmark of a typical aneurysmal bone cyst (Fig. 25-20). Microscopically, many blood-filled spaces are

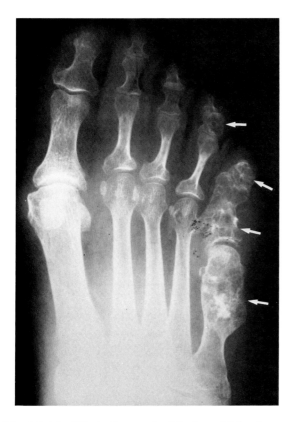

**Fig. 25-16.** Ollier's disease of a right foot with involvement of the fifth metatarsal and phalanges of the fourth and fifth toes. A chondrosarcoma has developed in the fifth proximal phalanx and has perforated the cortex on the medial basal portion of this phalanx, with extraosseous extension to the dorsal aspect of the distal portion of the fourth metatarsal. (From Wu KK: Secondary chondrosarcoma of the foot. J Foot Surg, 26:449, 1987, with permission.)

dral ossification (Fig. 25-17). Microscopically, the orderly arrangement of perichondrium, cartilaginous cap, and underlying bony spongiosa and cortex are continuous with those of the host bone (Fig. 25-18).

Hereditary multiple exostoses (osteochondromatosis) have a prominent hereditary incidence, which affects males more often than females. This disease is characterized by the presence of multiple exostoses, which are frequently bilateral and somewhat symmetrical and usually make their appearance during childhood or adolescence (Fig. 25-19).

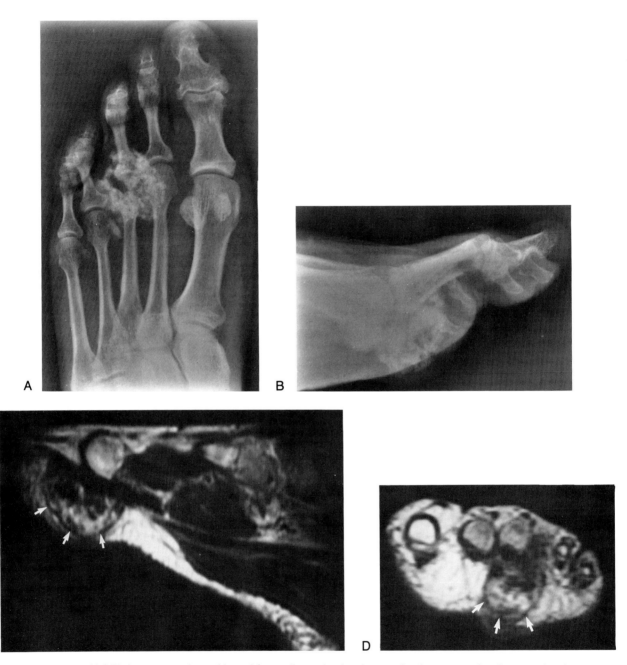

**Fig. 25-17.** (**A&B**) Anteroposterior and lateral foot radiographs showing a rather large osteochondroma under the left third metatarsal head. (**C&D**) MRI gives a sharp three-dimensional view of the osteochondroma. (From Wu KK: Osteochondroma of the foot. J Foot Surg, 29:88, 1990, with permission.)

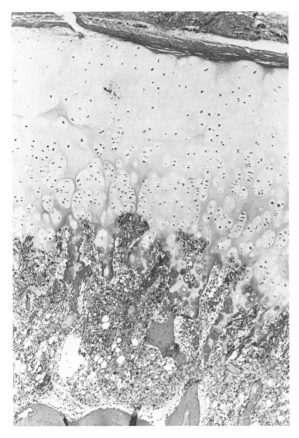

**Fig. 25-18.** Photomicrograph showing the orderly arrangement of perichondrium, cartilaginous cap, and the subchondral bone in an osteochondroma. (H&E, × 40.) (From Wu KK: Diagnosis and Treatment of Benign and Malignant Monostotic Tumors of the Spine. National Reproductions Corp., Detroit, 1985, with permission.)

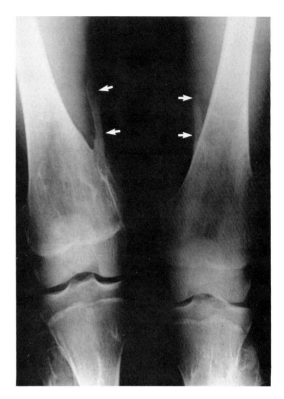

**Fig. 25-19.** Anteroposterior knee radiograph of a teenager with multiple exostoses showing the presence of multiple stalked exostoses.

separated from each other by interconnecting fibrous tissue, in which fibroblasts, collagen, thin osseous trabeculae, benign-looking multinucleated giant cells, macrophages with hemosiderin granules, and chronic inflammatory cells are among the structures found (Fig. 25-21).

## Unicameral Bone Cyst

Unicameral solitary bone cyst is a relatively common bone tumor, accounting for about 3 percent of biopsied primary bone tumors. It mainly affects patients in their first and second decades of life and shows a predilection for the metaphyseal and diaphyseal regions of long tubular bones such as the humerus, femur, tibia, and fibula, in order of decreasing frequency of occurrence. It should be noted that humeral and femoral cases alone account for approximately 70 percent of the reported cases, with an overall male to female ration of about 2:1. Clinically, a unicameral bone cyst may be completely asymptomatic or may produce localized pain and swelling, tenderness, joint stiffness, limping, and pathologic fracture. Radiologically, a unicameral bone cyst is a symmetrical, osteolytic, metaphyseal or diaphyseal, and slightly expansile lesion, with cortical thinning from the medullary side and no appreciable reactive periosteal new bone formation in the absence of pathologic fracture (Fig. 25-22). Microscopically, a unicameral bone cyst is usually lined by a thin fibrous membrane, which is made of a thin, loose-meshed fibrous tissue containing fibroblastic cells, collagen fibers, dilated thin-walled blood vessels, macrophages with intracytoplasmic hemosiderin granules or lipid, small multinucleated giant cells, a small amount of

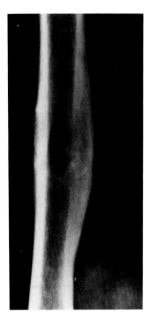
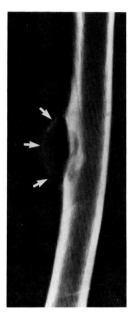

**Fig. 25-20.** An aneurysmal bone cyst of the femoral diaphysis has produced an eggshell-thin and balloon-like expansion of the femoral cortex. (From Wu KK: Diagnosis and Treatment of Benign and Malignant Monostotic Tumors of the Spine. National Reproductions Corp., Detroit, 1985, with permission.)

osteoid and thin osseous trabeculae, and some chronic inflammatory cells (Fig. 25-23).

### Fibrous Dysplasia

Fibrous (fibro-osseous) dysplasia is a relatively common bone disorder affecting patients from infancy to adulthood with a male to female ratio of approximately 2 : 1 or 3 : 1. Fibrous dysplasia can exist in both monostotic and polyostotic forms. Monostotic fibrous dysplasia has a predilection for the femur, tibia, rib, and jawbones. Polyostotic fibrous dysplasia tends to make its clinical appearance much earlier than the monostotic form and frequently affects bones of one limb, especially the lower extremity. It should be mentioned that Albright syndrome is clinically manifested by the presence of polyostotic fibrous dysplasia, precocious puberty, and multiple café-au-lait cutaneous spots.

Clinically, small, solitary lesions of fibrous dysplasia can be completely asymptomatic, whereas larger lesions can produce pain, swelling, visible deformities, and pathologic fractures. Radiologically, fibrous dysplasia tends to appear as a roundish or lobulated, somewhat expansile, osteolytic, metaphyseal or diaphyseal, concentri-

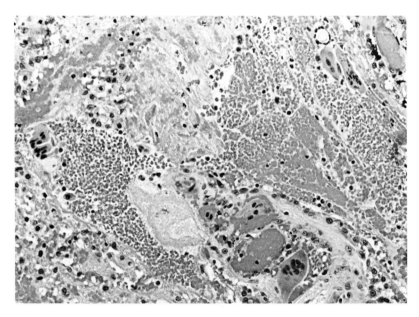

**Fig. 25-21.** Photomicrograph of an aneurysmal bone cyst showing several benign-looking multinucleated giant cells as well as large blood-filled vascular spaces that lack the endothelial lining of normal blood vessels.

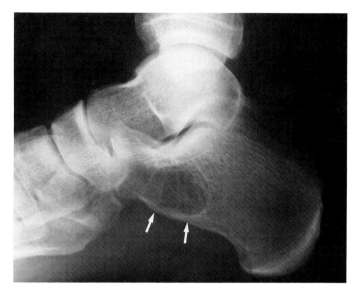

**Fig. 25-22.** Lateral hindfoot radiograph showing a unicameral bone cyst in the anterior portion of the calcaneus. Note its osteolytic appearance and well-defined tumor border and the absence of periosteal new bone formation.

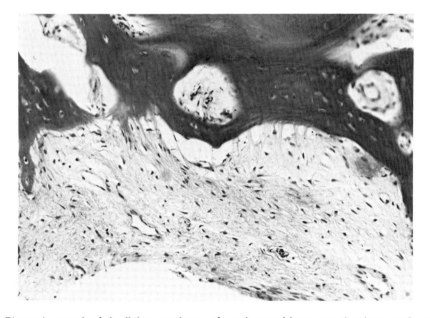

**Fig. 25-23.** Photomicrograph of the lining membrane of a unicameral bone cyst showing a moderate number of benign-looking fibroblastic cells in a loose and somewhat edematous intercellular matrix with a few vascular spaces. (H&E, × 160.) (From Wu KK: Diagnosis and Treatment of Benign and Malignant Monostotic Tumors of the Spine. National Reproductions Corp., Detroit, 1985, with permission.)

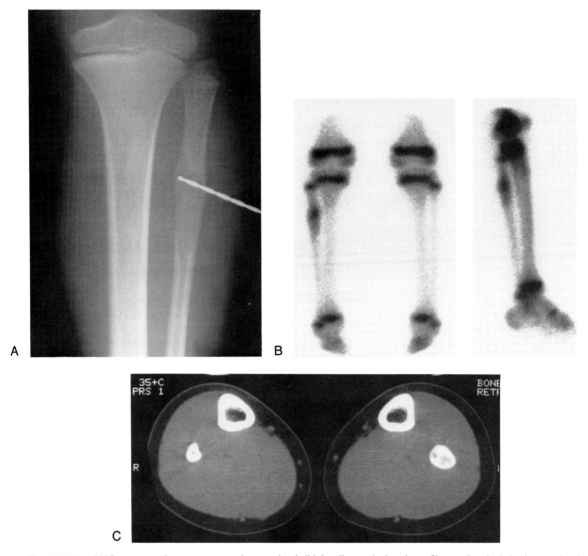

**Fig. 25-24.** (A) Intraoperative anteroposterior proximal tibial radiograph showing a fibrous dysplasia in the proximal portion of the fibular diaphysis which has a ground glass appearance and some cortical expansion. (B) Bone scan of the same leg showing an increase in radionuclide uptake in the proximal fibular diaphysis. (C) CT scan of the leg showing a significant enlargement of the involved fibular diaphysis with large amount of intramedullary new bone formation.

cally or eccentrically located, bubbly or trabeculated lesion, with a border of host bone sclerosis with or without the typical ground glass appearance (Fig. 25-24). Microscopically, the predominant cells of the lesion are oval or spindly fibroblastic cells, which are actively producing varying amounts of immature, irregularly shaped bony trabeculae of the type likely to produce the ground glass radiologic appearance (Fig. 25-25).

## Fibrous Cortical Defect and Nonossifying Fibroma

Fibrous cortical (metaphyseal fibrous) defect and nonossifying (nonosteogenic) fibroma are closely related bone tumors. Their common features are their predilection for the metaphyses of long tubular bones, tendency to undergo spontaneous healing, minimal or no clinical

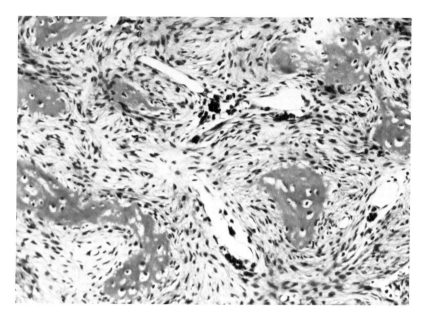

**Fig. 25-25.** This histologic section of a fibrous dysplasia showing many oval and spindly fibroblastic cells actively producing immature bony trabeculae. (H&E, × 160.) (From Wu KK: Diagnosis and Treatment of Benign and Malignant Monostotic Tumors of the Spine. National Reproductions Corp., Detroit, 1985, with permission.)

symptoms, and identical histologic appearance. Occasionally, a fibrous cortical defect is transformed directly into a nonossifying fibroma by growing into the medullary cavity. However, a fibrous cortical defect does differ from a nonossifying fibroma by its smaller size; its minimal perifocal sclerosis; the absence of medullary involvement and virtual absence of pathologic fracture; and its more or less constant distance from the epiphyseal line, higher frequency of occurrence, and predilection for young children instead of older children and adolescents, as is seen in nonossifying fibroma.

Radiologically, a fibrous cortical defect is an eccentric, well defined, radiolucent, metaphyseal cortical lesion, which usually measures less than 1 cm in its greatest diameter and does not normally cause significant bulging of the involved cortex or produce pathologic fracture. In contrast, a nonossifying fibroma is a sharply delineated, osteolytic, eccentric, multiloculated, metaphyseal or diaphyseal lesion, with a sclerotic border and intramedullary involvement. It usually measures 4 to 7 cm in its greatest diameter, which is oriented in line with the longitudinal axis of the involved bone and can produce a cortical bulge and a pathologic fracture (Fig. 25-26). Microscopically, both fibrous cortical defects and nonos-

sifying fibromas are characterized by the presence of many fibroblastic cells in a whorled or interlacing pattern associated with a moderate amount of collagen fibers. Benign-looking multinucleated giant cells, lipid-laden xanthoma cells, thin bony trabeculae, and the absence of cellular anaplasia are common histologic findings (Fig. 25-27).

## Fibrohistiocytic Tumors

The fibrohistiocytic tumors are characterized by the presence of many fibroblastic and histiocytic cells in association with a varying number of multinucleated giant cells. *Malignant fibrous histiocytoma* is a sarcoma with a propensity for producing local tumor recurrence and distant metastasis, whereas *giant cell tumor* is a locally aggressive tumor, which has a high incidence of local tumor recurrence but does not normally produce distant metastasis.

Malignant fibrous histiocytoma has a predilection for the metaphyses of long tubular bones (femur and tibia) of patients in a wide age range, with an average age of about 43 years, without any particular sex preference.

Giant cell tumor accounts for less than 5 percent of

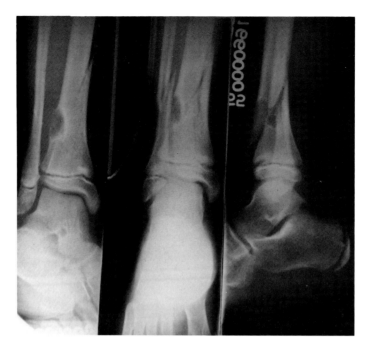

**Fig. 25-26.** Anteroposterior, lateral, and oblique ankle radiographs showing a nonossifying fibroma with an osteosclerotic border involving the lateral aspect of the distal tibia and producing an oblique pathologic tibial and fibular fracture. (From Wu KK: Surgery of the Foot. Lea & Febiger, Philadelphia, 1986, with permission.)

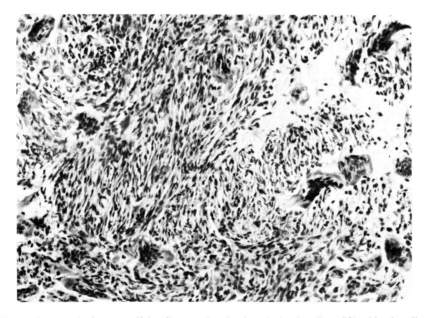

**Fig. 25-27.** Photomicrograph of a nonossifying fibroma showing interlacing bundles of fibroblastic cells in association with a few benign-looking multinucleated giant cells. (H&E, × 160.) (From Wu KK: Diagnosis and Treatment of Benign and Malignant Monostotic Tumors of the Spine. National Reproductions Corp., Detroit, 1985, with permission.)

biopsied primary bone tumors, and shows a predilection for the ends of long tubular bones of patients between 20 and 40 years of age, who account for about 75 percent of the reported cases. There is no apparent sex predilection.

## Vasogenic Tumors

Vasogenic tumors are derived from mesenchymal cells, which give rise to the different components of vascular tissues. *Malignant hemangioendothelioma* (angiosarcoma) is a frankly malignant bone tumor with a propensity to produce local destruction and soft tissue invasion and fatal distant metastases. In contrast, *hemangiopericytoma* can exist in both benign and malignant forms and has an unpredictable clinical course. *Hemangioma* is a benign bone tumor, which normally runs a benign clinical course.

Hemangioendothelioma is an uncommon bone tumor, which accounts for about 0.5 to 1 percent of all primary malignant bone tumors. It has a predilection for long tubular and flat bones (femur, tibia, humerus, and ilium) of patients in a wide age range, with an average age of approximately 45 years, with no particular sex predilection.

Hemangiopericytoma is a very rare tumor that accounts for only about 1 percent of all vascular tumors. It preferentially attacks the long tubular and large flat bones of patients in a wide age range, with no apparent sex preference.

Hemangioma is the most common form of intraosseous vascular tumor. It shows a strong predilection for the axial skeleton (skull and vertebral column) of patients in a fairly wide age range from the fourth to the seventh decade of life, with a male to female ratio of about 1:2.

## Neurogenic Tumors

Neurogenic tumors affect both the central and peripheral nervous systems and the tissues and organs supplied by them. *Neurogenic sarcoma* is a malignant tumor with a propensity to produce local bone destruction, neighboring soft tissue invasion, and fatal distant metastases, whereas *neurilemmoma* and *neurofibroma* are benign tumors which run a benign clinical course.

### Neurogenic Sarcoma

Approximately 50 percent of the reported cases of neurogenic sarcoma were produced by malignant degeneration of neurofibromatosis, especially in patients over 50 years of age and in large and deep nerve trunks of the extremities. The remaining 50 percent usually developed de novo. No apparent sex predilection has been identified.

### Neurilemmoma

Neurilemmoma shows a strong predilection for the head region, especially the mandibular site. Neurilemmoma less frequently affects the humerus, femur, ulna, scapula, tibia, fibula, patella, ribs, metacarpals, and phalanges without showing any particular sex or age range predilection.

### Neurofibroma

Solitary intraosseous neurofibroma unaccompanied by neurofibromatosis is an extremely rare bone lesion, and only a few cases have been reported. In contrast, neurofibromatosis is an autosomally and dominantly inherited disease, which causes disturbance of the supportive and neuronal tissues of the central and peripheral nervous systems, affecting both the neuroectodermal and mesenchymal tissues. The most common orthopedic manifestations of neurofibromatosis include scoliosis, kyphoscoliosis, rib cage deformity, and pseudarthrosis of long tubular bones, particularly the tibia (Fig. 25-28).

## Lipogenic Tumors

Lipogenic tumors are derived from mesenchymal cells with lipoblastic differentiation. An important feature of these lipogenic tumors is the presence of an abundant amount of intracytoplasmic lipid droplets, which can be clearly demonstrated by means of different fat stains or by electron microscopy.

Skeletal *liposarcoma* is a malignant bone tumor, which is locally destructive and invasive and can lead to distant metastasis and death; in contrast, skeletal *lipoma* is a benign tumor with a benign clinical course. Liposarcoma is an extremely rare and preferentially attacks long tubular bones of patients in a wide age range without any particular sex predilection. Lipoma is a rare lesion, which

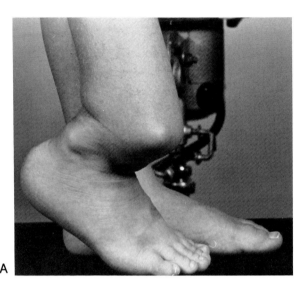
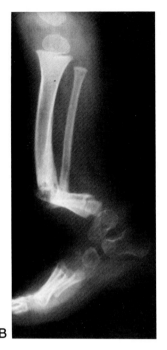
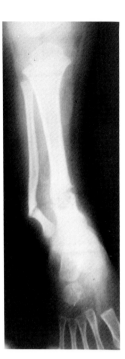

**Fig. 25-28.** (A) Four-year-old white boy with a neurofibromatosis-induced pseudarthrosis of his right tibia. (B) Anteroposterior and lateral lower leg radiographs of the same boy. (From Wu KK: Surgery of the Foot. Lea & Febiger, Philadelphia, 1986, with permission.)

shows a predilection for bones of the lower extremity such as the tibia, fibula, femur, and calcaneus, without showing any strong sex or age group preference.

## Ewing's Sarcoma

Ewing's sarcoma is a highly malignant bone tumor, which most commonly affects patients in their second decade of life. It has a predilection for the long tubular and large flat bones (femur, tibia, humerus, fibula, and ilium), with a male to female ratio of about 1.5 : 1. Clinically, increasing pain and swelling for a few months up to 1 year or longer are the most common major complaints. Limping, joint effusion, limited joint motion, muscle atrophy, palpable tender mass, prominent cutaneous veins overlying the tumor, local heat, and constitutional symptoms are other clinical symptoms and signs.

Radiologically, Ewing's sarcoma is a metaphyseal or diaphyseal lesion, with a mottled and "moth-eaten" appearance, poor tumor margin, frequent onion-peel periosteal bone formation, symmetrical fusiform swelling, and frequent cortical perforation and extraosseous tumor extension (Fig. 25-29). Microscopically, the tumor cells of a Ewing's sarcoma have fairly uniform, round or oval nuclei, with a finely divided or powdery chromatin, inconspicuous nucleoli, vacuolated and slightly granular cytoplasm, indistinct cytoplasmic borders, and very little intercellular matrix (Fig. 25-30).

## Malignant Lymphomas

Malignant lymphomas are a group of closely related lymphoreticular tumors that arise in lymphocytic cells. They are found primarily in lymph nodes, thymus, spleen, liver, bone marrow, and the submucosal region of the respiratory and gastrointestinal gracts. Lymphocytes and histiocytes in different stages of differentiation and maturation are the basic cell types. Malignant lymphomas can be subdivided into Hodgkin's disease and non-Hodgkin's lymphomas, both of which have an affinity for the vertebral column, sternum, ribs, scapula, ilium, and long tubular bones.

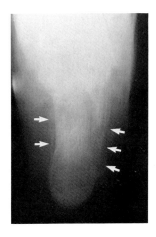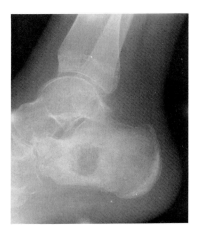

**Fig. 25-29.** Lateral and axial views of the calcaneus of a 13-year-old white girl with a calcaneal Ewing's sarcoma showing mottled bone destruction, an indistinct tumor border, and prominent periosteal new bone formation. (From Wu KK: Surgery of the Foot. Lea & Febiger, Philadelphia, 1986, with permission.)

## Multiple Myeloma

Myeloma is the most common primary bone tumor. It is caused by neoplastic proliferation of a single clone of plasma cells originating in the primitive marrow reticulum of bones with hematopoietic red marrow, such as spine, skull, ribs, and pelvic bones. Myeloma shows a strong predilection for the spinal column, especially the vertebral bodies of the thoracic and lumbar spine of patients between 50 and 70 years of age, with some male predilection.

## Leukemia

Leukemia is a systemic neoplastic disease characterized by abnormal proliferation of hematopoietic cells in the bone marrow and other organs. These cells eventually appear in the peripheral blood. Acute lymphocytic leukemia is the most common form of leukemia in children; it is also the most common malignant disease of children and the leading medical cause of death in children. Clinically, leukemia can produce bone pain, especially in the metaphyseal regions of long tubular bones. Joint effusion and tenderness, limited joint motion, muscle atrophy and other signs can also be present. The most common radiographic finding in acute leukemia in children is a transverse zone of increased radiolucency through the metaphyseal region of the most rapidly growing bones (Fig. 25-31).

## Metastasis

Metastasis is the most common cause of malignant bone lesions. Carcinomas of breast, prostate, lung, colon, kidney, stomach, bladder, uterus, thyroid, are among the most common sources of metastases. However, on a statistical basis different metastatic tumors have a predilection for different age groups. For example, neuroblastoma accounts for the majority of metastatic bone lesions in children under the age of 5. From age 5 to young adulthood, leukemia, osteosarcoma, malignant lymphomas, and Ewing's sarcoma are the most common causes of bone metastases. However, after the age of 40 metastatic carcinomas and multiple myeloma are usually responsible for producing malignant bone lesions.

## Other Malignant Bone Tumors

*Mesenchymoma* is a rare malignant bone tumor with a predilection for the long tubular bones of patients in a wide age range and no apparent sex preference.

*Chordoma* is a malignant primary bone tumor, which is most likely caused by uncontrolled proliferation of cell remnants of the primitive notochord. The axial skeleton from the skull to the coccyx is the exclusive primary tumor site for chordoma. The sacrococcygeal region, spheno-occipital synchondrosis region, cervical spine, lumbar spine, and thoracic spine, in decreasing order of frequency of occurrence, are the exclusive primary

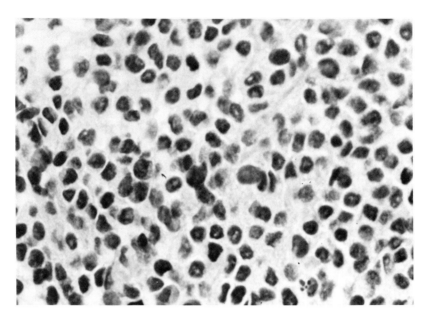

**Fig. 25-30.** Photomicrograph of a Ewing's sarcoma demonstrating that these tumor cells have fairly uniform and round nuclei, powdery chromatin, inconspicuous nucleoli, indistinct cytoplasmic border, vacuolated and granular cytoplasm, and a paucity of intercellular matrix. (H&E, × 600.) (From Wu KK: Surgery of the Foot. Lea & Febiger, Philadelphia, 1986, with permission.)

tumor sites. It should be noted that chordoma affects males twice as often as females. The sacrococcygeal chordomas usually affect patients between 40 and 75 years of age, whereas spheno-occipital chordomas tend to affect patients about a decade younger (age 30 to 60). Very rarely, chordoma can even occur in children and neonates.

## TREATMENT

### Surgical Procedures

The chief aim of bone tumor surgery is complete eradication of the neoplasm, with maximal preservation of all the useful function of the operated site. Various degrees of surgical resection are recommended for individual tumors based upon tumor type and staging. The following types of surgical resection may be recommended.

*Surgery with an intralesional margin:* The plane of dissection cuts through the tumor pseudocapsule, as in an intralesional curettage.

*Surgery with a marginal margin:* The plane of dissec-

tion is next to the reactive tumor pseudocapsule, as in a simple tumor excision ("shelling out the tumor").

*Surgery with a wide margin:* The plane of dissection includes a cuff of normal tissue that completely surrounds the tumor, as in an en bloc resection or amputation.

*Surgery with a radical margin:* The plane of dissection includes the removal of the entire bone, as in complete osteotomy or disarticulation.

### Chemotherapy

Chemotherapy usually employs nonspecific cytocidal drugs that are effective in destroying tumor cells engaging in mitotic division. However, normal tissues with high mitotic activity, such as bone marrow, hair follicles, skin, mucous membrane, enteric epithelium, and gonads, are similarly attacked by these cytotoxic drugs. By combining different cytotoxic drugs that attack different stages of the life cycle of the cells, the tumoricidal effects of chemotherapy can be enhanced and the chances of emergence of drug-resistant tumor cells by random cell mutations can be reduced.

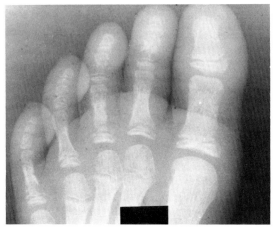

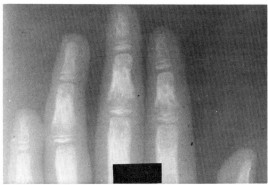

**Fig. 25-31.** Anteroposterior radiographs of the toes and fingers of a 4-year-old white girl with acute lymphocytic leukemia show a zone of increased radiolucency through the metaphyses of the phalanges.

## Radiotherapy

Ionizing radiation such as x-rays, γ-rays, electron beams, and neutron beams can produce ionization of cellular components and changes in cell membrane permeability. Ionization of circulating minerals can result in electrolyte and intra- and extracellular disturbance, as well as acid-base imbalance and blood supply disturbance. The above effects of radiation, as well as damage to DNA, RNA, enzymes, protein, and other organic and inorganic compounds, can all directly or indirectly cause cell death.

## Resection of Pulmonary Metastases

Since the lung is the most common site of metastasis of malignant bone tumors, pulmonary resections such as wedge excision (the most common procedure), segmen-

tectomy, lobectomy, or pneumonectomy have been shown to be effective in prolonging cancer victims lives and can even produce a permanent cure under favorable circumstances. These pulmonary resections can be repeated when the need arises. Pulmonary CT scans are very useful in detecting both large and small metastatic pulmonary nodules.

## SUGGESTED READINGS

Abrams HL: Skeletal metastases in carcinoma. Radiology 55:534, 1950

Aegeter E, Kirkpatrick JA: Orthopaedic disease. WB Saunders, Philadelphia, 1975

Akbarnia BA, Rooholamini SA: Scoliosis caused by benign osteoblastoma of the thoracic or lumbar spine. J Bone Joint Surg [Am] 63:1146, 1981

Appenzeller J, Weitzner S: Intraosseous lipoma of os calcis. Case report and review of literature of intraosseous lipomas of extremities. Clin Orthop 101:171, 1974

Batson OV: The vertebral vein system as a mechanism for the spread of metastases. AJR 48:715, 1942

Batts M Jr: Periosteal fibrosarcoma. Arch Surg 42:566, 1941

Benedict PH: Endocrine features of Albright's syndrome. Metabolism 11:30, 1962

Bertoni F, Campanacci M: Ewing's sarcoma of soft tissues: case report. Ital J Orthop Traumatol 2:413, 1976

Bhansali SK, Desai PB: Ewing's sarcoma. Observation on 107 cases. J Bone Joint Surg [Am] 45:541, 1963

Biesecker JL, Marcove RC, Huvos AG, Mike V: Aneurysmal bone cyst. A clinico-pathologic study of 66 cases. Cancer 26:615, 1970

Bloom MH, Bryan RS: Benign osteoblastoma of the spine. Clin Orthop 65:157, 1969

Bonakdarpour A, Levy WM, Aegerter E: Primary and secondary aneurysmal bone cyst. A radiological study of 75 cases. Radiology 126:75, 1978

Bose KS, Thakur S, Chakrabarty S, Banerjee S: Intraosseous malignant schwannoma. J Indian Med Assoc 54:328, 1970

Boston HD, Dahlin DC, Ivins JC, Cupps RE: Malignant lymphoma (so-called reticulum cell sarcoma) of bone. Cancer 34:1131, 1974

Bullough PG, Walley J: Fibrous cortical defect and non-ossifying fibroma. Postgrad Med 41:672, 1965

Buxton SJD: Tumours of tendon and tendon sheath. Br J Surg 10:469, 1923

Campanacci M, Boriani S, Giunti A: Hemangioendothelioma of bone: a study of 29 cases. Cancer 46:804, 1980

Campanacci M, Cervellati C, Donati V, Bertoni F: Aneurysmal bone cyst (a study of 127 cases, 72 with long term follow-up). Ital J Orthop Traumatol 2:341, 1976

Campanacci M, Giunti A: Periosteal osteosarcoma: review of 41 cases, 22 with long term follow-up. Ital J Orthop Traumatol 2:23, 1976

Cannon JF: Hereditary multiple exostoses. Am J Hum Genet 6:419, 1943

Caruolo JE, Dahlin DC: Lipoma involving bone and simulating malignant bone tumor: report of a case. Proc Mayo Clin 28:361, 1953

Cauble WG, Bowman HS: Dyschondroplasia and hemangiomas (Maffucci's syndrome). Arch Surg 97:678, 1968

Codman EA: Epiphyseal chondromatous giant cell tumors of the upper end of humerus. Surg Gynec Obstet 52:543, 1931

Cohen P, Goldenberg RR: Desmoplastic fibroma of bone. J Bone Joint Surg [Am] 47:1620, 1965

Dahlin DC: Bone Tumors. 3rd Ed. Charles C Thomas, Springfield, IL, 1978

Dahlin DC, Coventry MB, Scanlon PW: Ewing's sarcoma. A critical analysis of 165 cases. J Bone Joint Surg [Am] 43:185, 1961

Dahlin DC, Cupps RE, Johnson EW Jr: Giant-cell tumor: a study of 195 cases. Cancer 25:1061, 1970

Dahlin DC, Ivins JC: Fibrosarcoma of bone. A study of 114 cases. Cancer 23:35, 1969

Dahlin DC, Ivins JC: Benign chondroblastoma. A study of 125 cases. Cancer 30:401, 1972

Dahlin DC, MacCarty CS: Chordoma: a study of fifty-nine cases. Cancer 5:1170, 1952

Dahlin DC, Unni KK: Osteosarcoma of bone and its recognizable varieties. Am J Surg Pathol 1:61, 1977

Das Gupta TK, Bradsfield RD: Solitary malignant schwannoma. Ann Surg 171:419, 1970

Dickson AB, Ayers WW, Mason MW, Miller WR: Lipoma of bone of intraosseous origin. J Bone Joint Surg [Am] 33:257, 1951

Dorfman HD, Steiner GC, Jaffe HL: Vascular tumors of bone. Hum Pathol 2:349, 1971

Dunn EJ, McGarran HH, Nelson P, Greer RB: Synovial chondrosarcoma. Report of a case. J Bone Joint Surg [Am] 56:811, 1974

Elmore SM, Cantrell WC: Maffucci's syndrome. Case report with a normal karyotype. J Bone Joint Surg [Am] 48:1607, 1966

Enneking WF: A system for the functional evaluation of the surgical management of musculoskeletal tumors. p 5. In Enneking WF (ed): Limb Salvage in Musculoskeletal Oncology. Churchill Livingstone, NY, 1987

Eyre-Brook AL, Price CHG: Fibrosarcoma of bone. J Bone Joint Surg [Br] 51:20, 1969

Ewing J: Diffuse endothelioma of bone. Proc N Pathol Soc 21:17, 1921

Falconer MA, Cope CL, Robb-Smith AHT: Fibrous dysplasia of bone with endocrine disorders and cutaneous pigmentation (Albright's disease) Q J Med 11:121, 1942

Faucett KJ, Dahlin DC: Neurilemmoma of bone. Am J Clin Pathol 47:759, 1967

Fienman NL, Yokovac WC: Neurofibromatosis in childhood. J Pediatr 76:339, 1970

Fucilla IS, Hamann A: Hodgkin's disease in bone. Radiology 77:53, 1961

Gilmer WSJ, Macewen GD: Central (medullary) fibrosarcoma of bone. J Bone Joint Surg [Am] 40:121, 1958

Gisser SD, Moss EG: Solitary neurofibroma of rib. N J Med 77:115, 1980

Goldenberg RR, Campbell CJ, Bonfiglio M: Giant-cell tumor of bone. An analysis of 218 cases. J Bone Joint Surg [Am] 52:619, 1970

Goldenberg RR, Cohen P, Steinlauf P: Chondrosarcoma of the extra skeletal soft tissue. A report of seven cases and review of the literature. J Bone Joint Surg [Am] 49:1487, 1967

Green TL, Gaffney E: Desmoplastic fibroma of the mandible. J Oral Med 36:47, 1981

Gross P, Bailey FR, Jacox HW: Primary intramedullary neurofibroma of the humerus. Arch Pathol 28:716, 1939

Hart MS, Basom WC: Neurilemmoma involving bone. J Bone Joint Surg [Am] 40:465–468, 1958

Heard G: Malignant disease in von Recklinghausen's neurofibromatosis. Proc Soc Med 56:502, 1963

Heckman JA: Ollier's disease, Arch Surg 63:861, 1951

Higginbotham NL, Phillip RF, Farr HW, Hustu HO: Chordoma. Thirty-five-year study at Memorial Hospital. Cancer 20:1841, 1967

Hodges PC, Mosely RD Jr: Solitary and multiple osteocartilaginous exostoses and enchondromatoses. Postgrad Med 26:77, 1959

Hutter CG: Unicameral bone cyst. J Bone Joint Surg [Am] 32:430, 1950

Huvos AG: Primary malignant fibrous histiocytoma of bone. Clinicopathologic study of 18 patients. N Y State J Med 76:552, 1976

Huvos AG: Bone Tumors. WB Saunders, Philadelphia, 1979

Huvos AG, Higinbotham NL: Primary fibrosarcoma of bone. A clinicopathologic study of 130 patients. Cancer 35:837, 1975

Inagake J, Rodriguez V, Bodey GP: Causes of death in cancer patients. Cancer 33:568, 1974

Iwata S, Coley BL: Report of six cases of chondromyxoid fibroma of bone. Surg Gynecol Obstet 107:571, 1958

Jackson RP, Reckling FW, Mantz FA: Osteoid osteoma and osteoblastoma. Clin Orthop 128:303, 1977

Jaffe HL: "Osteoid osteoma": a benign osteoblastic tumor composed of osteoid and atypical bone. Arch Surg 31:709, 1935

Jaffe HL: Tumors and Tumorous Conditions of the Bones and Joints. Lea & Febiger, Philadelphia, 1958

Jaffe HL: Intracortical osteogenic sarcoma. Bull Hosp Dis Orthop Inst 21:189, 1960

Jaffe HL, Lichtenstein L: Benign chondroblastoma of bone: a reinterpretation of the so-called calcifying on chondromatous giant cell tumor. Am J Pathol 18:969, 1942

Johnson EW Jr, Ghormley RK, Dockerty MB: Hemangiomas of the extremities. Sug Gynecol Obstet 102:531, 1956

Kauffman SL, Stout AP: Extraskeletal osteogenic sarcoma and chondrosarcomas in children. Cancer 16:432, 1963

Keigley BA, Haggar AM, Gaba A et al: Primary tumors of the foot: MR-imaging. Radiology 171:755, 1989

Larsson SE, Boquist L, Bergdahl L: Ewing's sarcoma. A consecutive series of 64 cases diagnosed in Sweden 1958–1967. Clin Orthop 95:263, 1972

Larsson SE, Lorentzon R, Boquist L: Malignant hemangioendothelioma of bone. J Bone Joint Surg [Am] 57:84, 1975

Legge DA, Tauxe WN, Pugh DC, Utz DC: Radioisotope scanning of metastatic lesions of bone. Mayo Clin Proc 42:755, 1970

Lichtenstein L: Bone Tumors. 5th Ed. CV Mosby, St. Louis 1977

Luck JV Jr, Luck JV, Schwinn CP: Parosteal osteosarcoma, a treatment-oriented study. Clin Orthop 153:92, 1980

Mabrey RE: Chordoma. A study of 150 cases. Am J Cancer 25:501, 1935

MacIntosh DJ, Price CHG, Jeffree GM: Malignant lymphoma (reticulosarcoma) in bone. Clin Oncol 3:287, 1977

Mainer F, Minagi H, Steinback HL: The variable manifestations of multiple enchondromatosis. Radiology 99:377, 1971

Margolis J: Ollier's disease. Arch Intern Med 103:279, 1959

McCarthy EF, Matsuno T, Dorfman HD: Malignant fibrous histiocytoma of bone. A study of 35 cases. Hum Pathol 10:57, 1979

Mullins F, Berard CW, Eisenberg SH: Chondrosarcoma following synovial chondromatosis. A case study. Cancer 18:1180, 1965

Murphy WR, Ackerman LV: Benign and malignant giant cell tumors of bone. A clinical-pathological evaluation of thirty-one cases. Cancer 9:317, 1956

Neer CS II, Francis KC, Marcove RC et al: Treatment of unicameral bone cyst. A follow-up study of one hundred seventy-five cases. J Bone Joint Surg [Am] 48:731, 1966

Nilsonne U, Gothlin G: Desmoplastic fibroma of bone. Acta Orthop Scand 40:205, 1969

Nixon GW, Gwinn JL: The roentgen manifestations of leukemia in infancy. Radiology 107:603, 1973

Paul LW, Pohle EA: Solitary myeloma of bone. Radiology 35:651, 1940

Pear BL: Skeletal manifestations of lymphomas and leukemias. Semin Roentgenol 9:229, 1974

Perez-Soler R, Esteban R, Guardia J: Urinary monoclonal immunoglobulin in multiple myeloma. Ann Intern Med 94:140, 1981

Phelan JT: Fibrous cortical defect and non-ossifying fibroma of bone. Surg Gynecol Obstet 119:809, 1964

Redman HC, Federal WA, Castellino RA, Glastein E: Computerized tomography as an adjunct in the staging of Hodgkin's and non-Hodgkin's lymphoma. Radiology 124:381, 1977

Riccardi VM: Von Recklinghausen neurofibromatosis. N Engl J Med 80:1617, 1981

Samter TG, Velios F, Shafer WG: Neurilemmoma of bone. Report of 3 cases with a review of the literature. Radiology 75:215, 1960

Schajowicz F: Juxtacortical chondrosarcoma. J Bone Joint Surg [Br] 59:473, 1977

Schneider HM, Wunderlich T, Puls P: The primary liposarcoma of the bone. Arch Orthop Trauma Surg 96:235, 1980

Schutt PG, Frost HM: Chondromyxoid fibroma. Clin Orthop 78:323, 1971

Schwartz A, Shuster M, Becker SM, Amboy P: Liposarcoma of bone. Report of a case and review of the literature. J Bone Joint Surg [Am] 52:171, 1970

Selby S: Metaphyseal cortical defects in the tubular bones of growing children. J Bone Joint Surg [Am] 43:395, 1973

Sharpe WS, McDonald JR: Reaction of bone to metastases from carcinoma of breast and prostate. Arch Pathol 33:312, 1942

Sherman MS: Osteoid osteoma: review of literature and report of thirty cases. J Bone Joint Surg 29:918, 1947

Soule EH, Newton W Jr, Moon TE, Tefft M: Extraskeletal Ewing's sarcoma: a preliminary review of 26 cases encountered in the intergroup rhabdomyosarcoma study. Cancer 42:2569, 1978

Spanier SS, Enneking WF, Enriquez P: Primary malignant fibrous histiocytoma of bone. Cancer 36:2084, 1975

Staley CJ: Skeletal metastases in cancer of the breast. Surg Gynecol Obstet 102:683, 1956

Stark JD, Adler NN, Robinson WH: Hereditary multiple exostoses. Radiology 59:212, 1952

Stuhler T, Brocker W, Kaiser G, Poppe H: Fibrous dysplasia in the light of new diagnostic methods. Arch Orthop Trauma Surg 94:255, 1979

Thomas A: Vascular tumors of bone: a pathological and clinical study of twenty-seven cases. Surg Gynecol Obstet 74:777, 1942

Unni KK, Dahlin DC, Beabout JW, Ivins JC: Parosteal osteogenic sarcoma. Cancer 37:2466, 1976

Unni KK, Ivins JC, Beabout JW, Dahlin DC: Hemangioma, hemangiopericytoma and hemangioendothelioma (angiosarcoma) of bone. Cancer 27:1403, 1971

Vang PS, Falk E: Hemangiopericytoma of bone. Review of the literature and report of a case. Acta Orthop Scand 52:903, 1980

Warrick CK: Polyostotic fibrous dysplasia. J Bone Joint Surg [Br] 31:175, 1949

Warrier RP, Kini KR, Raju BU et al: Neurofibromatosis and malignancy. Clin Pediatr (Phila) 24:584, 1986

Wilber MC, Hyatt GW: Bone cysts: results of surgical treatment of 200 cases. J Bone Joint Surg [Am] 42:879, 1960

Wu KK: Diagnosis and Treatment of Polyostotic Spinal Tumors. Charles C Thomas, Springfield IL, 1982

Wu KK: Diagnosis and Treatment of Benign and Malignant Monostotic Tumors of The Spine. National Reproductions Corp., Detroit, 1984

Wu KK: Osteogenic sarcoma. J Neurol Orthop Med Surg 7:117, 1986

Wu KK: Chondrosarcoma. J Neurol Orthop Med Surg 7:265, 1986

Wu KK: Surgery of The Foot. Lea & Febiger, Philadelphia, 1986

Wu KK: Metastatic lesion of the foot. J Foot Surg 26:164, 1987

Wu KK: Osteogenic sarcoma of the foot. J Foot Surg 26:269, 1987

Wu KK: Chondrosarcoma of the foot. J Foot Surg 26:449, 1987

Wu KK: Fibrosarcoma of the foot. J Foot Surg 26:530, 1987

Wu KK: Malignant fibrous histiocytoma. J Neurol Orthop Med Surg 8:5, 1987

Wu KK: Fibrosarcoma. J Neurol Orthop Med Surg 8:113, 1987

Wu KK: Neurogenic sarcoma. J Neurol Orthop Med Surg 8:213, 1987

Wu KK: Malignant lymphoma. J Neurol Orthop Med Surg 8:317, 1987

Wu KK: Osteoblastoma of the foot. J Foot Surg 27:92, 1988

Wu KK: Hemangioendothelioma. J Neurol Orthop Med Surg 9:367, 1988

Wu KK: Chondroblastoma of the foot. J Foot Surg 28:72, 1989

Wu KK: Ewing's sarcoma of the foot. J Foot Surg 28:166, 1989

Wu KK: Osteogenic sarcoma of the tarsal navicular bone. J Foot Surg 28:363, 1989

Wu KK, Collon DJ, Guise ER: Extraosseous chondrosarcoma. Report of five cases and review of the literature. J Bone Joint Surg [Am] 62:189, 1980

Wu KK, Frost HM, Guise ER: A chondrosarcoma of the hand arising from an asymptomatic benign solitary enchondroma of forty years' duration. J Hand Surg 8:317, 1983

Wu KK, Guise ER: Chondrosarcoma of the foot: a report of three new cases plus a review of the medical literature. Orthopedics 1:380, 1978

Wu KK, Guise ER: Ewing's sarcoma: a clinical analysis of forty-six cases treated at Henry Ford Hospital. Orthopedics 2:237, 1979

Wu KK, Guise ER: Extraosseous osteogenic sarcoma: a clinical analysis of ten cases. Orthopedics 3:115, 1980

Wu KK, Guise ER: Pagetoid sarcoma: a clinical analysis of ten cases treated at Henry Ford Hospital. Orthopedics 3:410, 1980

Wu KK, Guise ER: Unicameral bone cyst of the spine. J Bone Joint Surg [Am] 63:171, 1981

Wu KK, Guise ER: Malignant hemangioendothelioma of bone: a clinical analysis of 11 cases treated at Henry Ford Hospital. Orthopedics 4:38, 1981

Wu KK, Guise ER: Synovial chondrosarcoma: a case report. Orthopedics 4:291, 1981

Wu KK, Guise ER, Frost HM, Mitchell CL: Osteogenic sarcoma. Report of one hundred and fifty-seven cases. Henry Ford Hosp Med J 24:213, 1976

Wu KK, Guise ER, Frost HM, Mitchell CL: The technique of hindquarter amputation. A report of 19 cases. Acta Orthop Scand 48:479, 1977

Wu KK, Guise ER, Frost HM, Mitchell CL: Chondrosarcoma: a report of 65 cases. Henry Ford Hosp Med J 26:39, 1978

Wu KK, Kelly AP: Periosteal chondrosarcoma. J Hand Surg [Am] 2:314, 1977

Wu KK, Mitchell DC, Guise ER: Chordoma of the atlas. J Bone Joint Surg [Am] 61:140, 1979

Wu KK, Ross PM, Mitchell DC, Sprague HH: Evolution of a case of multicentric giant cell tumor over a 23-year period. Clin Orthop 213:279, 1986

Zuelzer WW, Flatz G: Acute childhood leukemia. A ten year study. Am J Dis Child 100:886, 1960

# Index

Page numbers followed by *t* indicate tables; those followed by *f* indicate figures.